THE

LESSER WRITINGS

OF

SAMUEL HAHNEMANN.

COLLECTED AND TRANSLATED

BY

R. E. DUDGEON, M.D.

WITH A PREFACE AND NOTES.

BY

E. E. MARCY, M.D.

AUTHOR OF "THE HOMŒOPATHIC THEORY AND PRACTICE."

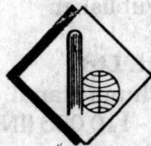

Printed in India

Price : Rs. 125.00

Reprint Edition : 1999
© Copyright with the Publisher
Published by :
B. Jain Publishers Pvt. Ltd.
1921, Street No. 10, Chuna Mandi
Paharganj, New Delhi - 110 055 (INDIA)

Printed in India by :

Unisons Techno Financial Consultants (P) Ltd.
522, FIE, Patpar Ganj, Delhi - 110092

ISBN 81-7021-124-7
BOOK CODE B-2268

AMERICAN PREFACE.

In presenting to the American public, at a very moderate price, a reprint of Hahnemann's Lesser Writings, the Publisher has been actuated by an earnest desire to make generally known to laymen, as well as to medical men, the vast knowledge, the genius, and the genuine philanthropy of the illustrious founder of Homœopathy. The present volume, comprising as it does, many clearly expressed articles of general interest to all classes, commends itself to the attention of all who feel a true interest in the advancement of the healing art.

On rising from the perusal of almost any portion of these pages, the reader will not fail to be impressed with the noble benevolence, as well as the natural and acquired talents of Hahnemann.

Commencing, as the volume does, with papers which were written while our author still belonged to the Old School, and at a period several years previous to the discovery of the homœopathic principle of cure, we are enabled to appreciate in the fullest manner his greatness even as an allopathic writer.

The most intelligent critics of all schools who are familiar with his literary works, entertain the opinion that he was one of the most profound thinkers, and one of the most learned and intelligent writers of his day, even when he is judged by those productions which have no special bearing upon Homœopathy. His descriptions of disease, his thorough knowledge of ancient languages, and of the medical literature of the past, his wonderful powers of observation, his critical acumen, and above all, his acknowledged benevolence and integrity, would have secured for him a position among the great men of his century under any circumstances. But as a reformer of the opinions and practices of a class of men whose influence has remained pre-eminent for more than two thousand years, he has met with the most violent and determined opposition from the commencement to the termination of his career. His *earlier* essays, however, published in

Hufeland's Journal, and in pamphlet form, attracted universal admiration from all sources, for their great originality, comprehensiveness, and justice. Eminent among his cotemporaries as a classical scholar, and for his profound knowledge of the lore of the ancients, his translations from the Syriac, Hebrew, Greek, Latin, French, and English, were looked upon as *beau ideals* of what such works should be, and were appreciated and used accordingly.

No sooner, however, had he announced a doctrine of cure which clashed with the stereotyped dogmas of his brethren, and which threatened to impair their pecuniary interests, than, a system of opposition and persecution of the most dishonourable character was instituted by both physicians and apothecaries. Not content with circulating bitter denunciations, and the most unfounded calumnies with respect to Hahnemann and his doctrines, they appealed to several European governments for legislative enactments, which should repress their promulgation and practice, in order that they might still continue to dictate to the public what should be their medical faith.

For a time, this arbitrary course was partially successful, and victims were drugged as usual with poisons, to swell the coffers of the doctors and druggists; but gradually honest minds were directed to the subject, and notwithstanding the almost certain risk of losing caste with their friends, and of sacrificing, to a greater or less extent, their general influence and their business interests, nearly all who had the candour to *investigate,* became convinced of the truth of the homœopathic theory and had the moral courage to adopt it in practice. As time has rolled on, the system has continued steadily to extend, always among the most intelligent classes, until at the present time, every civilized nation on the earth hails it as the most important discovery, and the greatest blessing to suffering humanity of modern times.

All must concede that but few medical writers have appeared since the days of Hippocrates, whose opinions have stood the test of half a century so triumphantly as those of our author. In a subject so extensive and difficult as that of the healing art, it is of course impossible for any single man, however exalted his genius and talents, to arrive at absolute perfection, or to remain entirely free from errors; but in the instance of Hahnemann, we might almost claim an exception to the rule, were it not for two or three minor, and really unimportant matters of opinion which are of but little importance in a practical point of view. His great law of cure *similia similibus curantur*, stands forth before the world, and will ever continue to stand, an immutable and glorious truth.

His doctrine of applying remedies which operate specifically upon *diseased parts alone*, rather than upon those which are *healthy*, must ever commend itself to the sound judgment of all thinking men.

In like manner, the discovery that the subdivision of crude substances, and the diffusion of their atoms through an inert vehicle, developed in them new and previously unappreciated curative powers, when properly administered, is in itself sufficiently important to immortalize its author.

So also, the introduction into medicine, of drug-provings for the purpose of ascertaining the pure specific action of each article upon the healthy organism and thus of enabling the practitioner to apply his remedies in disease knowingly and efficiently, is another feature in modern medical science which has already commanded the attention and admiration of the whole scientific world.

But while we claim for Hahnemann so exalted a position among the good, the wise, and the great benefactors of modern times, we are not so devoid of common sense as to claim for him *infallibility*. The wisest and best men of all ages, have had their faults and their errors, and it would be folly on the part of the homœopath, to attribute to the discoverer of *similia*, absolute perfection in every thing pertaining to the theory and practice of medicine. By so doing we should follow in the footsteps of the allopathists who for so many centuries have adopted the views and practice of Hippocrates, without question and without comment. Hahnemann has laid the foundation of the true healing art on a firm and incontrovertible basis. The great fundamental principles to which we have already alluded, have been thoroughly tested for more than half a century, with the most gratifying results; and it is now very generally conceded by impartial observers who have investigated the subject, that upon these principles alone can a rational system of medicine be founded.

But if this solid and glorious foundation has been laid for us, let it not be supposed that the edifice is complete, and that nothing more remains to be accomplished. Let it not be supposed, that with the death of the venerated Hahnemann, the genius of Homœopathy perished also; but let us give a just meed of praise to the many noble spirits who by their labours have contributed so much towards the vancement of our art. We need only mention the names of JAHR, RAU, BŒNNINGHAUSEN, NOACK, TRINKS, HERING, HENDERSON, HARTMANN, STAPF, GROSS, and RUCKERT, to call forth a cordial response to our sentiments. Our School at the present time, contains a large number of gentlemen of the highest order of talent, who are labouring assiduously to perfect the system in all its details, and it becomes us as seekers after truth, to avail ourselves of their experience and industry. We are aware that there is a limited number of intolerant and contracted persons, who would gladly repress all further original thought, and stifle all future iuvestigations upon the subject of Homœopathy. Bigoted, weak of intellect, and incapable of generating an original idea themselves, they have the presumption to set up a doctrine of infallibility, for the present as well as for all future generations, perfect in all respects, and ever to be blindly worshipped. Forgetting the old maxim that " to err, is human, but that perfection belongs only to God," they would inculcate a fixed standard of belief and practice for all coming time, regardless of all new discoveries and improvements. Such men are a curse to any system, and were the great Master himself living,—he who passed his whole life in patiently seeking after new facts, in order to modify and correct his erroneous ideas upon medical subjects—he would be the first to condemn such an illiberal policy. The author of Homœopathy, throughout the whole of his glorious carreer, was remarkable as a man of facts. Without a particle of bigotry or prejudice in his composition, and possessing no special reverence for the heathen dogmas which had been handed down from generation to generation, his aim was *truth* alone, to arrive at which, his efforts were untiring, as the manifold facts he has put upon record amply prove. May all of his disciples follow in his footsteps, and by exercising the same industry, the same liberality, and the same devotion to science, seek to advance Homœopathy to that state of perfection which it must eventually attain.

To form a just estimate of the genius and learning of Hahnemann, and of the gradual and laborious manner in which he developed and perfected his great Medical Reform, it is necessary to study not only his more finished and larger works, *the Organon, the Pure Materia Medica* and *the Chronic diseases*, but also his miscellaneous medical writings, which I have here collected into one volume. In these we trace the gradual and progressive development of the homœopathic doctrine, and of the peculiarities of its practice; we perceive that from the very earliest period of his career, Hahnemann felt dissatisfied with the practice of medicine as it had hitherto existed, and that, casting from him as much as possible the prejudices, dogmas and false assumptions of the schools, with which we know from his own confessions he was deeply imbued, he sought by various ways to improve the most important of all arts, that of medicine, until at length, abandoning the time-honoured by-ways of vain speculation, he entered on the only true but hitherto almost unbeaten track—of interrogating nature herself; with what success, the wonderful results furnished by the practice we owe to his genius and labours, testify.

It is not my intention to enter here into a critical analysis of the writings contained in this volume, they must be read by every student of homœopathy who wishes to become acquainted with the Master-mind; suffice it to say I have thought fit to include in this collection, an elaborate work (*On Venereal Diseases*) of a date antecedent to Hahnemann's first notion respecting the homœopathic principle, which will be found to contain many original ideas, and most important innovations on the common practice; the date of its publication sufficiently accounts for its old-fashioned pathology and chemistry. I have also included a work of a popular character, consisting chiefly of Essays on subjects connected with Hygiene, which will well repay a perusal. The remainder of the Essays in this volume bear more or less upon the reformed system of medicine, with the exception of the "*Dissertation on the Helleborism of the Ancients*," which could not have been omit-

ted from a collection of Hahnemann's works, as it shews the extent of
his acquaintance with the writings of the ancients, and is a masterly
specimen of critical acumen, medical knowledge and philological research. It will be observed that I have arranged the writings as much
as possible in the order of their appearance. I may mention, that
this volume, besides containing all the Essays in Stapf's collection,
includes upwards of twenty that are not to be found there, some of which
were only published after Stapf's volumes appeared (1829), but others
were either over-looked, or purposely omitted by that editor.

The notes I have added between brackets [ ] are simply such as I
have deemed requisite, in order to explain certain passages which
seemed to require elucidation.*

The remainder of Hahnemann's lesser writings which, from their
not referring strictly to the subject of medicine, from their antiquated character, or from other causes, I have not introduced into this collection, I shall now briefly enumerate.

I. ORIGINAL WORKS.—

1. *Dissertatio inauguralis medica, Conspectus adfectuum spasmodi-
corum aetiologicus et therapeuticus.* Erlangae, 1779, p.p. 20, 4to.

2. Some small writings in the second part of Krebs' *Medic. Beo-
bachtungen,* Quedlinburg, 1782. I have been unable to lay my hand
upon these, but from a reference in the next work, I find that one of
them relates to a mode of checking salivation at its commencement,
probably by means of liver of sulphur, or sulphuretted hydrogen gas,
as described in the *Venereal Diseases.*

3. *Directions for curing radically old sores and indolent ulcers, with
an appendix, containing a more appropriate treatment of fistulas, caries,
spina ventosa, cancer, white swelling and pulmonary consumption.*
Leipzic, 1784, pp. 192, 12mo. This work contains a good many useful observations on the management of the system in general, and of
old ulcers in particular: it shews up the absurdities of many
of the usual modes of treating disease, illustrated by exam-

---

* The "Case of Colicodynia" was translated by Dr. Russell, and the two Essays,
"Æsculapius in the Balance," and "On the Value of the Speculative Systems of
Medicine," originally appeared in an incomplete form in the *British Journal of
Homœopathy,* by whom translated I am unable to ascertain; I have adopted these
translations, supplying their omissions, and making many alterations so as to constitute them more exact renderings of the originals. For these translations, therefore, I
hold myself as much responsible as for the rest, which were entirely translated by
myself.

ples chiefly derived from the author's own practice at Hermanstadt in Transylvania. He gives a very naïve relation of several cases which he had treated according to the most approved methods of the schools, with no other result but that of rendering his patients worse, and he mentions how they were cured by some fortuitous circumstance, such as a total change in their habits of life, &c. In this work he mentions that he has invented a certain "strengthening balsam," for the treatment of old ulcers, whose composition he does not reveal, but which he offers to supply genuine to any one. Perhaps, like Shakspere's starved apothecary, it was his poverty and not his will that consented to this unprofessional bit of retail trade—but be this as it may, this is probably the circumstance that has given rise to the accusation, magnified by transmission through a host of eager calumniators, of his having sold a nostrum for all diseases. As regards the medicinal treatment recommended in this book, it is just what might satisfy the Edinburgh College of Physicians, but what Hahnemann himself, after a period of reflection and labour, some years of which were spent in retirement from practice, subsequently inveighed against with all his might; and we know that every discovery he afterwards made in medicine, and every improvement he effected in its practice, he immediately revealed to the world, so that all might derive from it the benefit it was capable of affording; though as he himself observes in his preface to the Chronic Diseases, with perhaps the slightest suspicion of a reminiscence of the old balsam speculation, his discoveries would have been much more profitable to himself had they been kept secret until after his death.

4. *On Poisoning by Arsenic, the remedies for it, and its medico-legal investigation.* Leipzic, 1786, p. p. 276, 8vo. This is a most learned work and displays great chemical knowledge. I would willingly have translated it for the present collection, but chemistry is a science that has advanced with such gigantic strides of late years, that a work upon the subject written upwards of fifty years ago would be scarcely intelligible now a-days.

5. *On the difficulties of preparing soda from potash and kitchen salt.* (In *Crell's Chem. Annal.*, 1787, pt. 2.)

6. *Treatise on the prejudices existing against coal fires, on the modes of improving this combustible, and on its employment in heating bakers' ovens. With an appendix, containing M. M. Lanoix and Brun's prize essays on this subject.* With three copper-plates. Dresden, 1787, 8vo.

7. *On the influence of some kinds of gas on the fermentation of wine.* (In *Crell's Chem. Annal.*, Vol. i, 1788, pt. 4.)

8. *On the tests for iron and lead in wine.* (In *Crell's Chem. Annal.*, Vol. i, 1788, pt. 4.)

9. *On the bile and gall-stones.* (In *Crell's Chem. Annal.*, Vol. ii, 1788, pt. 10.)

10. *On an uncommonly powerful means for checking putrefaction.* (In *Crell's Chem. Annal.*, Vol. ii, pt. 12, 1788.) This was translated into French by Cruet, in the *Journal de Médecine*, T. lxxxi, Paris, 1789, Nov., No. 9.

11. *Unsuccessful experiments with some pretended new discoveries.* (In *Crell's Chem. Annal.*, 1789, Vol. i, pt. 3.)

12. *Letter to L. Crell, respecting heavy-spar.* (In *Crell's Annal.*, Vol. i, 1789.

13. *Discovery of a new constituent in plumbago.* (In *Crell's Chem. Annal.*, 1789, Vol. ii, pt. 10.)

14. *Some observations on the astringent principle of plants.* (In *Crell's Beiträge zu den Chem. Annal.*, iv, x, 1789.)

15. *Exact mode of preparing the soluble mercury.* (In the *Neuen literarischen Nachrichten für Aerzte*, for the years 1788 and 1789, 4th Quarter, Halle, 1789; and in *Baldinger's Neue Magazin f. Aerzte*, Vol. xi, pt. 5, 1789.)

16. *Complete mode of preparing the soluble mercury.* (In *Crell's Chem. Annal.*, Vol. ii, 1790, pt. 8.

17. *Insolubility of some metals and their oxydes in caustic ammonia* (In *Crell's Chem. Annal.*, Vol. ii, 1791, pt. 8.)

18. *Means for preventing salivation, and the disastrous effects of mercury.* (In *Blumenbach's med. Bibliothek*, Vol. iii, 1791, pt. 3.)

19. *Contributions to the art of testing wine.* (In *Scherf's Beiträge zum Archiv der med. Polizei und Volksarzneik.*, Vol. iii, Leipzic, 1792.)

20. *On the preparation of Glauber's salts according to the method of Ballen.* (In *Crell's Chem. Annal.*, 1792, pt. 1.)

21. *Pharmaceutical Lexicon.* First vol., first part. A to E. Leipzic, 1793.—First vol., second part. F to K. Leipzic, 1795.— After the publication of these two parts the work ceased. It contains as far as it goes a great deal of useful information, though the plan adopted does not seem to me to be the most felicitous that could be devised : thus the objects of natural history, in place of being

treated of under their well-known scientific appellations, are arranged
alphabetically under the most barbarous, break-jaw compound German words, invented for the occasion : for example the *nux vomica*
here appears under the hideous name of *Krähenaugenschwindelbaum*,
the *filix mas* is metamorphosed into *Männleinwurmtüpfelfarn*, and the
mentha crispa into *Blumenfkopkrausemünze*, which nomenclature, although it may be very euphonious to a German ear, and very expressive to a German understanding, is certainly far from scientific, and
necessitates the separation of things that ought to have been found
together.   The principle of the arrangement will be best understood
by likening it to a Directory arranged alphabetically according to the
christian names in place of the surnames of individuals.

22. *Remarks on the Wirtemberg and Hahnemann's tests for wine.*
(In the *Intelligenzblatt* of the *Allg. lit. Ztg.*, 1793.   No. 79, p. 630.)

23. *Preparation of the Cassell yellow.* Erfurt, 1793, 4to. (It is
also published in the *Act. Academ. Scient.* Erford ad ann. 1794.)

24. *On Hahnemann's test for wine and the new liquor probatorius
fortior.* (In *Tromsdorf's Journal der Pharmazie für Aerzte.* Vol. ii,
pt. 1, 1794.)

25. *Fragmenta de viribus medicamentorum positivis, sive in sano corpore humano observatis.* 2 vols. Leipzic, 1805. This is the germ
of the Pure Materia Materia.

II. TRANSLATIONS FROM VARIOUS LANGUAGES, GENERALLY WITH ADDITIONS AND NOTES BY HAHNEMANN.—

1. *Physiological essays and observations, by John Stedman.* London, 1769.—Leipzic, 1777.

2. *Nugent's essay on the hydrophobia.* London, 1753.—Leipzic,
1777.

3. *W. Falconer on the waters commonly used at Bath.* 1775. 2
vols.—Leipzic, 1777.

4. *Ball's modern practice of physic.*—2 vols. Leipzic, 1777 and
1780.

5. *Procédés chimiques, rangés méthodiquement et définis par M. Demachy.* On y a joint précis d'une nouvelle table des combinaisons ou
rapport p. s. de suite à l'Institut de Chimie. 1769, réimprimé avec des
annotations de Struve dans les descriptions des Arts et Métiers. Neufchatel, V. xii, 1780.—In 2 vols. Leipzic, 1784.

6. *L'Art du destillateur liquoriste, par Demachy et Dubuisson, avec*

des annotations du Dr. Struve. Paris, 1775.—In 2 vols. Leipzic. 1785.

7. *L'Art du vinaigrier, par Demachy, avec des annotations de Struve dans les descriptions des Arts et Métiers.* Neufchatel, V. xii, 1780.—Leipzic, 1787.

8. *Les falsifications des médicaments dévoilées, ouvrage dans lequel on enseigne les moyens de découvrir les tromperies mises en usage pour falsifier les medicaments tant simples que composés, et où on établit des règles pour s'assurer de leur bonté. Ouvrage non seulement utile aux médecins, chirurgiens, apothécaires, droguistes, mais aussi aux malades.* A la Haye et à Bruxelles, 1784.—Dresden, 1787.

9. *The history of the lives of Abelard and Heloisa, comprising a period of eighty-four years, from 1079 to 1163, with their genuine letters from the collection of Amboise ; by Sir Joseph Barrington.* Birmingham and London, 1787.—Leipzic, 1789.

10. *Inquiry into the nature, causes and cure of the consumption of the lungs, with some observations on a late publication on the same subject; by Michael Ryan, M. D., F.R.A.S. Edin.* London. 1787.—Leipzic, 1790.

11. *Dell' arte di fare il vino ragionamente di Ad. Fabbroni, premiato della Reale Academia economica di Firenze.* Florence, 1787, 2d edit. 1790.—Leipzic, 1790.

12. *Advice to the female sex in general, particularly in a state of pregnancy and lying-in, to which is added an appendix, containing some directions relative to the management of children in the first part of life, by John Grigg, accoucheur and surgeon to the Bath Workhouse.* London, 1789.—Leipzic, 1791.

13. *Annals of agriculture and other useful arts, by Arthur Young. F.R.S.* London, pts. 1 to 30, 1786.—Leipzic, 2 vols., 1790 and 1791.

14. *A treatise of the materia medica, by William Cullen, M. D., Professor of the Practice of Physic in the University of Edinburgh.* Edinburgh, 1789.—Leipzic, 2 vols., 1790.

15. *A medical and pharmaceutical chemistry and the materia medica, by Donald Monro, M. D., physician to St. George's Hospital, F.R.C.I Lond. & F.R.S.* London, 1788.—Leipzic, 2 vols., 1791.

16. *Essai analytique sur l' air pur et les différentes espèces d'air par De la Metherie, doct. med., membre des Académies de Dijon e. Mayence.* Paris, 1788.—Leipzic, 2 vols, 1791 and 1792.

17. *Chemical observations on sugar, by Edward Ringby.* London 1788.—Dresden, 2 vols., 1791.

18. *Principes de J. J. Rousseau sur l'éducation des enfants, ou instruction sur la conservation des enfants, et sur leur éducation physique et morale, depuis leur naissance jusqu'à l'époque de leur entrée dans les écoles nationales. Ouvrage indiqué pour le concours, suivant le décret de la Convention nationale du 9 Pluviose dernier.* A Paris, l'an 2 de la République française.—This, which was published at Leipzic in 1796, under the title if *Handbuch für Mütter* (Mother's Manual), is usually inserted among the original works of Hahnemann, but a careful comparison with the work whose title I have given enables me to state that it is nothing more than a translation of that work, with a few additions and one or two alterations by the translator. It therefore properly belongs to this list.

18. *Thesaurus medicaminum. A new collection of medical prescriptions, distributed into twelve classes, and accompanied with pharmaceutical and practical remarks, exhibiting a view of the present state of the materia medica and practice of physic, both at home and abroad. The second edition, with an appendix and other additions. By a member of the London College of physicians.* London, 1794.—Leipzic, 1800. Hahnemann published this translation anonymously; I have given his preface to it, which is a masterly satire on the contents of the work itself, at p. 344 of this volume.

20. *The materia medica of Albert von Haller.* Leipzic, 1806.

Besides the above, many translations from the English and Latin were made by Hahnemann for the *Sammlung der auserlesensten und neuesten Abhandlungen für Wundärzte,* Leipzic, 1783, 1784, 1787.

London, July, 1851.

Appended as a fac-simile of Hahnemann's handwriting, which may be interesting to his admirers. The little note possesses no particular interest in itself, beyond being a good specimen of his minute and beautiful writing at the age of 86, and shewing the affectionate style he had of addressing his friends. The following is a translation of it.

" To Hofrath Lehmann,*

" Dear friend,

"I beg you to send me the third trituration in powder of the

---

* Dr. Lehmann of Cöthen, to whom Hahnemann entrusted the preparation of all his medicines up to the latest period of his life, and to whom I am indebted for this autographic relic.

medicines in the accompanying list, which you have not yet sent me, and to give them to Amelia,* she will bring them with her to me, along with a few lines from your pen, so that I may see that you are still alive, and that you are well and happy, and also how your dear family are.

" Both of us here are well, and send you all our hearty regards.

" Yours,

" SAM. HAHNEMANN.

" Paris, 23d March, 1841."

---

* One of Hahnemann's daughters, Madame Liebe, formerly Süss.

Fac-simile of Hahnemann's writing.

CONTENTS.

INSTRUCTION FOR SURGEONS

RESPECTING

VENEREAL DISEASES,

TOGETHER WITH

A NEW MERCURIAL PREPARATION.

By SAMUEL HAHNEMANN, Doctor of Medicine.

FIRST PUBLISHED AT LEIPZIG, IN 1789.

PREFACE.

My intention in this book is to make the medical public familiar with a wholesome theory and an improved treatment of the diseases herein spoken of.

Hunter, Schwediauer, Hecker, André, Simmons, Peyrilhe, Falk, and some other, known and anonymous, older and more recent authors have assisted me, partly by supplying me with what I did not know, partly by enabling me to arrange my matter. I have made grateful mention of their names or books.

I therefore trust my labour is not superfluous, for to the construction of a building belong not only beams and pillars, but also partition walls and buttresses; not only stone blocks, but small stones to fill up the intervening spaces; and well is it if they fit.

It is in every way a ticklish undertaking to propose a new remedy, or to bring again into notice a neglected or little known one. The person who attempts this must either be a man of high repute, or be entirely free from any suspicion of mean objects.

Although destitute of the former, I am quite at ease respecting the latter. I give an accurate account of the mode of preparing an excellent remedy. Any one who has been in the habit of preparing other chemical drugs, can unhesitatingly prepare this one, assured of the result; I conceal no step, no manipulation in the process. The excellence of the remedy is obvious from the very nature of the thing, and is further proved by the observations of myself and my friends, who have seen similar advantage from its employment. Any one who knows a better, is at perfect liberty to make it known and give it the preference to mine.

When I call it mine, I only mean thereby to say, that I show a purer and more certain mode of preparing it than my predecessors, and give more definite instruction regarding the precautions to be attended to in its use and its mode of action, and not that no one has ever thought of employing anything similar.

1

A precipitated mercury, very similar to the "soluble mercury," (*præcipitatum mercurii carnei coloris, qui ex solutione mercurii vivi in aqua forti paratur, affuso volatili urinæ spiritu*) was first used internally with the best effects in syphilis, 1693, by Gervaise Ucay, made into pills with equal parts of oxydised mercury and some honey—the dose, two or three grains several times a day. I refer the reader to his *Traité de la maladie vénérienne*, Toulouse, 1693, chap. 9, though the preparation could not have been entirely free from turbith and white precipitate.

This excellent remedy, however, subsequently fell into complete neglect, until in recent times the progress of chemistry suggested similar mercurial preparations; but we can hardly say that their employment was ever greatly in vogue, with the exception perhaps of Black's *pulvis cinereus*. Prepossession in favour of what was old, although less efficacious or even prejudicial, combined with no small prejudice[1] against all that could be called new and untried in mercurial preparations or other remedies for venereal affections, induced practitioners not to give the latter a trial, but rather to stick to their calomel, sublimate, and Neapolitan ointment.

And yet the more recent pharmacopœias furnish us with remedies which bear a striking resemblance to mine, and may have occasionally been used.

Such a preparation is the mercury precipitated from nitric acid by ammonia, *pulvis mercurii cinereus*, E., *turpethum album*, O., *mercurius præcipitatus dulcis*, O., as also the *turpethum nigrum* or *mercurius præcipitatus niger*, precipitated by ammonia in vapour from the same acid. I long made my preparation in the latter way, until I corrected its imperfections by the changes mentioned below.

Dr. Black is said to be the inventer[2] of the *pulvis mercurii cinereus*, which he directs to be made in the following way. "Take equal parts of weak nitric acid and mercury, mix together and let the mercury dissolve, dilute it with pure water, add ammonia until the mercury is completely separated, wash the powder with pure water and dry it."

I may here allude to the *mercurius præcip. fuscus Wuerzii*, a pre-

---

[1] The many disappointed hopes respecting the more recent specifics for syphilis, which their quackish vendors announced with the most exaggerated recommendations, and kept secret to the great advantage of their pockets, have served to render practical physicians very shy of such remedies. They did not observe any of the boasted effects of these costly nostrums, but often the injurious results from their use; and the discovery of their composition often revealed some mercurial preparation that had long been known.

[2] Gervaise Ucay, as I have shewn above, prepared it long before him for the same object.

cipitate from nitric acid by potash, merely because it bears some resemblance to mine.

All the authors of the remedies I have named sought to obtain a pure oxyde of mercury free from corrosive acids, especially from sulphuric and muriatic acids, and from the disadvantages of the white precipitate and turbith; let us see if they attained their object.

The purest saltpetre is never used for the preparation of nitric acid; it is always adulterated with earthly muriates or neutral salts. Even the most purified is not free from these. When mercury is dissolved in this, heat is usually applied by means of a sand-bath, in order to hasten the solution. The liquid is at first clouded white but soon afterwards all becomes clear, that is to say the white precipitate at first formed is redissolved and retained in solution in the acid in such a way that even dilution with water cannot precipitate it, and this can only be done by an alkaline solution. If the mercury be now precipitated from this solution by any alkali, the liberated white precipitate falls at the same time, and the precipitate is thus adulterated by no small quantity of a very poisonous medicine.

If we take any one of the mercurial preparations I have named, put it into a medicinal bottle of considerable size, and place this in a sand-bath in such a way that it lies almost inverted, but so that the powder rests upon the side; the neck of the bottle being completely buried in the hot sand, and the bulging out part of the bottle wherein the powder lies completely surrounded by the sand. If heat be now gradually applied, a white deposit will take place in the uppermost part of the glass, composed partly of corrosive sublimate, partly of calomel, these being the two preparations into which the white precipitate is resolved by sublimation. The weight of both together will indicate the quantity of white precipitate contained in the mercurial preparation, and every one can easily convince himself of the truth of my assertion. If we employed purified and redistilled nitric acid for its preparation, we should certainly be much more sure of the result, but greatly increase the price of the substance. But even this will not suffice to free it from sulphuric acid.

But as the ordinary nitric acid is procured by the action of ordinary vitriol on nitre, it has frequently an admixture of sulphuric acid. It must first be rectified over fresh nitre, before we attempt to purify it by redistillation, and this will increase still more the value of the dissolvent. Who could trust to avaricious apothecaries paying attention to all these particulars?

I now pass on to the precipitating agent, and it is a matter of indifference which of them be used, (whether volatile or fixed alkali or alkaline earths), provided only it be pure.

Common chalk, marble, oyster-shells furnish, when calcined and dissolved so as to form lime-water, a very good precipitant in many cases but I may here observe that all are products of the sea, consequently, as experiment likewise demonstrates, not free from muriatic acid.

Ordinary fixed alkali is usually obtained from potashes, which in many cases contain an admixture of sulphuric acid, (often designedly added to it for the sake of adulteration) but chiefly of magnesia, and also ordinary kitchen salt. The water usually employed for its purification contributes not a little to this impurity.

The potash prepared from tartar would be much more serviceable for the purpose, if it were prepared by burning pure crude tartar and extracting the salt therefrom by means of distilled water; but even this has the disadvantage of containing too much carbonic acid, and when, in a watery solution, it should precipitate the mercurial oxyde from the nitric acid, it redissolves the greater part of it again.

The carbonate of ammonia and ordinary spirits of hartshorn possess the same disadvantages, from their excess of carbonic acid. But caustic ammonia and that distilled with alcohol have not this fault, but both of them, as well as the dry carbonate of ammonia and the ordinary fluid spirit of hartshorn, contain no small proportion of muriatic acid; as we may perceive, by saturating them with acetic acid and adding nitrate or sulphate of silver, when the chloride of silver is precipitated.

It is not indifferent what water we employ for the necessary dilution. Well water almost always contains a proportion of muriatic acid and will not do for this purpose. Many spring-waters also are not free from it.

It is well known that much depends on the purity of the mercury, which is frequently adulterated with lead and bismuth. A mere distillation of the suspected metal will not suffice; much of the mixed metals would pass over along with it. Still less will the mere mechanical purification by squeezing it through leather suffice; a certain proportion of bismuth liquifies the lead in the mercury so much, that it will also pass through the pores of the leather. A much better plan is to get the metal by the reduction of cinnabar, especially that in the massive form, which may be mingled with potash, lime, or iron filings, and the metallic mercury obtained therefrom by distillation.

If a saturated solution of the mercury of commerce in nitric acid, diluted with equal parts of water, be boiled for half an hour with twice as much suspected mercury as there is in the solution, the mercury will lose all traces of foreign metals and be as pure as that obtained by reducing cinnabar.

Preparation of the Soluble Mercury.

Mercury purified in the latter manner I placed in a deep cellar,[1] and poured upon it as much nitric acid of an inferior kind (distilled with alumina or otherwise) as was necessary for its dissolution, and stirred this several times a day, for the heaviest portion of the solution floats closely above the mercury and soon puts a stop to its further dissolution unless we adopt this manipulation.

After the lapse of eight days we may be certain of the saturation of the acid, though there should always remain some undissolved mercury at the bottom.

This solution should now be decanted off from the sediment, evaporated and crystallized ; the crystals are to be taken out, the fluid shaken off them, and after being dried upon blotting paper they are to be dissolved in as small a quantity of pure alcohol as possible. By this means they will be completely freed from all admixture of turbith and white precipitate. The solution must now be filtered, and it will then be serviceable for use.

The precipitating agent is prepared in the following way : carefully washed eggshells are exposed to a red heat for a quarter of an hour ; they are then slaked like quick-lime, with distilled water, and the resulting powder is put into a well stopped bottle.

When we wish to prepare the soluble mercury, we take a pound of the fine slaked lime prepared from the eggshells, and mix it in a large new cask with 600 pounds of distilled water, heated to 100° or 150°, stirring well for some minutes till we are assured of the most perfect solution.

After allowing it to remain at rest for a quarter of an hour, by means of a tap two inches from the bottom of the cask, we draw off the pure and clear lime-water (if it be thought necessary through an outstretched woolen cloth of close texture) into a similar cask of equal dimensions, which must either be new or only used for this purpose, and which must be very even and smooth inside.

Into this clear lime-water we pour without delay, and stirring continuously, a quantity of the above mercurial solution, containing two pounds of the metal.

The black liquid soon settles, we then draw off the clear water, wash out the heavy black sediment with distilled water into glass jars, allow it to settle for twenty-four hours, pour off the water, mix up the sediment with as much fresh distilled water as we have poured off, let it again settle completely, decant the water, place the glasses in a large pot, (filling up the intervals betwixt them with ashes or sand)

---

[1] If the cold was intense (in winter), I let the solution take place at a temperature of 40° Fahr.

and put it in an oven just warm (200°) until the deposit is completely dry. This may be more quickly effected by spreading it out on white paper and heating it gradually on tin pans over a moderate charcoal fire, taking care not to singe the paper.

This dark greyish-black powder is the *soluble mercury*[1]; which name I give it because it is completely dissolved in all animal and vegetable acids, and in water impregnated with carbonic acid; also in the gastric juice with great speed, as every practitioner may observe from the rapidity with which it causes the mercurial fever.

Lockowiz, near Dresden,
    29th September, 1788.

Just as I had laid down my pen and was about to send my book to press, Girtanner's work (*Treatise on the Venereal disease,* by Christopher Girtanner, Göttingen, 1788) reached me and gave me great pleasure. He has well thought over his plan and his subject. I was glad to observe that he adopts Hamilton's excellent treatment of gonorrhœa in its essentials, and shews up the ordinary irrational mode in its true colours; that he combats the *à priori* dread of an obstruction after such a rapid suppression of the discharge, and denies the possibility of a metastasis of the gonorrhœal matter in sympathetic chemosis; he gives the distinctive signs of the various secondary gonorrhœas, shews where the venereal differs from other leucorrhœas, and the scrofulous from the venereal glandular swellings, and gives very useful instructions for preventing the suppuration of the latter. I was rejoiced to find that he perceives that the antivenereal metal can only destroy the venereal poison by a previous alteration in it, produced by the reactive powers of the animal digestive and assimilative functions; that is to say, not by mere contact or chemical affinity. I was pleased to observe that he is deeply impressed with the hurtful character of corrosive sublimate, a poison which has been so imprudently deified: that he strongly recommends the strengthening plan before, during and after the mercurial treatment, and generally rejects the French debilitating system, and that he convincingly exposes the harm of all excessive evacuations during the mercurial treatment. I was delighted to see that he unmasks so beautifully the absurdity of talking about "masked" venereal diseases, and shews up the worthlessness of preservative remedies against infection. I was glad to find that he refutes the assertion relative to the innocculation of the child by the semen and in the uterus, as also by the nurse's milk, and advises

---

[1] [For an improvement on the above mode of preparing the *Soluble Mercury,* see Postscript to the Venereal Diseases. This complicated preparation was afterwards superseded in homœopathic practice by the *mercurius vivus.* See *Reine Arzneimittellehre,* 3d edit., vol. i.]

the treatment of even children with the antisyphilitic metal—all maxims which are of the utmost importance for the weal of humanity.

How often have I wished for the concurrence of some physician of eminence on these very points! I always hoped to obtain it, believing that observations conducted by really practical minds must eventually unite in truth, as the radii of a circle though ever so far asunder at the circumference, all converge in a common centre.

What else I deemed it expedient to extract from Girtanner, as it was no longer possible to incorporate it with the text, I have subjoined in the form of notes.

14th October, 1788.

CONTENTS.

PART SECOND.
SYPHILIS.

APPENDIX.

INTRODUCTION.

1. THERE is much that is puzzling and inexplicable in the nature of the venereal virus.

2. It has this peculiarity, that once communicated to the body it increases indefinitely, and that the forces of the corporeal life of the human being possess no power of overcoming it, and of expelling it by their own effort, like other diseases and even gonorrhœa. Its seat appears to be in the lymphatic system.

3. We find that neither the breath, nor the perspiration, nor the exhalation, nor the urine of persons affected with the venereal disease are capable of communicating either the local or the general affection. The semen of a person affected with general syphilis does not, according to the testimony of the most experienced observers, beget syphilitic children; mothers affected with general syphilis only do not seem to have any power of infecting their offspring, nor can nurses affected with syphilis communicate the poison by their milk.

4. Usually the venereal diseases consist only of local affections; a general malady accompanying these is something merely accidental.

5. The most remarkable thing about them is the difference betwixt the first and the second infection.

6. The first infection gives rise only to independent local diseases or idiopathic venereal local affections, gonorrhœa and chancre; in their essential character buboes and condylomata belong to these, yet as regards the period of their occurrence, they constitute the transition into the second infection, in which the absorption of the hitherto merely local virus of the gonorrhœa, chancre and buboe into the general fluids, produces a state of the system that only makes itself known by local affections of another description, which may therefore be called *symptomatic venereal* disease, and the individual or collective phenomena of which are usually termed general venereal disease or syphilis.

7. Many experiments shew that true gonorrhœal matter when inoculated produces chancre, and that matter from the latter gives rise to true gonorrhœa, that consequently both of these affections apparently so different arise from the same virus, which only exhibits different phenomena according as it is applied to different surfaces. [1]

---

[1] [Hahnemann, in common with the whole medical world at this period, entertained the opinion that the syphilitic and gonorrhœal poisons were identical. His views upon this point, as well as upon others of higher importance, were subsequently changed.]—*Am. Pub.*

8. Parts of the body destitute of epidermis designed for the secretion of natural fluids, when the virus is brought in contact with them, become subject, as Hunter demonstrated, to abnormal fluxes of mucus and pus without loss of substance ; this phenomenon is called gonorrhœa. On the other hand when applied to, or rather rubbed into, surfaces of the body provided with epidermis, it excites specific ulcers, which on account of their corroding character are termed chancres (*ulcera cancrosa*). In agglomerated glands it gives rise to buboes.

9. As long as the virus continues in the form of these local affections at the seat of the first infection (or in its neighbourhood, as in buboes) it retains unaltered the power to cause local infections and to excite (*e. g.* by inoculation) similar idiopathic venereal affections according to the nature of the part acted on. Should, however, these local affections disappear without treatment, or should a small portion of their matter pass into the circulation (the second infection) this virus is thereby altered in such a manner, that along with the development of the general malady, besides other local affections, ulcers arise, the matter of which, according to Hunter's careful researches, can neither, when applied to moist surfaces, produce venereal gonorrhœa, nor when introduced into wounds develop chancre, and hence is incapable of producing syphilis in healthy organisms.

10. The matter absorbed by the lymphatic vessels from chancre gives rise to buboes, but the matter of the ulcers of the general affection when driven inwards produces none. As little can the virus of syphilis produce chancres on the genitals or gonorrhœa from within outwards ; if it break out on parts destitute of epidermis, as for instance on the alæ nasi, it forms only general venereal ulcers, whilst the chancre virus applied to the same part produces a nasal blennorrhœa.

11. The virus of chancre and gonorrhœa inserted into general venereal sores or into suppurating buboes, does not aggravate either of these, neither does the chancre become more malignant than it was previously by the application of gonorrhœal matter, nor the gonorrhœa by that of chancrous matter.

PART FIRST.
IDIOPATHIC LOCAL VENEREAL AFFECTIONS.
First Class.
IDIOPATHIC LOCAL VENEREAL AFFECTIONS ON SECRETING SURFACES
OF THE BODY DESTITUTE OF EPIDERMIS.

FIRST DIVISION.
PRIMARY GONORRHŒA.

CHAPTER I.
GONORRHŒA[1] IN THE MALE.

12. Ordinarily not long, often immediately after connection with a woman affected with venereal leucorrhœa, or who has in the vagina venereal matter, the male experiences a notable, not unpleasant[2] itching in the orifice of the urethra, sometimes resembling a flea-bite, accompanied by a not disagreeable sensation of heat in the genitals; a kind of formication is felt in the testicles; the lips of the urethral orifice become somewhat swollen. Every gonorrhœa is ushered in by this irritation,—the *first* stage of the disease.

13. The transition of the first into the second stage is accompanied by a greater or less degree of tension of the penis, the sensation of a constriction in the urethra, and of a twisting formicating motion in the testicles. By pressing in the region of the specific seat of the gonorrhœa, some mucus appears at the mouth of the urethra.

14. The *second* stage. The tickling sensation changes, usually after one or two days, into a painful feeling, into a shooting and intolerable burning in the urethra when the patient makes water, the usual seat of which is under the frænum, namely in the navicular fossa[3] of the mucous membrane, behind the glans (the usual primary seat of the gonorrhœa).

---

[1] The German name for this disease, *Tripper*, is derived from the principal phenomenon, the dropping from the urethra. Common people say, "es trippt," instead of "es tröpfelt"—it drops.

[2] Sometimes it spreads all over the glans, causing erection of the penis and seminal emission, and seems to incite to an abnormal excercise of the sexual function. But the sensation is sometimes less pleasant.

[3] I believe Cockburn, in 1717, was the first who demonstrated gonorrhœa to be an affection of the mucous follicles, and its original seat this spot; hence he explained the nature of the discharge much more correctly and naturally than his predecessors and many of his successors, who alleged that a large quantity (the gonorrhœal discharge sometimes amounts to 4 oz. in the twenty-four hours) of semen and prostatic fluid flowed from the seminal vesicles and prostate gland, thereby giving an explanation of this phenomenon directly opposed to all sound physiology.

15. As long as the gonorrhœa, as in this stage, retains its specific seat, the patient experiences no pain in making water until the urine comes to within an inch or an inch and a half of the orifice of the urethra.

16. The natural white viscid mucus of this canal, which is scarcely observable in health, now exudes by drops. The lips of the glans are more than usually congested with blood; the glans is shining, cherry-red, and transparent. The whole penis, or at least the glans, appears fuller and thicker than it is naturally when unerected; it seems half erected. The urine[1] commences to be of a dark-yellow colour. There occur frequent, painful erections,[2] especially at night, occasionally accompanied by emission of semen.

17. Usually a short time after the occurrence of the scalding[3] on making water, there occurs a discharge[4] of a watery white fluid, as if it were mingled with milk.

18. The patients point to just behind the glans[5] in the urethra, as the seat of their pains, which they feel most intensely when the penis is erected : on looking into it, we observe that is has a raw appearance near the orifice.

19. During the continuance of this discharge, the scalding diminish-

---

[1] On account of the swelling of the penis, probably also on account of contraction of the urethra by the inflammation, perhaps also because the patient, on account of the pain, dreads to let his water come freely, the urine flows in a smaller stream than usual; sometimes it splits on emerging from the urethra, probably on account of the unequal contraction internally.

[2] The painful erections and the scalding of the urine distinguish the primary from secondary gonorrhœa and other discharges from the urethra.

[3] Which, with its concomitant symptoms, continues until the irritating poison is expelled with the discharge, from a few days to several weeks. If it continue some time without any discharge, this troublesome and sometimes dangerous condition is usually denominated by the contradictory name of dry gonorrhœa.

[4] The interior of the urethra in the healthy state is always kept covered with a fine, mild, viscid transparent mucus, that spontaneously exudes from the exhalent vessels and from the excretory ducts of the mucous glandules, so that the acrid urine may flow over without irritating it. But when irritated by the venereal poison, these excretory ducts are compelled to pour out more of their moisture ; a bountiful provision of nature to dilute and carry off the injurious poison. The contractile power of the urethra suffices to expel the gonorrhœa matter by drops.

[5] The usual seat of gonorrhœa is from one to one and a half inches behind the orifice of the urethra, (in some anomolous cases of a worse description the inflammation extends throughout the whole urethra, and seems to be of an erysipelatous character.) How it is that the gonorrhœal matter should always find its way into exactly that spot of the urethra, it is not easy to determine ; perhaps it first lies at the orifice, and thence gradually runs backwards till it reaches the spot which is most susceptible of its irritation, and where it can be least readily washed away by the urine.

es gradually.[1] In the course of time, and often alternately, this watery milky discharge changes into a thicker fluid, resembling melted lard, becomes yellower, exactly like pus,[2] and has a peculiar disagreeable odour.

20. When the pains and inflammatory symptoms have subsided, the *third* stage commences. The simple gonorrhœa is then usually disposed to heal spontaneously without artificial aid ;[3] all pain ac-

---

[1] There are claps almost without scalding, in which the discharge is copious, and others in which the painful sensations precede the discharge some weeks. There are even some, although these are rare, where the disease remains quite stationary at the second stage (*gonorrhée sèche*), where the scalding and even some dysuria exists without being followed by a gonorrhœal discharge, and among these are some that are cured without this latter phenomenon ever occurring. If such a dry clap be of a bad kind, the membranous portion of the urethra may become inflamed, and if not speedily relieved, a perinæal fistula be the result.

[2] The purulent character of the gonorrhœal discharge seems to indicate the existence of an ulcer in the urethra ; this is not the case however, in the ordinary simple gonorrhœa. There are several instances in which pus is produced without loss of substance, without ulceration. The outer surface of the lungs, the costal pleura, also the abdominal viscera have been found surrounded by pus without the slightest trace of ulceration of these parts. In ophthalmo-blennorrhœa of scrofulous or other kinds, as also in cases of severe catarrh, there occurs a discharge of true pus, without a suspicion of the presence of an ulcer. Were we to attribute the ordinary yellow gonorrhœal discharge to an ulcer, it is obvious that if the whole internal surface of the urethra were ulcerated, the size of this suppurating surface would not suffice to produce the quantity of pus that sometimes comes away in gonorrhœa. And moreover as the ordinary gonorrhœa depends on a true venereal miasm, it is impossible, if it arose from an ulcer, that any case could be cured without mercury (without which no venereal ulcer can be radically cured); but we find that a simple clap is often cured by the power of nature or with some slight unmercurial remedy. In persons who have been cured of clap, the urethral mucus often suddenly comes away yellow and puriform after being heated, after the abuse of spirituous drinks, frequent sexual intercourse, &c. It is especially in the inflammatory stage of the clap that the discharge comes away of a purulent character, whereas ulcers only secrete pus after their inflammatory stage is past. What we have stated is superabundantly corroborated by innumerable dissections of the urethra, both in cases which died during the clap and in such as had clap long before their death. In the latter no cicatrices were found, with the exception of a few rare cases ; in the former, however, it was observed that the seat of the discharge was not ulcerated, but only very red and raw-looking, and the coloured matter could be often pressed out of the lining membrane, whilst the gonorrhœal pus lay free in the mucous cavities (*lacunæ*), that is to say in the depressions caused by the mouths of the excretory ducts of the urethral glandules, without the slightest loss of substance being discoverable ; the lymphatic vessels were congested, as if injected with a white fluid. Pott, Morgagni, Hunter, Stoll and others are the authorities for these facts.

[3] [The fact that simple gonorrhœa has a tendency to subside spontaneously, when not aggravated and complicated by drugs, is of much importance. If this opinion, which was announced by the founder of homœopathy more than fifty years ago, had been appreciated by his cotemporaries, and by his successors, a vast amount of unnecessary suffering would have been spared the human race.]—*Am. Pub.*

companying erections is gone; the power of retaining the urine, and of discharging it in a full stream and without discomfort, is restored; the acrid, coloured discharge takes on gradually a whitish colour, and at length becomes colourless (in rarer cases it remains yellowish to the last), similar in character to white of egg, viscid (it can be drawn into strings betwixt the fingers), transparent, mild.[1]

21. It continues to decrease more and more in quantity, accompanied by a tickling sensation and a sort of not disagreeable itching of the glans and urethra, exciting erections, until at length only fibrous flakes are perceived in the urine, and even these at last disappear along with the cessation of the tickling alluded to. The gonorrhœa is cured, usually from four to five weeks after it first broke out.

22. The above is the usual course of the gonorrhœa, but there are innumerable varieties.

23. When the irritation from the gonorrhœal matter advances nearer to inflammation, the sensations of the patient are not confined any longer to the original seat of the gonorrhœa.

24. Weakness in the whole pelvic region, disagreeable sensitiveness in the scrotum, testicles, breast, hips, shooting extending into the glans and great scalding on passing the urine, dark redness of the latter, frequent painful erections and difficult passage of the fæces are the general concomitant symptoms usually observed. The inguinal glands are often at the time swollen.

25. If the inflammation be more intense, the whole urethra seems to be affected in an erysipelatous manner; it is as if shortened, in consequence of which the frequent sometimes continued priapism crooks the penis downwards, (chordee), causing the most excruciating pain, and often the discharge of some drops of blood.[2] The emissions of semen that sometimes ensue are agony. The urine is dark red, acrid, hot; the patient is forced to emit it every moment by teaspoonfuls or even drops, accompanied by the most violent cutting and with involuntary contortions of the features, especially as the last drops flows out. Sometimes the patient cannot remain a quarter of an hour on his legs (and then complete retention of urine often ensues). The penis is externally very painful, the lips of the urethra gape; some swelling of the glandules along the urethra, and a painful tumefaction of the perinæum are observable, frequently conjoined

---

[1] This fluid seems to be coagulable lymph, and its innocuousness is known by this (besides the cessation of all painful sensations) that it dries only upon one side of the linen, and the spot it makes may be rubbed completely off without leaving behind a coloured place, while the previous, more acrid discharge, stains and sinks into the linen.

[2] Which comes from some distended or lacerated bloodvessel of the inflamed membrane of the urethra, over-stretched by the erections.

with tenesmus ; the gonorrhœal discharge is then acrid, discoloured, greenish, or greyish,[1] sometimes even mixed with streaks of blood ; it sinks into the linen where it makes marks of a similar colour. The pain is great, it excites the pulse ; rigour and heat are present, especially towards evening ; blood drawn from the arm presents occasionally the buffy coat.

26. The above course which is never the normal one, and whose violence is often dependent on a bad constitution, but more frequently on improper treatment of the patient by himself or his surgeon, or an accession of febrile disease, a chill, fright, anger, vexation, riding, dancing, coition, heating liquors, purgatives, corrosive injections, &c., does not remain stationary at these symptoms, but, if effectual aid be withheld goes on to the most dangerous results.

27. The priapism readily passes into mortification, the inflammation of the glandules along the urethra into suppuration, which opens into the urethra, more rarely outwards ; the tumefaction of the perinæum, probably in Cowper's glands, forms an abscess which in course of time gives rise to a fistula perinæi, whereby an abnormal outlet for the urine in this region is constantly maintained. The prostrate gland passes into inflammation and induration, less frequently into suppuration. The foreskin inflames, chiefly in consequence of the contact of the acrid gonorrhœal matter which penetrates betwixt it and the glans (chancres under the foreskin and gonorrhœa preputialis are not unfrequent consequences) ; it swells and gives rise to phimosis or paraphimosis. The discharge may sometimes stop suddenly (*chaude-pisse avortée*) and sympathetic inflammation of the testicles or inguinal glands ensue.

28. Along with the sensation of a colicky pain in the abdomen and a weakness in the loins and pelvis, along with the pains in the coccyx and the whole urethra, and along with inclination to vomit, the efferent duct of one testicle, then the epididymis, and at last also the body of the testicle, seldom of both testicles, begins to swell, accompanied by symptomatic fever, quick, full and strong pulse. The testicle gets soft, full and swollen, (*chaude-pisse tombée dans les bourses*), by and by it becomes hard, yet the epididymis on the top of it is harder to the touch ; it is sensitive, full of a dull pain, sometimes accompanied by shooting. It appears to the patient to be intolerably heavy.

29. The spermatic chord also frequently swells and its bloodvessels are distended so as to become varicose, the spermatic duct becomes hard and painful.

30. In the meantime the gonorrhœal discharge diminishes, and, except in a few cases, stops completely ; the scalding of the urine

---

[1] Both colours may be owing to the admixture of small quantities of blood.

ceases. On the other hand, there occurs a more frequent call to
urine, a strangury, as the region of the neck of the bladder appears to
be now affected; the formerly superficial inflammation penetrates
deeper into the substance of the urethral membrane. Sometimes the
swelling goes alternately from one testicle to the other.

31. Other viscera also suffer, as has been said, from sympathetic
irritation; indigestion flatulence, colic, tendency to vomit are the
usual symptoms.[1]

32. Resolution is the most frequent termination, scirrhus the more
rare,[2] and mortification or suppuation the most rare.[3]

33. In like manner, along with the cessation of the scalding and the
occurrence of strangury, as also of the most of the other symptoms,
there sometimes arises a swelling of the inguinal glands which has but
a remote resemblance to true venereal bubo, as it is only caused by
sympathetic irritation. (Slight swellings of the inguinal glands are a
usual and unimportant symptom in every gonorrhœa of any severity, without the discharge thereupon ceasing. They go off without
further inconvenience on the cessation of the urethral irritation.)

34. Resolution or scirrhus is the most frequent, suppuration the
rarest result.

35. Rare but much more dangerous is the ophthalmia that occurs
under similar circumstances.[4] After a diminution or sudden cessation

---

[1] Excitement of the nervous system by passions, over-heating of the whole body
or of the genitals in particular, astringent injections, the rude employment of bougies,
purgatives, perhaps also a not sufficiently understood predisposition of these parts
may give rise to these swellings of the testicles and inguinal glands, which with few
exceptions are not venereal [syphilitic]. A mere sympathetic irritation of the lymphatic vessels in the urethra and caput gallinaginis seems to excite the remote swelling of these glands. A proof of this is to be found in the frequent reappearance
and disappearance of these swellings, and in their curability by antiphlogistic, sedative remedies, without mercury, which is never the case with true venereal buboes
and swellings of the testicle. It is very rare that with moderate care either pass into suppuration, and if this do happen the ulcers formed are as Hunter has shewn,
not venereal, and may be cured by non-mercurial means without being followed by
syphilis. Not to mention that true venereal buboes and swellings of the testicles
produced by a real metastasis of the miasm are much larger and more painful than
those arising from sympathetic irritation in cases of suppressed gonorrhœal discharge.

[2] Induration occurs especially when the discharge cannot be re-established, and
the swelling of the testicle does not diminish.

[3] Girtanner says, "it never passes into suppuration," contrary to Hunter's observations.

[4] There is certainly a sympathy known to exist betwixt the visual organs and the
genital apparatus, but whether that is sufficient to account for this phenomenon I
cannot decide. Although this blennorrhœic ophthalmia is usually attributed to a
true metastasis of the gonorrhœal matter, this assertion remains improbable and unproved as long as the venereal nature of the matter discharged from the eyes is not

of the gonorrhœa (frequently from two to three days after its suppression) in consequence of severe chill of the whole body or of the genital organs, by the intemperate or excessive employment of cold applications, by draughts, &c., a violent inflammation attacks the eyes, which very soon (in a few days) usually inevitably results in incurable blindness. At first the conjunctiva becomes inflamed, swells and presents the appearance of a mass of raw meat, from which a copious purulent fluid runs, soon causing inflammation of the lower eyelid. Every glimmer of light is intolerable to the patient. Most of the conjunctiva of the sclerotic inflames and swells over the cornea to such an extent that the latter appears as if sunk in a pit. A production of pus is observed to take place behind the cornea, which becomes whitish and opaque, scales off, and at length projects forward and bursts from the pressure of the suppuration of the eye. The destroyed contents of the eyeball escape, and the visual organ is forever destroyed.[1]

36. Ulcers in the urethra are certainly of rare occurrence, at least they are far from being an essential portion of the ordinary gonorrhœa when left to itself. The end of the pipe of an injecting syringe of the catheter, or of a hard bougie in the hands of an incautious person, may readily cause a wound in the urethral canal; a chancrous ulcer is the consequence. The laceration of a bloodvessel in the urethra (by priapism, onanism, coition) may give rise to something similar. An internal ulcer may also often arise from the bursting of an abscess of the external urethral glandules.

37. A severe pain on passing water, in a circumscribed spot in the urethra, which is renewed on introducing a catheter or bougie, as also by external pressure on the same spot, betrays the presence of such an ulcer. Ordinarily some blood escapes before the ulcer occurs.[2]

38. In such a case though all the inflammatory symptoms of the gonorrhœa may have subsided, yet the pain persists in the suspected spot even during the secondary gonorrhœa, and does not cease until a proper course of mercury puts a stop to it and its source, the urethral ulcer. If, in place of the antivenereal specific, astringent injections are employed, general syphilis is the result.

39. Sometimes, though rarely, (almost never in those who have a short foreskin, and never in those who have got none) connexion with a diseased woman causes a sort of external gonorrhœa. With a tickling and burning smarting sensation, there occurs, chiefly in the region of

---

demonstrated, as long as chancres have not resulted from inoculating it. In the mean time we shall hesitate to allow it the name of eye-clap. I perceive that Girtanner holds the same opinion as myself.

[1] Sometimes in from four to five days after the commencement of the disease, as Girtanner remarks.

[2] And, as Girtanner alleges, sometimes true pus mingled with blood is discharged along with the ordinary gonorrhœal matter.

the junction of the prepuce and glans, on the corona of the latter and inside the lower part of the former, a secretion of an acrid viscid matter, without our being able to detect any abrasion of the skin, or visible ulceration; occasionally we may observe through a magnifying glass that the affected part seems as if covered with aphthæ. This abnormal secretion on the spot indicated, is termed *preputial gonorrhœa*.[1]

40. Sometimes it involves the whole inner surface of the prepuce and the whole extent of the glans, at least I have noticed it also on its apex.[2]

41. Indubitable observations shew that the gonorrhœal matter may in some rare cases be absorbed, and produce general syphilis.[3] But the special conditions under which this may occur are not very clear. That this may arise from urethral ulcers, which date their origin almost invariably from some violence from without or injury received, is self-evident and requires no further proof. But under what circumstances the gonorrhœal virus may, without injury of the lining membrane of the urethra, be absorbed into the general circulation, is all the more doubtful; whether by too full living, or on the contrary, by inordinate blood-letting and purgatives, or generally by a debilitating regimen and internal and external relaxing remedies, the local

---

[1] Sydenham seems to be the first that observed it.

[2] Perhaps this last phenomenon is a not unfrequent commencement of urethral gonorrhœa. The following case seems to throw light upon this assertion, and to give rise to some inferences. A man who had never had clap, after an impure, half-compulsory connection, was affected by an almost raw, dark red spot, three lines in diameter, at the distance of two lines from the orifice of the urethra, which exuded but little, and caused very little uneasiness; he was otherwise free from venereal disease. Under these circumstances he had connection with a lady who was quite healthy in every respect. She got from him a very violent clap, and a sympathetic buboe in the right groin, besides an abscess in the fold betwixt the greater lip and nymphæ of the same side. The man now ceased to have connexion with her, and commenced bathing the exuding spot with warm milk, whereupon the disease gradually changed its seat, and in a few days reached the orifice of the urethra, the lips of which commenced to inflame. Some fluid had already commenced to flow from the orifice of the urethra, when he first put himself under treatment, and in the course of six days he was perfectly cured without further accident *merely* by the rapid and vigorous use of the soluble mercury. Subsequently he did not again infect the lady, and he is still, (after one year and three-quarters) in perfect health. The lady recovered by the external and internal use of antiphlogistics, and her abscess yielded to mercury.

Preputial gonorrhœa seems to give evidence of a peculiar tenderness of the epidermis of the glans; at least it is never met with in persons whose prepuce is short, cut off, or always retracted behind the glans. The epidermis of such a glans becomes thicker, and is therefore only inoculable by the venereal poison with chancres. Perhaps the apthous coating of the glans in these external claps consists of small chancres. Many observers, among others Gardane, have observed an alternation of urethral and preputial gonorrhœa, the one appearing when the other ceased, and *vice versa*.

[3] [During the latter years of his life, Hahnemann abandoned this idea, and advocated the opinion that the two poisons were distinct and dissimilar.]—*Am. Pub.*

employment of mercurial ointments and plasters, &c. ? Perhaps sometimes by some peculiar morbid diathesis, an accidental fever,[1] or habitual general indisposition. All this lies in obscurity, and there is but little probability that any metastasis of the gonorrhœal matter is possible, except when there is a urethral ulcer.

42. Thus much is certainly true, that it is not so much the mildness or malignancy of the infecting matter, as the various susceptibility[2] of the constitution of the different subjects exposed to the infection, that makes slighter or more severe gonorrhœa; but still it is going too far[3] to deny all modifying power to the different degrees of the poison, as Hunter does, who also maintains that it is the same with respect to other miasms.[4]

43. In most persons the first gonorrhœa seems to be the most severe, especially when it occurs in a sensitive or ardent temperament.

44. Repeated attacks of gonorrhœa seem to fortify the urethra against a new irritation of the same kind; each time it generally becomes unsusceptible for a new infection for a considerable time (always longer and longer.)

45. Persons who have what is called an unhealthy skin, are not on that account more difficult to cure of gonorrhœa; and again, those who are insensible to many irritants have often the most obstinate gonorrhœas.

46. Long continued scalding of the urine without the occurrence of a discharge, indicates a bad form of gonorrhœa, which before it breaks forth is often preceded by an anxious sort of restlessness; and yet severe scalding does not always prognosticate a great discharge, nor slight scalding a moderate one.

47. Men rarely communicate gonorrhœa before the discharge appears; women do so more frequently. Yet the poison is not inactive between the period of infection and that of the appearance of the discharge; it always in the interim causes sensations in the urethra.

48. On surfaces of the body which are destitute of epidermis and which are naturally moist, the gonorrhœal virus can excite similar

---

[1] J. Foote saw on the occurrence of the small-pox a gonorrhœa disappear and general syphilis follow thereupon. Was it fairly ascertained that no urethral ulcer was present?

[2] Instances are not wanting where one woman has communicated clap of the most various degrees to several men, and yet has not given it to those with whom she was in the habit of having most frequent connexion.

[3] In this Girtanner agrees with me.

[4] Is it perfectly indifferent whether the variolous virus be taken from mild cases of small pox or from children who have died of confluent small pox? In an epidemic of putrid fever, I saw ten individuals who frequented the same room attacked with almost exactly the same symptoms, whilst in other families, including the domestics, quite different modifications of the disease obtained, and were transmitted from one member to another with almost no difference.

discharges. It must therefore be carefully kept from the anus,[1] mouth, nose,[2] eyes ;[3] but in such situations also, as it is constantly washed away and diminished, it cannot be easily absorbed, the same as when it is in the urethra (consequently it can rarely give rise to general venereal symptoms), and hence is not to be cured by mercury.

49. But when introduced into wounds, it seems to act exactly like the chancre virus, and to infect the body with the venereal disease[4] (which is curable by mercury only.) J. Hunter innoculated the glans of a healthy man with gonorrhoeal matter, who thereupon was attacked by chancre, then buboes, and, lastly, had general syphilis.

50. Who knows but that many chancres on the glans and prepuce might be avoided, if the gonorrhoeal matter that flows out were carefully kept from those parts ?

51. If the ordinary gonorrhoea be venereal, as cannot be denied, there are not a few other gonorrhoeas whose infecting properties cannot be disputed, which are of a gouty, scrofulous, or other nature. These latter can often be very quickly cured, and an inexperienced practitioner might be apt to suppose the remedy he employed to be a specific for gonorrhoea, until its inefficacy or hurtful character in true venereal gonorrhoea shall convince him and others of the contrary.

52. Any one who wishes for information upon the subject of the non-venereal ones, which do not fall to be considered here, will do well to consult Hecker's work.

53. The infecting power of a venereal gonorrhoea does not cease until the discharge has completely ceased, and erections and the emission of semen takes place without the slightest pain, scalding, or abnormal tickling sensation.

CHAPTER II.
TREATMENT OF GONORRHOEA IN THE MALE.

54. The mildest (rarest) kind of gonorrhoea requires, besides a good diet and regimen, almost no artificial aid, although the time required to effect the cure may thereby be much shortened.

55. The more severe (the ordinary) kind will no doubt ultimately yield in most cases to the efforts of nature, but it will give way more happily, more quickly, and more easily with some assistance ; the chief points to be attended to in furnishing that assistance being the

---

[1] I saw gonorrhoeal matter which had been introduced into the rectum by one of the most unnatural of vices, give rise to chronic gonorrhoea of the rectum.

[2] Duncan observed it accompanied by violent inflammation of the Schneiderian membrane.

[3] Swieten saw a true case of gonorrhoeal ophthalmia.—A common symptom in children, which during birth are infected by the local virus in their mothers' genitals, is among others a gonorrhoea of the eye.

[4 Hahnemann undoubtedly imbibed this erroneous notion from tradition.]— Am. Pub.

following: to allay the inflammation and pain; to check the consequences of the morbid irritability ; to second the efforts of nature in its endeavours to throw off the poison ; and in some cases to rouse to increased action the indolent fibres. We should not have so many points to attend to, did we know of any specific antidote to the gonorrhœal matter.

56. If we are consulted immediately after infection, or in the first stage of the disease, we may succeed in preventing many cases of gonorrhœa by counselling diligent ablution of the penis, and injections of tepid milk [1] into the urethra, which have often been attended with complete success.

57. But we are usually consulted only when the pains compel the patient to seek advice in the second stage.

58. Under these circumstances, we should advise a mild vegetable diet, forbid the employment of acrid salts, of spirituous liquors and spices, (especially pepper, brandy, pickled or smoked meat), of pork, of fat, and all indigestable articles, and all excess in eating. The penis should be frequently bathed or washed in tepid milk.

59. For the proper treatment of the gonorrhœa, however, in order to remove the superficial inflammation of the urethra and to make it insensible to the irritation of the venereal matter, (the most important consideration in the second stage,) we should inject as often as possible into the urethra as far as the seat of the gonorrhœa, a fluid which possesses the power of doing both these. Three grains of opium are to be dissolved in 30 drops of sweet spirits of nitre, and the solution mingled with an ounce of water which contains three grains of acetate of lead in solution. The thin tube, an inch and a half long, of

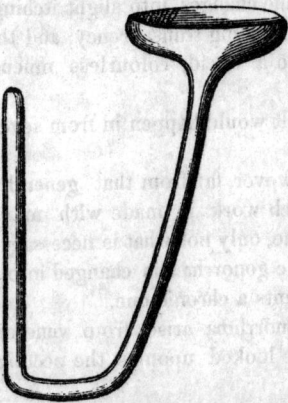

the small tin syphon here delineated, is to be carefully inserted into the fore part of the urethra, whilst the penis is allowed to hang down; the funnel shaped part of the instrument is to be held betwixt the fore finger and thumb of the left hand, and the tepid fluid above described dropped into the funnel-shaped opening of the small syphon, ten or twelve times a day, each time for a minute or longer. The fluid overflows out of the narrow end, exactly at the ordinary seat of the gonorrhœa, and forces its way down by the side of the instru-

---

[1] Or, still better, according to Girtanner, by injections of lime-water, whereby according to him, the gonorrhœa is stifled in its germ. Does the power posssessed by this remedy give evidence of an acid character of the venereal poison ? In place of lime-water, he employs also a weak solution of caustic potash.

ment, and out of the mouth of the urethra; whereby only those parts of it are moistened which require the application of the remedy. The patient performs this little manœuvre himself most readily when standding. He can thereby do no harm. All the inconveniences of the ordinary syringe are obviated by this contrivance. (The patient should previously make water each time.) Even when there is great sensitiveness of the urethra, so that the syringe dare not be employed, this operation may be performed, and that without difficulty. The rounded end of the tube should be moisted with milk or cream, before being introduced into the urethra. We may increase the opium and acetate of lead in the one ounce of water gradually to five grains of each.

60. Diluent drinks should at the same time be employed. An emulsion made with three to six pounds of water and six to eight ounces of hemp-seed, and sweetened with two ounces of syrup of poppies and an ounce of syrup of lemons, may be drunk daily; and this drink, in the inflammatory stage of the gonorrhœa, will do instead of any other internal remedy.

61. If the bowels are constipated, clysters of honey and water should alone be used, and to render these as seldom necessary as possible, fruit may be eaten.

62. In order to diminish the nocturnal erections, a tepid foot-bath for half an hour and a few drops of laudanum, taken just before going to bed, lying on the side upon an elastic mattrass, light bedclothes and a cool apartment will be found advantageous.

63. In the course of an ordinary gonorrhœa the patient goes on in this manner until the scalding of the urine changes into slight itching, until the glans loses its red colour and shining transparency, and the thin discoloured discharge changes into a viscid, colourless mucus, small in quantity.

64. Under such treatment, this result would happen in from seven to eight days.

65. This mode of treatment is, however, far from that generally adopted. In ordinary gonorrhœas much work is made with many different remedies and a great deal is done, only not what is necessary; and by a variety of manœuvres a simple gonorrhœa is changed into a complicated and malignant, or at all events a chronic one.

66. Judging from the maxim that gonorrhœa arises from venereal poison, mercury was from time to time looked upon as the peculiar antidote for gonorrhœa.

67. Physicians did not consider, and would not be taught by experience, that, there being no specific for gonorrhœa, mercury could not possibly be one, as long as this poison acts upon a moisture-secreting surface of the body, such as the interior of the urethra is, where it causes, so to speak, only a mechanical irritation, and on which conse-

quently, seeing that it lies as it were beyond the sphere of the circu
lation, the anti-venereal specific cannot act. (Gonorrhœa is a merely
local disease.)[1]

68. Some facts prove this superabundantly. A man that had just
got rid of chancres and a buboe by means of mercury, was infected
anew and got clap, which would not have been possible, if the gonorrhœal irritation could have been acted on through the circulation;
for as long as the juices are filled with this metal, there is no possibility of a penetrating venereal infection, such as a chancre, occurring.
During the mercurial treatment, cured gonorrhœa has been known to
break out again, and to remain for a long time as secondary gonorrhœa.

69. In cases of simple gonorrhœa, not the slightest use has ever
been observed from mercury; and, therefore, any unnecessary exhaustion of the patient's strength by this metal is quite contra-indicated,
often even hurtful: thus, for instance, a large dose of calomel, as of
any other drastic purgative, has often been found to be followed by
increased irritation in the genitals, wide-spreading inflammation, swelling of the testicles and inguinal glands, and so forth.

70. Peyrilhe has recommended his volatile alkali as a specific in
venereal diseases, and especially in gonorrhœa. Observations are
wanting to corroborate this statement: in the meantime, I may remark, that Murray has seen stoppage of the gonorrhœa and orchitis
strangury and hæmaturia follow its internal employment.

71. Now as we possess no specific remedy[2] for gonorrhœa, there
remains nothing for us to do but to remove all obstacles to, and to
second the efforts of nature, which generally performs the greater
part of the cure alone, though in a somewhat tedious manner.

72. Nature herself will usually establish a copious discharge of fluid,
probably for the purpose of gradually washing away the firmly adherent gonorrhœal poison, and of rendering it innocuous by extreme dilution.

73. This effort of nature is however often insufficient and difficult,
at all events disgustingly tedious, since along with the increase in the
secretion of the urethral fluid, the gonorrhœal poison is simultaneously
reproduced, and continues to exercise its specific irritation, until the
seat of the gonorrhœa, grown accustomed to the irritation, becomes at
length insensible to it, whereupon the poison (from want of the objective

---

[1] [This remark appears to clash with what has just before been advanced, thus
causing some confusion in regard to the real idea of Hahnemann at this period. It is
evident, however, that he is inclined to break away from the then prevalent belief
upon this subject.] *Am. Pub.*

[2] Otherwise the introduction of the before-mentioned (§ 59), or of some similar
fluid into the anterior part of the urethra, which has been employed by modern physicians with such incredibly rapid success, must be regarded as such a specific.

specific irritant) diminishes and goes away completely, whilst the sensitiveness in the urethra vanishes, and the discharge decreases or becomes mild.

74. Hence it is no wonder that this process of nature is tedious and accompanied by much pain, often by swelling, inflammation, and spasm ; symptoms that all demand the succours of art. It is only a pity that the best plan has not always been pursued in these cases, that the first of all the indications has been missed, namely to destroy the local irritation and the local inflammation at its very seat. The poison, or at least the inflammation, was short-sightedly enough sought for in the general circulation, in the primæ viæ, in the whole urinary system, &c.

75. It would occupy volumes to record the sometimes useless, often hurtful remedies, usually employed in this view.

76. Laxative salts, saltpetre, baths and venesections, appear at first sight to be advisable, and yet their employment cannot be allowed as a general rule, and only very rarely and exceptionally.

77. For since in the pure inflammatory state of a gonorrhœa, the whole mass of blood seldom takes part in the inflammation, it follows that it is only in these few cases that it is admissible and beneficial to open the vein, and none but an experienced practitioner can determine this.

78. Therefore, I know not what can be said for the frequently repeated venesections usually employed for every case of gonorrhœa ; but this I know, that in ordinary often mild-looking gonorrhœas, the system is thereby unnecessarily weakened, and the foundation for the most obstinate secondary gonorrhœas is laid ; and that in more severe cases, when irritabilty from weakness produces an accumulation of the most dangerous symptoms, venesections, and still more repeated venesections, usually increase the symptoms to the most frighful extent. Local blood-letting, on the contrary. can, as will be shewn below, be more frequently and certainly employed with benefit.

79. Warm baths, be they for the entire body or for the half only, should likewise not be uselessly lavished in simple gonorrhœas, as they rob the patient of much of his strength ; even in inflammatory symptoms, their employment is a matter of doubt, whenever these arise from pure morbid irritability.

80. Nitre is another favourite remedy of the French physicians in gonorrhœa ; every one that has a clap must swallow a quantity of the universal cooling remedy, nitre. Whatever truth or untruth there may be in the cooling virtues of this salt, experience teaches, that when taken in the inflammatory stage in considerable quantity, it invariably does harm, on account of the great irritation of the urinary passage it causes, not to mention that it is almost a specific weakener of the sys-

tem, and thus contributes to aggravate the symptoms due to that state. I have seen dyspepsia, low fever, and obstinate secondary gonorrhœa, result from its abuse in gonorrhœa.

81. Very nearly the same may be said of the other neutral salts. The use of laxative salts must, therefore, (likewise on account of the irritation to be feared and the weakness to be expected from their use,) be confined to cases in which clysters of honey-water fail to keep the bowels open. Glauber's salts given in drachm doses until an effect is produced, will suffice. In cases of impurities in the stomach, a moderate emetic will be serviceable, and diminish the irritation of the genitals caused by the use of laxative salts.

82. Still more dangerous are the drastic purgative medicines, so frequently used in gonorrhœa. Their usual effects are, — increase of the inflammation of the genitals, suppression of the gonorrhœa with all its dreaded concomitants, such as swelling of the testicles, inflammation of the perinæum, chordee, &c. Jalap root and resin, gamboge, scammony, agaric, colocynth, the purgative extracts (*extr. panchim. cathol.*), but above all, aloes and its preparation, are apt to produce these results.

83. Thre is still another sort of empirical remedies that are said to remove the gonorrhœal discharge rapidly. Such are, the *os sepiæ*, olive oil with citron juice, alum, sugar of lead, &c., given internally. These things must, on the one hand, be very injurious to the system, whilst on the other they can often do no good to the disease.

84. In like manner, in the second stage of gonorrhœa, all kinds of balsams, and all irritating and very astringent injections into the urethra, must be avoided, as hurtful and dangerous.

85. But more horrible still than all I have mentioned, is the mendacious counsel, which has been devised by wickedness, — that a person affected by gonorrhœa should have connexion with a pure virgin, and that he would thereby get quit of his disease. — In this case, the unhappy wretch inoculates the poor girl with the same poison that pervades his own genitals, and sensibly aggravates his disease by an accession of inflammation, while he has the fearful reflection that he has added a fresh crime to the original cause of his malady.

86. Finally, in the third stage of an ordinary clap, after the complete cessation of the scalding and all other painful sensations of these parts, especially the troublesome erections, when the discharge has become lessened, almost colourless, mild, and viscid so as to be drawn into strings betwixt the fingers, nature may be assisted in following manner.

87. I refer now to a gonorrhœa neglected under the ordinary treatment, which most certainly requires such aid, for if the best antiphlogistic and sedative local treatment have been vigorously employed

from the commencement, all the discharge ceases of itself either in a week or a little longer.

88. On account of their calefacient and stimulating, but at the same time also their diuretic, inspissating and strengthening powers, the natural balsams of Copaiba, Tolu, Canada, but especially the Rackasira-balsam[1] and the other turpentine-like substances are of use in these cases. They may be given alone, or rubbed up with sugar, or dissolved in water by means of yolk of egg, or in the form of pills to the extent of 50 or 100 grains daily.[2] Care should be taken not to give them before this stage, when the irritability has ceased.

89. This is the time when linseed tea, the Thebaic tincture, and the bathing of the genitals must be left off, but the diet must be allowed of stronger and more nutritive articles.

90. If, however, we have to do with very lax systems, or such as have been treated with remedies of a too relaxing character, in which the third stage of the gonorrhœa comes to be of a tedious character, and in which, though the disagreeable sensations in the urethra have all gone off, the discharge still continues in considerable quantity, yellowish and of some consistence, it is necessary to abridge this stage energetically, in order to avoid the occurrence of gleet.

91. Besides the internal use of tonics and balsams, the inner secreting surface of the urethra must be roused[3] from its inactivity, as old skin diseases are cured by blisters, chronic catarrhs by sternutatories, or habitual perspirations by a flannel shirt.

92. One, two or four grains of caustic potash or corrosive sublimate dissolved in eight ounces of water will form the best injections for this object. The frequency of their repetition should be regulated by the degree of irritation that these injections manifest on the affected parts;[4] if it be slight, they may be repeated the oftener.

---

[1] As early as 1695 Job. Vierzigman makes mention of these and similar remedies with the greatest approbation. See *Disp. de Phimosi*, Cor. 22.

[2] The most certain sign that the balsams have been given too soon is the occurrence of retention of urine, the renewal of the scalding, &c.; in that case their use is to be discontinued.

[3] These stimulating injections have many things in common with tonic remedies; when they rouse to activity the lax fibres, the latter gain a tone, whereby they are put on a par in point of strength with the unrelaxed fibres; they then react with a power peculiar to the natural tense fibres. We may therefore reckon these artificial stimulating remedies among the number of tonics, just as in certain respects cardamoms and ginger deserve to be called tonic stomachics, as much as the bitter and astringent vegetable substances.

[4] We should take care to ascertain beforehand that the organism has no tendency to morbid irritability and erysipelatous inflammation, which will be perceived from the characteristics of this kind of constitution given below, and will be known not to exist if the previous painful sensations in the urethra were confined to the actual seat of the gonorrhœa.

93. In this way we may eradicate this malady in a short space of time from those organisms that are apt to entertain chronic gonorrhœa (from five to seven days of injection usually suffice); we must only take care not to excite any inflammation by means of the instrument[1] used, by diluting or concentrating the injection to keep up the stimulation in a moderate yet sufficiently great degree. But this is a matter requiring some skill which the beginner is rarely possessed of.

94. These stimulating injections properly employed, are at the same time a good preservative against secondary gonorrhœa, which usually depends on weakness and laxity of the urethral fibres and of the excretory ducts or the mucous glands.

95. On the other hand, in those systems in which the inflammatory gonorrhœal symptoms were of an erysipelatous character, and which possessed a high degree of that irritability from weakness, they must not be used, nor yet in those cases where after a long-lasting dry gonorrhœal irritation the discharge is with difficulty established, or where tendency to strangury, to sympathetic buboe, and hernia humoralis, or to abscess of the perinæum exists; and in general not as long as the discharge continues thin and watery.

96. Along with these irritating injections and the internal use of the balsams, the part should be frequently bathed with cold water, and bark taken in order to aid in the complete recovery of the body.

97. By such means an ordinary gonorrhœa usually terminates soon and without further ailments.

98. But this is not always the fortunate result. A bad constitution of body and other circumstances often give rise to the above mentioned violent and even dangerous symptoms, the relief of which will now occupy our attention.

99. Persons who are of weakly constitution and who have a liability to a number of nervous complaints, spasms, and erysipelatous inflammations, are very often subject to the most severe gonorrhœas.

100. In such cases the malady is not limited to the special and ordinary seat of the gonorrhœal virus. The inflammation extends in an erysipelatous manner along the urethra, and frequently extends to a considerable distance over the adjacent parts, accompanied by the most violent and serious symptoms, such as I have described above (§ 23—25) as occurring in the worst form of gonorrhœa. The whole array of malignant gonorrhœal symptoms may ensue without the

---

[1] If the practitioner will not employ the small syphon (§ 59), but will make use of the unsafe syringe, he would do well to have the end of the pipe made quite round and two lines in breadth, increasing in thickness rapidly from the end backwards, so that it cannot be introduced more than half an inch; if this be done, no injury can occur to the internal part, without the greatest want of caution.

virus that entered the urethra necessarily being, as some think, of a peculiarly bad nature. The corporeal constitution which is so unfavourable in this case has besides other evils a peculiar morbid irritability resulting from nervous weakness, the characteristics of which I shall point out more accurately below.

101. In consequence of this kind of constitution, the frequent or even persisting erections (*priapism*) and curvature (*chordee*) of the penis, the pains in the whole organ on urinating and on being touched, the redness of the penis and of the perinæum and even of the adjacent parts, the strangury, the discharge of a green or grey matter, and all the other obvious inflammatory symptoms, have this peculiarity, that by the relaxing antiphlogistic treatment not only are they not removed, but they are very often thereby aggravated.

102. Repeated venesections, purgatives, nitre, and the other empirical remedies, do harm in such cases, even in those to all appearance most purely inflammatory; and laxative salts, relaxing fomentations and drinks, are not admissible.

103. The only things that do good in such cases, are derivative irritants applied at a distance, and tonic antiphlogistic sedatives employed locally and internally.

104. To this end we may, in a case where there is a constant increase in the violence of the erysipelatous inflammatory symptoms of the above described kind, apply a blister or mustard sinapism on the sacrum; bathe the affected parts with a lukewarm fomentation, made by boiling one-part of oak-bark in 30 of water, and on removing it from the fire, infusing in it half-a-pint of elder-flowers and a third of opium; and make the patient drink elder-flower tea, mixed with from 15 to 20 drops of *tinct. thebaici*. We should also use the injection into the urethra described in § 59, but should, according to circumstances, diminish the quantity of sugar of lead in it.

105. Rest on a horizontal hard couch, moderate coverings over the body, a well-aired not too warm room, and a nutritious easily digestible vegetable diet,[1] consisting of barley-water, oatmeal-gruel, sago, rice, groats, and farinaceous puddings, will be of use. Clysters of asafœtida, prepared by rubbing it up with water into the appearance of milk, will serve to keep the bowels open.

106. But if the morbid irritability of the body, its abnormal nervous weakness, and its tendency to this kind of bad inflammation, is

---

[1] We must take especial care to forbid the use of the very diuretic vegetables, as water-cresses (*sisymbr. nasturt.*), parsley (*ap petrosel.*), hops (*humul. lup.*), and an excess of asparagus; as also the hard husked seeds, as lentils, beans and peas, especially if cooked sour; and, as a general rule, much vinegar and strongly fermented liquors are to be avoided, on account of their irritating effects on the urinary organs.

developed in the highest degree[1] and if by this treatment the symptoms become if not aggravated at all events not ameliorated, we should adopt another method.

107. We must endeavour to discover if bilious impurities of the primæ viæ are not the cause of this aggravation (which is sometimes accompanied by febrile symptoms), in which case it will be necessary to give one, or, according to circumstances, several emetics.

108. Besides this, cold half baths, or foot baths, must be used once or twice daily for two or three minutes at a time, and cold compresses frequently renewed must be kept to the affected parts (of the same kind as the above described tepid ones, only stronger), and the employment of a sufficient quantity of bark in wine, in some cases, particularly towards night, combined with laudanum, as also the acid elixir of Haller taken several times a day in doses of 40 drops, are of the greatest service. The patient should lie only on the side, not on the back. Above everything, we should diligently employ the careful injection (§ 59) into the urethra of a fluid, which without possessing any astringent power, shall most rapidly remove the irritation. According to the experience of myself and others, from five to ten grains of opium, with as much gum arabic, dissolved by trituration in an ounce of water, is the most suitable preparation for this object. In addition to these means, clysters of a similar solution of opium in water are of excellent service, after we have procured a copious evacuation of the bowels, according to the counsel of Schwediauer.

109. Under such treatment all the bad symptoms usually yield, the gonorrhœal irritation commences to limit itself to its circumscribed specific seat in the anterior part of the urethra, and there again ensues a simple, mild clap, which is easily removable by nature or slight artificial aid. However, the patient must, during the remainder of the treatment, remain entirely in bed, or at all events confined to one room, he must not lay aside the suspensory bandage, and must keep to low diet, as the disease is very apt to return.

110. But as good and extensive acquirements are required in order to judge of the nature of the malady and of the patient's constitution, as well as of the suitable remedies, a physician will be required, and the attendant surgeon will not fail to call one in in such a case, for the sake of his own reputation. He will determine whether, opium, blisters, &c, are to be used along with the strengthening remedies.

111. Persons of strong, robust systems, with firm tense fibre, swart animated countenance, of violent disposition, and in the habit of

---

[1] In such cases there is generally rapid pulse, much pain, and copious thin discharge.

taking much exercise, are more disposed to pure inflammatory gonor-rhœa than others.

112. Moreover, violent and long continued exercise (especially during great heat and cold), dancing, riding, the ingestion of indiges-tible or strongly seasoned dishes (especially with pepper), and heating or spirituous liquors, anger, very hot rooms, late lying in bed, violent purgatives, irritating injections, the incautious introduction of bougies, onanism, coition, &c, especially in the above described constitution, are very apt to change a slight, mild gonorrhœa into a very inflam-matory one.

113. The symptoms, which in the above described constitution are to be regarded as purely inflammatory, and to demand antiphlogistic treatment, are : violent scalding on making water ; the escape of some drops of blood after the operation of urinating ; great pain on touch-ing the urethra, especially in the region of the peculiar seat of gonorrhœa, from one to one and a half inch[1] behind the orifice of the urethra; the discharge of a greenish or greyish thin ichor; frequent tension of the penis, especially its curvature downwards ; and some-times a febrile attack.

114. I put in the same class, because it demands the same treat-ment, the dry, scalding clap (*gonorrhee seche*), which occurs after an impure connection in some individuals, and often lasts several weeks before the discharge sets in, and may even be cured without any dis-charge occurring, especially by the diligent injection of a watery solution of opium into the urethra.

115. In general it will be found useful in all such affections to employ a tepid foot-bath, especially at night, emollient poultices of linseed meal, or bread-crumb with boiling milk, combined with a little saffron, well mixed together into paste and applied luke-warm ; as also injections[2] of warm milk, with infusion of saffron or opium ; together with the most cooling diet, linseed tea, strict abstinence from exercise, a horizontal, quiet, hard, cool couch; rarely venesection.

---

[1] The most characteristic pathognomonic sign that the gonorrhœal symptoms be they ever so intense, are of a purely inflammatory character, and do not depend on irritation from weakness or an erysipelatous constitution, J. Hunter rightly alleges to be the limitation of the scalding of the urine to the special seat of gonorrhœa ; a fact we would do well to remember in practice.

[2] The small syphon described at § 59 should be employed for the injection, or if there be a prejudice against using it, we may employ the syringe described in the note to § 93 with caution, taking care, while we regulate the piston-rod of the syringe with the right hand, to compress the urethra just in front of the scrotum with the left thumb and forefinger, so that the gonorrhœal virus may not be carried by the injected fluid beyond the special seat of the disease, and thus to give rise to fresh inflammation, which is dangerous in proportion as it extends nearer the bladder. Some deny that the gonorrhœal virus can produce inflam-mation beyond the proper seat of the disease.

116. The priapism, the painful curvature of the penis, the micturition of blood, the phimoses and paraphimoses, demand, in addition to the above, the application of leeches to the affected parts, a poultice with a good quantity of opium in it (often a fiftieth part), steam fomentations from an infusion of elder flowers, as also the internal use of laudanum, especially at night.

117. The same treatment is to be adopted for the violent pain in passing water, the painful inflammation of the perinæum, and the dry, scalding of urine. We may, in addition, employ in these cases frequent injections of equal parts of opium and isinglass, or gum arabic, dissolved in 60 parts warm (80° Fahr.) water.

118. The febrile symptoms decline spontaneously when the pain is diminished, so that we need not use any means specially for them.

119. If on the diminution or suppression of the gonorrhœal discharge (§ 28, 29), the testicles swell, they must be put in a suspensory bandage, and held up thereby sufficiently, yet gently. The testicles, in their suspensory bandage, should be dipped every half hour or every hour for some minutes in quite cold water,[1] and at the same time a tepid (§116) poultice should be applied around the penis. The same cold applications should be made to the inflamed perinæum, or the groin, when under similar circumstances the inguinal glands (§ 33) are swollen.

120. In these cases, a cautious injection into the urethra of warm infusion of saffron or of opium (§ 108) may be of great use in restoring the discharge, whereupon the tumefaction disappers spontaneously [2] We may for the same end employ as an enema half a drachm of opium dissolved in a pint of water, which is also often effectual in removing the accompanying strangury.

121. The repeated exhibition of a gentle emetic, even though the stomach be not affected with the bile or dyspepsia, in addition to the above mentioned topical applications, and an occasional opiate at night, will often succeed in restoring the discharge and dissipating the swelling of the testicles. But when all other means fail, a few doses of soluble mercury will often restore the discharge, as I can attest from experience. The introduction of a bougie covered with ammonia[3] will seldom be required to bring back the gonorrhœa.

122. Until this has taken place, there is always danger of the oc-

---

[1] Care should be taken not to use warm applications for sympathetic buboes.

[2] The swelling of the testicle is seldom capable of being resolved before the sixth day after its appearance.

[3] I would not advise (seeing that along with other irritations of the urethra, the mere introduction of a common bougie excites inflammation of the testicles,) this mode of restoring the clap, especially with fresh gonorrhœal matter, and in the inflammatory stage of the disease.

currence of complete retention of urine, which will demand immediate relief. The appliances described in § 120 being continued, we may order a tepid half-bath with chamomile and soap, and apply leeches to the perinæum, or a blister to the sacrum. Every thing of a diuretic character should be avoided in the food and drink.[1]

123. If, as seldom happens, the discharge cannot be restored, and swelling of testicles or inguinal glands continues, we must then change the compresses of cold water for vinegar and sal-ammoniac, or endeavour to bring about a revolution by rubbing Naples ointment into the scrotum or buboe, as soon as all the inflammatory symptoms of the gonorrhœa are gone; but not before, otherwise the irritation in the buboe is readily transferred to the testicles, or from one testicle to another, or we may expect other annoying symptoms.

124. Still more rarely do these sympathetic swellings proceed, under this treatment to suppuration; if this do take place, it is a simple abscess with usually nothing of a venereal nature in it. It will become quite healthy in character, if it be not so already, under the diligent employment of bark externally and internally. The inflammation of the perinæum also does not always yield to the repeated application of a cold (50°) decoction of oak-bark, which is usually so effectual, but sometimes passes on to suppuration. If the abscess be not connected with the urethra,[2] and no urine escape by it, it also is of a simple character, and curable without mercury.

125. It still remains to speak of the treatment of that rare but dangerous attendant of suppressed gonorrhœa—the purulent ophthalmia (§ 24), which goes on rapidly to complete blindness. The first and most important point is to restore the gonorrhœal discharge. We must make use of all the procedures spoken of (§ 119—121), except the cold compresses, as early and vigorously as possible; the tepid narcotic injections into the urethra, frequently repeated small emetics, the plentiful internal adminstration of opium, and even, if all other means fail, the introduction of a bougie covered with ammonia. At

---

[1] If notwithstanding all these means the retention of urine continues with its threatened fatal consequences, we should carefully introduce a catheter (a gum elastic one is preferable), and draw off the water. If this, perhaps in consequence of swelling of the prostate, be impossible, we must have recourse to perforation of the bladder through the rectum with the trocar (taking care to avoid the seminal vesicles), or to opening the neck of the bladder from the side.

2 In order to prevent this, it must be opened as early as possible; that is to say, whenever the inflammation presents a shining, soft elevation, in which the general pains are concentrated to a mere throbbing. If this he neglected, abscess usually bursts also internally into the urethra, whereby a serious disease, the urinary fistula occurs; which requires, besides the internal employment of mercury, good external applications and the use of the elastic catheter, through which we must allow the urine to flow each time it is passed until the cure is effected, which generally takes a long time.

the same time we must constantly apply to, or still better, bathe the eye in water cooled with ice, mixed with a thousandth-part of sugar of lead. Tepid foot baths, or half baths, venesections, blisters to the sacrum, scarifications of the conjunctiva, leeches to the temples, must not be neglected, nor incisions in the cornea if pus be accumulated betwixt its layers. But I will advise in preference to this operation, local fumigations with cinnabar,[1] and the application of a poultice of mandragora root. Some say they have seen advantage from the employment of hemlock and monkshood.

126. As regards preputial gonorrhœa (§ 39), the symptoms it occasions are of no great importance—sometimes a moderate degree of phimosis, and a slight discharge from the inferior part of the glands and prepuce; frequent washing with a mucilage of gum arabic is almost of itself sufficient to cure every case of this affection in a short space of time. But if it penetrate deeper, or if it be obstinate, it requires the internal use of mercury like other venereal affections, conjoined with cold and astringent applications.

CHAPTER III.
GONORRHŒA IN THE FEMALE.

127. As the genital organs of the female are less composite in their character, generally less sensitive and of laxer tissue than those of the male, it follows that gonorrhœa in the female should also present less complicated, less violent, indeed, often unrecognizable symptoms.— And such is the case.

128. The simple venereal leucorrhœa, when the vagina is only affected by it in a minor degree, is often so painless, and the functions as well as the appearance of the genitals appear to be so natural, that even experienced persons might often take the discharge merely for a symptom of weakness, scrofula, chlorosis,[2] &c., did not the general constitution of the patient testify plainly to the contrary, or should we not have ascertained that she infected one or more men with gonorrhœa.— Did we possess any specific antidote to gonorrhœa, its discovery would be very easy, and on the other hand the frequent spread of this affection occasioned by the difficulty of detecting[3] the venereal character of a simple gonorrhœa in the female, might be prevented.

---

[1] As long ago as 1556, Gabriel Fallopius (*De morbo Gallico*, Batav. 4to. 1564, cap. 69) observe this sympathetic metastasis of gonorrhœa (lippitudinem rebellem, quæ adnatam inflammat membranam et corneam excoriat), and cured it with cinnabar fumigations.

[2] A leucorrhœa arising from onanism is as obstinate as any of a venereal origin.

[3] Girtanner mentions some circumstances that should serve to distinguish the venereal from the unvenereal leucorrhœas; the latter appear at first only before the commencement of each menstrual flux, afterwards they also continue a few days after its cessation, and then cease for from eight to fourteen days; they cause the

129. But the case is quite different with the gonorrhœa of a complicated character in the female. It comes on with a sensation of warmth in the genital organs, and a tickling sensation causing desire for coition, with frequent erection of the clitoris. These premonitory symptoms, however, soon give place to pains accompanied by some discharge from the vagina.

130. The patient experiences in a few days a fulness, tension and burning in the vagina and labia, which along with increased heat and swelling, especially towards the lower commissure, are intolerant of the slightest touch. The urethra is inflamed at its orifice, in worse cases throughout its whole extent; the scalding on making water is as painful as in males. The clitoris is excessively sensitive. Coition or contact is impossible; walking, sitting and making water almost unendurable.

131. An acrid ichorous discharge of various colours issues from the whole inner surface of the vagina, or at least from beyond its sphincter muscle, and from the myrtiform rugæ, and in more severe cases from the urethra.

132. When exercise or over-heating of the body or of the genital organs is not avoided, or when injurious irritating remedies are given internally, there occurs also, as in males, sometimes a sympathetic swelling of the inguinal glands or inflammation of the perinæum, along with diminution of the discharge. In bad cases there may also occur retention of urine, likewise dependent on sympathetic irritation.

133. When the disease is of a more violent character, we perceive deep seated glandular inflammations in the body of the labia majora, which become painful, increase in size, and generally form abscesses betwixt their inner surfaces and the nymphæ[1] which burst.

134. Gradually the discharge from the vagina becomes thicker and more like pus; the scalding of the urine begins to diminish, and after a longer or shorter time at length ceases, along with the other troublesome and painful symptoms.

135. If the gonorrhœa be near its termination, (nature frequently takes many months to cure it), the discharge becomes, as in men, colourless, mild and viscid before it completely ceases.

---

diminution and at length gradually the total disappearance of the catamenia, whereupon the leucorrhœa begins to flow continually. They are also generally accompanied by pains in the loins, a dragging in the thighs, debility of the legs pale complexion, dyspepsia and hysteria, and at length sterility, all which serve to distinguish them pretty well from venereal gonorrhœa.

[1] De Horne observed almost in the same place in the internal surface of the great and small lips and in the vagina, occasionally some points (perhaps the orifices of similar glandular suppurations) which poured out a large quantity of watery pus, and might occasionally be regarded as secondary gonorrhœa in the female. He cured it by opening these small fistulous ducts.

CHAPTER IV.

TREATMENT OF GONORRHŒA IN THE FEMALE.

136. In general its cure is attended with fewer difficulties than in the male, but so much the more tedious is it.

137. In mild cases of gonorrhœa in the female, we have little else to do than to remove the irritation in the vagina and to strengthen the relaxed parts.

138. We fulfil all these indications by the simple treatment of making eight or ten times daily, repeated injections into the vagina of fifteen grains of sugar of lead, and eight grains of opium dissolved in an ounce of water. (§ 59.)

139. If this be not strong enough we may use in place of the sugar of lead, from 10 to 15 grains of sulphate of zinc, which will certainly prove effectual. About a fortnight is required to effect a cure.[1]

140. We must treat with contempt the old bugbear of the dangers of suppressing a gonorrhœa, which goes off without leaving behind it scalding of urine, strangury or other inconvenience. Everything that removes the local irritation and alters the specific gonorrhœal disposition, cures the ordinary gonorrhœa. But only locally, some one may retort; to which I reply, certainly, and most properly too, for it is merely a local malady.

141. These remedies will not be found to be too strong when compared with those for gonorrhœa in the male, more especially as the texture of the vagina, especially in the case alluded to, is astonishingly lax, spongy and unirritable, and not to be compared with any part of the male genital organs.

142. The more severe kind of gonorrhœa in the female, however, requires a different mode of treatment. Of the remedies proposed in the treatment of gonorrhœa in the male, the only admissible ones are the opiated linseed tea and the local sedative antiphlogistic compresses, as the excessive pain of the inflamed parts renders all injections impossible.

143. In this case we must make frequent applications of tepid poultices of linseed-meal, combined with saffron, to the external parts, and these must be repeated until the diminishing inflammation and tumefaction of the vagina admits of the injections at first of tepid and at length of cold infusion of saffron, which should be continued until the scalding of urine and the pain of the other parts of the genital organs

---

[1] Girtanner advises fresh lime water, or an equally strong solution of caustic potash to be injected from six to eight times daily into the vagina, by which process, he asserts, gonorrhœa in the female will be cured in five or six days; a period of time so short, as if experience corroborates the assertion, would point to an almost specific power of these antacid remedies against the gonorrhœal virus.

are completely removed. Injections of ten grains of opium with gum-arabic in an ounce of water, will also be of the greatest service.

144. On the occurrence of the glandular abscesses (§ 133) on the internal surface of the labia majora, we have nothing particular to do. The swelling will be resolved if that is possible by the external fomentations, or burst from the same treatment. We must in that case take care to keep open the ulcer, which is always somewhat deeply seated, and when the gonorrhœa has lost all its inflammation, give the soluble mercury till slight mercurial fever is produced, partly in order to prevent the serious effects of the absorption of the virus into the general circulation, partly to effect the most speedy healing up of the ulcer; which according to my experience is most surely and easily effected by this means.

145. During the inflammatory stage of the disease, we should prescribe, as in the case of males, a mild vegetable diet, a general cool regimen, and the strictest rest. The only other things required are an enema of honey-water to keep the bowels open, a mild opiate at night, and, in the purely inflammatory state, a few tepid foot-baths. Venesection is seldom requisite.

146. When the injections of the opium solution (§ 143) have removed the violent irritation, the inflammatory symptoms and the pains, we should go on with the narcotic astringent injections (§ 138, 139) until the cure is perfect.[1]

147. A syringe with a pipe at least two-thirds of an inch thick and with a rounded end perforated with several small holes, but having a narrow canal, is best for such injections; we are sure not to injure the internal parts with it, and the fluid is propelled far in and made to remain as long as possible. The thickness of the pipe dilates the myrtiform folds of the mucous membrane and the fluid comes in contact with the whole surface, thereby relieving the irritation and washing away the virus. The patient can herself most effectually perform the injections by lying on the back with the shoulders elevated, and the knees drawn up and separated; in this way the injected fluid can remain longest in the vagina, act longest on the affected parts and develope the greatest power.[2]

---

[1] Or we may employ for this end the lime-water so strongly recommended by Girtanner.

[2] Still more convenient is Girtanner's instrument, which consists of an india-rubber bag instead of the usual syringe, adapted to the cylindrical pipe.

SECOND DIVISION.
SEQUELÆ OF GONORRHŒA.

CHAPTER I.
CHRONIC STRANGURY AND ITS TREATMENT.

148. In cases of obstinate gonorrhœa, especially in the male, when the bladder and neighbouring parts have been implicated in the erysipelatous inflammation and unskillfully treated, there sometimes remains a frequent painful inclination [1] to make water, a burning or shooting pain in the urethra, often as far as the glans, pressure on the bladder after the evacuation of the urine, and a disagreeable sensation in the perinæum ; a pitiable disease that in course of time lays the foundation for thickening of the walls of the bladder, ulceration of it, urinary calculus, and even dilatation or suppuration of the pelvis of the kidneys.

149. If these symptoms be not owing to stone in the bladder, or stricture of the urethra, which may both be ascertained by means of the catheter, or swelling of the prostrate gland, which may be ascertained by the catheter and the introduction of the finger into the rectum, they depend on the above mentioned cause ; but the patient need not therefore fear, as he often does, that there still exist uneradicated remains of the venereal disease in his system, to occasion these sufferings.

150. These grave symptoms may often be removed by frequent bathing of the genitals in cold, and even the very coldest water, (whereby the weak parts are strengthened and their irritability diminished), and by the injection of a solution of opium. (§108.)

151. If this remedy be used for several weeks without effect, (which very seldom is the case), the employment of opium internally and externally (in topical applications and clysters) is, according to my experience, of excellent service.

152. If this do not suffice, besides the last named remedy, the application of a blister to the sacrum, or the introduction of a seton into the perinæum will produce the desired effect.

CHAPTER II.
CHRONIC CURVATURE OF THE PENIS.

153. The curved erection of the penis (chordee) sometimes persists after the removal of the gonorrhœa and its attendant symp-

---

[1] These sufferings are usually caused by a renewed irritation, resulting from spasm and weakness. and an irregular reaction of the bladder against the urethra. In the healthy state, before the evacuation of the urine, the neck of the bladder and the urethra are contracted and the bladder is relaxed, but when the urine is to be passed, the bladder contracts, and first the neck of the bladder and then the urethra relaxes, and after the urine has flowed out the two latter contract before the first becomes relaxed ; whereas in this case the natural operations of these parts are reversed, or at least take place in a perverted order.

toms. It renders coition painful, often impossible, or at all events un-prolific.

154. An induration of the membrane of the urethra, or thickening of a part of the corpora cavernosa is usually the cause of this affection.

155. Recourse is usually had to venesections and purgatives, although they cannot be of the slightest benefit, and often do much injury to the system.

156. The internal use of hemlock is said to be of use; the extract may at the same time be applied outwardly. If this do not succeed, mercury should be rubbed into the affected part, and bark taken internally as Schwediauer advises. Good results may be anticipated from the employment of electricity.

157. These things may prove serviceable when the symptom does not depend on too great induration and adhesions of the corpora cavernosa, or of the substance of the urethre. In worse cases, however, when the remedies just mentioned are inefficient against the cartilaginous adhensions, De la Peyronie has found the baths of Barèges useful. (These baths greatly resemble the other warm alkaline mineral waters containing sulphuretted hydrogen, at Aix, Baden, Töplitz, Kirchberg, Wolkenstein, &c.) In order that they may do more good than the other remedies, I believe they ought to be used in the form of douche on the affected parts.

158. Peyrilhe asserts that he has cured those almost osseous indurations by the internal employment of volatile alkali, and by applications of diluted soap lie.

CHAPTER III.
INDURATION OF THE TESTICLE.

159. In general this only remains after injudicious treatment, of the sympathetic swelling of this gland; it is worst when at the same time the spermatic chord is thickened, varicose and scirrhous. This affection is often very tedious, often incurable. If the epidydimis only be indurated, it is of less importance, it does not interfere with the reproductive faculty.

160. In cases of induration of the testicle that is not of too long standing, the application of a compress imbibed with a strong decoction of oak-bark has proved of excellent service in my hands. Others have recommended the internal use of hemlock and local fumigations with cinnabar, along with repeated emetics; I have never seen the slightest utility from any of these means in any kind of induration.

161. Some have advised, in addition, the rubbing-in of Neapolitan ointment [1] into the scrotum and perinæum, together with the internal

---

[1] Girtanner advises that ammonia ointment be rubbed in several times daily at the perinæum and scrotum. I have experienced its efficacy in other glandular swellings.

use of mercury (but as no lymphatics proceed from the scrotum to the testicles, this does no good, unless from the mere friction) and the external and internal employment of decoction mezereum. Poultices with belladonna leaves have also been enjoined. Where nothing else succeeded, good effects have been perceived from electricity (especially from the electrical bath and the simple spark, or very small shocks from the Leyden jar). Acrel has seen good results from the internal use of a decoction of an ounce of ononis-root in water.

162. Some reckon amongst the best remedial means the inoculation of an artificial gonorrhœa (by the introduction of gonorrhœal matter by means of a bougie, or by the injection of diluted ammonia[1]); others speak disparagingly of it.

163. Schwediauer advised a warm poultice of fresh mandragora root to be applied to the scrotum. Van Swieten trusted to a medicament composed of two ounces of crabs'-eyes and a pint of Austrian wine, four tablespoonfuls to be taken night and morning. Aepli of Diessenhofen completely cured a peasant of scirrhous and ulcerated testicles by the administration internally of fifteen or sixteen green lizards, raw, cut into pieces. We frequently have to alter the constitution before resorting to local remedies.

164. If the cure progresses favourably, the hardness of the epidydimis is the last to disappear. Before the body of the testicle decreases, it first becomes soft, and softer[2] than in the natural state, as Hunter observed and I can testify.

165. If all attempts prove fruitless, and the testicle remains very sensitive to touch, or traversed by agonizing shoots, grows rapidly in volume, &c., we may perform castration without tying the spermatic cord. If however the latter up into the abdominal ring be thickened, knotted and hard, this operation is inpracticable. Still it rarely passes into cancer.[3]

CHAPTER IV.

SECONDARY GONORRHŒA IN THE MALE AND ITS TREATMENT.

166. The mucous discharge[4] from the urethra, which continues undiminished from a primary gonorrhœa long after the cessation of the scalding of urine and of the painful erections, is termed secondary gonorrhœa (*gleet*).

---

[1] Girtanner recommends a simple, clean bougie for this purpose.

[2] Almos: pappy.

[3] Girtanner is of opinion that induration of the testicle never passes into cancer.

[4] Perhaps I should add "without venereal miasm," but the infecting power of clap and of gleet has not yet been accurately determined by observers, especially as in reality there are gleets whose continuance, as will be seen, depends on their venereal nature, I mean those arising from ulcers in the urethra.

167. The same appellation may be given to the discharge that recurs after excitation of the passions, after severe exercise, excesses in fermented liquors, or after repeated coitus. [1] All these re-exciting causes tend to change the mucous colourless gleet into a puriform discharge.

168. Seeing that there is no universally efficacious remedy for gleet, and seeing that things that do good in some cases, do manifest injury in others, it follows that this affection may arise from several causes.

169. Sufficient for practical purposes may be the division into gleet *from irritability*, gleet *from local or general weakness*, gleet *from habit*, gleet *from ulcers of the urethra*, and gleet *from strictures of the urethra;* although there may also be some from scrofulous and gouty causes, as would seem to be shewn by some cases.

170. The cure of these kinds of gleets would often not be attended with such difficulty if it were easy to ascertain the cause [2] in every case with certainty. But the following distinctive marks will suffice in most cases.

171. *The gleet from irritability* chiefly affects those persons who are subject to irritable weakness of the nerves and frequent indisposition, and in whom during the primary gonorrhœa the pains extend beyond the special seat of gonorrhœa to the neighbouring parts, and give rise to the above described bad symptoms.

172. Along with this gleet there is usually a disagreeable irritating sensation in the urethra, which however is not fixed to any particular spot; the distinctive features of the other gleets are not present, and their remedies manifestly aggravate it. [3]

173. It has this peculiarity, that when it is getting better it is aggravated by the use of mercury, irritating clysters and purgatives, by drinking much tea, by anger and other passions, or by slight excesses in venery, in eating and in drinking, and after it has ceased for some time is brought back again by such causes.

174. If we can remove the irritability from the system, or from the genitals if they only are the seat of irritability, then the gleet will go off of its own accord. Therefore the method I recommended (§150 —152) for the irritation of the bladder and the accompanying pains in the urethra remaining after gonorrhœa should be adopted.

175. The genital parts are to be bathed in cold astringent fluids, as

---

[1] That the gleet occasioned by excessive coition is not produced by a new infection, we know from this, that it comes on immediatly after the act, that it is accompanied by scarcely any pain, and from other circumstances.

[2] Sometimes it appears to be quite inexplicable, as is observed in those gleets that cease of their own accord after the fruitless employment of the most approved remedies.

[3] In this kind of gleet we must neither employ irritating nor styptic injections if we would avoid aggravating it and exciting erysipelatous inflammation.

a strong decoction of oak-bark, a solution of common vitriol or of alum in cold water, and the like, and a tepid solution of opium in water (in the proportion of one to sixty) should be injected[1] into the urethra, if that can be done without causing irritation.

176. Should there. be no opportunity of doing all this, the continued and repeated dipping of the genitals in plain cold water will often answer the purpose alone; especially conjoined with moderate exercise in the open air and a cold foot-bath for some minutes every day.

177. A general tonic treatment of the whole system, especially in obstinate cases, will contribute much, often more than anything else, to the removal of this kind of gleet, which is usually caused by an improper treatment of the original gonorrhœa by the abuse of Neapolitan ointment, venesections, purgatives and irritating injections during the inflammatory period.

178. *Gleet from habit.* Excessive coition and the unnecessary use of the bougie during the third stage of gonorrhœa, frequent infections, and other causes, may bring the excretory ducts of the mucous glands into a state of insensibility and induration, whereby they lose the power both of expanding and contracting themselves. Through their callous orifices they permit the escape of a quantity of the mucus concreted in the glands which would else be taken up again by the absorbent vessels. The discharge becomes almost like an issue, like that in chronic ophthalmo-blennorrhœa.

179. Astringent[2] or relaxing injections have no effect on this kind of gleet.

180. The discharge is not so copious or so watery as that in gleet from weakness: the urethra is painless and will readily bear the introduction of a bougie; but that arising from weakness may in course of time degenerate into this kind, if treated too remissly or not at all.

181. This kind of gleet must be treated, at least in the first place, with stimulating injections, for which a solution of a grain of corrosive sublimate in four ounces of water will suffice. The injection must be performed for the first two or three days, twice, afterwards three or four times daily. We may then, if the urethra bears this injection without any sensation, diminish the quantity of the water for the solution, in order to make it stronger.

182. If we suspect that the injection does not penetrate to the affected part (for the fluid rarely goes more than four or five inches into the urethra), we may introduce a bougie covered with onion-juice and dipped into the solution of sublimate. In obstinate cases we

---

[1] By means of a small syphon (§ 59).

[2] If this kind of gleet arises from long-lasting gleets from weakness, styptic injections may frequently cause inflammation of the urethra, sympathetic swelling of the testicles and other inconveniences.

may roll the bougie in finely pulverized red precipitate, and leave it but an instant in the urethra.

183. If, as ought to happen, the discharge hereupon increases, we cease and wait until the discharge diminishes to less than its usual quantity. We may then employ a solution of turpentine in water by means of yolk of egg, gradually increasing its strength until the cure is complete, or if it be delayed make use of strong astringent injections (§ 188).

184. These are the cases, especially when the disease is obstinate, in which the internal use of cantharides-tincture[1] has sometimes appeared to produce wonderful effects. We may try it in obstinate cases. Frequent horse exercise has also proved of use.

185. *Gleet from weakness*, notwithstanding its frequency, has been denied by some[2] who were unable to reconcile the idea of *weakness* with *increased secretion*, but as weakened glands and excretory vessels do not throw out an increase of humours from their own energy, but because, when weakened, they yield to the impetus of the bloodvessels, and are thus compelled, as it were, on account of the diminution of their reactive force, to receive a quantity of fluid, which they permit to flow in excess from their excretory orifices almost crude and but half concocted, in consequence of their inability to offer any resistance. We may therefore say that in this increased secretion they are rather passive than active. This is sufficiently evident from the mode of action of the remedies that are efficacious.

18 . Ordinarily this kind of gleet occurs in persons of phlegmatic constitution who have weakened the genital organs by excessive venery or onanism,[3] or by the abuse of relaxing drinks and baths, or in those in whom the primary gonorrhœa was accompanied by little irritation, but much discharge. Probably the relaxing method of treatment continued till the third stage, and the use of a quantity of laxative salts, or of saltpetre, and repeated venesections, contribute in no small measure to its production, as also the employment of sedative injections continued after the cessation of the scalding.

187. These gleets have this peculiarity, that almost no pain accompanies them, or at most only a sense of weakness in the loins and testicles, which hang down loosely. The discharge of a thin fluid is

---

[1] As early as 1698 this was recommended by Martin Lister (*Exercit. obs.* 12) in gonorrhœa, but if used at the commencement it might prove injurious.

[2] Particularly Hunter.

[3] The itching in the genitals that usually occurs towards the termination of a gonorrhœa, causes frequent erections, and if the patient, as might be anticipated, do not resist this sensation by abstinence, exercise and temperance, but if he rather obey what seems to him a healthy call of nature, by onanism or repeated coitus, he will often bring on this kind of gleet. We must take care to warn him against this erroneous conduct.

more copious than in the other kinds. It often diminishes and increases again almost without any cause, but the latter occurs usually after venereal excitement, the former sometimes after the inordinate use of wine, &c.

188. The genitals should frequently be bathed, for a minute at a time, in very cold water in which some common vitriol has been dissolved, and a similar footbath may be used for several minutes. Along with this, injections of a strong decoction of oak-bark may be employed, and the strength gradually increased. If all this fails, a solution of one part of white vitriol in thirty parts of water may be injected.

189. The internal administration of bark, horse exercise, the open air and nourishing diet, with a little wine, may greatly further the cure. Finally we may have recourse to electricity, *i. e.* small sparks drawn from the genitals.

190. *Venereal gleet.* Modern authors go too far when they allege the presence of ulcers in the urethra to be so excessively rare in gonorrhœa, although they are quite right in asserting that they are quite non-essential[1] to venereal gonorrhœas, and do not frequently occur.

191. These ulcerations may arise from the laceration of considerable bloodvessels in the urethra during spasmodic erections and coitus, from blows and other injuries from without, and from wounds of the internal lining membrane by the syringe, the catheter, or the bougie, &c. The gonorrhœal matter transforms these wounds into true chancres. In some rare cases they are formed by an abscess of an external urethral gland bursting into the canal.

192. We know this to be the cause of a gleet when during the gonorrhœa pure blood has flowed from the urethra, or when one or other of the exciting causes we have indicated above has occurred, but especially when, after the cessation of the inflammatory period of the gonorrhœa, the bougie touches a small raw, painful spot, causing a pain that is felt exactly in the same situation on touching the urethra externally. Hence it happens that even after the judicious treatment of the original gonorrhœa the discharge continues to flow, though in less quantity ; and it may occur that after the employment of astringent injections symptoms of lues venerea may begin to shew themselves.

193. It is self-evident that after the recognition of the cause of these gleets, the last-mentioned remedies should not be made use of. Even the internal employment of balsamic remedies is contra-indicated.

194. The only remedy we can have confidence in is a good prepara-

---

[1] It may well be that cicatrices are so seldom discovered in the urethra after death, for we often can scarcely observe in the glans or prepuce a trace of the chancres that formerly existed, provided they were not very large or deep, and were only cured by the internal use of mercury, and not by caustics.

tion of mercury (such as the soluble) given in gradually increasing doses until mercurial fever (§ 290) is developed. By this medicine alone, without the employment of any injection, this kind of gleet, with all traces of general venereal symptoms, will be easily, certainly and radically cured, and this remedy tends to aggravate every other kind of gleet.

195. *Gleets from strictures* in the urethra seldom occur immediately after the gonorrhœa; they often appear twenty or thirty years thereafter. They consist of a scanty, almost colourless, mild, mucous discharge, with retention of urine, or at least diminished size of the stream of urine.

196. The bougie is the only way to detect their cause, by revealing the strictured spot.

197. It ceases spontaneously after removing the stricture, without any additional aid, wherefore I must refer the reader to the treatment of the latter[1] affection (§ 207—245).

198. If the body have much predisposition to scrofula or gout, gleets often become complicated thereby.

199. The internal use of crude antimony, of burnt sea-weed, of purple fox-glove, and bathing in sea water, will perform in the case of the first what the remedies recommended for the other gleets are unable to effect, and extract of monk's-hood, cold baths and electricity will do the same for the last.

CHAPTER V.

SECONDARY GONORRHŒA IN THE FEMALE AND ITS TREATMENT.

200. The usual seat of this is the vagina, rarely the uterus, and still more rarely the urethra. To all appearance it does not differ from ordinary leucorrhœa; its very origin is undiscoverable if it have not continued to flow immediately after the venereal gonorrhœa. Its varieties are much less numerous than those in the male.

201. If it is already of long standing, it belongs to the gleets from habit, and must be treated entirely by stimulating injections (§ 181) gradually increased in strength.

202. After pursuing this treatment for ten or twelve days we should pause, in order to see whether the discharge will decrease in a few days; in which case, the strong astringent cold injections, recommended above for primary gonorrhœa in women, especially a strong decoction of oak-bark combined with alum, must be employed until the discharge ceases, and even for a couple of weeks thereafter.

203. But as in women we are unable to determine accurately in every case whether it be a gleet from habit or from weakness, we

---

[1] As urethral calculi only cause gleets when they have produced strictures in the urethra, as they often do, their treatment does not belong to this place.

would do well in most cases (seeing that on account of the loose texture and inferior sensibility of the parts we have less to fear than in
the case of the male urethra) to combat the malady at once with injections possessing both a stimulating and strengthening character.—
An injection of an ounce of blue vitriol dissolved in a pint of water,
or of three or even four ounces of white vitriol in the same quantity
of water, will be found very serviceable.

204. Should we, on the first injections of this fluid, meet with any
disagreeable, painful and inflammatory symptoms, we will know from
that that the gleet belongs to those arising from disability. We must
leave them off and treat the case only with injections of cold, even
ice-cold water; and at length we may have recourse to a decoction of
oak-bark. If the irritability be excessive (which will be ascertained
by other symptoms, the rapid pulse, the character of the primary
gonorrhœa, &c.) we may substitute injections with tincture of opium.

205. If along with gleet of this kind there be symptoms of a gouty
or scrofulous disposition, they must first be eradicated as far as possible by suitable remedies for these states, before we proceed with the
local treatment.

206. If, however, on the introduction of the syringe a painful internal spot should be observed, without any induration of the mouth of
the womb or other signs of internal cancer (the acrid nature, discoloured appearance or specific odour of the ichor discharged, the
shootings from the hips into the pelvis, &c.) being present, we may
suspect a venereal ulcer in the vagina; for which the internal use of
mercury (§ 614 et seq.) without any local means, is alone efficacious.

CHAPTER VI.
STRICTURE OF THE URETHRA AND ITS CURE.

207. All the phenomena of obstructed flow of urine, when no stone
was present, were formerly attributed to cicatrices and excrescences
in the urethra, which without examination were termed carunculæ
and collosities, and in conformity with the prevalent notion, were held
to be the relics of ulcers in the urethra, which were taken for granted
to exist in every case of gonorrhœa.

208. This opinion was for long the general one, until by an enormous number of autopsies it was proved that cicatrices and fleshy
excrescences in the urethra were of very rare occurrence, and that in
the great majority of instances all the symptoms ascribed to that
cause arose from narrowing and constriction of the urinary canal,
without actual thickening of its substance.

209. Although we do not allege that these strictures are always the
effect of gonorrhœa, this at least is certain, that they are chiefly to be
found in men who have been affected by this fashionable complaint;

but yet a disposition to rheumatism [1] may contribute not a little towards this, especially as they usually occur only in the middle or advanced periods of life (often 20 or 30 years after the patient has had gonorrhœa). What a distance betwixt the probable cause and the effect! Hence it happens that strictures are very rarely met with in the place where the gonorrhœa has its special seat; usually further backwards: whence we may infer, at least thus much, that it cannot be with propriety ascribed to simple ordinary gonorrhœa. Severe strictures have been met with in persons who had had very slight gonorrhœa) or even none at all), and those who have had the most violent gonorrhœas have remained free from strictures. Neither can they be ascribed, as it was formerly supposed they might, to the use of the bougie or of injections in the treatment of gonorrhœa; for, according to Hunter, strictures have occurred when gonorrhœas have been removed without these appliances. Be this as it may; as the actual exciting cause is still involved in obscurity, and as the general opinion has hitherto attributed strictures to a previous gonorrhœa, l feel myself necessitated to say what is essential regarding them.

210. Probably any severe irritation of the urethra (*i. e,* by urethral calculi) or any inflammation of it, more than merely superficial, is capable of making it liable to strictures.

211. Moreover it is subject to this affection in common with other canals of our body; as examples of continued strictures I may instance, constrictions of the œsophagus (I had recently an opportunity, at an autopsy, of observing a great contraction of the middle portion of the stomach) and those of the bowels, especially of the colon; the spasmodic strictures of the nasal duct at the lacrymal sack, of the gullet and of the bowels, have also some resemblance to urethral stricture.

212. *Strictures* are constrictions, or narrowings of the urethra as if it were drawn together by a thread, which are most frequently met with in the vicinity of the bulbus, much more frequently anterior to it, (from five to three inches from the orifice), and very seldom behind it; they either constrict the canal more or less uniformly all round towards the centre, or only at one side more than the other.

213. In consequence of the bladder reacting against the constriction of its excretory canal, and not being able to get rid of its contents easily, there often occurs a frequent anxious call to make water; the coats of the bladder become thickened, the posterior part of the

---

[1] A man, 58 years old, had for many years been troubled with pain in the hips, especially after drinking a little wine. His hitherto unnoticable urethral stricture once increased suddenly, and the most fearful retention of urine took place. Whilst this disease prevailed and I sought to relieve him from it, he had not the slightest attack of his rheumatic sufferings, not even when I let him drink wine; only the stricture appeared to be aggravated by it.

urethra, as far as the stricture, gradually dilates (often also the ureters up to the kidneys, sometimes the pelvis of the kidneys [1] themselves) in proportion to the degree of the stricture; and the internal membrane of this portion of the canal, distended and irritated by the stagnating urine, exudes a gleety looking mucus, or its coats inflamed or corroded by the acrid urine, if the stricture continue or contract still further, form an abscess which opens externally and usually gives rise to a perineal fistula, whereby nature is forced to provide a new passage for the urine.

214. The patient does not in general notice his malady, or think fit to seek advice for it, until the stricture has attained a serious height. The stream of urine commences to grow smaller and smaller, the desire to pass water more frequent, and still he apprehends nothing bad. Inflammation may occur, and even an abscess in the course of the urethra, still he regards it only as a local affection that will go off of itself, and does not suspect that it arises from the diminished flow of urine (which he may at that time have not deemed worthy of notice), or from the slow and unnoticed advance of the constriction of the urinary canal. It is often only when the urine passes by drops, or when complete ischuria has occurred, along with anxious desire to pass water, that he applies for aid; when inflammation, mortification and death are at the door.

215. *Strictures* that gradually increase to the highest pitch without intermission, in which the urine does not pass at one time more at another less freely, are termed *persistent* or *continuous*. On introducing the bougie we find at one time just the same amount of resistance as at another. The contraction remains under all circumstances, under every regimen the same, only that it goes on imperceptibly increasing until at last it will not permit even the smallest bougie to penetrate into the bladder. It is diminished neither by antispasmodic nor yet by derivative irritating remedies.

216. Externally the affected part generally presents a whiter appearance than the other parts of the urethra, and it frequently appears as if drawn together. The contracted part is seldom an inch in length, usually not more than a line; there is rarely more than one present in the urethra.

217. This persistent stricture never comes on immediately after gonorrhœa, and usually only attains its acmé at the end of the middle

---

[1] A pressive dull pain in the region of this organ (one kidney is usually the worst) indicates this affection, and the same pain with a roundish elevation in the side, speedily followed by the passage of a uniformly mixed whitish urine, with puriform sediment and diminution of the swelling, indicates an abscess of the renal pelvis common in severe chronic strictures, which often comes on in consequence of serious errors of regimen, as I have frequently had an opportunity of observing.

period of life (between 48 and 60). It alone is accompanied by that
sort of gleet (§ 195—197) that goes off spontaneously after the cure
of the stricture.

218. The *spasmodic stricture* is the very opposite of the persistent.
It does not remain in exactly the same spot, but sometimes moves an
inch forwards or backwards. The bougie that would formerly pass
easily, becomes all at once impeded in its passage or completely
stopped; occasionally also it is pushed back again, after lying there
for some time.

219. In these cases the urethra is very irritable and sensitive, and
with difficulty bears the introduction of the bougie or its continuance
in the urethra, but more readily after the passage of the urine, although
this is denied by Hunter, and after the local or internal employment
of antispasmodic remedies. It is increased by the use of astringent or
stimulating medicines.

220. It has the greatest similarity to the irritation of the bladder
(§ 148 *et seq.*), and the spasm of the neck of the bladder accompanying
that state, and apparently contributes much to aggravate that affection. It is the only kind of stricture that can occur soon after bad
gonorrhœas; it may also have much to do with the retention of urine
(§ 25) that often accompanies them.

221. Very rarely (at most only after the removal of persistent
strictures) it is the sole affection of the urethra; most frequently it is
merely the concomitant of the persistent contraction caused by an
urethral calculus, or of inflammation of the neck of the bladder. I am
unable to say with certainty whether it may not in course of time
assume the persistent form.

222. It almost never happens that a persistent stricture exists
without a spasmodic one, and if it do it can only be a very slight
one. The narrower the persistent one is, and the more it obstructs
the exit of the urine, the more frequently does the spasmodic one accompany it, and the more intense it is.

223. Hunter is unable to determine whether the spasmodic stricture
is *behind* or *in* the persistent one. I believe I have always noticed the
former; for I have frequently only required to press upon the stricture with a bougie too large to enter it, in order by this remote
irritation to remove in a revulsive manner the spasm behind it, whereupon I could easily penetrate through the spasmodic stricture with
a smaller bougie, which before this manipulation could not pass
through it.

224. We may always recognise the complication of the persistent
stricture with the spasmodic one in this way : a bougie not too large
for the first two or three inches of the urethra cannot penetrate to the
neck of the bladder, but when pushed in from four to six inches it

meets with an insurmountable obstacle (the persistent stricture) at all times, which, however, a smaller bougie (except in the worst cases) passes with ease, except occasionally (the spasmodic stricture) when its passage is more or less difficult.

225. Three modes are known of curing the persistent or permanent stricture (whereby no attention is at first paid to the accompanying spasmodic contraction), of which the two first are adapted to the case in which a small sound can still be passed, but the last is required when even the smallest bougie cannot pass. The first consists in the gradual dilatation of the stricture; the second in causing ulceration of it; the third in burning through it with caustics. • All three are practicable if the contraction be not seated exactly in the curvature of the urethra, in which case perhaps there is no remedy but the knife.

226. By the first method,[1] we endeavour to pass the largest bougie that can be made with a little force[2] to pass through the stricture, and allow it to remain a few minutes in the urethra, or as long as the patient can bear its presence there without great discomfort. If he can bear it for an hour at a time, we then take a larger one, with a point of a conical shape, and try to introduce it. We press it in cautiously, and for a short time also in an intermitting manner, and with a slight twisting movement. If it spring back, either we have not hit the opening of the constriction, or it is too narrow to admit the instrument, and we must use a smaller one. But if it penetrates in and remains fast we are certainly in the stricture, especially when the introduction has caused no pain and the point of the bougie is squeezed flat. We remove it again when the patient can bear it no longer, and endeavour on a subsequent occasion to make it penetrate further. If it pass through the stricture, we next try a larger one, and then again one still larger, until we have overcome the contraction; that is to say, until we are able to introduce into the bladder a bougie of from two to two and a half lines in diameter; for should there be obstacles farther backwards, we must proceed as with the first stricture.

227. The bougie must be neither too soft else it will easily bend, nor too hard, otherwise we might readily, as often happens with the catheter, especially when due caution is not exercised, push through a false passage near the stricture in the spongy body of the urethra.

---

[1] This mode of curing strictures of the urethra by the pressure of bougies, was known as early as the year 1560, when a physician of Nimes whose name has been lost, (see the 22d of the 37 observations appended to *Laz. Reverii Obs. Med.*, Lugd. 4, 1659,) cured them with leaden sounds.

[2] The stricture is often so narrow, that bougies sufficiently small to pass through it at first, and at the same time of adequate strength, cannot be procured: in this case we make use of catgut harp-strings of gradually increasing thickness, making their extremity round, and introducing them covered with oil.

4

We become aware of this having occurred, when, in introducing the instrument, we make way, with much suffering, to the patient, without at all facilitating the passage of the urine; and we avoid this accident in the case I speak of, by the employment of elastic bougies and carefulness. We ought also to withdraw the bougie from time to time, in order to observe whether or no its point be bent up. Should we allow the bougie to remain some time in the urethra, especially at night, it ought to be bent over about an inch at the top, and fastened with a thread behind the glans, in order to prevent its slipping into the bladder; an accident that could only be remedied by opening the bladder by the lateral operation to extract this foreign body, which is attended by much danger. The bougies ought not, as they usually are, to be made conical throughout their whole length, but they should be uniformly of the same thickness, consequently cylindrical, and should only be somewhat narrower at their point. The patient must soon learn to introduce the bougie himself; he will be best able to pass it with facility into himself; he will be best able to feel the part that is to be dilated, and will not be liable to make a false passage near the stricture, even with a harder bougie.

228. We should not discontinue the use of the bougie in consequence of the presence or occurrence of a swelling of the testicles, as in the case under consideration this swelling is usually the effect of the stricture of the urethra, of an urethral calculus, or of an abscess of the glands of the canal, and by the employment of the bougie would in the first case be removed, in the second relieved, and in the third not aggravated.

229. Sometimes, especially in cases of irritable nervous weakness, and when the stricture already causes troublesome symptoms, as difficult passage of the urine, irritable bladder, &c., there is usually present, along with the persistent stricture, as has been said, also a spasmodic contraction, generally behind the former. This is an obstinate and frightful malady. In this case, if the ordinary bougie will not pass, we must resort to all sorts of expedients in order to gain our object. We press a large bougie against the persistent stricture for a minute, and then try the smaller bougie which ought to be introduced. If this do not succeed, we must tickle or gently rub the perinæum, whilst with the other hand we press the bougie against it. If this too fail, we should try the immersion of the whole genitals in cold water, and the employment of a tepid foot-bath. If the spasm be frequently in the way, we may place a seton in the perinæum. In this case, certainly the best time for introducing the bougie is immediately after making water.

230. We must besides ascertain and make the patient avoid all that increases the spasm. In order more certainly to diminish the irrita-

bility, the patient should frequently pass his water, should use cold baths, take exercise in the open air, shun spices and heating, as well as relaxing drinks, and take internally quassia-powder. Astringent tonics, as bark, iron, &c., increase the spasmodic constriction in my experience.

231. This mode of removing persistent strictures by gradual dilatation, is certainly the easiest, but at the same time the most uncertain method. Even though by advancing to the very largest bougie, we have got so far that the dilated constriction of the urethra allows the free passage of the urine, the patient is notwithstanding not yet perfectly cured, nor guaranteed against a relapse. For a long time to come he must still introduce the thick bougie from time to time, every eight hours, at least, and let it remain there some hours, otherwise the place where the stricture is gradually contracts again, so as not to allow the passage of the largest bougie, and so on. He must never travel without providing himself with bougies in case of necessity, as the tendency of the dilated part to contract again is not radically cured.

232. If the patient take upon himself to assist in this dilatation, he can, after some smaller bougies have been passed, rapidly go to larger and much larger ones, and by means of the irritation produced in the affected part, create a small amount of inflammation and suppuration (the second method) which gradually rids him completely and radically of his malady. The texture of the contracted part is always a morbid abnormality, and hence it is much more readily brought into a state of inflammation and suppuration than the healthy portion of the urethra.

233. In order more certainly to attain this object, the forcible pushing through of the stricture with a bougie of large diameter has been advised, and this manœuvre has sometimes been wonderfully successful ; probably in this case a small part of the internal membrane in the stricture was thereby torn, and thus suppuration was produced, or the forcible stretching might have caused a contusion and thereupon inflammation proceeding to suppuration, or the circular fibres of the contracted urethral muscle might have been paralyzed by the force applied, or even torn, whilst the dilatable part of the stricture yielded. The last is the most probable, for cases have been observed in which, after this forcible manœuvre, the stricture disappeared suddenly and without relapse.

234. In spite of all this, this operation is attended with much uncertainty, and its performance is not advisable. With the force employed, it may easily happen, as we work in the dark, that we miss the stricture, or its central point, which is often far from being in the axis of the urethra, and so form a false passage.

235. In order to attain the same object with certainty, we take a horn staff, of the thickness of a bougie that fits the commencement of the urethra, we bend this by means of heat into a slightly curved form, and scrape down half an inch of its end, till it has almost uniformly the thickness of the bougie that hitherto readily passed through the stricture. This smaller end will form a sort of process to the rest of the staff (of which we smooth down somewhat the abrupt point of junction), just as if a smaller staff projected from a larger one. We first insert this smooth round horn staff into the urethra, in such a manner that its smaller end (up to the larger portion) passes through the persistent stricture, and if we can rely on the patient's steadiness, we allow him to push it in further himself, until the thicker portion passes through the stricture. It will at once be seen that in this way the smaller terminal portion shews the way, and guides the whole horn-staff, so that it must accurately follow the direction of the urethra, and cannot take a false direction. In this way we shall attain our object with much greater certainty. Should we think the horn-sound too inflexible, we may before using it let it soak for some time in linseed oil.

236. More peculiarly belonging to the ulcerating method is the destruction of the stricture with corrosive substances, with which we may arm the bougie we introduce, or the instrument itself may be entirely[1] composed of irritating matters.

237. For this purpose, we select the largest bougie of uniform size throughout that can pass into the anterior part of the urethra, in the abruptly truncated extremity of which we make a circular excavation, and fill this with red precipitate, firmly pressed in. This is to be moistened on the sides with oil, and passed up to the stricture, and pressed against it for a minute. This is to be repeated once daily, until the stricture, having gradually passed into suppuration, will easily admit the thickest bougie. Then, until the healing process is finished, we insert twice a day into the urethra, and allow to remain there a quarter of an hour, a large sized bougie, not armed with red precipitate, but moistened with a solution of myrrh in yolk of egg, in order that the cicatrix which is formed may be sufficiently wide. This troublesome operation is somewhat tedious, but it effects a radical cure.

---

[1] Philip, a Portuguese, (see A. Lacuna, *Method. Extirp. carunc. Rom.* 1551, 12, p. 34,) was the first who, in the middle of the 16th century, destroyed strictures of the urethra, by means of a corrosive mass, composed of verdrigris, orpiment, &c., wherewith he armed the end of a bougie. A similar treatment, variously modified, continued to be used from time to time, until Le Daran, a few years before the middle of this century, began to trumpet forth the excellence of his secret bougies, which were composed entirely of corrosive ingredients, and consequently they frequently excited inflammation and suppuration in healthy parts of the urethra, besides a number of other ill-effects, which rendered their use inadmissible, before his object, the destruction of the stricture, was attained. Guerin improved them.

238. By this method we may in most cases (even in those in which the smallest sound or harp-string cannot get through the stricture) be independent of the *third mode*, which Hunter teaches, for *burning through* the narrowest strictures, and which, as far as my experience goes, may be best performed in the following manner.

239. We take a tube of fine silver of the size of the thickest bougie and slightly curved, and we introduce this, the opening at its extremity being closed by a plug at the end of a wire, which runs backwards and forwards in the cavity of the tube, so that we may remove this plug whenever the extremity of the tube has reached the stricture. Were the tube unprovided with this plug, the mucus of the urethra would enter its cavity. As soon as we have removed the wire with the plug, we push in, in place of it, another wire of fine silver, at the end of which a piece of lunar caustic is fastened in a small forceps.[1] By means of the wire we press this caustic into the stricture for a couple of seconds, draw it back into the tube, and remove both; and this operation we repeat every second day,[2] until we can pass through the stricture with the tube. It is well to inject tepid milk immediately after the operation, in order to avoid the irritation which the caustic that flows from the cauterized part might produce on the adjoining healthy urethra. It is obvious that this method needs great caution.

240. Both these latter methods are of service when there is scarcely any opening remaining in the stricture, and where consequently the first method is not suitable. In case of inflammatory symptoms manifesting themselves, we ought to allay them by means of cold applications, tepid foot-baths, &c.

241. When an urethral calculus may have occasioned the stricture, a passage for it outwards may be made in either of the two last mentioned ways. If the stricture be still permeable, and if the stone be seated in the region of the scrotum, the symptoms it gives rise to might easily be confounded with those of a spasmodic stricture, if we neglect to ascertain its presence by the use of a metallic sound, which as soon as it touches the stone, communicates to a delicate touch a peculiar grating sensation. I have seen, after retention of urine from strictures owing to this cause, the urethral calculus discharged by the efforts of nature through a dangerous abscess in the perinæum.

242. It is rare that the spasmodic stricture (§ 218—224) remains long after the destruction of the permanent one, so as to demand special treatment. On the other hand, in the treatment of strictures

---

[1] In the mode in which a small piece of drawing-chalk is fastened at the end of a porte-crayon; a simall pair of pincers, which embraces the caustic or chalk in its hollow blades, whilst a ring pushed from behind effects the approximation of the blades, and holds fast the substance they enclose.

[2] In most strictures we do not require to do it more than twice.

of the urethra merely by dilatation, the spasm persists as long, and recurs from time to time, until all the tendency of the part (where the permanent stricture was seated) to contract again has gone off; which may sometimes last all the patient's life, if we do not perform the radical cure of the stricture after the second or third manner.

243. Before the spasm after the destruction of the persistent stricture goes off, we would do well, especially if it closes the urethra very suddenly after the withdrawal of the bougie, to employ a hollow catheter of gum-elastic,[1] which the patient should bear about with him, in order to draw off his urine at any time.

244. Frequent immersion of the genitals in cold water will completely dissipate the spasmodic stricture, especially if we endeavour to remove the morbid irritability of the organism by the use of external and internal tonic remedies. If it be already of long standing and if this method do not succeed, a seton introduced into the perinæum will greatly diminish and in course of time remove the malady.

245. Those subject to this affection must frequently pass their urine, and never retain it long. They must guard against chills, excessive passions, heating liquors and spices, and debauchery.

CHAPTER VII.
INDURATION OF THE PROSTATE GLAND

246. When neither paralysis of the bladder nor inflammation of its neck (in bad cases of gonorrhœa), nor a stone in the bladder, is the cause of the retention of urine, and when the introduction of the bougie or sound into the urethra detects no stone nor stricture, and yet the urine will not flow in spite of every effort, we may suspect a morbid condition of the prostate gland.

247. A finger moistened with oil is to be introduced into the rectum and directed towards the pubic region. If this be the cause of the retention, we shall here detect a hard body pressing in upon the rectum, often of such a size that we are obliged to pass the finger from one side to the other in order to ascertain the whole magnitude of this indurated prostate gland.

248. We may easily imagine to what a considerable extent this tumefied body must compress from both sides, and block up the commencement of the urethra, and how dangerous retention of urine may result therefrom.

249. In such cases the ejaculation of the semen is very painful.

250. A bougie[2] or catheter carefully introduced will easily draw off

---

[1] These are also the best we can use when a retention of urine is produced by a merely spasmodic stricture. It should be introduced by suitable manipulations into the bladder, and helped into the neck of the bladder by a finger placed in the rectum.

[2] The urine usually flows off by the side of it, but not without some effort of the bladder.

the urine; but this is only a transient remedy. The best plan is to insert an elastic catheter and to assist its passage through the neck of the bladder by introducing a finger into the rectum.

251. If we could with certainty disperse this glandular induration, we should then be able to promise ourselves permanent benefit, a cure. But as yet we know no remedy that can be relied on.

252. The internal use of hemlock has sometimes been of use, also burnt sponge, but especially burnt sea-weed and sea-bathing, as this affection is often of a scrofulous nature. Poultices of mandragora root frequently applied to the perinæum are said to have proved very efficacious in dispersing this indurated gland. Purple foxglove, crude antimony, hartshorn and electricity, perhaps also local fumigations with cinnabar, might be tried.

253. A seton inserted and long maintained in the perinæum the openings of which were two inches distant, once succeeded in reducing to a great extent an indurated prostate.

254. The best palliative remedy is, immediately after withdrawing the bougie to insert in the bladder, according to Pichler's plan, a catheter of gum elastic (without any spiral wire in its cavity) to let the urine flow through it, to fasten it in front of the glans and close up its extremity, only removing it about once a week in order to remove the calculous concretion that may be attached to it.

255. If, in a case of swelling of this sort, the urine do not flow on the introduction of an ordinary catheter, and if the instrument encounter an obstacle just behind the neck of the bladder (a rare affection which Hunter has best described), it is to be apprehended that a small swollen portion of the indurated prostate projecting into the bladder forms here a sort of valve, which lies upon the mouth of the bladder and obstinately prevents the egress of the urine.

256. In this case a very much curved, large-sized bougie introduced into the bladder has sometimes proved serviceable, the urine flowing past it. If this should not be effectual, we should carefully introduce a catheter, and whenever it has reached this valve-like projection, press it with the handle downwards, whereby its further bent extremity will almost always slip past and to the outside of the abnormal body into the bladder, and permit the urine to flow off.

Second Class.

IDIOPATHIC LOCAL VENEREAL AFFECTIONS ON PARTS OF THE BODY
PROVIDED WITH EPIDERMIS.

FIRST DIVISION.
CHANCRE.

CHAPTER I.

CHANCRE IN GENERAL AND ESPECIALLY THAT IN MALES.

257. The venereal infection is most readily communicated to surfaces of the body that are destitute of epidermis; hence the much
greater frequency of gonorrhœa than all the other venereal symptoms.
Next in point of frequency are the affections that occur on parts of
the body provided with a delicate epidermis; in the latter case there
occur ulcers which are termed *chancres*. The thinner the epidermis
the more easily does the infection take place and the more does the
chancre thus produced extend.

258. The most usual seat of the venereal infection is the genital
organs; hence chancre in the male generally makes its appearance in
the fossa where the glans unite with the prepuce, especially on either
side of the insertion of the frenum, next in point of frequency on the
internal surface of the prepuce and its border, on the glans, and sometimes on the external surface of the genitals, *e. g.* on the scrotum.

259. Should the lips of the mouth, the nipple, or a wound on any
other part of the body be touched with this virus, chancre will be the
result in either sex.

260. A small dark-red elevated spot appears, in some cases thirty-
six hours, rarely several days after the impure coitus, and with painful
itching it forms a hard, inflamed pimple filled with pus, that rapidly
developes itself into an ulcer. When the chancre first appears it is
raised above the surface of the skin; but its hard, light-red (or dirty
yellowish-white) base is a little sunk below the suety whitish borders
whose periphery is inflamed and indurated, but very defined. When
touched the patient experiences severe pains, and we can feel that the
hardness of the whole ulcer extends very deep. The matter that
exudes is of a greenish yellow colour. Such is the chancre, which
gradually increases in superficial extent and depth, accompanied by
pains more of a gnawing than shooting character.

261. Those chancres that have their seat in the inner surface of the
prepuce are much more painful and inflamed, and generally larger
than those that occur on other parts; the induration in and surrounding these chancres is more perceptible and more considerable than
when they occur on the glans.

262. At the junction of the prepuce with the glans they are at first

often no bigger than millet seeds; their most frequent seat is on either side of the frenum, where they readily eat around them and rapidly destroy this part.

263. Chancres on the glans are rare; the inflammation, pain and hardness of the small abscess is not so great as in those on other parts; their borders do not usually project like those on the prepuce for example, but the whole ulcer is as it were excavated in the body of the glans.

264. More painful and more inflamed are the chancres occurring on those parts of the genitals covered with a thicker epidermis, on the penis, or on the anterior part of the scrotum. In these situations they appear in the form of pimples that become covered with a slough, on the falling off of which a larger one is produced. The same is the case with chancres produced by the inoculation of the virus in wounds or parts covered by a firm epidermis.[1]

265. All chancres on a given spot would probably always present the same phenomena,[2] as the inoculating virus is perhaps of only one and the same nature, and seldom milder or more malignant in itself, if the various corporeal constitutions did not themselves cause those great varieties in the malignancy of the chancre (gonorrhœa, buboes, &c.), by the numerous modifications of their reaction.

266. It follows from this, as experience also teaches, that to treat these idiopathic veneral ulcers with the greatest success, we should pay particular attention to the peculiar constitution of the body in every case, which with proper attention we can soon learn from the course of the chancre and its accompanying symptoms.

267. In a diathesis that has a more than ordinary tendency to inflammation, the chancre will inflame to a considerable extent round about, and acquire great depth; the reverse will happen in cases of an opposite character. In a system peculiarly liable to irritability, the chancre will cause great pains, will have a blackish and discoloured appearance, and excrete a thin ichor.

268. The earlier the chancre begins to form sloughs, the greater is the tendency to sphacelus,[3] whereby the whole penis is often lost. We may apprehend great hæmorrhage in such ulcers, when they erode the parts about them much.

---

[1] The inoculation with chancre virus on parts covered by a thick epidermis (by means of wounds in the arms, thighs, &c.) produces more painful and serious symptoms (inflammation, swelling, violent pains) than in the glans, lips, prepuce, &c.

[2] André observes that the worst chancres affect in a very mild degree those persons who are only liable to the mildest infections, and that the interval betwixt the infection and appearance of the chancre is of the same length in most persons who have been several times inoculated with very different viruses.

[3] The inflammation of the chancre is usually of an erysipelatous character, hence the great tendency to sphacelus, as Girtanner has also observed.

269. In general the chancre appears later than the gonorrhœa from the same infection (perhaps they often are primarily caused by the gonorrhœal discharge remaining on those parts), and its virus may therefore be frequently removed by merely wiping the part or washing it with lime-water; they also appear more rarely, for we may reckon that gonorrhœas occur four times as often as chancres. They occur more rapidly on the prepuce; still more rapidly betwixt the junction of the prepuce and glands, especially at the frenum; most slowly on the other parts, probably because the epidermis is thicker.

270. The earlier a chancre breaks out after infection, the more is it disposed to inflammation; the later it appears, the more readily will the blood be inoculated by the poison, and lues venerea produced.

271. There are but few diseases of the body that have not been occasionally overcome by the efforts of nature. Chancre and lues venerea are to be reckoned amongst those few. If circumstances do not occur to produce the absorption of the virus out of the ulcers into the general mass of the circulating fluids (whereon buboes and lues venerea, diseases of still greater gravity than chancre, ensue), they may remain in the same place for several years without the least change, except perhaps growing somewhat larger.

CHAPTER II.
ON THE ORDINARY TREATMENT OF SIMPLE CHANCRE.

272. It is generally asserted that next to inveterate syphilis that has fastened on periosteum, ligaments and tendons, no veneral affection is more hard to cure than a chancre of considerable size and depth. The most skilful practitioners rejoice if they are able to cure a deeply rooted chancre within four to six weeks, by means of a host of external and internal medicaments, that inconvenience the patients not a little, and if they can be certain that in the course of treatment the virus has not slipped into the general mass of the circulating fluids, wandering about there undestroyed.

273. The most distinguished masters of our art are unable to promise to themselves that they will succeed in expelling it from its intrenchment in less time, assuredly not without the local employment of corrosive remedies. Without the latter, which are regarded in the light of an open assault, whilst the treatment by inunction or the internal use of the ordinary mercurial preparations is looked upon as an attack from behind, without these local corrosives, I repeat, they consider the art as impotent to eradicate this virulent ulcer.

274. How uncertain they are upon the subject, is evident from this, that some hold the local employment of mercurials as useless, whilst their opponents know besides the antivenereal metal no efficacious

topical application for chancre, but yet neither can adduce sufficient reasons based upon facts for their contradictory assertions.

275. Did the latter know that their local mercurial remedies have no effect on chancres if they be not of a corrosive nature, or at least become such in the sore, that consequently no form of mercury unprepared in the general circulation is capable of eradicating the venereal virus ; and were the former aware that their non-mercurial sceptics, equally with their mercurial caustics, possess the undoubted power of exciting the lymphatic glands to absorb the local venereal poison (and thus give rise to general lues, which can then only be eradicated by the internal use of mercury), that they moreover cause much pain without being of any material service, they certainly would not at the present day be quarrelling with one another, they would amicably discard their errors on either side.

276. All the objects we would propose to obtain by the employment of local caustics would certainly be best obtained by the use of lunar caustic. It coagulates and destroys with the rapidity of fire, and with the least possible inflammation, all moist animal parts. But how much pain does not the use of even this substance occasion ! It makes a slough, beneath which the remainder of the virus cannot escape ; when this falls off the ulcer looks clean ; we flatter ourselves that recovery is at hand ; it dries up, and behold the inguinal glands becomes painful, a buboe appears—the premonitory symptom of lues ; or suddenly the curative process is arrested, the pain the caustic occasions prevents its further use, proud flesh shoots up, which must now in its turn be destroyed. Frequently things do not go on so well with the employment of caustics ; under this treatment the edges of the chancre we wish to destroy turn over, tubercles appear round about it, the ulcer commences to bleed readily, it is the seat of constant pain, it eats all about it incessantly, and become a true cancerous sore.

277. Instances are recorded of small chancres having been burnt away by the repeated vigorous application of nitrate of silver, without being followed by lues venerea ; but so rare as such cases (Simmons has observed some, I confess I have not been so fortunate), that it is highly dangerous to reckon on such a piece of good luck.

278. But even let us take for granted that with proper care no evil results ensue. Supposing the chancre to disappear without these bad effects, still (I need only refer adepts in the medical art to their own experience) caustics are cruel remedies in chancres, which from the torture they occasion in most cases, change the local virus into a general affection,[1] consequently do more harm than good.

---

[1] Girtanner asserts that the absorption of the virus is so rare an event under merely local treatment, that I can scarcely believe my own eyes when I read the following words of his : "Of the many chancres," says he, "which I have treated

279. If my enemy remains in front of me, I remain always on my guard, I am convinced I have not yet conquered him; but I cannot be said to overcome him if I drive him into an inaccessible corner.

280. There is not a single one of all the so-called corrosive sore-cleansing remedies,[1] from calomel to blue vitriol, from lunar caustic to sugar of lead, which does not at the same time possess astringent, vessel-contracting properties; that is to say, the power of exciting the lymphatic vessels to absorb, and which does not display all this power in the local treatment of chancre. Could we find any remedies that would more certainly transform a chancre into lues venerea than these ?

281. The universal embarrassment that prevails in the treatment of a chancre concealed beneath a phimosis, when the patient will not submit to theof ten dubious operation, shews how ill ordinary practitioners can dispense with the employment of caustics.

282. But in order to cure chancre, local caustics are not the only things they use, they have recourse also to the internal employment of the antivenereal metal! That this is done proves that the former are insufficient of themselves; perhaps, also, it is had recourse to because experience suggested that the ill effects of the local applications should be prevented by the internal remedy. Of a truth they required to introduce all the larger quantity of mercury into the interior of the body, in order to endeavour to destroy the virus that had been driven into the system by these local applications (for that this takes place all are agreed); and on the other hand they found it necessary

---

merely by local remedies, without employing any internal medicines, not more than two cases have occurred in which after the treatment was completed, lues venerea broke out." Truly an incredibly small number only to be accounted for by a perhaps almost specific power in the caustic potash, which was his local remedy (which I confess I have not yet tried); but still too large, when we consider that under the appropriate treatment by the best preparation of mercury given internally, it is impossible that in any case lues can occur after the chancre has disappeared under its use. I do not therefore understand what he says further on : " Supposing the virus were absorbed (from the chancre), the mercury would not prevent this absorption, and could not hinder the occurrence of the general disease. Mercury *never* prevents lues venerea; but it cures it when it has occurred : it *never* destroys the latent virus, (is it more latent in idiopathic chancre than in general syphilitic ulcers?) but it eradicates the poison when it has developed its external effects." As if it did not exhibit its effects in cases of merely local chancre. In what a dilemma does he not place himself also with his lime-water or solution of caustic potash in phimosis ! Still I have such confidence in the unprejudiced mode of thinking of this author, that I am sure he would strike out the greater part of this chapter, if he had for some time cured chancres with the mercurial fever produced by soluble mercury. No external treatment cures so easily, certainly, and quickly.

[1] Pulverized glass even, certainly a powerful remedy for cleansing sores, which acts by mechanical irritation without any corrosive power, scarcely forms an exception, but it has not yet been employed in chancre

to come to the aid of the slow, sleepy efficacy of the mercurial treatment hitherto employed, in order to do something for it in a reasonable time.

283. But when are we sure that we have conquered the enemy by this double assault ? We are answered : 1st, when the local affection is gone and the chancre cured ; 2d, when as much mercury has been introduced into the body as will suffice to affect the mouth, until the commencement of ptyalism, and a little beyond ; 3d, if after this, signs of syphilis appear, we must have recourse to a new course of mercury.

284. The third point shews sufficiently the want of confidence to be placed in the ordinary mode of treatment ; the second is undecided as we sometimes witness a very rapid action of mercury on the mouth, and on the other hand there are cases in which it is impossible to cause salivation by the greatest amount of mercury, (sooner would the vital powers succumb), and yet neither in the one case nor the other is the venereal virus eradicated. The first is of no value as a diagnostic sign, for every chancre disappears when its poison has receded into the body by the use of external, astringent, irritant, or corrosive substances. The mere application of blotting-paper will cure chancre equally well.

285. I shall shew further on, the great disadvantages attending the concomitant employment of the different mercurial preparations in this case, the danger of the salivation accompanying them, that can never properly be guarded against, and the ruinous effects on the system of the long continued use of mercury, (until the mouth is affected.)

286. Could we discover an easier and surer mode of curing chancre with certainty, I imagined it must supersede that hitherto in vogue, and be much more acceptable both to physicians and patients. I hope to be able to shew such a method in the following pages; but I have my doubts whether the prejudice in favour of the old method will allow it to gain a footing.[1]

CHAPTER III.

TREATMENT OF SIMPLE CHANCRE.

287. I shall be very brief on this point, as I would be merely anticipating what I have to say when treating of syphilis, were I now

---

[1] The mechanical expulsion of the venereal virus by the infinitely divisible and excessively heavy globules of mercury is a whim long since exploded, which is forced to take for granted that the hurtful salivation is alone efficacious ; it is completely refuted by the power of a few grains of oxydised mercury in deeply rooted syphilis, and by the efficacy of as few grains of sublimed mercury in the less severe venereal symptoms.

to describe the better mercurial treatment. I shall, therefore, say nothing more than this : in order to cure a chancre radically, the soluble mercury must be given in increasing doses, until the mercurial fever that supervenes has completely cured the chancre, without the employment of the slightest topical application. From seven to fourteen days are sufficient in ordinary cases.

288. I shall merely mention what I mean by mercurial fever, and what is the appearance of a cured chancre. The special method of using the mercury to be employed for chancres, is the same as that for syphilis, to which I refer the reader at § 614—635, and which should be followed in every respect, even in regard to the removal of all unfavourable symptoms that should be avoided during mercurial treatment.

289. I am unable to determine whether the eradication of the venereal virus by mercury depends on a chemical decomposition,[1] or perhaps I should say *neutralization* (something after the manner in which the corrosive oil of vitriol instantaneously becomes tasteless and mild when combined with lead, or like arsenic with sulphur), or as the expression is, on the specific irritation which it excites in our body— which is not to be confounded with the injurious irritation (irritability from weakness, chronic trembling, &c.) which the long continued use of mercury creates, even without destroying the venereal poison ;— but this is certain, that the true destruction of the miasm depends neither on stuffing the greatest possible amount of mercury into the body in the shortest space of time, as has hitherto been imagined, nor in the affection of the mouth (in salivation, which often does so little good, it is certainly affected), nor on any other copious evacuation that the metal is liable to produce in some cases, as ptyalism, diarrhœa, diaphoresis (as Sanchez alleges), or diuresis, but rather on that specific alteration of the body which may not inaptly be termed *mercurialfever*, in which a disagreeable sensation in the mouth is a common but only accidental symptom.

290. The following is a description of the mercurial fever. — The patient gets a metallic taste in the mouth, a disagreeable smell in the nose, a painless, audible rumbling in the bowels, an earthy complexion, a pinched nose, blue rings round the eyes, pales leaden-coloured lips, an uninterrupted or frequently recurring shuddering (always getting stronger) that thrills deeply, even into the interior of the body. His pulse becomes small, hard and very rapic ; there is an inclination to vomit, or at least nausea at everything, especially at animal diet, but

---

[1] In imitation of Schwediaur, Harrison repeatedly inoculated recent chancrous matter which he had previously mixed with Plenck's mucilaginous preparation of mercury, in different parts of the body of a healthy person, without ever being able to cause a venereal ulcer or lues venerea.

chiefly a very violent headache of a tearing and pressive character, which sometimes rages without intermission in the occiput or over the root of the nose. The nose, ears, hands and feet are cold. The thirst is inconsiderable, the bowels constipated, great sleeplessness, the short dreams of a fearful character, accompanied by frequent slight perspirations. The weakness is extreme, as also the restlessness and anxious oppression which the patient thinks he never before felt anything like. The eyes become sparkling as if full of water, the nose is as if stuffed from catarrh; the muscles of the neck are somewhat stiff, as from rheumatism; the back of the tongue is whitish. At this period the patient experiences, if all goes on well, some discomfort in swallowing, a shooting pain in the root of the tongue, on both sides of the mouth a looseness or setting on edge of the teeth (the gums recede a little towards the root of the teeth, become somewhat spongy, red, painful, swollen); there is a moderate swelling of the tonsils and sub-maxillary glands, and a peculiar rancid odour from the mouth, without the occurrence, however, of a notable increase in the secretion of saliva, and without diarrhœa or immoderate perspiration. Four days seems to be the usual favourable period of duration of a fever of this sort, and its best crisis consists only in the permanent disappearance of every venereal symptom and the complete extirpation of the miasm. This picture is taken from an exquisite case of very severe mercurial fever.

291. For the eradication of the venereal poison a sufficient amount of the febrile action just described, in degree proportioned to the obstinacy of the venereal affection, is required. The result of the treatment depends on this, not on the copiousness of the evacuations. Accompanying slight, inconsiderable febrile action, there may often occur uncontrollable perspirations, a flow of fetid urine, a choleraic diarrhœa, or a salivation to the extent of ten pounds daily; the venereal symptoms cease for the time, but they return again, not because the latter are too strong, but because the former was too weak. We may always pronounce such evacuations during the mercurial fever as injurious, but only as regards their debilitating effects on the body, for they cannot prevent the cure of the venereal affection, if there have only occurred febrile action of the kind alluded to, of sufficiently strong character, on which all their efficacy depends. If we can prevent the violent evacuations, as I will attempt to shew how when I come to speak of the treatment of syphilis, we shall thereby increase the intensity of the fever which is so efficient, and spare the patient's strength.

292. While giving the soluble mercury for the cure of chancre until this action is developed, we should dress the ulcer with tepid water or leave it without any application.

293. Whilst the above described affection of the organism, the mer-

curial fever, pursues its course, the chancre commences without the aid of local remedies to assume the appearance of a clean suppurating sore, and heals up in a few days, that is to say, there is formed (without subsequent occurrence of lues, and without pain or swelling of the inguinal glands) a healthy cicatrix, of the natural colour and consistence of the neighbouring parts ; it presents indeed at first a somewhat deeper red colour, and on several parts small elevations if the chancre was very old, but gradually both these appearances disappear. In general the ulcer is healed up before the mercurial fever is completely gone. It is a matter of indifference whether there were one or several chancres, whether they were old and large or small and recent, if only the intensity and completeness (§ 290) of the mercurial fever be proportioned to them.

CHAPTER IV

CONTRACTION OF THE PREPUCE (PHIMOSIS] AND CONSTRICTION OF THE GLANS (PARAPHIMOSIS).

294. Phimosis is not a frequent symptom accompanying gonorrhœa if the prepuce was not previously naturally too narrow, in which case the gonorrhœal matter that insinuates itself betwixt it and the glans can readily produce inflammation or chancre.

295. This symptom occurs most generally when one or several chancres seated on the inner surface of the prepuce become considerably inflamed, thereby violently irritating the loose cellular tissue, and causing it to swell and become thickened, and its occurrence, if it be not evidently produced by other violent causes (such as over-heating the parts by walking, dancing, riding, coitus, onanism, ardent drinks and spices), always depends on a particular predisposition of the system to irritability, as this inflammation is usually of an erysipelatous character.

296. In this affection the prepuce projects over the glans in the form of a shining, transparent, inflamed,[1] tense, painful swelling, so that the dilatation and retraction of this skin, and the exposure of the chancres for the purpose of their local treatment is impossible, and even passing water is a matter of difficulty in consequence of the narrowing of the urethral opening; this condition is termed *phimosis*.

297. The matter from the ulcer becomes accumulated in the interior, and increases still more the swelling, irritation and inflammation ; it may even, if not relieved, bore through the prepuce, and thus effect a passage outwards. The abscess thus opened outwardly is often so

---

[1] And at the same time it is of a pale colour. This circumstance should not allow us to regard the danger as less, as Girtanner rightly remarks.

considerable in size that the glans forces itself out through it, and the remainder of the prepuce at the opposite side forms a distinct swelling.

298. This catastrophe will be so much the more rapidly brought about, when, as is sometimes the case, there was in the healthy state a natural contraction of the prepuce, consequently an impossibility of retracting it behind the glans.

299. But if the prepuce be accustomed to retract itself easily, spontaneously, behind the glans, or to remain habitually behind it, and if in this state of affairs it be affected by the chancrous inflammation; or if, when the prepuce is already contracted by inflammation, we bring it behind the glans, regardless of the impossibility of again drawing it over; or if, after retracting the prepuce affected by chancres, for the purpose of dressing the ulcers on it or on the glans, we imprudently leave it so retracted until the inflammation and distention render its replacement impossible; or if under similar circumstances the act of coition be performed, there will occur the troublesome and dangerous affection termed *Spanish collar, paraphimosis*, or *constriction of the glans*.

300. We can easily perceive that it must be accompanied by much more violent symptoms than phimosis (which is often its producer), for in it the prepuce compresses itself, and its tension and swelling are soon so increased that it, together with the glans whose afferent vessels are thereby completely constricted, is affected by gangrene. It resembles a tumour composed of several rings.

301. This gangrene not unfrequently extends to a part of the corpus cavernosum of the penis.

CHAPTER V.
TREATMENT OF PHIMOSIS AND PARAPHIMOSIS.

302. If chancres be the cause of either of these two affections, it will be requisite while resorting to external measures, even though we should be called in late [1] to the case, immediately to commence the chief means, which is to destroy the poison as quickly as possible by the internal use [2] of soluble mercury.

303. As soon as the mercurial fever commences, which may be brought about on the second, third, or at latest the fourth day, all the inflammatory swelling caused by the chancre poison disappears, in consequence of the miasm being exterminated, as also what there is

---

[1] I have found the beneficial effects of rapidly employing soluble mercury even when gangrene had already commenced, if the most powerful local means were at the same time made use of.

[2] In urgent cases we should commence with half a grain of soluble mercury, and increase the dose by a grain every twelve hours until the artificial fever sets in. We would do well to combine the mercurial with half its weight of opium.

of an erysipelatous character in it, by the revulsion caused by the febrile commotion. In the case of paraphimosis the mercurial fever also removes the chief stumbling-block : the chancres heal.

304. I said, this should be done during the employment of external means. Before the soluble mercury can perform even its most rapid service, the most powerful local means must be used as soon as possible, in order to avoid the urgent danger.

305. In all cases of inflammatory contraction or retraction of the prepuce, we must enforce strict rest, lying on one side on a horse-hair or straw mattrass in a cool room and with light coverings, and the abstinence from all exciting passions, drinks and spices.

306. In phimosis we should frequently inject with caution beneath the prepuce tepid milk in which 100th part of saffron has been steeped for some time, in order to bring away or at least dilute the acrid pus, so as to prevent it bursting through the substance of the prepuce like a pent-up abscess. To the base of the inflammatory swelling we should apply several leeches, and therewith draw off an adequate quantity of blood. Some advise the application of warm emollient poultices ; but they are injurious : they relax the part, and make it less able to resist the pressure of the blood ; the swelling and inflammation are thus increased. We should rather apply to the affected part, immediately after the leeches are removed, ice-cold water mixed with a twentieth part of extract of lead or sugar of lead and a fiftieth part of laudanum, renewing the application every minute. A few tepid footbaths may not be disadvantageous.

307. We should proceed in very much the same manner in cases of constriction of the glans by the retracted inflamed prepuce. We may omit the leeches, but the ice-cold compresses or immersion of the penis in water of that temparature should be repeated as frequently as possible. After a few hours, when the greater part of the inflammation has subsided, we must grasp the swollen glans in the hand, and by means of a gentle gradual pressure, attempt to press back the blood accumulated in it, and thereby diminish its size to such a degree that, seizing the prepuce with the nails of the thumb and forefinger of both hands, we may, by exercising some force, be able to draw it over the glans. This will succeed in most cases.

308. It is only after we have several times tried this manœuvre without success that we should proceed to the operation. In order that we may not be induced to have recourse to it at first, before every other means has been tried, we should consider that there are very few cases in which the operation is indispensable, partly because it cannot be done without great care and difficulty, partly because it usually increases the irritation still more, and usually is followed by sloughing, partly because the patient rarely submits to it at the right

time. In simple gonorrhœas it is also injurious for this reason, that the wound is almost inevitably infected by the miasm, and turns into a chancre.

309. In all cases where the operation is unavoidable, we must search at the neck of the swelling for the part of the prepuce that presents the greatest resistance to dilatation. which will be found to be its anterior border ; beneath this we insert the point of a curved bistoury, and slit it up to the extent of a quarter or a third of the whole length of the prepuce. Having removed the constriction in this manner, if the prepuce cannot be easily drawn over the glans we may leave it behind the glans until the cure is completed.

310. If it can be drawn over, we must take care, during the healing-up of the chancre under the mercurial course, and during the closing-up of the wound, to push it frequently backwards and forwards over the glans, partly in order to prevent the prepuce uniting with the glans, partly also in order that the orifice of the prepuce may not contract during the healing, and thus form a phimosis. A similar manœuvre is necessary also in the case of venereal phimosis, when the chancres beneath it commence to heal under the internal use of mercury, in which case the prepuce is apt to unite with the glans if this movement be not employed to prevent this taking place. The œdema often remaining after the operation is best dissipated by a strong saturnine lotion or decoction of oak-bark.

311. If however, in the case of paraphimosis, gangrene have already set in, relief must be given as speedily as possible. In such a case the following mode of procedure affords almost immediate relief; at least it is the best of all expedients.—Two ounces of finely powdered oak-bark are to be boiled slowly in two pounds of river-water for five hours, down to one pound of fluid, strained through a cloth, the strained sediment diluted with four ounces of white wine and this also strained ; the two fluids are then to be mingled together, and soft rags moistened with the decoction when perfectly cold, to be applied cold and fresh every half hour. I have observed that by this procedure all odour has gone off by the fifth hour. From that moment the gangrene ceases and the sphacelated part will be thrown off by healthy suppuration in the course of four days. The requisite manual aid should not be neglected, the operation on the prepuce will sometimes be indicated if there be still time for it. The same decoction, only ice-cold, may also be employed when, after the operation for paraphimosis (§ 309), the prepuce cannot be drawn over the glans.

CHAPTER VI.

CHANCRE IN THE FEMALE.

312. In the case of women we may very readily convince ourselves of the truth of Hunter's maxim, that the idiopathic venereal poison produces gonorrhœa when applied to surfaces of the body destitute of epidermis that in the healthy state secrete moisture, and chancres when applied to those parts that are naturally dry and covered by epidermis. We cannot find any chancres in the female genital organs where no epidermis exists.

313. The ulcers that occur on the inner surface of the genitals of females when they are affected by gonorrhœa differ very much from chancres. They are usually seated in the folds betwixt the labia majora and nymphæ, are formed slowly out of inflamed hard swellings, have a deep, concealed seat in the body of the labium, probably in its glandular parts, and have very minute openings which must be artificially enlarged and kept open. They always secrete a muco-purulent fluid until they heal up; in all their external characters they differ from the chancre. They resemble the ulcers of the glands along the urethra in gonorrhœa in the male. They have only a partial resemblance to chancres in this, that they cannot be cured without mercury, because by the contact with the gonorrhœal matter they become venereal.

314. Chancres,[1] on the contrary, are seated, in their usual form, only on those parts of the female genitals which are invested with epidermis, and generally just where that is about to cease; in persons who do not make a trade of voluptuousness, right in the border of the labia majora, at the inferior commissure and on the prepuce of the clitoris in rarer cases, and in such as have a more delicate skin, also on the external surface of the larger lips, on the mons veneris, on the anus and the perinæum. In public prostitutes, on the other hand, and other persons of a similar description, the chancres are seated from the above reason sometimes deep in the vagina, on the nymphæ, &c. Large chancres on the labiæ cause these to swell considerably.

315. The chancres on the external parts invested with a thicker epidermis, as the mons veneris, perinæum, &c., resemble those of males which are observed on the penis, scrotum, &c., and are, like these, usually covered by a scab, beneath which a larger one is always formed when the first falls off; they are excessively painful.

316. Probably the latter sometimes arise when the matter from chancres on the internal border of the genitals, where they always remain moist, repeatedly comes in contact with these external parts,

---

[1] They are of the same nature and same appearance in the female as in the male sex.

and thus gradually complete the innoculation through the thicker epidermis. At any rate, this is often the case with respect to those on the fourchette and on the anus.

317. The simple construction of the female genital organs, in those parts where the chancre can occur, does not allow of any such complex symptoms as occur in the more complicated male genitals.

318. The only chancres they are subject to that men are not, are those on the nipples, which they generally get by suckling those children whose lips are affected by true chancres. They eat rapidly about them, and if not speedily checked by the anti-venereal specific, they soon destroy the nipples.

CHAPTER VII.

TREATMENT OF CHANCRE IN FEMALES.

319. As the parts are not of so complex a character as in the male, we have as a general rule less serious symptoms to combat.

320. The external treatment has hitherto been the same as that of chancres in the male, by local remedies of corrosive, astringent, irritating character, precipitate ointment, saturnine lotions, solution of corrosive sublimate, &c. Such treatment is as prejudicial in females as in males, and even more so, because the absorbing surface is larger, and they have frequently several chancres at the same time. Just as, in males, the employment of irritating and corrosive remedies, whether mercury enter into their composition or not, always increases the absorbing power of the lymphatic vessels, so from the same reasons this happens all the more readily in females; perhaps also because the whole vascular system in females is more irritable. Astringent substances[1] are injurious in proportion to their energy. These topical applications, moreover, cause a great deal of local mischief: they alter the chancre, as in males, into ulcers that eat round about them, into spongy excrescences, into sycotic condylomata, &c.

321. We ought, therefore, to abandon this destructive method, and during the proper treatment by internal mercurial remedies dress the chancre, either not at all, or with something quite indifferent.[2]

322. As regards the internal treatment, practitioners are much more at a loss than in the case of chancres in the male. We are advised to

---

[1] Experience teaches that of all remedies that promote the absorption of the poison in chancres, none act so powerfully as the preparations of lead; they are therefore of all the most hurtful in such cases.

[2] André also advises that nothing but tepid water be applied to chancres during his alterative mercurial treatment.

continue the treatment an extraordinary [1] long time, and to use twice as much mercury as we do for the male sex.

323. This destructive method will be easily superceded by the employment of a better mercurial preparation and the requisite circumspection. I have not found it necessary to employ longer time nor to use more soluble mercury for the cure of chancres in females than in males. [2]

324. Attending to the rules to be hereafter (§ 591 *et seq.*) laid down for preventing violent evacuations, (ptyalism, diarrhœa, &c.,) I likewise in their case rose from a very small to a larger dose of the soluble mercury, in order if possible to bring on a sufficiently strong mercurial fever betwixt the fourth and seventh days, reckoning from the commencement of its employment; and during that time I caused the chancre to be dressed only with tepid milk or water. In ordinary cases from ten to twenty days sufficed to complete the cure.

325. If the chancres spread very much, and extend deep into the vagina, we should fill that part with charpie during the treatment, so that the granulations, when they cicatrize, shall not contract the vagina.

326. We should proceed in the same way with chancres on the nipples, that is to say, we should treat the body only internally, without the employment of any external means; but here we must endeavour to produce the mercurial fever as quickly as possible, in order to prevent, if possible, the rapid destruction of these soft parts by the virulent ulcer.

CHAPTER VIII.

TREATMENT OF THE ACCIDENTS RESULTING FROM IMPROPER TREATMENT OF THE CHANCRE.

327. The chronic phimosis (from induration and thickening of the prepuce) that remains after the cure of the chancre, especially when

---

[1] André and some others advise the use of internal mercurial remedies for nine or ten weeks before we can with certainty pronounce the chancres in the female cured, and all the virus eradicated out of the body. It would probably be a matter of difficulty to determine when this had occurred, if they employed local remedies. The best indication would be wanting to them (the spontaneous cure of the chancre) if they repelled it locally. Moreover, the weakness and uncertainty of their mercurial preparations required that they should employ *for so long such a large quantity of mercury*, frequently without any real result, and to the certain injury of the constitution.

[2] A woman who for some days had a bubo, and for a year several chancres on the inner border of the labium majus of the same side, the largest of which measured from four to five lines in diameter, but who was otherwise healthy, took, without employing any local remedy, three grains of soluble mercury in five days. The artificial fever came on strongly and characteristically; four days afterwards, after all the pains in the head and all the fever were gone, the chancres, together with the small bubo, had completely disappeared; for a year and a half she has remained perfectly free from all complaints.

performed in the ordinary manner, increases with the lapse of time, especially if the orifice be too small for the full stream of urine. It becomes schirrhous, and lays the foundation for a number of disagreeable symptoms.

328. In order to remove this evil, we draw the thickened portion of the prepuce over the glans, grasp it tightly, and cut it off cautiously, without injuring the glans. While the wound is healing, the prepuce must be frequently pushed back over the glans, in order to prevent the cicatrix, and thereby the orifice of the prepuce, from contracting again.

329. Where the scirrhus pervades the whole prepuce, it must be cut away entirely, or it may be merely slit up at a convenient point in order to allow the patient to perform the act of coition.

330. Hunter alludes to a kind of false chancre, that seems to result from the previous improper treatment of a true one. Its diagnostic marks are as follow :—It is only met with in persons who have previously (frequently only four to eight weeks before) been affected with real (idiopathic venereal) chancres ; it never occurs exactly on the cicatrix of the healed up chancre, but close beside, or at least not far from it ; it does not extend so rapidly nor so extensively as the true one ; is not so painful nor so inflamed ; has not such a hard base, and does not cause buboes by absortion, like the true chancre.

331. Of quite a different nature are those chancres that by a long abuse of mercury, and perhaps also by the use of improper external remedies, have degenerated into malignant ulcers. Such ulcers secrete much thin acrid ichor, are excessively sensitive and painful, their borders are very elevated, violet-coloured, and hard ; in a word, they resemble old scrofulous ulcers, and are of a similar nature.

332. In these cases there may be no longer any venereal miasm in the system. The abuse of mercury and other debilitating methods have caused the whole body to take on the scrofulous disposition, and have produced a cachexia of morbid irritability, and the ulcers do not effectually heal up before this condition of the organism is improved.

333. A further employment of mercury aggravates them perceptibly. The most powerful antidotes to this cachexia, cold baths, country air, bark, opium,[1] exercise, ammonia, and local tonics are of service.

334. When, in cases where there is an original predisposition to debility, nervous diseases and erysipelas, the chancres, which have in such states of the constitution already a tendency to abnormal inflam-

---

[1] It is in such cases that Turnbull's external employment of the opiate solution in (degenerated) chancres has such excellent effects.

mation, are treated with irritating local remedies and with an excessively long employment of mercurials, purgatives, and tepid baths, it sometimes happens that the morbid irritability of the system increases to such a degree, that even after the healing up of the chancres, inflammation of such intensity is developed on the genitals, that a dangerous affection occurs, which some have improperly termed cancer of the penis.

335. The swelling of the whole organ is great, the heat considerable, the colour bright red. Suppuration beneath the whole of the skin and prepuce rapidly ensues, and ulcerations break out here and there. In such cases a portion or the whole of the glans is not unfrequently lost; sometimes also the urethra, and even the whole of the penis, are destroyed by the suppuration, if the disease be not arrested in time.

336. Here also mercury will be found injurious. I have found no good results from anything besides the free internal employment of bark with ammonia and opium, and a very strong and ice-cold decoction of oak-bark, (if we are called in good time, strongly impregnated with opium) applied fresh every hour or half hour. When the danger is past and the ulcer commences to heal, we must, in order to prevent a relapse, make use of the other remedies usually employed for irritability with weakness.

337. Those chancres which have only been aggravated by the abuse of corrosive remedies, of which the borders become suddenly everted, very sensitive and excessively painful, which bleed easily, eat around them, and are beset with tuberculous indurations (a sort of cancerous ulcer), demand speedy aid. The affected part is to be constantly bathed with a lotion composed of one part of laudanum with twenty or ten parts of water, and bark largely combined with opium is to be given internally until the pain begins to yield. The ulcer will then begin to assume a more healthy character, and may now be cured generally with mild digestives (of cocoa-nut oil, yolk of egg and Peruvian balsam, &c.), if the venereal miasm have been previously destroyed by an appropriate mercurial course.

338. It is usual to stop the profuse hæmorrhage of an old chancre (when the miasm has not yet been destroyed from within) when it throws off an artificial or self-generated thick slough, by means of applications of turpentine. In many cases the local employment of opiates as palliatives is indispensable, especially when the recurrence of hæmorrhage is kept up by irritability from nervous weakness.

339. The spongy excrescences that protrude from chancres that have been treated with local remedies of an irritating character belong to the class of degenerated chancres among which I reckon the sycotic condylomata, of which I am about to treat.

CHAPTER IX.
VENEREAL WARTS AND EXCRESCENCES.

340. Very little of a positive character has been written concerning the nature of the condylomatous warts, and the place they should hold among venereal affections is still so undetermined, that I must take leave not to regard them as a symptom of syphilis, but to place them among the idiopathic venereal affections.

341. They certainly never appear, like gonorrhœa and chancre, immediately after local inoculation, but in this they resemble buboes; but still the humour they exude possesses, like the pus of inguinal buboes, the power of producing local infection,[1] a property that seems only to belong to the idiopathic venereal symptoms.

342. Their power to cause local inoculation, and the fact that when not of a horny hardness, the internal use of mercury can alone eradicate them as I have frequently observed, amply suffice to refute Hunter's opinion, that they are mere consequences of the venereal malady, and not themselves of venereal nature.

343. Thus much is certain, that they are not a primary symptom of immediate infection, but that they only appear from the neglect or improper treatment of the proper chancre. Usually when the latter are treated only by external remedies of an irritating and astringent character,[2] the chancre, without losing its idiopathic venereal virus, gradually changes its appearance, the irritated sensitive fibres attain a luxuriant growth, and excrescences arise on the former seat of the chancres; at least I have never seen a case where the chancres were healed according to my plan, only by the internal employment of the best mercurial preparation without the slightest topical application, where any such excrescence remained. We would therefore not be wrong in regarding this as a degeneration of the chancre, standing in the same relation to that as a gleet does to the primary gonorrhœa.

344. Their seat therefore is the locality where chancres may occur after an impure coitus; the prepuce, glands, clitoris, the orifice of the urethra, the labia, &c., and in those places most generally where the epidermis is thickest, round about the anus, in the perinæum, on the scrotum, &c.

345. Their appearance is various; they are sometimes broad and furnished with a pedicle, in which case they are termed *fig warts;* or they are long-shaped, and resemble a cock's comb; or their head sprouts out enormously, giving them the appearance of cauliflowers, &c.; and writers have classified them according to their resemblance

---

[1] André saw a venereal wart upon the glans communicate genorrhœa to a female.

[2] The power these remedies possess of causing the lymphatic vessels to absorb is the reason why we seldom observe condylomata unaccompanied by some symptoms of syphilis.

to buttons, onions, strawberries, mulberries, and so on, without reflecting that these names indicate no difference of nature, but only depend upon an accidental conformation, consequently are of no essential utility and cannot influence the mode of treatment. More interesting is a knowledge of their nature and of their course.

346. The warts on the prepuce, glans, clitoris and labia, are generally harder and drier than those on other parts; sometimes they are painless, and then they not unfrequently wither and disappear spontaneously (probably when the venereal poison they contain retreats inwardly into the general circulation); sometimes they inflame, and then usually degenerate into cancerous ulcers.

347. In addition to these, immediately after improper treatment of chancres with local irritating substances, spongy growths shoot out rapidly on the penis and in the vagina, which sometimes have little or no sensibility.

348. The condylomata on the nates and perinæum are also spongy, and the hollows and furrows in the skin betwixt them are usually ulcerated and painful. In this condition their surface appears full of chaps, which exude a fetid ichor. They are attended by gradually increasing inflammation and painful burning, until they in the course of time degenerate into fistulous ulcers of the rectum, &c.

349. But hard growths of this kind are also met with in this position, which are often covered with scales and inflamed, and even accompanied by violent pains; injudicious local treatment (without efficient internal assistance,) readily transforms them into cancerous ulcers.

350. The non-venereal warts and excrescences on the genital organs of both sexes are distinguished from the venereal ones by this: that the former have their roots in soft healthy skin, that they are usually of soft texture, dry and flesh-coloured, also that no venereal symptoms either have preceded or accompany them; whereas the base of the venereal ones is upon a hardened part, they are inflamed, and are always preceded by other idiopathic venereal affections, and generally accompanied by several symptoms of syphilis; more particularly there usually exist betwixt them ichor-secreting venereal fissures.

351. If the excrescences are only seated on the anus, before we can pronounce them venereal, or treat them as such, we must pay attention to their diagnostic marks, and also endeavour to ascertain whether they do not result from sodomy, or from some acrid discharge from hæmorrhoids, or from leucorrhœa, as not unfrequently happens, or whether they are not relics of external piles.

CHAPTER X.
CURE OF VENEREAL WARTS AND EXCRESCENCES.

352. If we have convinced ourselves of the venereal nature of the condylomata, from the above signs and from the history of the case,

we proceed to the treatment, which divides itself into external and internal.

353. As a general rule, these excrescences must not be primarily treated by local remedies,[1] for the same reason as I have given for condemning the topical treatment of chancres. If, as we have every reason to believe is the case, these excrescences be malignant transformations of the chancre owing to local treatment, the injudiciousness of such appliances will be more palpable, and the usual bad effects of their employment afford ample corroboration of this assertion.

354. We must consequently discard what made them from chancres into condylomata—the irritating and styptic local remedies, and make use of a judicious and internal administration of mercury,[2] unless which had been neglected they had not degenerated into that condition; in a word, in order to cure them radically, we must do what ought to have been done long ago.

355. The administration of (soluble) mercury serviceable in this case, and the rules for its employment, are the same as for the more remote degree of syphilis (for they belong to the most obstinate local affections), to which latter I refer the reader, in order to avoid unnecessary repetition.

356. I may merely observe that a properly developed (and rather strong) mercurial fever (§ 290) cures all true venereal warts and excrescences; that is to say, they dry up and fall off whole or in fragments, or (but this is rare) they put on a healthy suppurative process and ulcerate away.

357. Those warts that do not fall off nor suppurate away, nor gradually disappear by this internal destruction of the virus, are usually of a horny character; at all events are innocuous and non-venereal.

358. If, notwithstanding, we wish to get rid of them, they may, like all other non-venereal warts, according to circumstances, be removed by tying them with a wax thread and gradually drawing it tighter, or they may be burnt off with lunar caustic, or cut off with the scissors. Some have also advised to apply onions boiled in oil until the warts become soft, and then sprinkle over them powdered mezerium, whereby they are changed into mucus, that may easily be scraped off.

359. But as it nevertheless sometimes happens (although very

---

[1] They produce syphilis, if that be not already present, or cause them to degenerate into spreading ulcers.

[2] When Dease adduces as proof that mercury is of no use for warts, and that they consequently contain no venereal virus, that they sometimes have remained uncured although the patient has long used the metal and been salivated almost to death, he should have remembered that such abuse of mercury often leaves uncured other local affections evidently dependent on the venereal poison, which a rational administration of mercury eradicates rapidly and radically.

rarely in the case of the non-venereal remains of formerly venereal excrescences) that they again grow after removal by the ligature or scissors, we would do well, immediately after their removal by these instruments, if we observe any disposition on their part to grow again, to touch the part once or twice with lunar caustic; except in such cases, when, in spite of the radical destruction of the venereal miasm by the mercurial fever, such a wart still remains inflamed and painful, in which very rare case[1] we must abstain from all topical applications, and content ourselves with destroying the cancerous or scrofulous constitution of the humours by hemlock, cold baths, opium, ammonia, setons in the neighborhood, &c.

360. Peyrilhe recommended, in order to destroy the large spongy excrescences in the vagina, to apply butter of antimony with great caution, and immediately thereafter to cleanse with injections of lime-water the parts where this easily spreading caustic may have touched the healthy tissues. He prefers it to the lunar caustic, because the slough formed by the latter does not fall off under 36 hours; which would allow sufficient time to renew the excrescence beneath it. We may act in a similar manner by excrescences on the male genitals. I would not however advise any beginner in surgery to resort to this method. The judicious internal employment of mercury must always precede it.

361. The rectal and perineal fistulæ arising from condylomata, are hardly ever benefitted by the ordinary employment of mercurials in the shape of calomel, Neapoliian ointment, &c. The soluble mercury is, as it generally is, more powerful in such cases, when all the morbid irritability of the body, which is almost always present, is subdued before its employment, and when at the same time topical fumigations with cinnabar, &c., are not neglected.

SECOND DIVISION.
BUBOES.
CHAPTER I.
DIAGNOSIS OF INGUINAL BUBOES.

362. The swelling produced in the inguinal glands by the dessication of a chancre that has been treated only locally, that is to say by the absorption of the idiopathic venereal poison, is the most ordinary kind of buboe. We need not here dwell on the diagnostic marks of the swellings in the groin occasioned by the sympathetic irritation of the gonorrhœal inflammation, as they are not of a venereal nature, and have been already discussed when treating of gonorrhœa.

---

[1] Morbid irritability must be the cause of this phenomenon.

363. Seeing that the lymphatic system consists partly of single absorbent vessels and trunks, partly of glands, that is, as far as we at present know, of the division, reunion and interlacing of their smallest branches, we might easily suppose, *à priori*, that the former would be less frequently affected, irritated and inflamed, by the passage through them of the virus after its absorption from chancres than the glands.

364. And this opinion is corroborated by experience, which teaches us that the simple lymphatic vessels are seldom affected and almost only after the small glands along their course have already been swollen.

365. When such an occurrence does take place, if, for instance, the seat of the absorption was a chancre on the prepuce or the glans, a lymphatic vessel in the neighbourhood along the dorsum of the penis will be found thickened and indurated, apparently terminating at the root of the penis beneath the pubis, or it will be felt to run into the inguinal region, interrupting in its course by elevated tubercles (small buboes).

366. Something similar, it is alleged, occurs from the absorption of gonorrhœal matter. A cord-like thickening of a lymphatic vessel with small knots upon it is formed upon the penis, usually taking its origin from an indurated part on the prepuce, which frequently presents a raw appearance on the inner surface, a sign that it should be regarded as something more than an immediate metastasis of the gonorrhœal matter)which appears to me to be quite incomprehensible). The same thing happens, though more rarely, from the absorption of the chancre virus from the female genitals. The vessel leading to the gland feels like a cord, and is painful ; small glandular swellings are also produced in its course.

367. Usually however, as has been said, this does not occur ; the absorbents opening into the chancre generally convey the poison, without being affected themselves, to the nearest larger gland, where the angles of the anastomoses and the interlacings of the finer lymphatic branches retard the passage of the humours, and thereby allow the poison time, and give it the opportunity of exercising its irritant power.

368. Here the idiopathic venereal virus is arrested [1] on its way to mingle with the mass of the blood, whilst it, without in the meantime

---

[1] The glandular swelling however does not appear at any time to arrest with certainty the venereal poison from passing into the mass of the fluids, not even when it goes on to suppuration ; which fact may be alleged in opposition to those who say we should regard the bubo as a critical metastasis, and who therefore direct all their efforts to cause it to suppurate ; certainly in most cases a measure of very doubtful utility.

altering its nature, develops that specific painful inflammation and tumefaction in the lymphatic gland, termed buboe, the immediate result of the absorption of the virus from a chancre, more rarely from a primary gonorrhœa, and still more rarely from the uninjured skin, and the proximate source of lues venerea by its further absorption by the lymphatic vessels into the general circulation.

369. The absorbed poison usually settles in the nearest gland towards the centre of the circulation; in the case of chancres on the prepuce or the glans, ordinarily in the groin of the same side; from chancres of the frenum however, and from absorbed (gonorrhœal?) virus from the urethra, on either side without distinction, and often on both sides. But as the situation of these glands varies, so there are buboes which are seated pretty deeply under Poupart's ligament in the thigh, others close to the os pubis, and others again that are located in the abdomen right over or above the ligament indicated. If the absorbed poison be in greater activity, several glands may be affected at once.[1]

370. In women affected with chancres of the genitals on the clitoris, on the mons veneris, &c., they occur also on the same side, but at the commencement of the round ligament of the womb, whence they pass into the abdomen; probably these are lymphatic vessels inflamed by chancre-virus only. If the chancres be seated quite far back, at the posterior part of the labia or on the perinæum, buboes are developed along the furrow formed betwixt the greater labium and the thigh. The other seats of buboes in the female are the same as in the male.

371. If the chancres be seated on the hand or arm (by the introduction of the chancre-virus into wounds, ulcers, &c.), the absorbed virus is also transplanted into the nearest lymphatic gland towards the heart, usually not far from the elbow at the inside of the biceps muscle, but also occasionally in the axillary glands.

372. Chancres on the lower lip in one instance gave rise to buboes on both sides of the neck over the submaxillary glands.

373. The infection of the glands proceeds rather slowly; they have been observed to swell after from six days to several weeks subsequent to the local destruction of the chancre.

374. Chancres that are not treated at all impart their poison much more rarely and slowly to the glands than those treated by local corrosive, irritating substances. Of twenty chancres treated solely

---

[1] Some chancres on the prepuce of an officer of very dissolute habits, who had at the same time gonorrhœa, were merely covered by him with blotting-paper, and not otherwise attended to. He continued his dissipation, and got not only a buboe in both groins and suppuration of Cowper's glands, causing a perineal fistula, but also a similar affection in each axilla.

topically,[1] probably not one case occurs in which absorption does not take place; whereas I have seen many chancres that were subjected to no treatment persist for years on their seat, without the occurrence of buboes or lues venerea.

375. Venereal buboes commence with a slight pain in the groin an almost characteristic anxiety in the chest, and a small, hard swelling, which if it be not restrained by a scrofulous diathesis, by external remedies, the inunction treatment, &c., soon rises up (and then the swollen gland is from the first very painful), inflames, and passes on to suppuration.

376. At first and when still small, this venereal glandular swelling may be pushed hither and thither in the cellular tissue; we observe that but a single gland is affected; its boundaries are very circumscribed. It is only when inflammation has perceptibly set in (the inflamed part is bright red) that its size increases considerably, and then suppuration soon ensues.

377. An abscess occurs, which only differs from the chancre as to size, in other respects its nature is exactly the same.

378. Occasionally an erysipelatous inflammation accompanies the swelling, or watery fluid accumulates there (œdema), and the suppuration advances tardily.

379. If we take into consideration all these signs, and if we are convinced by the history of the disease of the venereal origin of the buboe, we shall very readily be able to distinguish it from others of a similar character.

380. Buboes from other causes are usually softer, and generally more easily dispersed. There are usually several glands swollen at once; in scrofulous affections, glands in other parts of the body are likewise affected. Non-venereal buboes are commonly less painful, and often complicated with catarrhal or hectic fever, in such a way, that the fever was already there before their appearance. They are so far from being amenable to mercury, that they are rather aggravated by its use (and can only be combatted by means of tonics, especially the cold bath, rubbing in of volatile ointment, burnt sea-weed, small doses of ipecacuan not pushed to emesis, shower baths, &c.) Non-venereal buboes increase more slowly, or even should they swell more rapidly, they do not readily pass into suppuration. If they do suppurate, more than one gland takes on the process, and sinuses are more apt to be formed, which is not the case with true venereal buboes.

381. A species of unhealthy suppurating venereal buboes sometimes remains after the treatment by mercurial inunction; the irritating qualities of the large quantity of mercury rubbed in seems to be the

---

[1] Girtanner's caustic alkali must be considered an exception, and must possess a specific antivenereal power which destroys the poison, and thus eradicates it directly.

cause of this phenomenon. A more dilatory employment of the inunction treatment, on the other hand, is apt to change enlarged but not suppurated inguinal glands into scirrhus.

382. In young persons buboes are apt to become scrofulous, in old persons they tend to become cancerous.

383. A surgeon who exercises a due amount of attention will not easily mistake a hernia, an abscess in the groin, or aneurism in the thigh for a venereal buboe.

CHAPTER II.
OBSERVATIONS ON THE ORDINARY MODE OF TREATING BUBOES.

384. When satisfied from the symptoms present of the real venereal character of the buboe, it is almost universally the custom to attempt to disperse the inguinal swelling, discarding the ancient notion that they are critical metastases of the poison and real beneficial processes of nature, and that the way pointed out by nature ought to be followed, which seeks to convert them into abcesses, in order thereby at once to get rid of the venereal virus in the best manner.[1] This delusion has, as I have said, been discarded and it is now sought to disperse them.

385. To accomplish this object no better method was known than to rub in mercurial ointment (lard rubbed up with an equal weight of the quick metal) in the region situated betwixt the place of absorption (the chancre) and the deposit in the gland (the buboe); that is to say, the mercury was introduced into the system in the same way in which it had received the poison, in order that this metal should pass through the gland, and thus, as was imagined, destroy the poison at the diseased place.

386. This treatment, founded merely upon the course of the lymphatic vessels, seems highly advisable in an anatomical point of view, and Hunter takes great credit to himself for the discovery; it involved the à priori unproved (and certainly groundless) supposition that mercury (it mattered not whether in the form of oxyde, solution or salt)[2] chemically destroys, as mercury, the venereal poison by mere contact; and if under the inunction treatment it passed through the swollen gland, it must necessarily come in contact with all the poison, and therefore destroy it in its seat.

387. I admit the propulsive power of this metal, whereby it removes mechanically some obstructions of the glands—for in truth perhaps not above the two-hundredth part of the metal is oxydised in

---

[1] Hence the injurious advice given by ignorant practitioners even of the present day, as soon as an inguinal swelling appears to indulge in dissipation, drinking and venery, to ride, and in a word to do every thing to cause these parts to inflame and suppurate. Nothing could be advised more repugnant to sense.

[2] Or united with the fatty acid in the form of a salt.

the Neapolitan ointment, the result of the inunction treatment more. over shews that the virus located in the inguinal gland really yields to this ointment; but the inefficacy of all applications of mercurials to chancres, and their injurious power (especially that of the mercurial ointment) in hastening the absorption of the poison from chancres into the general circulation, might have taught that the mercury does not destroy the venereal poison as mercury, not *ex opere operato*, but that a previous reaction of the powers of the whole system (the mercurial fever) is required to do that, either by directing the action of the mercury dissolved in the fluids of the body to lay hold of the poison, or by extinguishing the venereal irritation through the instrumentality of the specific irritation excited in the whole sensitive system, or by means of a peculiar change effected upon the metal during its concoction in the secundæ viæ (probably by its combination with some assimilating substance from the animal juices) to render it capable of effecting a chemical neutralization of this virus.

388. This preparatory action of the animal organism on the metal before it is capable of eradicating the venereal virus, should not have been overlooked; its oversight has been the cause of so many false steps in the treatment of venereal diseases, that the history of this divine antisyphilitic specific leaves us in uncertainty whether it have hitherto done more good than harm to suffering humanity.

389. The innumerable instances of buboes and of general lues caused by the merely local treatment of chancres by mercurial topical applications,[1] and of buboes by the merely propulsive force of the quick mercury contained in the ointment, would have diverted the observer from a prejudicial theory to one of a more beneficial character, had he not been led astray by certain accessory circumstances.

390. The internal employment of the mercury, namely, was combined with its external application (to the chancre); hence it followed as a natural consequence, that from the efficacy of the former, the injurious character or inefficacy of the latter could not be perceived. Buboes were dispersed by rubbing Neapolitan ointment into the groin. but the effects of the propulsion of the venereal virus into the general circulation which inevitably follow this treatment were not waited for, but the rubbing-in process was persisted in much longer, and in some cases the patient was actually cured, and thus general (undeveloped) lues was produced, to be cured if so be it might.

---

[1] If the virus be not absorbed into the circulation from the chancre under the application of the mercurials, it will remain for ever undestroyed under their local employment; this is an incontrovertible maxim of experience: otherwise the infinitely rare case must occur, in which the mercurial applied to the small surface would be absorbed in sufficient quantity to produce the same effects as arise from the internal use of the metal (mercurial fever, &c.)

391. If it were possible for the general lues venerea to break forth during the employment of the very minutest portion of mercury, it would certainly always be observed in the interval betwixt the disappearance of the buboe and the termination of the rubbing-in treatment; and in truth it was always noticed, if any considerable period of time were allowed to elapse after the disappearance of the buboe before resuming the rubbing-in (a convincing proof that the virus was not destroyed by direct contact with mercury as mercury); or if after ever so long a continuance of the rubbing-in, the action of a sufficiently intense mercurial fever did not ensue, consequently the treatment was left incomplete, the lues broke out some time thereafter; in this case the buboe had long disappeared, and yet the lues broke out.

392. The observation, that the same quantity of mercurial ointment rubbed into parts whence the lymphatic vessels do not pass through the swollen inguinal glands, although it did not dispel the latter so rapidly, yet effected a cure as often, might have taught medical men that as in these cases the disappearance of the buboe depended on the radical destruction of all the venereal poison, it was foolish to deprive themselves of this most certain criterion of the true destruction of the virus contained in the inguinal tumour, by the useless local dispersion of the buboe. For immediately after the local dispersion of the buboe by the Neapolitan ointment, the venereal virus still exists in the system as intact as when during the internal mercurial treatment the venereal inguinal buboe is still present, only that in the latter case the persistence of the buboe gives me the full assurance that the cure is not complete; but this is wanting in the first case, and the physician deceives both himself and his patient with a vain hope. For how is it possible to demonstrate to both immediately after the inunction treatment that the patient is not cured? It is only after the lapse of several months, that the breaking out of the lues venerea will shew them how greatly they have been deceived; every unprejudiced person will perceive how foolishly the physician has acted, in himself extinguishing the light which alone could guide him along the dark path to this desired goal.

393. Let it not be alleged that recent lues venerea requires no more time nor mercury for its cure than buboes and chancres, and that, consequently, it is a matter of indifference whether we have to destroy the local or the general virus. For even though it should in general require less time and mercury for the cure of lues, it will always be much more difficult (at all events for the ordinary treatment) to cure lues, when it presents itself under such an obscure form, and often takes such a long time before its presence can be ascertained by *indubi'able* signs; and even these indubitable signs are often removed from the observation of the physician by the smallest dose of mercury,

long before we can entertain an idea of the radical cure of the disease. The employment of mercury should be persisted in until the complete cure is accomplished. But when is it accomplished? by what sign shall we recognise the extinction of the virus?

394. How then can it be a matter of indifference whether the venereal virus be treated in the form of lues or of buboes and chancres, seeing that the latter especially and only [1] draw the infallible boundary-line betwixt the complete and incomplete extinction of the miasm, when without local treatment and by the sole internal employment of mercury they are cured and disappear without leaving a trace behind, whereas the undeveloped or concealed lues has nothing of the sort to shew.

395. But on the other hand, how useless was the anxious direction of those who insisted on the necessity of rubbing in the mercurial ointment exactly upon the part where the metal must by means of the absorbent vessels pass through the swollen gland, seeing that in many cases there does not exist a sufficiently extensive surface of the kind required for effecting this rubbing-in; as, for example, when the bubo is seated near the body of the genital organ or close to the pubic region in males, or on the round ligaments of the uterus or betwixt the labia and thigh in females.

396. But even this result of doubtful value could often not be effected by the rubbing-in process performed on the most convenient spot, (for example, on the thigh when the buboe was seated below Poupart's ligament), it often remained hard and swollen without going on either to resolution or suppuration; lues venerea might thereupon ensue or not. The virus often only lies latent in this indurated gland, and often breaks out visibly when the inunction treatment, which debilitates by long-continued irritation and violent evacuations, is discontinued, and the scrofulous diathesis excited by it is removed.

397. If however it be frequently powerless to cure a single buboe, how often must this be the case where there is a buboe on each side, where even the most zealous advocate for the rubbing-in system would not venture to rub in as much mercury as would suffice to disperse the buboes and destroy the virus in the whole system, as the quantity of mercury that would be required for such a purpose would ruin the constitution.

398. Moreover, the rubbing-in of the Neapolitan ointment at a distance[2] will at the utmost only succeed in dispersing a slightly in-

---

[1] I have elsewhere shewn the deceptive character of the sign of the extinction of the virus drawn from the severe affection of the mouth by mercury.

[2] In cases where there is no surface of the body betwixt the place of absorption of the poison and the buboe fitted for the rubbing-in, it has been the custom of some to perform the operation on the buboe itself; but they did not consider that the

flamed buboe, but not one of any considerable size that is on the point of suppurating, far less one that is already in a state of suppuration; on the contrary, a long continuation of the inunction not unfrequently, makes the buboe, when at length it suppurates, an unhealthy, fistulous, corroding ulcer.

399. Now as every physician who has skill in his profession has recourse to the internal exhibition of mercury when there is betwixt the place of absorption and the buboe no suitable place for rubbing in the ointment, or when two buboes are present at once, when suppuration has already commenced in the buboe, or when after repeated employment of the inunction method for buboes and their consequences there still ensue symptoms of lues, what is it that prevents him from employing it alone at the very commencement, in every case of buboe[1], if it be not partly that he has overlooked those objections to the rubbing-in system, partly that he has sometimes found his calomel, his corrosive sublimate, &c., inefficient and uncertain, or in a word, if it be not because he has not been acquainted with such an excellent preparation as the soluble mercury is?

CHAPTER III.
TREATMENT OF BUBOES.

400. The same reasons[1] that have induced me when treating of chancre to refer to the treatment of lues, lead me to do the same in the present case in reference to the employment of the soluble mercury, as neither more nor less is required for the cure of the one than the other, namely, a sufficiently severe mercurial fever (§ 290), taking care to avoid all the hindrances to the cure, as I shall hereafter (§ 573 —613) endeavour to show how.

401. For the reasons given above we must avoid all external remedies, all rubbings-in of ointment; we must discard all other mercurial preparations which are either inefficient or uncertain in their operation, and make use of the soluble mercury in preference to all others. We can employ it in all stages of the inguinal swelling, at its onset, when

---

ointment cannot in such a case penetrate through the lymphatic vessels directly to the empoisoned gland, and that the friction on this place would tend to promote that inflammation and suppuration that was sought to be avoided.

[1] In order to maintain the excellence of the ointment at the expense of the internal employment of the mercury, instances are adduced where, during the use of the latter means, buboes are said to have appeared, without the chancre being removed by local remedies. A careful examination of such cases, however, will shew that the chancres were not left without local applications, to which however the injurious power of increasing the absorbing faculty of the lymphatic vessels was not considered to be attributable.

[2] In order to avoid repetition.

it swells, and even when it is suppurating.[1] In the first and second case, on the occurrence of the factitious fever the buboes decrease and disappear (the sole and most certain sign of the true cure and complete extinction of the miasm); in the third it has often, contrary to all expectations, produced its dispersion,[2] and even when this was no longer possible it hastened the concoction of the pus, and the abscess was a pure healthy ulcer that soon healed up, almost without pain and without any ulterior consequences, for in this case the virus was at the same time destroyed, which is the final aim of all treatment for venereal maladies.

402. When, in such cases, I was convinced of the impossibility of resolution, I first excited a slight commencement of mercurial fever. I then discontinued the medicine, and as soon as the buboe, after having burst in a healthy manner, commenced to heal up, I excited by means of rapidly increased doses of soluble mercury, a second more severe mercurial fever, which effected the cicatrization and the complete eradication of the virus. Lint dipped in milk is the best compress to employ.

403. If called on to treat a buboe of long standing that is already in a state of unhealthy suppuration,[3] we must first ascertain the cause of its malignant character before we proceed to the administration of the soluble mercury. If it have been mistreated with emollient local remedies, we must employ balsamic digestive remedies (composed of myrrh, yolk of egg and cocoa-nut oil) or a mixture of decoction of oak bark with wine; if the ill-effects were caused by irritating and corrosive substances, we must have recourse to the local use of opium;

---

[1] When Girtanner says, "During the suppurative process mercurial preparations are highly injurious. As long as the patient is taking mercury, not only does the ulcer not heal up, but it becomes aggravated and more virulent", he either means—but this construction the sentence will not bear—an ancient buboe degenerated under an excessive employment of mercury, or, as that cannot be his meaning, he intends to discountenance an irritating, ineffectual mercurial treatment of the ordinary stamp. He would *invariably* have seen the reverse from a mercurial fever rapidly developed by soluble mercury. In that case he would not have needed to expose his patients to the risk of having lues venerea, as he now does, when he forbids the employment of mercury not only during the suppurative process, but even after the buboe is healed up, "until symptoms of syphilis display themselves." Why this delay if his former maxim (p. 250) be correct, as it undoubtedly is, "that syphilis always supervenes if we allow the buboe to come to suppuration"? If given before this period (previous to the appearance of the syphilis)," he says further on, "it has absolutely no other effect than to debilitate uselessly the patient's system." How I pity every honest man whom the badness of his mercurial puts in such a fright that may be so prejudicial to his patients.

[2] Certainly the most desirable termination of the venereal glandular swelling, if it can be effected along with the simultaneous eradication of the miasm (§ 420).

[3] In all cases of abscesses of glands, especially in unhealthy ones, we should take especial care to avoid the use of emollient and relaxing applications.

but if the whole constitution be ruined, this obstacle must be previously removed as much as possible, in the manner detailed below (§ 573—585), if we would obtain rapid and radical aid from the mercurial treatment; above all we should seek to remove the debility and the irritability, which has probably been caused by the long-continued employment of an excessive quantity of mercury and by the accessory treatment usually employed in conjunction with it.

404. We have to remove almost the same obstacles, and to employ almost the same preliminary treatment, where a long-continued inunction of Neapolitan ointment or other inappropriate external remedies have produced induration of the inguinal tumour. We should endeavour to remove the irritable, weak and scrofulous disposition by means of bark, opium, cold bathing, exercise in the open air, gentle emetics, burnt sea-weed and volatile alkali, and we may employ externally with advantage douches of sal-ammoniac dissolved in vinegar, dry cupping, and sea bathing,[1] in order to disperse the induration. If there be still relics of the virus present, the internal administration of the soluble mercury, after the system is improved, will hasten the resolution.

405. Multiplied observations have established it as a maxim, that it is best to let a buboe that has suppurated[2] burst of itself. It is the least painful process; the opening that is formed allows a free passage to the pus, prevents the suppurating buboe from closing up too soon, and leaves the most inconsiderable cicatrix.

406. Should we deem it advisable to make an artificial opening, we ought, according to the advice of the most eminent authors, to give a preference to the caustic potash, which is said to give much less pain and to make an opening of a more lasting character than the knife. The wound that remains is said to degenerate into an unhealthy state much more readily when the knife is used than when the caustic is employed. But be that as it may, the caustic makes an opening much more suitable for the discharge of the pus, and one through which we can more readily observe the internal character of the abscess, and manage it more conveniently, as Franz Renner[3] long ago taught.

407. It is only in cases where the opening of the buboe from other

---

[1] Girtanner recommends volatile ointment to be rubbed in.

[2] We may hasten the process, if it should advance too slowly, by applying warm roasted onions, boiled in soap water; or where the inflammation is greater by vene-sections, leeches to the part, and emollient fomentations impregnated with saffron.

[3] "When the buboe is red and soft to the feel it should be opened. I seldom do this with fleam, lancet or knife, but generally by the application of lapis caustic, so as to make a pretty large opening, in order to allow the waste and impurity to be the better discharged; and in this way we can obtain a much better view of what is going on in the interior than by any other method, and can evacuate and cleanse the abscess more conveniently," &c. (*Ein new Handtbüchlin*, 4to., Nürnburg, 1559, p. 94.)

important reasons becomes a matter of urgency, and when the abscess is ripe and ready to burst, that the knife should be preferred to the caustic.

408. But as the suitable employment of mercury often succeeds in re-solving buboes after suppuration has commenced, or when that is not possible, facilitates and hastens their bursting, I scarcely ever find it requisite to open them.

409. I have never required to make use of the resolvent power of emetics, useful though they undoubtedly are, along with the soluble mercury.

410. When it is doubtful whether a buboe arises from the sympa-thetic irritation of a declining gonorrhœa or from the true metastasis of the venereal poison from chancres, it is always advisable, before resorting to the employment of mercury, to try the effects of com-presses moistened with ice-cold water, which speedily disperse that arising from the sympathetic gonorrhœal irritation, but have no effect on the true venereal one, or at most will prevent it from anticipating the resolvent powers of the soluble mercury by too rapid inflammation and suppuration. If we should consider it still practicable to disperse a venereal buboe, we may employ some other expedients in addition to the administration of the soluble mercury. A cool, hard couch, leeches applied near the swelling,[1] and ice-cold water compresses will be found serviceable.

PART SECOND.
SYPHILIS.

FIRST DIVISION.
DIAGNOSIS OF SYPHILIS.

CHAPTER I.
INTRODUCTION TO THE DIAGNOSIS OF SYPHILIS.

411. When the virus that produces the local affections of chancres gonorrhœa and buboes, is absorbed into the general circulation, it gives rise to an universal disease of the body, whose visible effects may shew themselves on all the external parts; with the exception probably of the seat of the previous gonorrhœa and the situation of the former chancres and buboes.

412. When thus assimilated to the body, the virus changes its nature almost entirely: from being previously a violent, rapid, pain-ful, inflammatory (very infectious) virus, it becomes (with the excep-

---

[1] Girtannier advises the rubbing-in of volatile ointment beneath the gland.

tion of the affections of the tendons and bones) almost painless, slow and insidious, and the more insidious the longer it has lain latent in the body ; it no longer gives rise to chancre, gonorrhœa or buboe,[1] either in the same body or in that of another individual, by innoculation.

413. The venereal virus cannot be communicated to and incorporated into the general fluids of the body otherwise than by absorption from one of the two local affections that are caused directly by local infections (gonorrhœa ? and chancre), and from them alone can buboes (the precursors of lues) arise ; some rare cases excepted, where the absorption occurs from an unaffected part, that is to say, where the chancre-virus penetrates into the circulation without injury to the epidermis.

414. According to Hunter, out of 10,101 persons affected with lues, in one case at the very most might the virus applied to the glans have been absorbed into the system without giving rise to local symptoms. A hundred of these might be infected by the absorption of the poison from gonorrhœa, whilst 10,000 receive the lues venerea by the absorption of the virus from chancres, almost always in consequence of their merely local treatment.

415. In the stomach the chancre virus is digested without infecting the system, as Hunter found. Neither the breath nor the perspiration of individuals affected with the venereal disease communicates syphilis to healthy persons.

416. Where the disease has been communicated to mothers by persons employed to suck out the milk, and to nurses by strange infants, this happened by means of chancres on the lips, which produced similar ulcers on the nipples, then buboes in the axilla, and thence syphilis. Nurses, by giving their breasts on which are chancres or the chancre virus to their infants, cause the latter to have chancre on the lips, &c. Mothers inoculate their children in the act of parturition ; the chancres or gonorrhœal matter in their genitals is rubbed in through the tender epidermis of their bodies, or penetrates into the genitals, mouth, eyes, nose, or anus of the little creatures. The virus of general lues is not communicated to the fœtus either by the semen of the father or by the blood of the mother ; and just as little is the pus from general venereal ulcers capable of producing either syphilis or idiopathic venereal local affections by inoculation, according to the observations and experiments of Hunter and some others.

417. Simple wounds in persons affected with syphilis may be treated and cured by the ordinary vulneraries ; the general venereal virus in the system apparently does not complicate them, perhaps because the syphilitic poison itself determines the places where it shall break out.

---

[1] The cases that seem to shew it can do this are not quite clear ; on the contrary they admit of a good many objections and doubts.

418. The nature of syphilis consists in a peculiar irritation of a specific character distributed throughout the whole organism,[1] which gives rise to divers local changes and symptoms that are accompanied by an insidious, scarcely observable inflammation, and which shews itself, but only in sensitive individuals, by a slight fever with uneasiness,[2] sleeplessness, anorexia, headache, and so forth. This fever appears at first to be of a rheumatic character, and then gradually degenerates into hectic. The fever may be present before the local affections break out (and then it is easily curable by mercury), or *vice versa*.

419. Syphilis may be disposed to break out more rapidly by all sorts of derangements of the system, chills, overheatings, fevers, and the like ; and on the other hand, scrofula, gout, rheumatism, erysipelas, &c., may be excited by its irritating action.

420. The tendency of this disease to be roused into activity and to have its symptoms aggravated, in an especial manner, by cold, is shewn partly by this, that in hot countries it is far from spreading so rapidly, and does not attain nearly the height, and can also be more readily cured than in colder climates; partly also by this, that the symptomatic venereal local affections appear only on the external surface of the body, and chiefly on those parts that are most exposed to the cold air.

421. Although, as has been observed, all parts of the body seem to be infected by the lues venerea at once, yet some local affections appear usually sooner than others. The former may be called those of a *proximate*, the latter those of a *more remote* kind ; the latter generally occur at a much later period than the former, often only after these are healed, and then the susceptible part is probably, before their outbreak only, in a state of simple infection.

422. Before proceeding to an enumeration of the local affections, I must observe that the older authors, and even those of the most recent period, indicate such a large number of symptoms and modes of breaking out of syphilis, that one is uncertain whether they have been deceived or have sought to deceive others. All kinds of cutaneous eruptions, ulcers, indurations and swellings of the fluid, soft and firm parts of the bones and ligaments, all conceivable diseases of the brain, nerves and viscera, in a word, all maladies of the body that did not yield to a slovenly system of treatment were pronounced to be venereal.

---

[1] Perhaps only in the lymphatic system?

[2] There is usually an anxious solicitude about the incurability of the enemy within and its devasting progress. With grief they see the poison that nature is unable to eradicate gradually preying upon their organism, nor is it possible to allay their anxiety by reasoning with them, nor to comfort them.

423. This multiplication of pretended venereal symptoms dates from that remote period when no proper attention was paid to the course of this disease, and when ignorance of the diagnosis and treatment of chronic diseases was concealed under an array of names that were either pure inventions or had no definite meaning attached to them: they were attributed to magic, to the omnipotent influence of sidereal influences or of the Archæus, to the morbific principle of the acids, to hypochondriasis, to piles, to spasms, to the venereal disease, to infarctus, &c., for the purpose of enabling physicians to include them, with a good grace, in the list of diseases excessively difficult to cure, and so to obtain for an uncertain art a surer footing with the uninitiated, to give it a more important air and to increase the profits of its professors.[1]

424. In addition to this, everything that did not yield to the general mode of treatment by purgatives and venesections, but was cured by salivation, was said to be of a venereal character, because it was assumed that the latter alone were amenable to salivation.[2] Dropsies, hydrocephalus, cutaneous affections, old scrofulous ulcers, pulmonary consumptions, inveterate agues, &c., were cured by salivation, and thereupon these maladies, by this mode of reasoning, were pronounced to be venereal affections.

425. In order to escape from this labyrinth of opinions which complicated to such an extent the true nature of syphilis, and so effectually effaced the boundary line betwixt truth and error, we shall proceed upon the safe path of scepticism, and only describe those symptoms of syphilis the genuineness of which is not called in question by any writer of eminence or practitioner of experience, but shall pass over in silence all other alleged symptoms, until indubitable facts shall remove all doubts as to their hitherto assumed origin.

CHAPTER II.

DIAGNOSIS OF SYMPTOMATIC VENEREAL LOCAL AFFECTIONS OF THE MORE PROXIMATE KIND.

426. The most certain symptoms and local affections of syphilis of the more proximate kind are the *venereal spots*, among which we may include venereal pimples, ulcerations of the skin and mouth, onychia and rhagades on the hands.

427. From six weeks to several months, at most—and that rarely

---

[1] [These remarks indicate the lack of confidence entertained by Hahnemann, at this early period (1789), respecting the value of allopathic theory and practice.]—*Am. P.*

[2] Hence the work made about so-called masked syphilitic diseases and their vaunted cure by mercurials, generally by salivation. How were they recognised beneath this mask ? Was not the inference drawn from the efficacy of the remedy ? By a similar process of ratiocination obscure diseases may henceforth be considered of a scorbutic character if they are curable by water-cresses.

six months after the presumed absorption of the idiopathic venereal poison, the skin of the anterior part of the body, first on the pit of the stomach, then on the forehead, face, and so on, is observed to present a bright coloured, spotted appearance. These spots become in course of time of a definite form, rose-red and darker. On those parts the skin shines through the epidermis as if semi-transparent, especially in warm weather or when the body is otherwise very warm. These spots do not however project above the general surface of the skin where they are located, nor do they occasion pain or itching. There the lightest coloured spots gradually disappear, the darker ones remain and assume a round form of from four to ten lines in diameter. In course of time the epidermis covering them scales off, and the spot seems to be scarcely red any more. We might suppose it was going away entirely. But soon afterwards it appears again, the epidermis again scales off, and this takes place several times successively. The more frequently this takes place the more elevated (though but slightly so) the rougher, the more yellowish red[1] and hard is the epidermis that comes off; the spots then begin to be surrounded by a whitish circle. The warmer parts of the body, betwixt the nates and betwixt the legs, present redder spots than those exposed to the air.

428. The more frequently the spot throws off its epidermis, the rougher, harder and thicker does it become, and then it is termed a scab (schorf).

429. Every scab that comes off is replaced by a new one of larger size.

430. At first the spot beneath the scab that falls off is dry, but at last, when it becomes too thick to allow the exhalations to escape, a humour is formed beneath the scab, which rapidly dries and forms a scaly base.

431. Beneath the latter the skin becomes corroded by the acrid humour, and after several scabs have been thus thrown off there occur *open venereal ulcers*.

432. These spots are frequently seated at the borders of the hairy parts of the body, on the chest about the hairy part of the axilla, on the temples, round the forehead and behind the ears, at the border of the hairy scalp, at the circumference of the hairy parts of the genitals, and so forth; also betwixt the shoulders, and then the hairs fall out from those parts; also on the beard, the eyebrows, &c.

433. In the palms of the hands and soles of the feet they also throw off one layer of epidermis after another; on account of the natural thickness of the latter no scabs are formed in these situations, but the furrows in the skin termed the lineaments at last crack, the epidermis splits and forms raw chaps, which go by the name of *venereal rhagades*.

434. On other parts of the body also, as has been said, there occur no dry scabs of the above described kind. If, for instance, the spots

---

[1] They are then called rust spots (copper-coloured spots).

are on parts that are usually covered by other parts of the body opposite to them, betwixt the nates, betwixt the scrotum or the labia majora and the thigh, in the popliteal space and under the arms, where the transpiration is more copious, they do not become covered by a dry bark, but are invested with a moist greyish white substance, through which a humour exudes.

435. When, as is not unfrequently the case, venereal spots occur beneath the nails of the fingers, they also shine through of a red colour. Gradually the root of the nail is affected, the nails fall off, and a new, irregular, imperfect one appears. If no remedial means are used, then venereal ulcers are formed at the root of the nails, which are called *venereal onychia*.

436. All these cutaneous affections, even after their transformation into scabs and ulcers, are wonderfully free from pain.

437. The so-called *venereal pimples* or *venereal itch* are just as little sensitive ; they arise from small, reddish spots, much less raised above the skin than other pimples ; they have not such dark areolæ, and neither itch nor burn. They appear mingled with the copper-coloured spots on the forehead and other parts. Some are deeply seated in the skin, and these produce bran-like scales ; others, though also seated deeply in the skin and in like manner small and red, possess a hardness like small buttons, and there exudes from their apices a small drop of reddish coloured lymph.[1] It is only on those parts of the body that are covered by other parts, in the fiexures of the elbows and knees, &c., that they are somewhat painful and exude more moisture. Just as, on the external surface of the body, the general venereal ulcers above mentioned gradually arise from venereal spots, so is it with the ulcers in the throat and mouth,[2] which on account of their earlier appearance I shall treat of before the ulcers of the skin, although they resemble each other in their essential nature.

---

[1] They may be distinguished from so-called heat-spots and other pimples on the skin by the latter forming small abscesses, or soon dispersing and disappearing without causing any change in the skin, as Girtanner rightly observes.

[2] André does not regard ulcers of the tonsils as a sign of general lues, but as an idiopathic venereal affection or something similar, that, is to say, as a transference of the chancre to these parts, because he says that the chancre on the genitals manifestly declines when the ulcers on the tonsils appear ; that the latter occur soon after the disappearance of the former ; that tonsillar ulcers frequently occur without any other symptom of syphilis, and that, like chancres, they are capable of producing local infection, as for instance by kissing. The first proofs are of no value, even though they were correct, if the power of causing local infection be not certain which we have great reason to doubt. Moreover, this does not agree with the observation that chancres, whenever the poison for the production of a buboe (most assuredly an ulcer very analagous to the chancre) has been absorbed, are not always thereby in the least ameliorated ; they may cause all this and still go on increasing. Now as all

438. The dark-red, painless spots on the tonsils of the throat, at the back part of the inside of the cheeks, on the palate, on the lateral aspect of the tongue(in the angles of the lips?) are often, on account of their want of sensitiveness, not observed, until, after frequent, generally unnoticed throwing-off of the thin epidermis, they become somewhat elevated, and until a moist, whitish crust covers the part, which cannot be wiped off, becomes thicker and thicker, and eats more and more into the subjacent substance.

439. In these soft, warm, moist parts covered with such a thin epidermis, the venereal spots pass much more rapidly into ulcers than when they are seated on the more external surface of the body, and their transition into *tonsillar ulcers* is at first so little observed, both on that account and because they are not particularly perceptible to the feeling or the sight.

440. When their tough crust falls off from the motions of these parts, swallowing, &c., or from an impulse from within, we observe somewhat excavated round ulcers, with well-defined whitish borders.

441. These venereal ulcers of the throat are so little sensitive that they do not cause any actual pain, but only on swallowing a feeling of rawness and slight shooting as if the outer skin of that part had come off; the part whereon they are seated too is neither swollen nor hot, their circumference and base is not hard, as is the case in other ulcers of the tonsils, quinsy, &c. Still these ulcers spread more rapidly and are a little more sensitive than the other general venereal cutaneous ulcers on the surface of the body. In some few cases they impede speech a little.

442. The tonsils[1] are usually the first (and in most cases the only) parts of the mouth that are affected by venereal ulcers.

443. Sloughs or ulcers in the throat that do not occur till a year after the disappearance of the idiopathic venereal local affection (*e. g.* a chancre) do not seem to be of a venereal character.

444. Venereal spots on the skin last several months before they form scabs, and these again some months before they penetrate suffi-

---

the circumstances whence the physician must draw his inferences of this kind, in general involve to such a degree the honour of the patient, our inquiries will often elicit the most downright falsehoods on the part of persons otherwise of most trustworthy character. The ulcers of the tonsils are of the same nature as other symptomatic venereal ulcers, whose great difference from chancres may be readily perceived by comparing the description of chancres (§ 260) with that of ulcers of the tonsils (§ 438—447).

[1] Scorbutic ulcers usually attack first the gums, which then bleed very easily, before they reach the tonsils; they are not like the venereal ulcers of a defined round form, they have no whitish borders, no whitish grey excavated bottom; on the contrary, they are angular, bluish and filled by spongy looking flesh; scorbutic ulcers are accompanied by other symptoms of scurvy, and venereal ulcers usually by symptoms of syphilis.

ciently deep to constitute open *cutaneous ulcers,* so that the latter often only appear from ten to thirty months after the absorption of the chancre poison into the general circulation.

445. Although the venereal cutaneous ulcers usually arise only from the scabs of the venereal spots and from the venereal pimples, appearing as discrete ulcers, from six to ten lines in diameter, chiefly confined to the anterior surface of the body, first in the forehead and top of the head; in the face, alæ nasi, on the muscles of the neck, &c., but afterwards also on the legs, principally over the tendinous expansions (fasciæ) ; yet this is not always the case, for when the spots are seated very closely together, the small ulcers unite to form a larger one which has sometimes a diameter of six inches, as I have not unfrequently observed upon the vertex and forehead, on the sides of the neck and other parts, as also on the legs. But even when as large as this they retain as much as possible the rounded form.

446. On other parts also where spots are but rarely observed, *e. g.* on the body of the penis, we see venereal ulcers occur, which however differ from those lying on muscular parts or bones in being somewhat more sensitive and painful; they increase more rapidly in extent, and their red bottom, covered with small elevated fleshy granulations, becomes raised, like a cancerous growth, almost above the borders, which are however neither everted nor discoloured, nor hard, as they are in cancer.

447. On the other hand, the other general venereal ulcers on firmer parts already alluded to, have some, though but a shallow depth, often only one line,[1] still oftener but half a line of depth. Their bottom, which is rose-coloured, smooth and firm, spreads out in an undulating manner, is raised slightly towards the borders, that are almost level with the sound skin ; there is no perceptible inflammation nor hardness about the borders nor surrounding them. They have this peculiarity, that they almost always retain their round form. They are distinguished by the indolence of their course : they arise gradually, without any previous symptoms of inflammation, itching, burning, &c., out of copper-coloured spots and venereal eruptions, are accompanied by very insignificant pains, even when of considerable extent ; they secrete a thickish not viscid matter, like melted tallow, and of a pale green colour ; they are sometimes covered with a cheesy substance. They may sometimes be healed up by means of astringents ; but then others occur in other parts. As a general rule the general venereal

---

[1] Besides the skin they appear to destroy only the cellular structure containing the fat, at all events the depressed, hard, shining cicatrix appears to be closely united to the underlying solid parts, *e. g.* the muscle, and the latter loses its power of movement. The hairs upon the seat of the ulcer do not again grow, as their roots are destroyed.

ulcers on the head, &c. (the parts nearest the heart), heal up before
those on more distant parts, e. g. the legs, just as at first they appeared
sooner on the former than on the latter parts. Does the healing up
of a portion of such ulcers give evidence of a diminution of the syphilitic virus (I believe it remains the same), or does the cause of the
phenomenon consist in this, that these parts have at length become
insensible to the venereal irritation, whilst the newly attacked parts,
unaccustomed to this irritation, have more susceptibility for it? The
first general venereal ulcers, for example those on the tonsils, are
more sensitive and spread more rapidly, and the other symptomatic
venereal ulcers become all the more indolent in their extension, and
all the less sensitive the longer the virus has existed in the body.
(Even gonorrhœas become all the milder the oftener they occur in
the same individual, and he becomes less susceptible to infection.
These are facts that demonstrate a predisposition for the poison, which
the above serves to explain, at least to illustrate). General venereal
ulcers do not propagate by inoculation either idiopathic venereal virus
or lues venerea. All these circumstances are sufficient to distinguish
them from all other kinds of ulcers.

448. Pulmonary phthisis occuring without hæmoptysis and during
the existence of evident local affections of syphilis that has not been
treated medicinally,[1] should be regarded as venereal in its nature.—
When I said that lues venerea only attacks external parts (according
to the best observations), venereal phthisis is no exception to this.
The lungs have, in reference to the air that surrounds us, a great resemblance to the external cutaneous surface; their transpiration is
even greater, and they are oftener exposed to the cold of the atmosphere
(on account of the frequent respirations) than the skin; why then,
seeing that the lungs are obnoxious to similar diseases,[2] should we
hesitate to believe that in this case they will also follow the nature of
the skin, and on account of their frequent exposure to the cold air be
liable to venereal eruptions and ulcers ?[3]

---

[1] We might add: which, along with the syphilis may be rapidly and radically
cured by simple mercurial fever, without any need for salivation. It has also sometimes cured non-venereal phthisis by revulsion.

[2] Various cutaneous eruptions are accompanied by chest diseases, and the driving-
in of the former is often followed by the occurrence of the latter.

[3] A poor woman, forty years of age, had had for some years several venereal ulcers on the hairy part above the forehead and on its upper part, also occasionally a
dry cough. In the year 1787, these ulcers having been healed up by means of mercurial plasters, the anterior part of the thigh and leg became affected with many ulcers of the same kind. She also applied various things to these parts, and a number
of them healed up. She now became affected by a more violent cough, great dyspnœa and moderate fever, that was ameliorated on the occurrence of purulent expectoration. The expectoration was very copious; her strength did not, however

CHAPTER III.

DIAGNOSIS OF THE SYMPTOMATIC VENEREAL LOCAL AFFECTIONS OF THE MORE REMOTE KIND.

449. I have already stated that these affections usually occur many months and even some years after the absorption of the idiopathic venereal virus, often after all the affections of the proximate kind are healed and gone, sometimes by topical applications, sometimes by the internal employment of mercury in quantity sufficient to cure them, but not to eradicate the infection in distant parts. Sometimes they occur along with affections of the proximate kind, seldom without any pre-existence of the latter so as to constitute the sole local symptoms of lues venerea.

450. In all cases the symptoms of the more remote kind testify to the greatest obstinacy of the syphilitic virus, which has become as chronic and insidious as possible.

451. In this case also the nature of the poison betrays itself by its usual course of selecting those parts of the body for its seat which lie nearest to the cold atmosphere.

452. The tendinous expansions (fasciæ) and the periosteum on those bones that are of the hardest structure and not covered by muscle (consequently the coldest), on the bones of the skull, especially the most projecting parts of the parietal and frontal bones, on the dorsum of the nasal bones, on the anterior flexure of the clavicle, on the coracoid process, on the external protuberance of the elbow (more rarely on the internal one), on the anterior surface of the tibia, seldom on the ribs, become gradually enlarged by a hard swelling, which either extends without any well-defined limits, or is of a circumscribed round shape (venereal nodes). It is, especially in the former case, so hard, and is so closely attached to the bone, that one would take it and it has been considered as an osseous tumour.

453. These tumours and nodes are at first unaccompanied by pain, and are usually not noticed until with the lapse of time pains occur in them, that gradually increase in severity, so that it seems to the patient as if the bone were hacked to pieces or crushed, as if it consisted of two dry pieces that were rubbed against one another, or as if

---

diminish proportionably; the ulcers on the legs were still present in considerable numbers, but, as she said, without pain. I made her lay aside the plasters and take in the course of eight days six grains of soluble mercury in increasing doses. She became affected by severe sickness, disgust at food, and a feeling of illness that she could not describe, but without a trace of ptyalism. She was at the same time costive in the bowels. In the mean time the cough and expectoration went off, the breathing became as free as if she had never ailed anything in that respect. The ulcers were healed up in the course of fourteen days after the first dose of the remedy, and for fourteen months she has been quite free from all venereal and chest affections.

something were gnawing therein. They occur in greatest intensity at night, especially towards the morning, but in some rare cases they are equally severe during the day.

454. At this period the swelling is very painful on being touched. At first there does not seem to be any inflammation; but in this later stage it sets in and increases ever more and more, until at length the swelling gradually—often some years after its first appearance—bursts and discharges an albuminous-looking matter.

455. In these circumstances the subjacent bone is almost always corroded, on account of the destruction of the periosteum, or at least it is very nearly approaching to a carious state and is swollen.[1]

456. It is, however, difficult to determine the time when the node

---

[1] In order that we may be able to treat these swellings in time, we must be satisfied of their venereal nature, which is sometimes difficult. In order to aid our diagnosis, the following circumstances should be attended to.—Rheumatic swellings of the bones, and pains, usually occur at the joints where the osseous structure is spongy; they are preceded by redness and inflammation of the superincumbent soft parts, pain and fever, and when these symptoms, which are usually of a sudden character are past, then only does the node commence to deposit its calcareous matter in the ligaments; gradually it becomes free from pain. Cold baths, frictions and aconite diminish and remove commencing rheumatic nodes. By warm applications to parts affected with rheumatic pains, the pain is ameliorated; cold baths are a good remedy for them. They are not only not diminished (permanently) by the most violent mercurial fever, on the contrary, they are thereby aggravated and rendered more obstinate and incurable. Distilled spirits cause fever, but no pain in the rheumatic nodes.

Venereal nodes and periosteal swellings, on the other hand, are seated in the parts indicated above (§ 452) of the bones of densest structure, probably never on the capsules of the joints. At their first appearance they are quite destitute of pain; it is only afterwards that they are accompanied by it, without any perceptible local inflammation, without swelling of the skin, and it increases so progressively that it attains at length such a degree of severity that the pains of the nodes not only continue to gnaw uninteruptedly (especially after midnight) but even merely touching the part becomes quite intolerable. The contents of the swelling, when it is cut into are of an albuminous character. External warmth increases these pains in the bones; they are also aggravated by cold baths, by friction, and by partaking of spirituous liquors. Aconite and bitter vegetable extracts afford no relief. An adequately strong mercurial fever removes the pain speedily and permanently.

If a faithful confession of the previous infection be made, or if there are present several symptoms of syphilis, we can the more speedily become convinced of the true nature of these nodes and pains in the bones.

The barometrical pains of the elevated cicatrix (callus) of an old fracture of a bone cannot easily be confounded with the pains of venereal nodes, partly on account of the difference in the shape of the swelling, partly because the history of his case given by the patient helps us in our diagnosis, partly also because the pains of the callus usually occur when the weight of the atmosphere is diminished, and are more of a tearing and drawing than of a gnawing and boring character, and are besides ameliorated by the cold shower-bath, which increases those of venereal nodes.

7

changes into the abscess which is fraught with so much danger to the bone beneath. There is little inflammation present, and that which may exist is too slight to produce a properly elaborated pus; a thick mucous albuminous matter is formed that lies close upon the bone and corrodes it. This circumstance and the hardness of the node prevent us perceiving any fluctuation.

457. But if we carefully consider the inflammation, slight though it be, and the throbbing and shooting pains experienced by the patient in the centre of the node, it will not be impossible to discover the formation of this kind of abscess.[1]

458. On no part of the body do the bones lie nearer to the atmospheric air, in other words are covered with so little and such soft parts as in the nose. Hence the delicate nasal bones are usually the first that are acted upon by the venereal virus after the soft parts covering them (the Schneiderian membrane) are completely or partly destroyed. Generally the ethmoidal and turbinated nasal bones, that is to say the most delicate ones, are the first destroyed; then the vomer, the palatial bones, and lastly the maxillary bones.

459. But as has been said before, the bones beneath the venereal nodes become also corroded, and necrosis is the result, which does not differ from ordinary caries from other causes, except that it is more rapidly cured by the aid of mercury.

SECOND DIVISION.
ANTIVENEREAL REMEDIES.
CHAPTER I.
MERCURIAL PREPARATIONS IN GENERAL.

460. Ever since the wide diffusion[2] of the venereal disease, immediately after the discovery of America, when mercury was apparently at the first used for this disease, no one has been able to deny with reason the specific curative powers of this metal in that fearful disease; although from the year 1515 until the middle of that century, medical men having been frightened by the murderous employment of

---

[1] Gardane includes among the symptoms of syphilis that sensitiveness of the mouth of the womb which is increased to intolerable pain on the occurrence of the catamenial period, on the introduction of the finger or of the male organ, and which is frequently the cause of miscarriage (probably also of cancer of the womb.) I myself have frequently observed this affection, but am unable to determine if it is venereal as I have had no opportunity of treating it. Gardane recommends the use of cinnabar fumigations for it.

[2] Girtanner, by adducing the original authorities, renders it highly probable that it first came from America in the year 1493, and was first brought to Barcelona by the ships of Columbus.

that drug by empirical practitioners, sought to replace it, first by guaiac, then by sarsaparilla and bark.

461. But as this liquid metal can only be brought by artificial preparation into a fit state to be taken into intimate combination by the fluids of our body[1] in sufficient quantity, so an infinite number of mercurial preparations were invented, the almost endless list of whose names in the ancient dispensatories, especially those of Falk and Baldingen, and in the London pharmacopœia, fills us with astonishment. It would be sad indeed if only those who had extensively tested all these mercurial preparations in their own experience were qualified to treat the venereal disease properly. A long series of generations were not sufficient to do so. Strictly speaking, we require but one, the best preparation. Had medical men always had in view the attributes of such a one, based on true physiological and therapeutical principles, they had not fallen into such adventurous speculations.

462. Now, how can we ascertain which among the innumerable mercurial preparations is the most efficacious, the most certain, and the mildest, seeing that in this pitiable disease we should regard Celsus's maxim of *cito, tuto et jucunde* as our highest aim, much more than in almost all other corporeal ills, which beneficent nature alone is often able to conquer without any aid from man?

463. I think I do not err, if, as an answer to this, I lay down the following maxim, *that that mercurial preparation is the most efficacious, the most certain and the mildest, which is completely soluble in our juices, can readily be taken up by the system of absorbent vessels, and not rendered corrosive by combination with any chemical substance, is capable of exciting the pure and simple specific powers of this metal.* Such a preparation will possess the virtue of producing definite effects, which it will be in the power of the physician to regulate, diminish and increase with certainty.

464. The farther all known preparations diverge from these attributes, so much the more inefficacious, so much the more injurious are

---

[1] Mercury does not act on the venereal virus until it is dissolved in our juices, and then it develops its effects in a pretty uniform manner in the secundæ viæ. Mercurial preparations that are not powerless all act upon the mouth, but with different degrees of intensity; pure quicksilver and corrosive sublimate less powerfully than the others. All produce the same taste when dissolved in the saliva; the saliva of those that are salivated has a similar odour, by whatever preparation the ptyalism may have been produced. The greatest difference among them that is noticed by the superficial observer, consists partly in their greater or less solubility in water, which differs widely from the property they possess of being assimilated by our juices, as they possess this property in very various degrees, quite independent of their solubility (thus the sublimate is much less assimilable by our juices than oxydized mercury); partly in their action on the primæ viæ (thus corrosive sublimate, the yellow, white and red precipitates act chiefly in a poisonous manner on the stomach, calomel chiefly on the bowels.)

they ; cinnibar and turbith may serve as examples. I shall briefly pass in review the most ordinary preparations judged by this standard.

465. As regards the corrosive mercurial medicines, it will readily be granted that it is impossible there can exist in the mineral acids to which they owe their excessive acridity, anything curative of the venereal virus (for the dessiccant and antisceptic power that they display in wounds and elsewhere does not come into play here.) Among these corrosive preparations I include the nitrate of mercury, the corrosive sublimate, the various white precipitates,[1] the red precipitate,[2] calomel and turbith.[3]

466. If greater efficacy in this disease has sometimes been observed from the use of these preparations than from the less active ones, this arose from the accidental irritant qualities of the acids combined with them, but only in the same manner as other not specific irritant remedies act, such as the volatile alkali, the acrid resin of guaiac, mezereum, lobelia and cantharides—also from their exciting an accidental fever, which sometimes promotes the cure of syphilis by mercury, by rousing the activity of the nervous power, increasing the force of the circulation, and thus as it were facilitating the detection of the recondite virus by the only specific drug, or because, by setting up an irritation of a different kind, they silenced the venereal irritation, as rheumatic pains are subdued by blisters, dysentery by ipecacuan, or intermittent fever by arsenic; these substances thus remove affections without possessing any specific action upon the diseases just named.

467. But, as I have said, the borrowed irritation of these preparations is far from contributing materially to the cure of the venereal affections ; it often smothers the specific power of the metal to such a degree, and is so uncertain in its action, that it not unfrequently happens that we may kill, but are unable to cure a patient affected by inveterate syphilis, with calomel, sublimate, nitrate of mercury, white and red precipitates and turbith.

468. Were it easy to prepare mercurial salts with vegetable acids in a ponderable definite form, it would be much preferable to administer these than those just described. But this cannot be done, and, moreover, such salts in a concentrated form have something in them that excites the sensitive fibres of the primæ viæ much more readily to evacuations upwards and downwards than to absorption into the

---

[1] Mayerne, was, I believe, the first who in 1659 recommended the internal use of ordinary white precipitate.

[2] About the year 1535, Matthioli first recommended the internal use of red precipitate (calcined and washed a second time) five grains for a dose. According to Girtanner, it was Joh. Vigo who first employed it as early as 1513.

[3] William Cowes, was, I imagine, the first who in 1575 counselled the internal use of turbith in syphilis.

secundæ viæ, where alone the mercury is truly efficacious. Experience also shews that they readily cause salivation, and still frequently fail to effect the cure.

469. On the other hand, as might be supposed, it is inadvisable to employ internally for the treatment of syphilis the almost insoluble mercurial preparations, such as cinnibar, Ethiops mineral, prepared by the humid process, (*pulvis hypnoticus*) or by the dry process, for they usually produce no perceptible action, and then perhaps all at once, though rarely, cause ptyalism.

470. The cause of this uncertainty may be, either that we are unable always to determine how much there is in these preparations capable of being taken up by our fluids, or what quantity there is in them capable of penetrating into the secundæ viæ; but this well-grounded objection of uncertainty of action applies also to Plenck's mucilaginous preparation of mercury, and to those preparations in which the quicksilver is extinguished by sugar, honey, crab's-eyes, fatty substances, balsams, &c.

471. If it is sought to lay the blame in such cases on the great variety in the susceptibility of the absorbent vessels of the primæ viæ, I reply that this very circumstance is to be attributed to these preparations, that they are not of such a character as to enable them to be uniformly received into the system by every degree of susceptibility of these vessels, and I am fully convinced that the fault of this occurrence lies in the infinite variety of the solubility of these preparations in the gastric juice, and the extraordinary variety of their capability for being taken into the secundæ viæ, and not in the great difference of the solvent and absorbent powers of our system, (which it is not possible to conceive can exist to such an extent.)

472. What there is of a servicable character in these latter preparations, consists in the proportion of mercury that has been oxydized in them during their preparation; but as this varies so much (according to the nature of the medicine, the temperature of the atmosphere, or the force, time and skill of the preparer) that sometimes the twentieth part, but often scarcely the two hundredth part of the metal employed is oxydized, it follows that we can never reckon confidently on obtaining a certain effect; these preparations must sometimes be almost inert, while at other times, when the physician expects a moderate effect, he finds the most violent action occur from their use.

473. Of equally uncertain effect are the mercurial fumigations, whether cinnabar, calomel, or amalgam be employed for this end, partly on account of the difficulty of applying them equally to all parts of the body at once, whilst avoiding a respiration of them, partly on account of the very various absorbent power of the cutaneous vessels. In the employment of this, as in that of the other mercu-

rials we have mentioned, we are not in a position to calculate the quantity of the metal introduced into the body, and yet we should have a positive knowledge of the dose of the remedy as well as of its potency, in order to allow us to make an accurate repetition of a medicinal experiment.

CHAPTER II.
PARTICULAR MERCURIAL PREPARATIONS.

474. *Mercurial ointment* has been employed since the thirteenth century in various forms, and with various admixtures, for the cure of leprosy, itch, and other cutaneous diseases. At the end of the fifteenth century it was at once employed to combat the venereal disease that had then gained a fearful height, as it was held to be a similar cutaneous disease.

475. Its use has never been quite abandoned; and notwithstanding that attempts have been made from time to time to replace it by some better internal remedy, as occurred in preceding centuries as well as especially about the middle of the present century, yet it has at all times been resorted to in extreme cases. In recent times also, after the fond dream of the omnipotence of corrosive sublimate was dispelled, the ointment was again promoted to the rank of an antisyphilitic remedy.

476. The chief reason for the preference given to it, I believe, lies in this, that it is imagined; "1. That the greater the quantity [1] of mercury that can be introduced into the body in a given time, the greater is the certainty of curing the venereal disease. 2. That the metal when rubbed into the skin does not incommode the primæ viæ like the preparations of mercury given internally: and, 3. That by means of frictions we can apply the mercury exactly to the spot where its presence is most required, in order to be efficacious."

477. It is very easy to refute these three maxims that have served to obtain for inunctions such a great preference in practice. The first is overthrown by the experience that the smallest quantity of mercury, if it do but excite a sufficiently strong mercurial fever (§ 290) is capable of eradicating the greatest degree of the most deeply rooted syphilis, and that the subtle exhalation proceeding from the saliva of a salivated person, which is certainly impregnated with a scarcely ponderable quantity of the metal, has sometimes succeeded in curing the venereal disease. On the other hand, we often find that some almost incurable diseases are the result of a larger quantity of mercury gradually introduced into the body; such as, irritability from weakness, hectic fever, chronic trembling, scrofula, caries of the bones, and

---

[1] No other way was known of introducing the largest quantity of mercury into the body but by means of the ointment.

so forth, without the venereal poison being thereby eradicated. The second point is weakened by the observation that colicky diarrhœas not unfrequently result from frictions with mercury. As regards the third maxim I have already expressed by opinion (§ 387), where I shewed that the mercury must first permeate the whole mass of the blood, and undergo a sort of digestion or intimate assimilation, before it is capable of overcoming venereal affections, that, consequently, the local power of this metal over the venereal poison is illusory, and often does more harm than good.

478. But the following maxims, deduced from experience, irrefragably demonstrate the doubtful propriety of employing frictions. 1. The quantity of metallic or oxydised mercury that can be introduced into the body by rubbing in the ointment can not be determined, and is entirely uncertain. 2. There are often obstacles that prevent the rubbing-in. 3. The frictions are often not suitable for the disease. 4. They are frequently injurious.

479. In reference to the first point, it should be remembered, that the power of the person who rubs in the ointment can never be determined, can never be relied on. If strong rubbing-in favours the the absorption, if it be done more weakly the absorption will be much less. But if, as some allege, stronger friction prevents the absorption, the same variety in reference to the quantity of mercury that penetrates into the body will occur, but in the inverse ratio of the force employed in the rubbing-in.

480. Be this as it may, however, this at least is certain, that when the force employed in the rubbing-in is less, the oxydation [1] of the minute mercurial globules, and consequently the solubility of this metal in our juices, is not favoured to such an extent as by stronger frictions. The same undeterminable variety in the demetallization [2] of the mercury occurs also in the preparation of the ointment itself, which is considered good when we can no longer see metallic globules in it. How deceptive is this sign! There are ointments of exactly the same appearance which, according to the different manner in which

---

[1] I cannot say with certainty whether the rubbing employed in the preparation of the mercurial ointment oxydises the metal, or whether a combination of the latter with the fatty acids occurs; the latter appears to me the more probable. This however is certain, that it is only that part of the mercury that has become non-metallic in the ointment that is the really serviceable part against the venereal virus.

[2] The warmth or coldness of the ingredients, the hardness or softness of the fatty substance, the purity of the mercury or its adulteration with other metals (in the latter case it is more easily rubbed down), the employment or withholding of turpentine, the force exerted by the preparer, his skill, and the time he expends on its preparation, render different specimens of the Neapolitan ointment extremely different, although they have all the same appearance.

they are prepared, contain from a two-hundredth to a thirtieth part of the metal in the non-metallic form. But in the Neapolitan ointment it is only the mercury that has been oxydised by friction that is efficacious against the venereal poison, whereas the metallic globules, even though they be invisible to the eye, are absolutely insoluble in our juices, and only possess a mechanical propelling power. Who can fail to perceive here an infinity of unavoidable causes which may render the power of the ointment on our system extremely various?

481. The absorbing power of the cutaneous vessels is inconceivably various, and cannot be relied on. There are skins so constituted that they will not take up the ointment at all, and yet the physician is unable to detect them accurately; and on the other hand there are some individuals on whose skin if we but lay the ointment,[1] we cause the most severe ptyalism. Even in the same individual the skin is more susceptible to the ointment under certain circumstances than under others; and even one part of the skin may be more susceptible than another.[2]

482. But admitting we always knew with certainty (although this is incredible) what proportion of oxydised mercury the ointment contained, and what quantity of it entered the system, how can we know what length of time the vessels of the skin will take to deliver up their contents into the general circulation, seeing that they are more active at one time than at another, in order that, when the absorbent vessels have scarcely brought their contents that just suffice to produce salivation into the general circulation, we may not, by a fresh rubbing-in of the ointment excite an uncontrollable attack of this fearful excretory process, before the mercury first rubbed in has commenced to act?

483. With regard to the second point (§ 478) the frictions not unfrequently cause, especially in delicate and sensitive individuals, erysipelatous inflammations, desquamation of the epidermis or painful itching herpetic eruption,[3] rendering their further employment impossible.

---

[1] A healthy, very sensitive man was affected with pediculi on the hairy parts of the genitals, and anointed that portion of his skin with a piece of Naples cintment, the size of a hazel nut, only once, and that quite superficially, without rubbing it in in the least. Soon afterwards he had to make a journey during the prevalence of a cold, moist wind. After the lapse of twenty-four hours he was attacked by uncontrollable ptyalism that lasted four weeks.

[2] What a quantity of ointment must remain on the patient's linen, and on his skin, and on the hand or glove of the person who performs the frictions, that we cannot weigh, and that must differ in every case.

[3] These effects are not produced only by ointments mixed with turpentine. Rancid fatty matters produce them; and in all mercurial ointments the fatty matter is already rancid, probably because the metal absorbs its acids. The sudden occurrence of ptyalism prevents their further employment, and not less frequently are we obliged to desist on account of their long continued inutility.

484. But even were this not the case, the circumstances of every patient do not admit of our using this method. Not only its troublesome and repulsive character, neither of which are inconsiderable, but also its suspicious character often forbids its employment, for the process of rubbing-in and the presence of venereal disease are so intimately associated in people's minds, and this operation is so difficult to be concealed from all observation, that it exposes every patient, whose good name should be a matter of inviolable sanctity to the physician, to injurious reports of this kind.

485. With respect to the third point (§ 478); in cases of deeply rooted syphilis that has existed a long time, whose symptoms have become in the highest degree insidious and chronic, and are seated no longer in the soft superficial parts, but in the tendinous expansions, or have even attacked the periosteum or bones themselvss, where the virus is obstinately concentrated, the rubbing-in of the ointment is very rarely able to extirpate the disease.

486. In reference to the fourth point, or the injurious effects of the mercurial ointment, we must bear in mind, that the frictions must be continued for a long time in order to be of any considerable service; and in that case the long-continued irritation exercised by such a large quantity of mercury on the fluids and solids of the body, gives rise to a number of chronic and often incurable diseases, that are sometimes worse than the venereal disease itself.

487. The fluids of the body become acrid, its fibres are thrown into abnormal vibrations and relaxed, and the vital force is gradually melted down to such a degree, that impaired digestion, sleeplessness, debility, flying heat, hectic fever, chronic ulcers, caries of the bones, tumours, scrofula, irregular rheumatic pains, and chronic trembling, are the most ordinary results of this employment of mercury.

488. The equivocal repulsion of the local virus from buboes into the general circulation, and the lues venerea that not unfrequently thence arises may justly be attributed, as experience shows, to mercurial ointment, when it is rubbed into parts where, as has been shewn above, the mercury must be conducted by the absorbent vessels through the buboe.

489. It is by no means a rare thing in practice to meet with buboes that, by the long-continued employment of such frictions, have become schirrhous, and ultimately cancerous.

490. According to Fabre's observations, of twenty patients treated with frictions, fifteen became affected with ptyalism, which often comes on so unexpectedly, and in spite of every precaution is so uncontrollable, that either the life of the patient is thereby endangered, or those parts that are affected by this disgusting, weakening and painful discharge are seriously injured. Corroding ulcers in the mouth and on the

tongue, loss of the palate and uvula, caries of the alveoli and of the spongy bones of the nose, are common results. The more modern, almost playful employment of the ointment seems to be a modified copy of this frightful picture; but it is on the whole the same thing; the terrors of the salivation are somewhat more carefully avoided, without on that account curing more cases of the venereal disease, and the terrible effects (§ 649) are almost more frequent than before.

491. Inunctions of the ointment when gonorrhœa is present frequently transform the latter into an almost incurable gleet, probably in consequence of the excessive relaxation of the lymphatic system and the morbid irritability they occasion.

492. What can I say of the hurtful nature of frictions when they are employed in those cases in which a previous injudicious employment of mercury has already complicated the venereal affection with an accession of those chronic non-venereal diseases (§ 487)?

493. The treatment of venereal diseases by frictions is usually commenced[1] with venesections, purgation and tepid baths. By these means it is imagined that the system is best prepared for this mode of using the mercury. Then two drachms or a dram and a half, seldom only one drachm of the ointment (composed of one drachm of the fluid metal, rubbed up with the same quantity by weight of lard) is slowly rubbed in beside a coal fire, upon the lower extremities, usually every other day; by and bye the same process is repeated on the upper extremities; the patient is required to keep his room and drink frequently of some thin warm drink. This process is continued until salivation commences, which is sought to be checked by discontinuing the medicine and by the employment of the purgatives, baths, diuretic remedies, ptisans and clean linen. When the mouth has again returned to a state of quiescence, the frictions are again continued with the same or even increased quantities of the ointment, until fearful symptoms forbid their further employment, or until the venereal symptoms disappear and the patient appears to be cured. Finally, venesections, purgatives and baths are again made use of. During the whole treatment no solid food is allowed. However great the hunger may be, the patients dare not partake of anything but soups.

494. On an average, thirty-two drachms of ointment and about forty-five days are required for a moderate degree of lues venerea, but sometimes forty-eight drachms[2] of ointment (three ounces of mercury!) have been rubbed in, and above three months employed in the treatment.

495. The treatment of syphilis by *fumigations with mercury* is,

---

[1] In accordance with the alterative method usually adopted at Montpellier.

[2] Girtanner says from twelve to thirteen ounces of ointment; six and a half ounces of mercury!

after the rubbing-in treatment, the most ancient[1] mode of treating this disease, and for this purpose cinnabar is used. In later times it fell into oblivion, except that it was still employed by some rude people (as I found to be the case among the Wallachs of Transylvania).

Recently experiments with it have been instituted (Lalouette[2] is the principal person who has revived it), expedients being devised for keeping the vapour away from the mouth during its use, and in place of cinnabar, the vapour of volatilized calomel, or of mercury amalgamated with tin, has been selected.

496. Although this vapour is very penetrating, wound-cleansing and dessicative, and moreover when the inspiration[3] of it is avoided, does not readily cause salivation or diarrhœa, yet its employment for the complete eradication[4] of syphilis is scarcely advisable.

497. It should be borne in mind that the quantity of mercury that on each occasion penetrates into the organism in the form of vapour is quite undeterminable, and can never be relied on, as will be sufficiently obvious without my testimony; experience also shews that this method of treatment is only of some utility in slighter cases of syphilis, in cutaneous affections and the like, as an accessory means along with the employment of other mercurial remedies; and it not unfrequently becomes injurious when there is too great sensitiveness and inflammation of the sores, in dry and spasmodic asthma, great emaciation of the body, in ulceration of the womb and the like.

498. I have also sometimes noticed, from its local employment, chancres pass into buboes, and the local virus thereby driven into the general circulation. An immense number of authors[5] have observed convulsions, general trembling and fatal apoplexies result from the use of cinnabar fumigations.

499. In the modern employment of mercurial fumigations, it is the custom to prepare the system, as in the case of frictions, by baths, venesections and purgatives. Then according to Lalouette's method the patient is placed in an apparatus (usually a box made expressly, where the head of the person who is seated therein, in a state of nudity, projects through the lid, and his neck is so enveloped and all apertures are so closed that no vapour can escape) in which the whole body is played on by the vapour, but the mouth is not touched by it. The

---

[1] Cataneus first brought it into use in 1505.

[2] He has however had few imitators.

[3] Which the older physicians did not always employ proper precautions to prevent, and by the dreadful accidents that their rude practice gave rise to, they brought this means into great discredit.

[4] The local employment of mercurial fumigations with proper care will always remain one of the most excellent remedies for the removal of obstructions and the improvement of malignant diseases.

[5] From Joh. Benedict (1510) up to the most recent times.

calomel is made to evaporate in a sublimating apparatus introduced beneath the seat.

500. The fumigation is repeated usually every other day, and from half a drachm to one drachm and a half of calomel is employed (cinnabar or mercury amalgamated with tin is seldom used), and the patient is at the same time made to drink frequently some warm thin ptisan.

501. On an average about three ounces of one of these substances are required to complete satisfactorily the treatment of a moderate syphilis (with symptoms of several kinds) in thirty days or thereabouts.

502. Attempts are often made with success to cure or to ameliorate malignant venereal ulcers or slight pains in the bones by means of small local fumigations.

503. The employment of *corrosive sublimate* in venereal diseases is also pretty ancient,[1] but it was previously avoided by regular physicians as a dangerous method of treatment, or it was confined chiefly to the practice of the mystic physicians, until, about the middle of the present (18th) century, a more convenient mode of administering it with safety was discovered.

504. It has this advantage, that it can be introduced into the system in a determinate small quantity, that it does not frequently excite salivation, at least not long-continued salivation, and in obstinate gleets does more good than harm. It has often succeeded in curing children affected with slight symptoms of syphilis, in whom the other preparations of mercury could not be employed with safety. It has also proved of service in some slight symptoms of syphilis in adults, and another especial advantage it possesses is that during its use patients do not require to be so strictly confined to their room as during the employment of frictions and calomel, because it seldom excites salivation, and because it does not produce such excessive debility as

---

[1] Richard Wiseman (*Sev. chir. treatises*) was the first who in 1676 alluded to the employment by empirical practitioners of a watery solution of corrosive sublimate in water for syphilis; and according to Malouin it was about that time very much used as an internal remedy under the name of *remède du cavalier*. Stephen Blankaart in 1690 also made mention of its employment. Thereafter, in 1717, Turner alluded to its empirical employment against this disease. The better method of using it, however, remained unknown until in 1742 Sanchez heard from a German physician who had been some time in Siberia that it was the custom in that country (as travellers have mentioned since 1709) to give in syphilis sublimate dissolved in brandy, conjoined with the use of vapour baths. Sanchez instituted experiments with it, and a few years afterwards communicated the results to the celebrated Van Swieten, who promulgated this method about the year 1754 in letters to Benvenuti and Hundertmark, and subsequently at greater length in the fifth volume of his Commentaries, and, without making mention of the vapour baths (according to Sanchez the most efficient part of the treatment), praised it above its merits, having been deceived by the mendacious eulogiums of his flatterers.

the other ordinary mercurial preparations, with the exception of the mercurius nitratus and the oxyde of mercury.

505. This is, however, all the good I can say of it, for on the other hand it is, 1st, often inefficacious to effect any considerable amelioration, and 2d, its use is attended by peculiar ill effects and disadvantages.

506. As regards the first point, it has seldom, when given internally, been of much use in chancres, in buboes, especially such as are of long standing and have hard borders and a cancerous appearance, in condylomata and other venereal growths, in swellings of the bones, and generally in inveterate symptoms of syphilis. I have employed it without success in chancres and general syphilitic ulcers, notwithstanding that I have gradually increased it to the very largest doses.

507. It has besides this deceptive character, that the adventitious acridity it derives from the muriatic acid combined with it, enables it to excite an irritation foreign to the mercury it contains, which (by counter-irritation), lulls for a time the venereal symptoms; which, however, when the patient thinks himself cured, usually again burst forth with redoubled violence. During its use the ulcers in the throat are cured in an almost miraculously short space of time; but this cure is generally of a deceptive character, for on leaving it off, similar symptomatic venereal affections arise, or the same disease appears and spreads with greater rapidity than before.

508. With regard to the second point (§ 505), it is one of its great faults, that its acrid character[1] obstinately prevents its entrance into the lymphatic vessels of the primæ viæ. Besides this, its taste is horrible; a sensitive stomach cannot bear it at all. Oppression of the stomach, inclination to vomit, colic, inflammatory eruptions on the skin, are often the accompaniments of its use. Hectic fever has been laid to its charge, which is produced by small ulcerations in the stomach caused by its corrosive properties. Brambilla, a respectable witness, has observed it give rise to blindness and deafness, spitting of blood, phthisis, hectic fever, and abortion.

509. As a general rule, its employment is contraindicated where there are, slow fever, derangement of the alimentary canal, tendency to hæmoptysis, fluent hæmorrhoids, melancholic temperament, dispo-

---

[1] Barchusen has misled Girtanner to apprehend the presence of arsenic in the corrosive sublimate made in Holland. I doubt if arsenic be more poisonous than corrosive sublimate, but still more do I doubt (although Bergman has shewn the *possibility* of the union of these two substances in the process of sublimation) if corrosive sublimate be ever really adulterated with arsenic. With the exception of Barchusen, whose chemical knowledge cannot be very implicitly trusted to, no chemist has observed this mixture. The modes Girtanner employs for detecting the presence of arsenic in corrosive sublimate are either dangerous or unsatisfactory. Those mentioned in my work *On Arsenical Poisoning* are easier and surer.

sition to violent mental emotions, gout, spasmodic affections, or other symptoms of an irritable, nervous system, and a dry constitution.

510. After preparing the body in the good French style, by means of purgatives, venesections and baths (but these are not so absolutely insisted on for the corrosive sublimate treatment, as for that with other mercurial preparations), it is usual to commence the treatment with the daily dose of a quarter[1] of a grain dissolved in two pints of fluid, and to increase the dose until it amounts to one grain in the day. In the case of children an eighth of a grain is at first given daily, and increased to one fourth of a grain in a pint of fluid.

511. On an average, twenty-eight grains and about forty days were required to remove moderate venereal symptoms in adults. From six and a half to ten grains were sufficient for children.

512. Sanchez, who revived the use of corrosive sublimate, employed conjointly with this remedy, after the Siberian method, frequent Russian Vapour-baths, and by this combination he cured an immense number of internal and external chronic maladies, which he, without any proof, asserted to be masked venereal affections, (for there is scarcely any tedious or complicated malady that he does not consider as a consequence of syphilis). These affections were usually cured,[2] as might be expected, from the powerful diaphoretic means (the vapour baths) alone; but they were not always venereal diseases because a plan of treatment succeeded wherein a mercurial remedy was at the same time used. He makes infinite confusion with the symptoms of syphilis; it is certain that the maladies so cured were seldom of that nature, or only a small proportion of them, in which corrosive sublimate and diaphoretic remedies can, as is well known, prove serviceable, or if they were syphilitic then the cure was not permanent, and only in appearance.[3]

513. *Calomel* has for a long time,[4] but especially since the commencement of this century (the 18th), been one of the most frequently used mercurial remedies for syphilis, and that especially on this

---

[1] Swieten gave twice a day a fifth of a grain dissolved in half an ounce of brandy. I may mention here, incidentally, that Girtanner is wrong when he says of this solution, that corrosive sublimate does not dissolve well in brandy.

[2] The sublimate did not need to contribute more than its irritating powers.

[3] I do not make mention of the corrosive sublimate clysters of Royer, or of the analogous baths of Baumé, as the former caused painful tenesmus, and both are unserviceable, as experience has shewn.

[4] The surgeon David de Planis Campy (*la verolle recogneue.* 8. Paris, 1623) seems to be one of the first who gives the recipe for the *Pilules de la violette* (p. 174), which along with purgatives, were at that time much used in syphilis, and he lauds in rather an empirical manner their efficacy in this disease; they contain calomel, a scruple for a dose. Mayerne followed in 1650 with his *pulvis colomelanicus.* (Oswald Croll, in 1608, was perhaps the first who described, though obscurely, the mode of making this mercurial preparation.)

account, that the supposed poisonous acridity of the metal was presumed to be corrected and sweetened[1] in it, and experience taught that this preparation, of all the internal remedies then known, had the least corrosive qualities.

514. The following maxims, deduced from experience, however, are opposed to its reputed mild nature and much vaunted efficacy in the treatment of syphilis. 1. The ordinary semitransparent lanceolated calomel in the form of cakes contain no mean proportion of sublimate. In this form it often occasions violent vomiting. If this be not the case, and if it be purer, still it causes almost specifically enormous alvine evacuations, which are accompanied by pains and great weakening of the body. 2. If it be quite pure, it is an almost insoluble mercurial salt, in which the small quantity of muriatic acid (often less than a sixth of the whole) is saturated with so much mercury, that but very little of it is dissolved in the gastric juice and passes into the absorbent vessels, the whilst coliclike irritation of the bowels it produces expedites its expulsion. 3. The portion of it that penetrates into the secundæ viæ excites almost uncontrollable ptyalism, a fault that seems to be most peculiarly attached to it of all mercurial preparations next to the ointment. It possesses all the powers inherent in the latter, of causing weakness of the body and innumerable chronic maladies thence accruing (§ 649); or if possible it even excels the ointment in this.

515. Attempts have been made in vain to deprive calomel of its irritating effects on the bowels, by subjecting it to repeated sublimation. The excess of its purgative property is best removed by boiling it in a large quantity of water along with a tenth part of sal-ammoniac, as has been the custom in recent times, or by mere boiling in water (as F. Hoffman used to do), with the intention of thereby depriving it of the corrosive sublimate adhering to it; it is also sometimes combined with opium.

516. Of late years[2] it has been used as a chief remedy for syphilis in combination with some earthy powder, or made into pills with diascoridium. After a methodic preparatory treatment by venesections, purgatives and baths, the patient being strictly kept to one well warmed room, and partaking especially of warm drinks, first, two grains were given, and the dose increased daily by about a grain, and if still no ptyalism occurred the dose was elevated to a scruple

---

[1] The white precipitate sweetened by boiling with sal-ammonic has the same action as the calomel. Girtanner gives the preference to Hermbstädt's white precipitate before all others (I do not know why), and proclaims him as the discoverer of the sweet mercury prepared from turbith and kitchen salt, although he has done nothing more than make some improvements on the mode pointed out in the *Laborant* (2d pt. pp. 155, 156).

[2] In olden times it was sought to remove the disease by large doses, often from a half to a whole drachm given at once. A dangerous procedure!

daily, and thereafter the dose was decreased daily in the same manner in which it had been increased.

517. If it was wished to perform the treatment without salivation, as has been atterly the custom, either the doses were not increased so rapidly, or when the disgusting evacuation occurred, strong purgatives were given, which often did not, but sometimes did, stop it, though with but small advantage in regard to the eradication of the venereal virus, but with such manifest loss of strength (§ 648, 649), that this so-called *alterative* method of treating syphilis usually lasted longer than that by salivation, and was often not so efficacious in destroying the virus as the latter.

518. All the ills that can arise from the employment of any irritating, debilitating mercurial treatment (§ 648, 649) have been observed from even the gradual administration of calomel; the production of scrofula and erysipelas, the gouty diathesis, obstinate ulcers in the mouth and on other parts of the body, caries of the nasal bones, wasting fever, and, in short, every malady that can be produced by long-continued mercurial irritation and depression of the strength. Even in this case physicians failed to perceive that mercury loses its effect upon the venereal virus in proportion as it causes any increased evacuation, be that ptyalism or diarrhœa, or whatever other inordinate excretion.[1]

519. Still more celebrated in modern times is the so-called *mixed method*[2] of curing syphilis by means of frictions and corrosive sublimate at the same time; whereby it was thought to unite the advantages of both, after the frequent insufficiency of both used separately had been perceived.

520. I shall not dilate upon its disadvantages, as they are the same as I have pointed out relative to both methods separately; except that they affected the system more severely than the employment of a single mercurial preparation, and that less of the ointment was used, consequently the excessive salivation caused by it was to a certain extent avoided. Indeed it was often possible to do more by the combination of the two than by either separately.

521. For this purpose it was usual, after the ordinary preliminary treatment, either to give these two remedies in alternation, administering at one time the corrosive sublimate alone, and at another the frictions without the corrosive sublimate, or both were employed at once, from one to two drachms of ointment every third or fourth day, and from a quarter to a whole grain of corrosive sublimate dissolved in two pints of water daily.

---

[1] Clare's method of rubbing-in the calomel on the interior of the mouth does not, it is true, incommode the bowels, but it readily produces salivation, and is incapable of curing syphilis of any great intensity.

Gardane is said to have invented it.

522. In order to remove syphilis in this manner, twelve drachms to four ounces of ointment, and from one drachm to fifteen grains of corrosive sublimate, according to circumstances, and a period of from thirty to one hundred days were required; on an average, nineteen drachms of ointment and twenty-eight grains of corrosive sublimate in forty-eight days, in moderately deep-rooted cases.

523. To gain the same end, especially for symptoms of the proximate kind, recourse was also had to *fumigations* combined with frictions; in which case a smaller quantity of ointment, or less calomel for fumigating was required than when either process was employed alone.

524. Three ounces of ointment and twelve drachms of cinnabar, or calomel, were on an average the quantity required for the eradication of moderate venereal affections.

525. I shall not describe the still more mixed methods, in which more than two different mercurial preparations were given at once, plainly proving, if I mistake not, that frequently neither the employment of a single one of the mercurials ordinarily used, nor yet the mixed employment of two of them at once, sufficed to cure a high degree of syphilis.

526. I may here mention the not very new preparation, the so-called *Mercurius nitratus* [1] (*Solutio mercurialis*, Edin., *Mercurius liquidus, Aqua mercurialis*, Paris), or the solution of mercury in nitric acid. I admit that in some cases it acts in a milder and more antiseptic manner than corrosive sublimate, and for that reason sometimes does more for the cure of syphilis than the latter; also that it equally seldom excites ptyalism. I will also admit, that by employing it we can substitute the uncertain form of the mere solution for the more defined one of the crystallized nitrate of mercury; also that it has this advantage, when the solution has been prepared by the heat of a sand-bath, that it is not decomposed by the muriatic acid in the primæ viæ into the pernicious white precipitate, like that dissolved in vegetable acids; certainly a great recommendation! But all this does not make it into a good preparation; it always remains a corrosive metallic salt, with which we must, as with all the preparations of mercury with mineral acids, on account of its accidental corrosive properties, frequently go much more cautiously to work than the obstinacy of the venereal affections will admit of. Its acridity easily excites vomiting

---

[1] As early as 1676 Charas employed a similar solution of mercury (*essentia mercurialis*), respecting which it has been asserted, without reason, that it was powerless, and resembled a weak dilution of aqua fortis, because the greater portion of the mercury has precipitated from it by the large quantity of water used; distilled or pure spring-water has not this effect; well-water precipitates white precipitate and changes the liberated nitric acid into nitrate of soda, but not into aqua fortis.

8

in sensitive stomachs ; colics and oppression of the stomach are no unusual concomitants of its employment, and if we are thereby necessitated to give it in smaller doses we shall seldom obtain our object of a radical cure. Profoundly rooted syphilis is as seldom cured by it as by corrosive sublimate, because, like every other mercurial salt formed by a mineral acid, it is, on account of its irritating property, taken up by the absorbents of the bowels and brought into the general circulation, only in the smallest undeterminable quantity. It deceives us by the adventitious irritation it excites, which smothers the venereal symptoms by its greater intensity, or by a mere superficial cure, as, for instance, a deceptive amendment in the ulcers of the mouth.

527. A third of a grain is given at first and the quantity gradually increased until from two to three grains are given daily, dissolved in two pints of liquid.

528. Mercury changed into powder by laborious [1] shaking, then calcined, dissolved in vinegar, and made into pills with manna, was the composition of *Keyser's Dragées*, of which from 1000 to 3000 often had to be taken before the desired effect ensued. This expensive [2] remedy has gone out of fashion, as it also occasions diarrhœa and salivation, and is very often unable to cure deeply-rooted syphilis. From forty to seventy days were usually required for the treatment.

529. The limited character of my design does not require that I should attempt the thankless task of describing the remaining mercurial preparations of this kind, which bear a great resemblance to those already treated of.

530. More nearly allied in nature to the best preparation of mercury is on the one hand, *Plenk's mucilaginous mercury*, a remedy that is indebted for the efficacy it possesses to the oxydation of the mercury, by being rubbed up with mucilage.   In this oxydised state the metal is very mild and not at all irritating, at least to the primæ viæ; it is readily dissolved by the gastric juice, and brought without difficulty into the general circulation, where it destroys the venereal poison with the greatest power.   This is the ideal excellence of this remedy.

531. We may bestow the same commendation on Belloste's pills,[3] the mercurial pills of the London and latest Edinburgh pharmacopœia, or the trituration of mercury with honey, sugar, or crabs' eyes. These preparations owe their mildness to the absence of mineral acids, and

---

[1] Keyser's remedy is nothing new. Bernhard Penot had (before 1613) a shorter mode of preparing this remedy. *Theatr. Chym.* lib. I, p. 654.

[2] Twenty-seven livres' worth of these pills were required for the (often fruitless) treatment. *Paralléle des diff. méth. de tr la mal. vén.* Amst. 1794, p. 178—272.

[3] The first pills of this sort that were used in Europe (in 1537) for syphilis were the Barbarossa pills (almost the first preparation that was much given internally for this disease), the dose of which was one pill daily, which contained about four grains of mercury, extinguished by rubbing.

their efficacy to the portion of oxydised mercury they contain that is so soluble in our fluids, and that is produced by rubbing up mercury with any of these substances.

532. But how much is the value of such preparations diminished when we know how unequal, how indefinite is the small portion of oxyde of mercury that is produced by rubbing up with mucilage, &c. The temperature during the operation, the strength of the mucilage, but more than all the strength and skill exercised by the operator during the rubbing-up process, are subject to such great varieties, and render these and the other preparations I have mentioned, such uncertain, I had almost said such useless, remedies, that we may well hesitate before bestowing on them even a moderate amount of praise.

533. I shall not dwell upon the fact, that in Plenk's solution the greater part of mercury falls again to the bottom, and that it cannot be kept above eight days in summer ; for this objection he has obviated by his pills, which, however, on the other hand, become excessively hard, and pass undigested through the bowels if they be not prepared fresh every day. The greatest disadvantage attendant on the employment of these preparations is, that they sometimes cause sudden salivation, sometimes diarrhœa, sometimes they produce no effect, and seem to be quite powerless; a plain but unnecessary proof of the truth of my assertions. They contain often scarcely the eightieth, but sometimes again the twentieth part of the mercury rubbed up in them, in the oxydised form.

534. *Pure oxyde of the mercury alone, without the slightest admixture of anything acrid, that, without causing any inconvenience to the primœ viœ, is unobservedly, easily and certainly assimilated by the juices of our body, and may be given in determined quantities,* is the most powerful and surest mercurial preparation, and is superior to all others, which, either from the quantity of active matter they contain being undeterminable, or from their corrosive acridity, or also from their insolubility, are injurious or untrustworthy.

535. In this important respect the *mercury oxydised*[1] *per se*, has become justly celebrated, and it is certainly among the preparations hitherto employed, the one best calculated, with proper precautions, for removing the highest degree of inveterate syphilis, speedily, easily, and surely.

536. Of this oxydised mercury, (*merc. calcin.*, Lond.) one grain is given daily, and the dose gradually increased up to three grains daily, until amendment ensues or the mouth becomes affected. It does not

---

[1] There is an extremely ancient though previously seldom used remedy that was highly recommended for the treatment of syphilis by Anthony Gallus, in 1540, under the name of *præcipitatum rubrum solare*, but its mode of preparation was first made known in 1693, by Gervaise Ucay.

so readily (for what reason is not known) produce true salivation, and seldom diarrhœa or vomiting, if it do not encounter any muriates in the stomach. As this last circumstance was not understood, it was usual to mix it with some preparation of opium in order to guard against this effect.

537. The mode of preparing this substance is well known, but the experienced professional man must be aware how extremely difficult, intricate and tedious is its true preparation. These difficulties in its manufacture are so excessive that it is one of the dearest medicaments. Now, as in the matter of pharmaceutical preparations the frequency of the adulteration of a remedy is always in the direct ratio of its price, I shall not be discredited in asserting that this drug is very seldom to be obtained genuine. The corrosive red precipitate[1] is probably the substance most frequently used for its adulteration.

538. I cannot tell why such an expensive, untrustworthy and circuitous mode of preparing a pure mercurial oxyde has been sought to be retained. I know not why medical men did not undertake more frequently to precipitate a pure metallic oxyde from the solution in nitric acid, and to bring it into general use in the treatment of venereal diseases. It has been prepared, but assuredly a number of serious accidents[2] have been observed from its administration, the source and remedy of which it was thought impossible to discover.

539. Chemistry should have taught them that their solvents, as also, all their precipitants, were contaminated with muriatic or vitriolic acid which imperceptibly adulterated their precipitate with those dangerous mercurial precipitates (see preface). As regards turbith, it is well known to have frequently caused death, and I once saw a strong person die in strong convulsions from taking two grains of white precipitate.

540. We can expect the best effects only from a mercurial oxyde precipitated from pure nitrate of mercury by lime free from all admixture; we may expect that well-prepared *soluble mercury* will remove the most deeply engrafted syphilis easily and surely. But of this more below.

CHAPTER III.
NON-MERCURIAL REMEDIES.

541. The dreadful effects of injudicious mercurial treatments, and

---

[1] We may convince ourselves of its presence by boiling with acetic acid; it remains undissolved whilst the oxydised mercury is taken up in solution.

[2] The *merc. præcip. fuscus Wuerzii* has, according to Girtanner, fallen into disuse. Black's *pulv. mercur. cin.* (certainly one of the best of the ordinary preparations) still retains its position. It is given at first in from one to two grains daily, and gradually increased to six grains. It is far from being free from faults, as I have shewn in the preface, but it approaches near to my soluble mercury.

heir frequent inefficacy, has from time to time diverted the attention
f practitioners from the divine metal, the true antisyphilitic specific,
nd their conscientiousness led them to resort to remedies from the
egetable and animal kingdoms, in order to avoid the poisonous effects
hat, according to them, every medicine in general, and mercury in
particular, exercises on the human body.

542. It is probable that the venereal disease at the commencement
of its extension over Europe spread much more rapidly, and in its rapid course produced more disastrous symptoms than are now observed.
The inexperience of physicians that then prevailed might have rendered them unable to meet the horrible effects of the virus, and patients were readily abandoned to the practice of rash empirics; the
disgrace of the disease also might have the effect, as is still the case,
of driving the sufferers to these nameless vagabonds, partly seduced
by their wonderful promises, and partly in order to recover their health
in privacy. These unconscientious advisers, who were always provided with the most active medicines, had as usual no object but to
fill their purses quickly, and in a short time to bring about the deceptive semblance of a cure without caring for the after effects. Hence
it happened not unfrequently that from their furious salivation the
most dangerous dilapidations and maimings of the body resulted,
which were often more horrible than the venereal disease itself; many
died from these effects, whilst the lues venerea more rarely proved
fatal. What could be more natural than that physicians generally
laid the blame upon the mercury, and hesitated to employ it? What
could be more natural than that from an early period (from 1515[1])
they looked about for non-metalic remedies, which, as they believed
were more suited to the human body?

543. Guaiac wood was the first lucky hit in this way, which the
Chevalier von Hutten, before any one else, undertook to praise in a
book specially written for that purpose,[2] alleging that it had worked
miracles on him after the fruitless employment of the most dangerous
mercurial treatment. He died nevertheless of syphilis.

544. The antivenereal plants probably first derived their reputation
from America; for want of mercury the inhabitants of that continent
tried their most potent plants for this disease, and in many respects
they may have caused at least alleviation of the disease.

545. After guaiac wood, cinchona bark,[3] sarsaparilla,[4] and, finally,
ceanothos and lobelia, gradually obtained a reputation in Europe.
From the resemblance of their mode of action to that of these plants,

---

[1] Girtanner says as early a 1509.
[2] After him an enormous number of others.
[3] According to Girtanner in the year 1525.
[4] According to Girtanner in 1530.

we added to them mezereum, conium, walnut-husks and dulcamara. Ammonia, opium and lizards completed the list.

546. Guaiac wood was and is still given in a strong decoction in water of from one to several ounces per diem, drunk warm; it is an acrid vegetable substance, possessing much power to act on the skin and urinary secretion. The small green twigs of this tree, which the Americans use, are probably still more powerful than the hard, dry wood employed by us. It is most useful in soft, spongy systems.[1]

547. Sarsaparilla fell gradually into complete disrepute, until later[2] physicians again commenced prescribing it to the extent of three ounces daily in strong watery decoction.[3] Cinchona bark underwent the same fate, but has as yet found no resuscitator.

548. Of lobelia, which was so much recommended by the North Amerians, a handful of the dried roots is boiled in twelve pints of water down to six or nine pints, and half a pint of this is given to the patient, at first twice, thereafter four times a day, until the diarrhœa it causes becomes intolerable. It is then left off for three or four days, and again given until the cure is completed.

549. Mezereum[4] has been considered to possess similar properties.[5] Two drachms of this were boiled in three pints of water down to two pints, and half a pint drunk from twice to four times daily. The stalks of dulcamara were prescribed to the extent of two drachms daily, boiled in water, and mixed with milk. A much larger quantity could be given by increasing the dose gradually.[6] The green husks of walnuts are said to have been not less efficacious.[7]

---

[1] Girtanner alleges that it speedily causes incurable consumption in weak and thin persons.

[2] Especially W. Fordyce. Girtanner has never seen any good effects from its use.

[3] As much as fifteen pounds of this dear medicament were used for one treatment.

[4] I find as early as 1553, in the works of Augerius Ferrière of Thoulouse (*De pudendagra lue hispan. lib. duo.* Antwerp, 1564, p. 26), this shrub much recommended for this disease in the form of decoction.

[5] Especially in pains of the bones and venereal cutaneous diseases.

[6] So that it shall not occasion convulsions or vomiting, as Girtanner remarks, who recommends this plant highly in this disease.

[7] Girtanner speaks very highly of this remedy, to the extent of two ounces daily in decoction, when it is fresh, and in the form of extract for the most inveterate symptoms. This writer also recommends a perfectly new non-mercurial remedy, the *Astragalus exscapus* (he gives an engraving of it), from the reports of his friends in nodes of the bones, venereal cutaneous eruptions, venereal warts, &c. Winterl first mentioned it as an ordinary domestic remedy for this disease in Hungary; after him Quarin spoke highly of it; Huncczovsky has seen good effects from it in gout, but not in venereal affections. It causes purging, diueresis, most frequently copious diaphoresis, and a kind of cutaneous eruption. One ounce boiled in a pint of water down to three-fourths is given daily.

The *ledum palustre* may probably act in a somewhat similar manner, especially in venereal skin diseases; of this we should give, daily, at first half an ounce, gradually increasing the dose to an ounce in infusion.

550. I have elsewhere observed that many very different irritant substances are capable of producing amelioration in venereal affections, inasmuch as the counter-irritation caused by them alters the morbid disposition of the primarily affected parts, and the pains they are subject to (e. g., the venereal pains in the bones) are alleviated by the greater irritant effects of the drug.

551. It is in this way that the most of these plants appear to have acted when they have done any good; at all events, this is the case with the purgative herbs, lobelia and mezereum, and the diuretic and diaphoretic ones, guaiac, walnut shells and dulcamara. In this respect this good effect resembles that of turbith, corrosive sublimate and blisters (applied to swellings of the bones. The mucilaginous diuretic sarsaparilla, may contribute not a little to the diminution of the morbid irritability.)

552. If they be given in conjunction with the mercurial treatment, their irritating power may also assist the action of the metal, but only in the manner in which ginger assists in strengthening the stomach when given along with bitters, which it is unable to do of itself. Perhaps also, when by a long-continued, fruitless use of mercury, the body has become insensible to the curative stimulus of this metal, the new, unaccustomed irritation of these drugs may have caused amelioration, and on this account they were regarded as antivenereal.

553. The last-mentioned plants may often, when given quite alone. in consequence of their great depurative power, have cured a number of external diseases, even such as are of a painful character, which from want of pathological knowledge had been considered as venereal. With respect to mezereum and guaiac, at least, it is certain that they cannot cure the most indubitable incipient sign of syphilis, e. g., the copper-coloured spots; how then could they remove inveterate lues?

554. But more than this, it was the custom formerly (and is so still) for physicians, in ignorance of venereal semeiotics, to look upon diseases arising from the long use of mercury, such as caries, tumours, rheumatic symptoms, scrofula, &c., as of a true venereal nature, and when guaiac, mezereum, and the like, removed these affections, to laud these plants, as antisyphilitic remedies.[1] The foreign irritation of these drugs, especially of guaiac, has not unfrequently been of great service in those after sufferings resulting from the long-continued use of mercurial treatment, which had arisen from morbid irritability and dissolution of the humours: obstinate ulcers, trembling, febrile states, and the like, the first of which are still sometimes mistaken for venereal.

---

[1] Some of the ancients were more discerning than these short-sighted persons when they said: *luis veneræ mercurius antidotum, mercurii guaicum.*

555. I may be permitted to entertain almost the same notions respecting Peyrilhe's[1] antidote to venereal disease, ammonia. With the exception of caries and nodes of the bones, aphthæ of the vagina, schirrhous buboes and urinary fistulæ, he alleges that it is specific for all other venereal symptoms. Of ammonia obtained from sal ammoniac by means of potash, he directs from fifteen to eighteen grains (and in bloated individuals as much as thirty grains) dissolved in four or five ounces of fluid, to be taken early in the morning and four hours after dinner, and this to be continued for about eight days, then to be left off for the same time and again used as long, again omitted and again used, until the affection is removed. I believe this substance to be really a powerful adjuvant in the treatment of venereal diseases, and I go so far as to believe, that if any medicine can be of use in syphylis, besides mercury, this is the one.

556. Plenk, Murray and others affirm that they have seen following its employment increased inflammation of the venereal ulcers, inflammatory suppression of gonorrhœa with swelled testicle, strangury with hematuria, and several other disagreeable effects. It has proved of much service in my hands in chronic affections resulting from a long course of mercurial treatment, and has materially aided in diminishing the morbid irritability.

557. Before all other remedies, however, opium[2] owes its reputation to this virtue. Hunter could not succeed in curing the slightest venereal symptoms with opium, although he gave it in increasing, and at length in the very largest doses, whereby he once killed a man without previously curing his disease. He and Grant, like myself, found it a chief remedy in the morbid irritability resulting from the abuse of mercury.

558. Hemlock has probably just as little specific virtue in syphilis, and all the action it has may be owing to its peculiar irritant power, and even when it has proved serviceable for supposed venereal after-sufferings, it might have acted by virtue of its sedative and anti-scrofulous powers.

559. The lizard, which was first employed in America, and subsequently also in Europe, according to report with extremely happy effects, in inveterate syphilis with nodes, pains in the bones, ulcers and slow fevers, besides other diseases, is the *lacerta agilis*, L., a large (greenish coloured) species; the smaller varieties also are useful, though in a less degree. They reside in old walls, and prey upon spiders, flies, ants, earth-worms, crickets and locusts.

---

[1] Lemery and Sylvius had already recommended ammonia in syphilis, as Girtanner remarks.

[2] It is no novelty to give it in venereal diseases. I found that Fernel frequently employed it in syphilis as early as 1556. Willis and Simon Pauli followed his example, as Girtanner observes.

560. We take the living animal, quickly cut off its head, tail and legs, extract the viscera, skin it, and cut it into a number of small bits, which we make the patient swallow with some liquid, while still alive and warm, either alone or covered with liquorice powder, or rolled up in a wafer, but without further preparation. Of the larger kind, the flesh of one or two is to be swallowed daily; of the smaller kind that of several. From twenty to one hundred are required to complete the treatment.

561. The chief effects resulting from their use are, increased heat of the whole organism, a certain amount of nausea, a (frequently copious) flow of yellowish opapue saliva, occurring after twelve or twenty-one have been taken, sometimes sooner, a (sometimes profuse) fetid diaphoresis, fetid urine, and also occasionally copious bilious alvine evacuations.

562. According to the observations of some writers, they are probably not less efficacious when the flesh is minced fine, made into pills by means of flour, and so swallowed. This, however, remains to be determined by experience. This remedy deserves attention, as it is in itself so harmless. Its chief efficacy seems to reside in the volatile alkaline component parts. It may be very powerful, but we are unable to determine if it can radically cure true syphilis.

563. But whilst the other reputed antisyphilitic remedies are for the most part only able to cure accessory symptoms, heterogeneous remnants of the venereal disease, and the various affections produced by the irritation occasioned by the abuse of mercury, all of which have been considered to be venereal merely on account of their coexistence with syphilis, it always remains an established fact that mercury is the only thing that removes all sorts of venereal affections with certainty, so that we have no need to look about us for any other remedy for venereal diseases, provided the preparation we possess be of the very best kind.

THIRD DIVISION.

REMOVAL OF THE OBSTACLES TO THE MERCURIAL TREATMENT.

CHAPTER I.

OBSERVATIONS ON THE ORDINARY PREPARATORY AND ACCESSORY TREATMENT

564. Those to be subjected to the mercurial treatment (with very few exceptions) are prepared, after the French fashion (§ 493), by purging,

venesections and tepid baths ;[1] the last, moreover, are employed often during the whole treatment and during the after treatment (Haguenot was the first who sought to make their use general), but the first are used at various intervals. At the same time a watery, non-nutritious diet is given, consisting chiefly of a multitude of tepid and warm drinks ; and all this is done in order to guard against any symptom of the venereal disease inimical to the cure, and to make the mercury all the more efficacious.

565. I have often puzzled myself in vain to determine how this preparatory treatment could have the effect of preventing all ill consequences during the treatment, and I believe I have found that all this is done under the erroneous impression that all possible disagreeable symptoms occurring during the mercurial treatment, even the salivation that especially ensues under this method, are of a purely inflammatory nature, and depend solely on tension of the fibres and an excess of red blood. This must have been the indication that guided the originators of this method, or they must have chosen it for want of something else to do, for in no other case, except to remove the most violent pure inflammatory diathesis of the organism, is it capable of doing the slightest good ; in all other states of the body whatsoever it is quite the reverse of beneficial.

566. Now as pure inflammatory diseases and symptoms are rare amongst us now-a-days, especially among the inhabitants of large towns, and all those symptoms in this kind of diseases that can be regarded as inflammatory are chiefly of scorbutic, erysipelatous, scrofulous, rheumatic, or of that character which I have termed irritability from nervous weakness, and as all strength-destroying, debilitating and enervating treatment aggravates all the symptoms in the latter case, as experience teaches, we perceive on the one hand how inappropriate that common treatment by the so-called alterative, emollient, attenuating, relaxing and antiphlogistic method is, and on the other hand how much of the frequently disastrous results of that French plan of treating lues venerea must be ascribed to this abominable weakening system.

567. There are few constitutions so good as to be able to bear up against the force of this strength-wasting method,[2] and not very many in which the amendment produced by the mercury does not suddenly

---

[1] The number used in the preparatory treatment at Montpellier is usually thirty, without reckoning what are employed when salivation sets in and after the treatment.

[2] This method, which in the opinion of its defenders is best calculated to check the salivation and to point out to the mercury the direct way of eradicating the virus, is termed the *alterative treatment*. The Spanish physician Almenar, as Girtanner observes, was one of the first to insist on the use of purgatives and baths for this purpose ; Chikoyneau reiterated his maxims, and Haguenot increased the number of baths to be used.

come to a stand-still in the middle of the treatment, in which an enervating, uncontrollable salivation[1] does not occur, which eats away the
nasal and palatial bones and gives rise to corroding, often sloughing
ulcers of the mouth and tongue; in which the borders of bubonic abscesses do not suddenly become everted, spread in a cancerous manner, pour out fetid corrosive ichor, and terminate in mortification; in
which cutaneous ulcers and condylomata do not take on an unhealthy
suppuration, become painful, and degenerate into deep sinuses and
fistulous ulcers; in which swellings of the periosteum do not occasion
more speedy caries of the bones beneath, and in which sinking of the
strength, uncontrollable diarrhœas, debilitating perspirations, and the
whole array of symptoms of hectic fever, do not occasionally effect
the deliverance of the unhappy sufferer from the methodical, artificially produced disease, by conducting him prematurely to the final goal
of all mortals (§ 648, 649).

568. This French folly of pretending to assist the action of mercury
by enervating the body is carried to such a height, that when in the
treatment of venereal diseases the last named disagreeable symptoms
occurred, which were chiefly produced or at least aggravated by the
debilitating accessory treatment, frequently nothing more was done
than to renew[2] or to increase the anti-phlogistic method, to the destruction of the patient.

569. Physicians did not observe that the serious symptoms that
occur during the use of mercury in this disease are seldom of a purely
inflammatory character, and that when they will not yield to the antisyphilitic metal, an excess of corporeal strength and of pure strong
blood is certainly not the cause of this phenomenon; in a word, they
imagined they had to do with savage Gauls and rude Germans whose
seething blood required to be drawn off, whose flaming nervous force
had to be smothered by pouring in streams of water, and whose over-
tense fibres needed to be relaxed by soaking in a succession of warm
baths, so as to prevent the irritating metal exciting the most uncontrollable inflammatory symptoms; whereas they really had only to
deal with their degenerate descendants, their mere shadows, whose
already weak blood they draw off in large quantity, in order to make
it still more watery by deluging it with ptisans; whose delicate
stomachs and bowels they weakened into dyspepsia by mucilaginous
fluids and laxatives, and whose skin, that was already frequently too

---

[1] Astruc mentions that Morand employed on five soldiers the same kind of frictions; of three of these who got no baths one only had slight salivation, but the two
others who daily employed baths at the same time were salivated violently and for
a long time.

[2] As may be seen in the fourth part of *Observations faites et publieés sur les
différentes méthodes d'administrer le mercure dans les maladies véneriennes, par de
Horne.*—Paris, 1779.

sensitive to every change of weather, they weakened by heated apartments and repeated baths, to the highest degree of irritability and extreme susceptibility to take cold. Experience teaches often enough that those cases in which this method was employed to its full extent on the most approved principles had almost always the saddest termination. We cannot readily conceive of anything more inappropriate than to weaken fibres that ought to be strengthened, to abstract vital force that ought to be multiplied, and to diminish the tone of the nerves that require strength for the due performance of their operations!

570. If it be alleged that this method is directed more against the venereal affections than against the symptoms to be dreaded from the employment of the mercurial treatment, why, it may be asked, should the venereal disease, whose nature is the very opposite of purely inflammatory, be combatted with antidotes calculated for subduing the most violent inflammatory fever of a sunburnt savage?

571. If it be contended that the bad symptoms and obstinate after-sufferings during the treatment of venereal diseases may arise from the irritating metallic poison used, I will readily grant that they occur even where the French preparatory and accessory treatment has not been employed, but I am all the more astonished that the latter can be prescribed along with the mercury, seeing that it is productive of equal injury, and thus lends a helping hand to the devastations of the mercury.

572. If it be asserted that the venesections, the confinement to a heated room, the streams of warm drinks, and the baths, constitute a diaphoretic treatment, which is to keep the mercury from irritating the bowels and salivary glands, I ask, what is the object of the anti-diaphoretic purgatives? I ask, has not experience shewn that such a sudorific treatment most frequently creates a tendency to take cold, whose effects are worse in proportion to the weakening tendency of the diaphoretic treatment?

CHAPTER II.
PREPARATORY TREATMENT.

573. If there be any general method whereby those who enter into a venereal hospital must be artificially prepared for the mercurial treatment, the very nature of the thing shews us a directly opposite system should be adopted, since laxity of fibre and nervous weakness have come to be the chief ingredients of all the chronic diseases of our age.

574. In most cases of old-standing syphilis[1] we observe a general weakness of the body, a pale countenance, a dull eye, relaxed muscles,

---

[1] Also in cases of idiopathic venereal diseases, especially those for which mercury has already been employed in vain.

and frequently, on account of the low fever kept up by the venereal irritation, a weakened digestion, a small, unsteady, very rapid pulse, tendency to cramps, and all the signs of increased morbid irritability of the whole nervous system.

575. All these symptoms indicate tonics for the preparatory treatment, which are all the more necessary because without them the mercury increases the delicate state of the constitution, or thereby is prevented from exercising the requisite power over the venereal virus.

576. If they be neglected, then the low fever and tendency to scrofulous inflammation increases, and, what is worst, on the administration of the smallest quantity of mercury a dysenteric diarrhœa, an uncontrollable diaphoresis, or most commonly an irrepressible salivation, breaks out, that consumes all the strength, and frequently leaves behind it the after-sufferings often alluded to, frequently without having eradicated the syphilitic virus.

577. Not unfrequently a tendency of the system to rheumatic and gouty acridities, to scrofula and to scorbutus, forms an impediment to the mercurial treatment; and these diatheses must previously be removed if we would not see these affections uncommonly aggravated during or after the venereal treatment, or if we would employ the mercury with certainty and efficacy.

578. Accordingly, in order to diminish beforehand the morbid liability to the above (§ 576) evacuations, and to eradicate the unfavourable diatheses alluded to, it is, for the reasons given, indispensably necessary to employ the strengthening preparatory treatment according to circumstances, with special regard to the removal of the scrofulous, scorbutic or other disposition, according as the one or the other betrays its presence by its diagnostic marks.

579. Among general tonic remedies I reckon footbaths, half, and at length whole baths of cold (50°) water, each used for a few minutes, once or several times a day, combined with energetic friction[1] of the parts bathed. For internal remedies, at first the bitter vegetable extracts (if the morbid irritability is very great), before proceeding to the astringent bitter medicines, as cinchona and the like. If the body is bloated and full of indolent juices, we may at first combine them with carminative and stimulating things, as cardamoms, peppermint oil, and so forth, in order to accelerate their action. Among the best of strengthening remedies I reckon the use of moderate exercise in the open air. Great irritability from weakness, with urgent, painful symptoms, demands the cautious external and internal employment of opium, combined with the strengthening treatment. But if the irritability from weakness be not excessive, we may soon have recourse to bark, iron-filings and sulphuric acid as internal tonics. I now come to

---

[1] With woollen towels.

the accessory treatment of the prevailing morbid concomitant diathesis.

580. It is only in the case when previous to or during the employment of the strengthening method the tongue becomes white, and thirst for cold water, severe headache, a full, hard pulse, &c., occur, without any bad taste in the mouth, fulness of the abdomen, indigestion, or commotion of the bile, then and then cnly must we make a moderate bleeding, which paves the way for the tonic treatment, which may then be gradually increased.

581. If we combine the tonic treatment with the fresh expressed juices of the cochleara, the arum root, and the water-cress, and aid it by fermented liquors, fresh fruits, and exercise in the open, dry air, we shall subdue the scorbutus, which offers the greatest impediments to the cure of syphilis. For if, without this precaution, we proceed at once to the employment of the mercurial treatment on a scorbutic venereal patient, there occur, in the midst of the most energetic action of this metal, rapidly spreading foul ulcers, which give sufficient evidence of their non-venereal nature by their being worst at this particular time.

582. The strengthening method alluded to, combined with the employment of carbonate of ammonia and small doses of ipecacuan[1] or burnt sea-weed, will prevent the scrofulous diatheses interfering with the cure of syphilis.

583. In like manner guaiac resin dissolved by the combined action of potash and alcohol, but especially the extract of aconite conjoined with the tonics indicated above, more especially with the cold bath, is generally sufficient to destroy the gouty diathesis in the system.

584. Steel filings will remove the chlorotic disposition, and along with the other tonic remedies, help to increase the red parts of the blood.

585. A tendency to erysipelas demands great moderation in the use of meat and similar articles of diet, and the plentiful use of fruit and whey combined with the general strengthening method.

586. Haller's or similar acid elixirs will moderate or remove inflammatory dispositions of unknown, indefinite or composite character.

587. It is only after having strengthened the fibres in this or some similar manner, thereby bringing the tone of the nerves into more uniform and powerful vibrations, and after having dimininished or removed the obvious accessory disease,[2] that we should undertake to attack the syphilis with mercury.

588. Let it not be objected that such a preparatory treatment would

---

[1] So that for a couple of weeks every forenoon is passed in constant nausea and slight heaving.

[2] Also where hysteria is present we must adopt some similar preparatory treatment, or at least be always on our guard for fear of the occurrence of couvulsions. The occurrence of the catamenia demands the intermission of the mercury until it is past; bleeding hemorrhoids demand a similar precaution.

consume much time and put off for a long period the employment of the mercury.   If the morbid accessory diathesis be strong, and the chief ingredient of the composite disease, then nothing more expedient, nothing more appropriate can be conceived, let it last ever so long. But even in the very worst cases we shall 'have advanced so far with the general or special strengthening treatment (if it were at all applicable) in from three to five weeks, that we shall be able to commence the use of the metal.

589. Sometimes it is requisite to continue the tonic treatment along with the mercury, which, with the exception of the cold baths, may be done without restriction[1] in the most of such cases.

590. It is only when the symptoms of syphilis are very violent and urgent, and when they constitute the major part of the composite disease, whilst the accessory morbid diathesis constitutes its minor part, only in such cases can we employ the mercury at once, combined with the tonic treatment.

CHAPTER III.

PREVENTION OF THE DISAGREEABLE EFFECTS OF MERCURY.

591. It has been proved by thousands of observations that no deeply rooted venereal virus can be expelled by any visible, far less excessive evacuations, diarrhœa, salivation,[2] diuresis and diaphoresis, and that these rather have the effect of palpably hindering[3] the metal in its antisyphilitic action, and ought consequently to be avoided.[4]

592. Whether the threatened *salivation* can be kept back by the use of powdered sulphur, my experience has not yet taught me ; still the trials of others lead us to anticipate much advantage from it, as also the expectation deduced from chemical science, that the sulphur, penetrating the mass of blood, effects a mineralization of the dissolved metal (Ethiops mineral), and suddenly renders it inefficacious.

593. Some advise that the patient should be exposed to severe cold, others that he should be kept very warm, both with the view of checking the salivation ; but both frequently fail of their object, especially when the exciting cause that could indicate one or other of them is lost sight of.

---

[1] Only that the strengthening remedies should not be given all day, but only two hours before and two hours after dinner.

[2] It is remarkable that as early as the commencement of the sixteenth century (1502) the Spaniard Almenar sought to prevent and remove salivation by every possible means, in order the better to cure this disease.

[3] At all events by diminishing the mercurial fever.

[4] Sydenham says, in his *Epist. resp. ad Henr. Paman,* that a remedy must destroy the venereal poison in the body directly, without evacuation, in order to deserve the name of an antisyphilitic specific.

594. If a previous chill have caused an inconsiderably small quantity of mercury, that has been given, to act on the salivary glands without there being present any plethora, a diaphoretic, moderately warm treatment may be of service. If plethora and an inflammatory fever be the cause of the rapid salivation, then sometimes a venesection, but most certainly a general cool treatment, cold air, &c., will tend to check it.

595. But what are chiefly relied on are drastic purgatives,[1] under the supposition that the salivation will thereby be suddenly brought to a stop, although many thousands of cases demonstrate the impropriety of this treatment. The salivation is not thereby restrained ; on the contrary, it often increases still more when the action of the purgative is over, especially when, as is often the case, irritability was the cause of the sudden ptyalism. Moreover, who is ignorant of the debility that such a powerful evacuant medicine, or the repetition of such purgatives as are usually prescribed, leaves behind it, each of which is equivalent to a venesection in its weakening effects ? In a word, experience and reflection are equally opposed to this proceeding, as hurtful as it is useless.[2]

596. Were we better acquainted with the nature of camphor than we are, much might be expected from its use. But both the constitution that indicates it in this case, and the dose in which it can be of service, are still uncertain. I have often experienced the opposite from its use, and sometimes maintained in full force, for certain purposes, ptyalism persisting from irritability, by the daily administration of six grains of camphor; but the salivation that occurred was destitute of smell. Perhaps it is most powerful as an antidote to salivation, when the latter has resulted from suppressed perspiration.

597. Linnæus observed chronic salivation cured by an infusion of white horehound; the infusion prepared with wine likewise merits attention. Sanchez lauds the efficacy of vapour baths for preventing salivation; they do not, however, prevent it, as the Chevalier von Hutten piteously relates.

598. Morris found contrayerva, in the dose of two scruples twice a day, efficacious in obstinate cases. Others have advised blisters to the nape.

599. I mention these things in their proper place, but believe that we shall always meet with more success if we prevent the ptyalism beforehand, than if we rely upon checking it when it has already commenced.

---

[1] Desault brought them into great repute for this evacuation, about the year 1730.

[2] [It is interesting to remark the dissatisfaction of our author, respecting most of the prevalent notions of this period, upon medical topics. From the multitude of empirical methods, he is earnestly seeking for something of reason and truth.]—*Am. P.*

600. For this end it will be most expedient, in all the states of the system above spoken of, whether a general weakness and irritability, or any other accessory disposition, constitute the obstacle to the mercurial treatment, to regard the general (§ 578, 579) or specially directed (§ 580—585) tonic treatment as the chief preventive remedy of salivation, and by no means to neglect its employment. Still we would do well, in obstinate cases of composite venereal disease, to precede the use of the mercury by a local treatment of the mouth, which shall communicate the greatest possible tone to the salivary glands, and give them sufficient firmness to resist the too facile penetration of the mercurial irritation.

601. For this purpose I have found in my experience that the best thing to do, is for some days previously to hold in the mouth or move them frequently hither and thither, substances that are strongly astringent without causing nausea. I have often found of service an electuary of catechu or kino, mixed with a portion of alum, and with the addition of some syrup. I have employed a cold solution of sulphate of zinc, and also alum and sulphuric acid, with much benefit, to gargle or rinse out the mouth.

602. If we have to do with some (rare) cases of syphilis accompanied by such urgent symptoms as to require the immediate use of the mercury, we must immediately after the first dose of the mercury, proceed to strengthen the mouth (§ 601), and if that will not suffice to prevent those hurtful evacuations, we must have recourse to external remedies also. A strong solution of alum or sulphate of zinc in water, frequently applied, quite cold, (or cooled by ice), round the whole neck, has proved uncommonly useful to me.

603. In very irritable, emaciated, debilitated subjects, especially in such as have already suffered salivation from a previous employment of mercury, the early administration of this metal is always of doubtful propriety. In spite of every precaution we shall sometimes, especially if the obstinate symptoms of syphilis demand large doses of the antivenereal metal, be completely unable to prevent salivation by these external remedies.

604. If this take place we must immediately discontinue the mercury, and besides the external use of the ice-cold compresses (§ 602) frequently renewed, we should uncover or shave the head, pour over it cold water, and again dry it, whilst we envelop the feet in warm coverings, or place them every four hours in a tepid (96°) foot-bath for a quarter of an hour. The patient must rest in a cool dark room, in a sitting posture, with a light covering over him. His attention should be engaged with amusing stories, with music, &c.

605. As chewing greatly excites the salivary glands, we should not allow at this time any other articles of diet besides thin soups, or

9

easily digestible vegetables in the form of purée, with beer, milk and
the like; but solid food, tasty and sweet things, especially coffee, as
also everything that excites disgust, must be avoided. If the thirst is
great, we may give sour drinks and food.

60 5. We may at the same time continue assiduously the use of the
astringent electuary gargle (§ 601), combined with an eighth part of
laudanum. It is under these circumstances that I have also found
good effects from the internal employment of opium [1] (sometimes
combined with Minderer's spirit.)

607. If the bowels are constipated, they should be opened by one
or several clysters of vinegar.

608. I think I have been able to convince myself, by some experiments I have instituted, that drinks saturated with sulphuretted
hydrogen gas do in a short time remove all the irritation produced by
the presence of mercury in our fluids, as this remedy rapidly penetrates
all the vessels. and instantaneously mineralizes the mercury wherever
it encounters it. We should give from six to eight grains of some
good preparation of hepar sulphuris in the form of pills within twelve
hours, and cause the patient to drink thereafter a large quantity of
warm tea, made sour with lemon juice or cream of tartar.

609. But the surest way to prevent salivation is always a gradual,
cautious employment of mercury, and especially the selection of such
a preparation from which such an injurious effect is least to be apprehended. I have already sufficiently pointed out that the ordinary
mercurial preparations (especially the insoluble precipitates combined
with mineral acids, the turbith mineral, the red and white precipitates,
and calomel, as also Keyser's dragées, frictions, &c.) possess this
disadvantage in a high degree, with the exception of corrosive sublimate
and nitrate of mercury, also Plenk's mucilaginous mercury, but almost only when it is least powerful, but especially the mercury
oxydized *per se*, partly because it is not very apt to excite this evacuation of itself, partly and chiefly however because it can be given in
determinable small doses that we may rely upon penetrating into the
fluids, which is not the case with the mucilaginous. I have found that
the soluble mercury uncommonly seldom produces salivation, not only
on account of its peculiar nature, but also particularly because it acts
in such small, such definite doses, so very uniformly, and far more
certainly and mildly than that oxydised *per se*. If we commence its
use in very small doses, and only increase it gradually, paying great
attention to the state of the mouth, and if we employ at the same time
the accessory treatment pointed out, we shall *very rarely* be surprised
by salivation, even in those urgent cases in which it is requisite to
give it at the very commencement, or if it do come on it may readily

---

[1] According to the experience of Hunter, Girtanner and myself, it has certainly
great power in salivation, although Bloch denies it.

be checked by some of the means indicated.   So much is this the case that when I deemed salivation of use in certain non-venereal affections, I never thought of employing the soluble mercury for its production ; in such cases calomel best answered my purpose.

610. Violent diarrhœas are not easily avoided during the employ-ment of the ordinary mercurial remedies, for either the preparation itself is a purgative, such as calomel, or it becomes such from the muriates that are present in the primæ viæ (white precipitate), like the mercury introduced into the system by the rubbing-in process, the nitrate of mercury prepared in the cold, Keyser's dragées, and Plenk's preparation ; substances of which the first and last, if perchance they be very well prepared, contain an unexpected quantity of oxydised mercury, which may be transformed by the muriates in our system into a quantity of white precipitate sufficient to excite all at once vio-lent diarrhœa ; the other preparations named are always ready, the moment they come in contact with a gastric juice impregnated with muriates, to change *entirely* into that strong, noxious purgative, white precipitate.   The addition of opium to these remedies is of little use.

611. Regarding the soluble mercury we may be sure, that even though we neglect the rules for diet given below, it will excite no purgation, but only one or a couple of loose stools, because the small dose of it prescribed, even were it all changed in the stomach into white precipitate, is not sufficient to cause drastic evacuations.

612. If, as sometimes happens, a violent continued perspiration disturb the action of the mercury, a cool regimen and the employment of sulphuric acid, will speedily check this evacuation.   Some have found bark very useful.

613. The diuresis that is more rarely observed, may be stopped by a diaphoretic regimen and the intercurrent exhibition of cinchona bark, as long as we know of no remedy that possesses the power of speci-fically checking this evacuation.

FOURTH DIVISION.

THE NATURE OF THE SOLUBLE MERCURY AND ITS EMPLOYMENT IN VENEREAL DISEASES.

614. Well prepared soluble mercury (see Preface) is of a blackish grey colour and tasteless.   It may be dissolved in vinegar, and in water impregnated with carbonic acid, without leaving behind a trace of turbith mineral or of white precipitate.

615. The rapidity of its action shews that it is almost instantly dissolved in the gastric juice.   It very quickly combines with the

saliva in the mouth, and then immediately produces the peculiar mercurial taste.

616. When the proper diet is observed (§ 619) it causes no disagreeable sensation in the stomach or in the bowels, no vomiting, no diarrhœa, but passes directly, and in the course of a few hours, dissolved by the process of digestion, into the mass of the fluids.

617. It is only when there are muriates in the primæ viæ that there is an exception to this; in that case there occurs slight nausea, or one or two loose stools. But it is usually taken so rapidly into the general mass of the fluids, that even in this case there is seldom time for its complete conversion into white precipitate.

618. As it is in every case the duty of a patient to avoid overloading his stomach, which he cannot transgress with impunity under any moderate treatment, we may safely expect from any man whose nature is not quite bestial, that in the treatment of such an important disease as syphilis is, he will observe a slight restriction in diet which will cost him such a small sacrifice and have so much influence on the well-being of his future days.

619. In order to obtain this object and to remove all traces of muriates from the primæ viæ, if the antivenereal remedy is to be taken, as is usually the case, in the morning, we let the whole supper of the previous evening consist of some uncooked fruit. The following morning we allow the dose of soluble mercury to be taken as early as possible in some distilled water, and nothing to be partaken of for four or six hours thereafter; then if there be great thirst [1] the patient should take a little more distilled water, or cow's milk, or if there be weakness, a draught of good wine; so that during a period of twenty hours nothing shall enter the stomach that contains a trace of muriate of soda. At dinner time (noon) he makes an ordinary or moderate meal of anything [2] that comes to table, excepting the flesh and fat of geese, ducks and pork. We may allow those accustomed to it a glass of wine.

620. We may give the soluble mercury either alone, or in order to make the dose appear larger, rubbed up with some liquorice or mallow root. If we have to do with persons who are not to be trusted to in the observance of dietetic rules, we may add a half or whole grain of opium.

---

[1] This should be endeavoured to be avoided; for during its continuance there seems to be developed in the gastric juice, or to be deposited therein from the blood, an ammoniacal or muriatic acridity. The distilled water may be used either cold, or in the form of tea, made with liquorice and linden flowers, provided we dispense with the use of sugar. The thirst may also be quenched in the morning by means of fruit.

[2] Meat may be partaken of along with the vegetables as long as the former is not contraindicated by the advent of the mercurial fever or any other inflammatory state.

621. Although in the case of very sensitive but healthy persons who are very obedient in respect to diet, I have sometimes not had occasion to use more than *one* grain of soluble mercury in all, in order to cure moderate idiopathic venereal symptoms and commencing syphilis, yet I have met with cases in which sixty grains were necessary.

622. This extreme variety depends, as far as I have been able to observe accurately, on this, that in the first case the mercurial fever (§ 290) occurred as rapidly as could be wished for. But when I was forced to use such a large quantity, the reason was, that either some circumstance suddenly occurred that frequently interrupted the employment of the medicine, or that previouslymuch mercury had been used in vain, or that (in the case of persons of good constitution who could not, on account of their avocations, omit appearing in public every day) I had to excite and maintain a gradual (slow) mercurial fever.

623. On an average however I have found, that in order to eradicate a moderately severe syphilis, not more than eight grains were required, while for a severe and deeply rooted case, about twelve grains were needed.

624. But if we wish and are able to excite, 1st, a rapid mercurial fever (*febris murcurialis acuta*), a still smaller quantity is necessary in the very severest cases; but if, 2dly, on account of the circumstances that may arise, we must divide the mercurial fever into two or three small attacks, then more, sometimes much more, than the quantity indicated is required; but much the largest quantity is necessary when from the above reasons we have to excite, 3dly, an unnoticeable mercurial fever (*febris mercurialis lenta*). I beg that these three cases may be carefully distinguished.

625. In the first case I must be satisfied that no tendency to salivation exists, or that the patient has previously used mercury without having incurred this evacuation. In that case I gave from the very first large doses of the soluble mercury, and increased them rapidly, in order to excite quickly a severe mercurial fever,—(probably from a half to one, two, three grains; or in robust subjects and severe cases of lues, one two, three, four grains.)

626. In the second case (§ 624), usually when there was present a tendency to salivation, or when this evacuation had already occurred during a previous employment of mercury, I increased the quantity of the soluble mercury very gradually, so that I could leave it off on the slightest appearance of salivation, employ measures to combat it (in the progressive scale of from $\frac{1}{4}$ to $\frac{1}{3}$, $\frac{1}{2}$, $\frac{3}{4}$, 1, $1\frac{1}{4}$ grain). I calmed the irritation of the mouth and recommenced after an interval of from eight to fourteen days, to increase the dose (from about $\frac{1}{2}$ to 1,

1½ up to 2 grains), and so on until the syphilis had completely disappeared.

627. In the third case (§ 624) I used for eight or ten days only one quarter of a grain[1] daily, then for about the same period one grain, then two, then four grains, until all traces of the lues were destroyed. Patients of this sort must either be otherwise of very healthy robust constitutions, or else they must be unremittingly treated with tonics at the same time, in order that the long continued irritation shall not injure them. On the slightest affection of the mouth the mercury was discontinued for one or even several days, and the precautions I have described employed to combat this accident.

628. As a rule it is good, after the complete disappearance of the venereal symptoms, and the occurrence of a proper mercurial fever, especially in the rapid treatment (to which, when it is admissible, I give the preference), at once to discontinue the soluble mercury, and to wait and see whether or no the same symptoms do not reappear after four or five weeks. If nothing occurs we may, even in cases of deeply rooted syphilis, rest assured that a cure has been effected (even without waiting till this time has elapsed, we can be *perfectly sure* of the cure, if a sufficiently severe mercurial fever made its appearance) ; but should the same symptoms shew themselves, the mercurial fever must have been too weak, an error we must seek to repair by endeavouring, after the lapse of this time, to develope a new and much more severe mercurial fever than the first was (which is done with more trouble and by means of doses increased more rapidly), whereby all remains of the venereal poison will be certainly eradicated to the very last trace. But this is a very rare case, that can only happen to an inexperienced practitioner.

629. Recent buboes, simple chancres, and commencing lues, require almost the same degree of mercurial fever ; but lues with symptoms of the more remote kind, with nodes, &c., as also condylomata and old degenerated chancres and so forth, require the more severe fever.

630. If we wish to prevent a painful and inflamed buboe from suppurating, by the speedy destruction of the venereal virus, or timeously avert the threatened danger in phimosis and paraphimosis from chancres, a severe mercurial fever must be quickly excited. Accordingly directing our attention to the preservation of the salivary glands, of which I have treated in the previous chapter, we should here increase the doses of soluble mercury from 2 to 3, 4, 5 grains, and whenever the fever shews itself of sufficient severity, call a halt, and then terminate gradually what we were forced to commence violently.

---

[1] This dose given for four or five successive days without increase, frequently sufficed with sensitive individuals to produce an adequate artificial fever, and thereby to effect a perfect cure.

631. All the doses spoken of in this chapter are to be understood as daily doses, as it is well always to wait for twenty-four hours, and during that time to observe the effects of each dose.

632. In cases where I have found no special preparatory means requisite, *e. g.*, in otherwise healthy, robust subjects, not only are no venesections, baths, or diet drinks prescribed, but not even a dose of laxative medicine, even should there be plenty of time for all this, for in the medical art nothing unnecessary should be done. When circumstances demand it, I prescribe not only every one of them, but I even give previously, or during the course, emetics, when obstinate impurities of the stomach, derangements of the bile, and so forth, present obstacles to the treatment.

633. As mercury does not cure syphilis by causing evacuations (§ 591) (but often thereby makes it more obstinate), but as it rather only cures the disease by the gradual or sudden antipathic irritation of the fibres of a specific nature (I do not deny that there may be a chemical neutralization or destruction of the venereal virus by the mercury dissolved and assimilated in the fluids of the circulation); it follows, that the physician, carefully avoiding all severe mercurial evacuations (salivation, diarrhœa, &c.), should direct his especial attention to develope the above (§ 290) described mercurial fever[1] in the manner indicated, in a degree accurately proportioned to the intensity and age of the lues, and of the idiopathic venereal affection.

634. Thus, when all circumstances are favourable, the most inveterate lues may be radically removed in the course of a few days by a severe mercurial fever, while a slighter degree of recent syphilis, a single chancre, &c., may require a long time for its cure (let alone an old standing case of syphilis) if we do not produce an obvious mercurial fever, but administer the mercury in too weak doses, and do not increase them sufficiently when the symptoms are about to disappear.

635. If during the latter mode of treatment, which is of very doubtful propriety, the system should, from the long-continued mercurial irritation, have become very sensitive and weakly, as often happens if the tonic treatment have not at the same time been employed, it must be resorted to immediately after the termination of the mercurial treatment, or still better, immediately on the appearance of the debility and symptoms of irritability, and be energetically continued until the body can be pronounced sound in every respect.

---

[1] I lay it down as an already proved axiom, that the effect of the mercury on the venereal poison stands in direct relation to the intensity of the mercurial fever, and is diverted by any attack on the mouth, the bowels, and other excreting organs ; but the mercurial fever is so much the greater, the less mercury there has previously been used: and the milder and more soluble the mercurial preparation employed is, the more rapidly it is introduced into the system, and the more completely all evacuations are avoided during its use.

On this account also we must beware of a too sleepy employment of mercury, as it only tends to make the virus more obstinate, and even disposes the system to let it break out still more virulently,[1] when the metal is no longer in the fluids.

FIFTH DIVISION.

LOCAL AFFECTIONS AFTER THE TREATMENT OF SYPHILIS.

CHAPTER I.

LOCAL AFFECTIONS THAT REMAIN AFTER A SUITABLE TREATMENT OF SYPHILIS AND THEIR REMOVAL.

636. There are few local affections dependent for their morbid character on the virus of syphilis that should remain in the body after a rational employment of soluble mercury.[2] I shall only make mention of the warts, the periosteal and osseous swellings, and the caries of the bones.

637. The venereal warts must be uncommonly hard and old if they

---

[1] I gave a peasant, who was affected with some condylomata on the anus, scarcely observable pains in the bones of the shoulder, and small ulcers in the tonsils of the throat, in the course of seven weeks, 12½ grains of soluble mercury, divided into equal small doses. In the first two or three days all the symptoms were alleviated, without his having experienced the slightest mercurial fever: the ulcers had disappeared from the mouth, the pains in the bones were gone, and the condylomata were painless and dry. His amelioration remained in this state until after this small number of powders had been used. He thought he required no further aid, discontinued attendance, and only returned after the lapse of four weeks. His mouth was now covered to the lips with ulcers; an ulcer 2½ inches in length and half as broad, had eaten away the upper surface of the penis, the anus was beset with similar ulcers, humid fissures, and a number of moist condylomata; the pains in the bones were intolerable, and the patient seemed to be weary of life. I now gave him 12 grains of soluble mercury, to take the first day 3, the second 4, and the third 5 grains. He had a very severe fever without salivation, and after five days not a trace of his venereal malady remained. The ulcers were healed, the pains gone, and the warts dried up and gradually fell off. At the present time, after 2½ years, he is as well as ever. From this it appears 1st, that a sleepy employment of mercury rather excites than cures the venereal disease ; 2d, that the point of importance is not the quantity of mercury introduced into the system, but the adequate intensity of the mercurial fever.

[2] We have still greater advantages in the treatment of chancres and buboes ; for if we have once cured them by internal mercurial remedies only, we may be assured of the eradication of the idiopathic virus. But in syphilis, especially when it is of long standing, the local affection is often so masked, so very similar to other diseases, that we cannot be immediately certain of the cure, if we cannot be convinced of the intensity of the previous mercurial fever ; but especially difficult is it to decide, when local affections remain that present the appearance of uncured venereal ones, for then the eradication of the virus becomes a matter of only doubtful probability.

do not wither and fall off, or otherwise disappear, under a mercurial fever of due intensity, or, as more rarely happens, terminate in healthy suppuration.

638. If after complete extinction of the virus there remain some old, horny, large warts, they may be removed by surgical means. They may either be tied with a waxed thread, by drawing which daily tighter and tighter, they will be gradually perfectly dried up and so fall off, or they may be cut off close to the root, and the wound touched once or several times with lunar caustic, and when the last slough falls off the wart is completely removed.

639. But if they are in situations where they do not cause any inconvenience, if they are not very large or elevated, we may in many cases allow them to remain. They are innocuous, and generally disappear gradually of their own accord.

640. It is almost the same with the periosteal and osseous swellings. They usually diminish gradually of themselves after the complete eradication of the lues venerea. The parts exposed to the more remote kinds of local diseases are affected by a perceptible swelling whose removal we should not attempt to obtain by pushing the employment of the mercury too far. Even were the virus not completely eradicated in them, it cannot be again absorbed into the system from them, and so cause fresh symptoms of syphilis; but it will be destroyed, provided the mercurial fever was of sufficient intensity. In the latter case the swelling and induration will usually remain stationary, shewing that the virus has been destroyed; after some time it declines spontaneously if it be not too hard, and if the patient be not too aged.

641. I have already said that such nodes usually pass spontaneously into a mucous suppuration, which on account of the ensuing destruction of the periosteum, becomes dangerous for the bone beneath Under the adequate mercurial fever the unhealthy pus already formed becomes changed, and not unfrequently resolved; a true cure, which at the most only leaves behind it a painless elevation of the node. If the result be so fortunate, it often remains a matter of uncertainty whether an abscess was previously formed, as its existence is so difficult to discover while the lues is still uncured. It is however a matter of great indifference; it suffices if the cure is effected.

642. But if the abscess have gone too far, if the mercurial fever have indeed deprived it of its venereal character, but is unable to effect its resolution, then there is always danger of the bone being corroded after the destruction of the periosteum. We must ascertain the existence of the abscess in order to be able to treat it locally.

643. It is moreover not difficult to discern the presence of this non-venereal abscess (however difficult the discovery of the venereal abscess may be), as its existence cannot be doubted if during the adequate

mercurial fever, or a few days thereafter, a throbbing pain continues or occurs in the centre of the periosteal node ; a sensation that differs widely from the agonizing pains of the still venereal node.

644. We should then make a sufficiently deep and extensive incision, evacuate the pus, clean the ulcer, taking care not to remove any of the sound periosteum, and we should treat the wound like an ordinary ulcer.   When we make this opening we perceive a pus of a mucous character certainly, but mostly well concocted, whereas what existed before the mercurial treatment was merely an albuminous fluid.

645. This it is that after corroding the periosteum causes caries of the bone.   If the mercurial treatment is at an end, and the node, on account of the persistence of the pains, opened and cleaned, we shall soon be able to discover the caries, if it exist.   It is now no longer venereal, if the mercurial fever was of sufficient intensity, and, like all other caries from external causes, it will take on the healing process, and will require to be treated by similar remedies.

646. If the caries be superficial, advantage will be derived from scraping the bone, from the employment of the actual cautery, from sprinkling it with euphorbium powder, from touching it with a solution of nitrate of silver, and so forth.   If it penetrate more deeply, and be already seated in the interior of the hard tubular bone, it is generally accompanied by slow fever, brought on by the acrid ichorous secretion.   We should bore holes in different parts of the bone, and deep enough to allow of the escape of the matter, and then treat the interior with a solution of lunar caustic or nitrate of mercury,[1] &c. Caries of the spongy bones, *e. g.* of the nose, requires a cautious injection of the latter remedies,[2] and the moderate introduction of the vapour of a small portion of cinnabar into the nose.[3]   If all these kinds of caries are mere remains of the cured syphilis, they will be susceptible of cure without much difficulty ; but much more destructive and obstinate, as also more frequent, is the caries produced by the irritation of mercury and from the morbid condition of the fluid and solid parts thence resulting, of which more anon.

647. The swellings of the ligaments, tendons and tendinous aponeu. roses that remain are very obstinate.   If, as is however seldom the case, they have not yielded on the extinction of the venereal virus by mercury, we must combat them by the application of blisters.   If this prove ineffectual, and they still remain painful after the mercurial fever

---

[1] One part of each dissolved in from 300 to 400 parts of water, to which should be added thirty parts of tincture of myrrh or aloes.

[2] Girtanner recommends strongly the repeated injection of a solution of caustic potash, or the same remedy used as a gargle.

[3] Without however drawing in air by the nose, in order to prevent the vapour from getting into the lungs.

(a sign that they have become non-venereal abscesses), they must be opened. They must then be treated with proper vulnerary (one part of corrosive sublimate dissolved in from 400 to 500 parts of water) and balsamic remedies.

CHAPTER II.

LOCAL AFFECTIONS AND SECONDARY SUFFERINGS THAT FOLLOW THE ABUSE OF MERCURY.

648. We might *à priori* suppose that a drug like mercury, which produces such tremendous effects on the body (such as mercurial fever, salivation, &c. are), must by a long-continued and too frequent employment weaken the strength to a great degree, and set the fibres into morbid, irritable vibrations, the source of all sorts of chronic diseases that are difficult to cure, of rheumatic, erisipelatous, and especially of scrofulous (scorbutic) and chlorotic character, of trembling, of low, wasting fevers, of malignant, corroding ulcers of the soft and hard parts of the human body, &c. And this is just what we find from experience, which presents us with thousands of lamentable instances of this sort, produced by the immoderate use of inunctions, mercurial plasters, calomel and the like.

649. Gonorrhœas are transformed into gleets, and those already cured again commence to discharge ; buboes take on an unhealthy suppuration, become deep and excavated, excrete a large quantity of acrid fetid ichor, evert their hard borders, and eat about them in a cancerous manner, accompanied by agonizing pains ; close to the seat of the previously healed chancre numerous ulcers break out ; the constitutional syphilitic ulcers break out again, or become altered in their nature ; they inflame, excrete much matter, get a hard base, a cancerous look, and are painfully sensitive ; condylomata discharge•much ichor, and are corroded into deep, painful fistulous ulcers ; others grow into sensitive, spongy swellings, almost impossible to be got down ; we perceive on different parts the periosteum thickened and painful ; venereal ulcers in the throat that have healed up again break out ; the tonsils swell again and become sore ; the palate also becomes affected by intolerable shooting pains, studded over with small ulcers, and at length perforated ; the uvula sloughs off, a fetid smell proceeds from the nose, which, along with the antrum Highmorianum (in the worst cases) are gradually eaten out ; the body becomes pale and lax, the digestion is deranged, the catamenia disappear, the legs swell sometimes, the patient is excessively sensitive to all impressions, to heat and cold ; there is great weakness and despondency ; his nights, full of pains and restlessness, are martyrdom to him ; the bowels are at one time constipated, at another purged : towards evening he has transient debilitating heats, and his pulse usually ranges from 100 to 130

in the minute; only for a few, often fixed, hours during the day do his agonizing pains lessen somewhat; at other times they prevail constantly, especially during the night. There are stiffness of the joints and chronic trembling. One or both eyes are affected by amaurosis.

650. There are various causes for these ill effects of mercury, which have mostly been already mentioned in the former parts of this book. It has been usual to lay down the following pernicious maxim for the treatment of venereal disease: that as much mercury as possible must be introduced into the system—though modern physicians have wisely added this limitation (which however is unsatisfactory and, on account of the nature of the ordinary mercurial preparations, impracticable)— in as short a time as possible without causing salivation. Had they been aware that success depends upon the adequate intensity of the mercurial fever, and not on the introduction of an enormous quantity of the metal into the system, they had forborne to lay down this pernicious rule. Moreover, as the nature of the ordinary mercurial preparations rendered it impossible to know whether much or little of the active part of the metal got into the circulation in a given time, it could not but happen that sometimes too much was imperceptibly dissolved in the juices, and occasioned horrible devastations. Besides this it has hitherto been the custom to employ the irrational French weakening system, both during and after the treatment, which did all that was possible to assist the irritating and debilitating power of the mercury.

651. But what did more than all the causes I have mentioned to render the ordinary mercurial treatment so injurious, was the unpardonable inattention to the connexion betwixt cause and effect, for the symptoms that arose during the treatment from the mercurial irritation were considered to be genuine venereal symptoms, and were combatted anew with a still longer continuance of the mercury, to the injury of the patient, who thus became the victim of stupidity. Weak, chlorotic, scrofulous, or scorbutic subjects, those, namely, who had become affected with spreading ulcers in the mouth, from the quantity of mercury they had taken, were dosed with still larger quantities of this irritating metal, and caries took possession of the nasal and palatial bones; these were still held to be venereal, the consequence of which was, that the malady increased to the most horrible, often fatal extent. Buboes that had, by a succession of errors, degenerated under the long continued employment of mercury into spreading ulcers, were treated by an increased administration of mercury, and mortification or cancer (or whatever this sloughing diathesis may be called). hectic fever, hemorrhages, diarrhœas, night sweats and death, were the result.

652. And yet what opportunities presented themselves for deducing

this maxim, *that the very first day when the amendment of the venereal symptoms stood still under the judiciously increased administration of the mercury—that the very first hour, when, under the mercurial treatment, new affections, new pains, new abnormalities presented themselves, or the previous genuine venereal symptoms were aggravated—we should pause ; and that state of the body that presented these obstacles to the venereal treatment, be it scrofula, chlorosis, erysipelas, gout, scorbutus, or only weakness and irritability, should be combatted, and the (frequently irritating) mercurial preparation, the usual exciting cause of such morbid diathesis, should be discontinued immediately.* All the pains that remain, increase, or arise during the mercurial treatment, all local affections, further, swellings, ulcers, caries of the bones, &c., that break forth anew, increase or occur for the first time during the use of mercury, are no longer of a purely venereal nature, they are often of a totally non-venereal character, and can never be cured[1] by the further administration of ever so large doses of this metal—but will, on the contrary, be aggravated. If this maxim had been kept in view, there would not assuredly be so many unfortunate beings whose health has been undermined and destroyed by misdirected mercurial treatment.

653. I say, *no longer of a purely venereal nature,* for all those whose sufferings have been aggravated by the continued or renewed mercurial treatment, are not therefore free from all taint of the venereal virus. In deeply rooted syphilis occurring in scrofulous, scorbutic, gouty, erysipelatous, chlorotic, or otherwise weakly irritable individuals, the ordinary inappropriate mercurials may, after a debilitating preparatory treatment, or along with a similar accessory treatment, be given in such a drowsy fashion, that this metal can scarcely do more than exercise its weakening irritation, but not its antisyphilitic power ; and then it will happen that the concomitant morbid diathesis gains so much the upper hand, that when we would endeavour to destroy the venereal virus (which is now almost concealed beneath symptoms foreign to it, so as scarcely to be cognizable) by means of a further or increased employment of mercury, the slow fever, the scrofu. lous ulcers, &c., arising from the concomitant diathesis, increase to such a height that the patient is in danger of losing his life, or a chronic dyscrasia is the result, and still all remains of syphilis may not thereby have been eradicated.

654. The traces of the venereal virus in the system are not at once cognizable amid these exacerbations, and amid these obvious injurious effects of the mercury. It is only when, by an energetic (often tedious and lengthened) treatment of another kind, the patient has *perfectly* recovered from his accessory diseases, and has regained his

---

[1] A cure might occasionally have been effected by a dangerous salivation.

health, then only does the syphilis again rear its head in an unmistakeable manner, the symptoms proper to it still remain, which may not be removed by any remedy in the world, any tonic, anti-scorbutic, anti-scrofulous, and anti-chlorotic drug—but only, and that easily, by the renewed employment of a good mercurial preparation alone. This event alone (we have no other mode of proving it) demonstrates by the result, that during the former unfortunate mercurial treatment the syphylitic virus was still undestroyed.

655. This is the place to dispel the delusion that after such an excessive administration the mercury still remains almost ineradicably in the system, and gives rise to all the horrible devastations, the hectic fever, corroding ulcers, caries of the bones, trembling, wandering pains, &c.

656. The metalic mercury occasionally found in the cavities of the bones proves nothing ; we may carry this about with us without our health being thereby affected. How can an insoluble substance beyond the circulation act upon the latter ? But, it is replied, this fluid metal is a proof of the probable coexistence of a dissolved portion of mercury in our fluids ! As long as we are unable to prove its existence in our fluids more accurately than by supposition in those chronic diseases, so long may we be allowed to ascribe their obstinacy to other causes, which as I have shown in many places, are not far to seek.

657. The fact of gold growing pale and brittle when worn by those who have this metal in their fluids, the destruction of the vermin on their head, but chiefly the non-infecting power of their chancres, &c., gives us distinctly to understand that where these phenomena are wanting, there can be no question of the existence of mercury in the circulation. According to accurate observations we may with certainty assert that the portion of mercury dissolved in the circulation to-day will be no longer present after the lapse of four weeks, but will be indubitably expelled by its own constant irritation through some excretory channel. We may perhaps[1] at first find traces of the metal in the saliva of a person undergoing ptyalism ; but shall we be able to detect any after the lapse of three weeks from the last dose of mercury ?

658. Should it be still time to suspect an excess of this metal in the secundæ viæ, in order to remove the secondary sufferings from a mis-directed mercurial course, sulphuretted hydrogen as a drink (§ 608), or used as a bath in a similar form, may prove of service.

659. The removal of the other symptoms, occasioned or aggravated by the mercurial treatment, is to be conducted on nearly the same

---

[1] Cruikshank's experiments do not allow that any mercury exists either in the saliva or in the urine of a person undergoing salivation.

principles as I have laid down in regard to the preparatory treatment (§ 579 – 586). We may employ in addition, country air, sea voyages, the diligent use of cold bathing, especially in the sea, and in many cases the use of the Pyrmont waters. The sores should be dressed with cleansing and strengthening remedies, especially with a solution of lunar caustic, with the addition of essence of myrrh and tincture of opium, the latter of which, both externally and internally, must be the chief remedy in many of these cases.

660. This same medicament, consisting namely of one part of nitrate of silver dissolved in from 500 to 600 parts of distilled water, to which is added 30 parts of laudanum, and 40 parts of essence of myrrh, will be the very best injection[1] for the caries of the bones, produced or aggravated by the same cause. All that surgery requires to do besides, consists in an appropriate extension of the fistulous orifices that occur, in order to remove the dead pieces of bone conveniently and without employing any force, and in making suitable openings at the most dependent points, in order to allow the matter to escape. A numb sensation of the external integuments of the cheeks, and the severe pain inwardly at that part, enables us to discover a collection of matter shut up in the antrum Highmorianum, which we should endeavour to let out by extracting the third molar tooth of the same side, and boring through the alveolar cavity, and through this hole the injections should be performed.

661. But besides these operations the chief thing we have to attend to in such cases of caries of the bones, which are generally kept up by irritability from weakness, is the general constitutional treatment. If any other accessory diathesis be present at the same time, we should bear it in mind. The remedies serviceable for the latter should therefore be continued with the general tonic treatment, which should be gradually increased to the very utmost extent. Cold steel baths for the whole body, exercise in the open air, bathing the shaven head in ice cold water, general frictions, steel, bark, wine, &c. With these tonics we must combine opium, wherewith we shall best be able to soothe the sleepless painful nights, and we should also give it in combination with tonics as a general rule, in order to moderate the irritability for which it is almost specific in this combination, as Grant has remarked, and I have had opportunities of observing. In this combination I have also employed ammonia with the best effects.

662. Sarsaparilla in strong decoction, taken to the extent of three ounces daily, and large doses of assafœtida or hemlock, are said to be of great use in this caries of the bones.

---

[1] Should the disease, as usually happens, have its primary seat in the back of the palate, the nitrate of silver mixed with 3000 parts of water, and used as a gargle (also combined with laudanum), will prove the best remedy.

APPENDIX.

VENEREAL AFFECTIONS OF NEW-BORN INFANTS.

663. The venereal affections of new-born infants have very rarely been an object of investigation on the part of medical men, partly because they have seldom come under their cognizance, partly because these poor creatures often survive their birth but a few months, partly because their disease has often been mistaken. Doublet[1] has given us the best information on this subject; I shall follow him in many of the subsequent remarks.

664. Most authors hold them to' be an infection in the mother's womb; others, but few,[2] consider the venereal affections of infants to be local inoculation,[3] and degenerations and extensions of the disease. I must confess that I incline to the latter opinion, for several reasons.

665. That the cure of the pregnant mother of the venereal disease is followed by the birth of healthy children proves nothing, as no one can be cured of syphilis without at the same time losing the local and idiopathic venereal affections. On the other hand, syphilis may seem to be born with the children, because in them all symptoms follow each other more rapidly, and local affections pass so rapidly into general maladies; their bodies are more tender and irritable, their skin is much more delicate, and the circulation twice as rapid as that in adults. But has any one ever observed in infants immediately after their births, the copper-coloured spots or the ulcers of the tonsils, or genuine open syphilitic ulcers on the surface of the body, or even the venereal itch? That these are found after several weeks or months proves nothing. On the other hand, we find those parts of the bodies of new-born infants affected with the venereal inoculation, which, either on account of their being destitute of epidermis, are capable of being inoculated in adults also, or are most pressed upon or rubbed in their passage through the female parts. Their epidermis is still so delicate (so much the more so, as these children on account of the mother's indisposition can seldom be carried to the full term, or are otherwise weakly and delicate), that on those parts the poison can penetrate through the

---

[1] And now Girtanner.

[2] Among these, more especially Girtanner.

[3] The inoculation of healthy nurses by venereal infants is no rare occurrence. How could the latter however communicate chancres to the nipples when sucking, if they had not themselves chancres seated on the outer or inner surface of the lips, that is to say, idiopathic venereal ulcers, which constitutional syphilis can never produce?

epidermis, which, from an opposite reason, cannot occur in adults. But I shall admit all these affections to be of a general syphilitic character, whenever any one shall shew me such a child was born of a mother that had been infected with syphilis, but who was completely free from all local idiopathic venereal affections on and in the genitals, from gonorrhœa, chancres, and condylomata.

666. We find, 1st, the following affections on parts where adults also may be inoculated without any previous injury. The eyelids, especially the upper ones, are swollen ; the eyes are at first affected by dry inflammation, subsequently they usually discharge an acrid, purulent whitish-green, often copious matter (blennorrhœa of the eye from local inoculation) ; during sleep the lids stick together. (This is one of the chief diagnostic marks of this sad disease in children.) Spots on the cornea, hypopyon, blindness, are not very frequent effects of it. The ears also are apt to discharge similar matter.

667. The corners of the mouth, the frenulum of the tongue, the anterior part of the gums, are studded over with small ulcers, which are very hard at their bottom and all around them—true chancres. Buboes in the parotid gland, at the angle of the lower jaw, &c., ensue.

668. The nostrils discharge a purulent matter (nasal blennorrhœa) they are also stopped up with masses of hardened pus.

669. Inflammation of the genitals, chancres in the glans and labia; strangury, swelling of the scrotum and of the external labia, and fissures and pustules at the anus, are common symptoms. Gonorrhœa, however, is not found in male children ; but from the female genitals there exudes a yellowish matter, that may easily be distinguished from the discharge of a natural fluid, to which all new-born female infants are subject.

670. The affections of new-born infants, 2dly, on parts where adults are not infected without being wounded, are most frequently regarded as signs of syphilis communicated to them in the womb, although they are manifestly quite the reverse ; they are inflammations of the skin on parts of the body where the skin alone is stretched over projecting bones, which have been during delivery particularly rubbed against the genital parts of mothers that are covered with the chancrous discharge, and thus have been inoculated (*per diapedesin*) through the thin epidermis. They are of the following kinds :

671. The region of the coronal suture, the protuberance of the parietal and occipital bones, the shoulders, the region of the sacrum and hip bone, the ankles and the heels, are externally reddened and inflamed The epidermis soon falls off, the sore places extend and become covered with a white crust, beneath which an acrid fetid ichor exudes.[1]

---

[1] Or these parts rise up in inflamed, brown, soft swellings, which usually p??? dangerous suppuration.

When these parts become black, mortification is nigh, the sign of approaching death.

672. A similar inflammaiion of the skin and ulceration attacks from the same cause the neighbourhood of the navel, in consequence of this part being very much strained during the process of delivery; and moreover the natural inflammation that takes place in infants before the navel string falls off may favour the action of the virus on that part.

673. The affections that constitute the transition of the idiopathic virus into the general circulation in adults are also not unfrequently met with in infants some time after birth, I mean the glandular swellings. These buboes occur in them in the cervical glands, in the parotid gland, and in the auxiliary glands, either from the chancres on the lips or from similar ulcers (§ 671) on the head and shoulders— in the groins from chancres on the genitals or from similar sores on the sacrum and hip bones, the ankles, &c.—or also, in any of these situations, from the direct penetration of the chancre poison through the external integuments, without any previous chancres; and this occurs much more frequently in these delicate creatures than in adults. These glandular swellings, like those in adults, usually terminate in suppuration if the virus be not destroyed by mercury. The suppuration of the parotid gland has a great tendency to involve the bony structure of the mastoid process.

674. The symptoms of general lues *always* occur only after several weeks,[1] sometimes (according to some authors) not before eight months after birth. The skin becomes covered with bluish spots, which, as in adults, become in course of time somewhat elevated, and gradually are covered with a greyish dry crust. Or there are at first merely excoriations. Subsequently there are formed at these parts venereal ulcers, which arise most rapidly in the axilla, betwixt the thighs and betwixt the nates, and have a white, suety-looking appearance. The whole skin is also sometimes covered with bran-like points. General venereal ulcers also appear in the mouth and on the tonsils. Single elevated pustules are formed on the dorsum of the fingers and toes, which rapidly pass into ulcers and cause the nails to fall off by the roots. Running chaps appear at the anus. Swellings of the bones, however, and gonorrhœa in the male, are not met with in infants.

675. Such children are usually very weak and emaciated; their skin, especially that of the face, is of a bluish colour, shrivelled and full of wrinkles, like an old person's.

676. The usual mode of treating the venereal diseases of new-born infants at Vaugirard consists in treating the mothers before they are

---

[1] Girtanner says, in from ten to fourteen days.

born or while they are at the breast.   None of the metal is given to the infant directly.[1]

677. If the mother be subjected to treatment before her confinement, she is treated with diluent drinks, bitters, mild purgatives, baths and mercurials, so as to alleviate her disease and to facilitate her delivery; but after delivery, from the twelfth day onwards, she is made to rub in every other day from one to two drachms of mercury at a time, so as that she shall use from three to four ounces in the course of five, twelve, or even twenty weeks.   During this course she suckles the infected infant, or even a couple of them, in order to impregnate them with the antisyphilitic specific along with the milk.

678. It is observed that children whose mothers have been treated with mercury before their confinement suffer little inconvenience from the mercurialized milk (they are already used to the metallic impression); those, however, who have experienced none of the influence of the mercury on their fluids before their birth, on using this milk become pale and get belly-ache, heat and loss of appetite, especially if they are kept not warm enough or too warm.   In this case the frictions are discontinued, and soothing medicines, mucilaginous drinks and clysters are employed.

679. Very soon the putrid hospital apthæ attack and carry off a large number of these children.

680. In course of time, about the sixth week, slow fever, diarrhœa, &c., usually set in, whereby many are destroyed.

681. The rest gradually escape the danger; the venereal symptoms disappear, and there only remains a greater or less liability to the common diseases of children.

682. From all this we learn nothing more than that the venereal affections of new-born infants are curable, for as regards the mode of treatment, it is burdened with such a vast number of evils that it cannot be recommended for imitation.   Let us for a moment consider how much injury the health of the pregnant woman must at first suffer from the five to twenty weeks of mercurial irritation, and how aimless such a treatment is, as not only are they not cured by it, but it is not intended for their cure!   If the mother have syphilis in a great degree, this treatment, continued for a considerable time, affords no relief either to the mother or to the infant; the latter usually dies. Rendered liable to various diseases from the treatment during pregnancy, or from ordinary ailments, or from other circumstances, the mother is often not in a position to suckle her child, and then the wet-nurse who takes it gets venereal fissures and ulcers on the nipples

---

[1] Now, according to Girtanner, they are subjected to the fumigation treatment—or they get eighty drops of Swieten's solution of corrosive sub'imate every night both of these are either useless or hurtful procedures.

from the chancrous mouth of the child, whereupon inflammation of the mamma, stoppage and drying up of the milk, usually ensue. The chancres on the lips and frenulum linguæ of the infant impede or prevent its sucking. But besides this, how tedious is this treatment, how often does not the death of the little sufferer anticipate its termination, or if that does not happen, how many are carried off by the hospital air, how many (if some few do go through all this), how many, I repeat, of these few, by the instrumentality of this long-continued mercurial irritation that makes their fluids acrid, their fibres weak and irritable, are rendered liable both to dangerous maladies and to chronic dyscrasias, to which death itself is often preferable! Of the injury that accrues to the mothers and nurses from such a treatment I shall say nothing further, as I have already spoken of the disadvantages attending the inunction treatment.

683. From an institution so conducted I can imagine no real advantages to society which could outweigh all the sacrifices connected with it; but this we see, that the French nation [1] probably surpasses all other civilized [2] people in delicacy of sensibility for suffering mankind.

684. I shall not stop to consider the other mode commonly practised of curing children of the venereal disease, as they usually only come under treatment when they are a year and a half old or still older, and are treated with sollution of corrosive sublimate, as in adults, only with smaller doses. A tenth, an eighth, a quarter, and at length as much as half a grain is given them daily in different kinds of mild fluids, frequently with greater success than in adults. But how many of them die before they attain this age, before they are brought under the action of this remedy, be it ever so efficaciously administered! Besides, my business at present is with new-born infants.

685. The medical police could arrive at a much shorter way for attaining this object [3] of preserving these young citizens of the state, if they kept in view the maxim that I have been induced from a multitude of observations and reasons to propound as an axiom; if they were convinced that syphilitic children have only become so by their

---

[1] The only hospital for syphilitic children that I know of is the *Hospice de Charité* of Vaugirard, which requires enormous sums of money for its maintenance.

[2] Germans.

[3] Girtanner says, "a venereal mother is generally (on account of the bad state of her lymph, whereby she is unable to nourish the foetus) confined in the sixth or seventh month, without any other exciting cause, and the child is usually dead: or the movements of the foetus cease in the sixth or seventh month, and at the end of the pregnancy the child is born dead and half decayed. If it is alive it has a very thin and emaciated appearance, and soon dies." What a loss for posterity! How necessary is the cure of the syphilitic mother in her pregnancy, to prevent the state experiencing a great loss!

local infection in the genitals of their mothers during parturition,[1] and that pregnant women are not more difficult to cure of their venereal affections, without injury or premature labour, than other weak persons are to be freed from this disgraceful malady.

686. If the first point is conceded to me, all the greater objections are made to the last. Let it be remembered however that to dread ill effects from a radical mercurial treatment for pregnant women and their offspring, and on that account to leave both uncured till after birth,[2] implies that the treatment is more dangerous than the disease itself. If the inunctions, calomel, &c. are of this character, I am sorry for it. As far as I am aware the cautious administration of soluble mercury indicated in this book is not so; I am indebted to it for the lives and health of many mothers and their offspring. I must refer to what I have already said as regards its employment in this case. A physician who is such in the true sense of the word, will understand how to supply what is necessary for the accessory circumstances.

687. If however we are called on to treat a new-born infant affected with venereal symptoms, there is very little hope for it if the symptoms are in their highest degree, if the child is much emaciated and cannot take the breast, or if its mother cannot suckle it. But even in such circumstances we ought not to despair.

688. In the last case we shall not be able to do much without a wet nurse, as the poor creature will hardly be able to contend with the process of accustoming it to unnatural food and the attacks of such a dangerous malady, without succumbing. We may however attempt to nourish it (and this we must at all events do if it be unable to suck) with goat's milk for drink, and in the commencement without any other food, until the case takes a favourable turn (and then it will be able to partake of pounded biscuit, &c.), and on the very first day we are called in, after purging the primæ viæ of their impurities, commence with the soluble mercury,[3] which is the only preparation that from its mildness, certainty and rapidity of action, holds out to us any hope, where no other remedy is admissible.

689. In most cases not more than one grain of soluble mercury will

---

[1] In public lying-in institutions no woman affected with syphilis should be allowed to be confined without being cured of all her venereal symptoms. If little can be done, we should at least treat and cure their genitals by the local application of a strong solution of lead, in order to prevent the child being infected during delivery. The syphilitic virus can afterwards be eradicated by an appropriate mercurial treatment after parturition. But the latter may also be done during pregnancy, and that is the preferable course to pursue.

[2] Who can reckon the number of abortions that occur in those unfortunate beings who are with methodical over-cautiousness designedly left uncured of their syphilitic complaints until after delivery.

[3] Girtanner also considers it best to give the child mercury.

be required. We may rub it up with a drachm of liquorice root powder, and of this mixture give the first day (for we should give but one dose daily) five grains, the second seven grains, and so on, until we observe a marked alteration in the complexion, restlessness, rumbling in the bowels, fetor of the breath, heat in the eyes, &c., the signs of the mercurial fever. If the signs are but of moderate intensity, and the change in the venereal symptoms not striking, we may repeat the last dose; otherwise not, for if the mercurial fever was sufficiently strong it would fully perform its service, and remove the venereal affection. The infant may take the medicine in its goat's milk, and not partake of anything else until the cure is effected.

690. If the child can, immediately after birth, take its infected mother's breast, we should only treat the latter with soluble mercury, in the doses above indicated for adults; but we should commence immediately after being called in and attend to the accessory treatment and precautions[1] required in such cases. The child will recover by partaking of her milk, if any adequate mercurial fever is developed in her.

691. Similar doses of the antisyphilitic metal and similar precautions must be employed in the case of the nurse (even though she be perfectly well) who suckles the child in place of its mother, partly in order that she may not be infected herself, partly in order that the child may be restored to health by partaking of her medicated milk, which will be the case if she get a sufficiently intense mercurial fever.

692. If the child cannot or will not take the breast, or if there be none to give it, we must endeavour, after its recovery, to send it into the country and allow it to be reared by some experienced person.

693. During the treatment the child must be bathed and gently washed twice a day in a tepid decoction of marsh-mallow root, for a few minutes. The sores and excoriations should be dusted with lycopodium powder, or dressed with lint. Its linen should be changed twice a day until it is quite recovered; it should be carried about, and the air in the apartment should be renewed as often as possible. If there be constipation, soap and water injections should be used; the aphthæ may be cured by frequently touching them with water acidulated with from $\frac{1}{100}$th to $\frac{1}{50}$th part sulphuric acid.

---

[1] If the circumstances are not urgent we may delay the treatment until the twelfth day after confinement.

POSTCRIPT.

(Whilst these sheets were going through the press I have been enabled to make the following additions and corrections.)

As regards the preparation of the soluble mercury (see Preface), I have found that in order to deprive the nitrate of mercury of all traces of muriate of mercury, there ought to be no free acid at all in the metallic salt before the precipitation is performed. Accordingly I find it requisite to wash the crystallized mercurial salt with about a tenth of its weight of distilled water, and then dry it on bibulous paper before proceeding to dissolve and precipitate. I have further observed that ammonia carefully prepared contains but an inconsiderable quantity of muriatic acid, and may consequently be appropriately used instead of the egg shell lime to precipitate the (in this case white) soluble mercury. But as no acid is more frequently met with in nature than this muriatic acid which is so prejudicial to our object, and as it may, in spite of the greatest carefulness on the part of the operator, exist in a small proportion in our preparation, we would do well to change by a simple operation the white precipitate that may be present into the much more innocuous calomel. For this end we boil the crude precipitate, in place of sweetening it, in fifty times its weight of distilled water for an hour, then pour off the water and dry the sediment on bibulous paper for use.

If it be objected to (§ 619) that muriates exist even in the cleanest stomach, which, let the oxyde of mercury thus prepared be ever so free from white precipate, would soon decompose it, and change it in the alimentary canal into something similar, my observations teach me, that the ingestion of white precipitate already prepared, in consequence of its forming small, insoluble, corrosive masses, causes much more poisonous effects than that which is only changed in the stomach, by decomposition, into amazingly fine heavy particles of white precipitate, which only cause a slight griping, and enveloped in the mucus of the bowels are soon expelled. But even this need not be dreaded, if in place of any other fluid, a couple of glasses of Selters or Pülna water be drunk, for as I have found by numerous experiments, the carbonic acid redissolves the white precipitate that has already been formed, and even the turbith mineral, and retains it in solution until this gas is driven off by a considerable amount of heat, so that the metal (in that case it must have been prepared with lime-water, or with caustic potash) cannot be precipitated from the fluid. If this precaution be adopted in taking the medicine, even the inconsiderable griping that occurs from the oxyde of mercury may be prevented, if that be deemed necessary.

Among the most powerful antidotes to the ulcers that degenerate into corroding sores (§ 331, 381, 403, 648, 649,) or are caused by the abuse of mercury, I must, from my experience since the foregoing was written, place the sulphuretted hydrogen gas, spoken of at § 608, as it is preferable to all other remedies for removing all affections arising from the long continued irritation of mercury, the pains in the limbs, the low fever and night sweats, and the exhausting salivation.

A young man was, on account of a gonorrhœa and small chancre, so mistreated by a barber-surgeon with enormous quantities of calomel for six weeks, that besides having an immoderate salivation, he got also severe hectic fever, profuse night sweats, tearing pains in the limbs, trembling, and large pustules all over the body, which, being aggravated, (and these aggravations the quack considered to be venereal symptoms) by additional quantities of mercury, degenerated into large deep ulcers (some were an inch and a half in diameter,) surrounded by inflamed elevated borders, and covered with a suety looking substance. The worst symptoms were the ulcerations in the throat, at the posterior nares, in the tonsils, on the palate and uvula; in this situation one large ulcer seemed to be eating away all the parts; from the mouth and nose bloody pus flowed; he could not utter any intelligible sounds; he was emaciated and excessively feeble. All the remedies used were of no avail until I gave him ten grains of hepar sulphuris[1] within twenty-four hours, which produced a rapid amelioration of all the symptoms, so that the other remedies required, the sulphuric acid for the low suppurative fever, and a solution of lunar caustic for the foul ulcers in the mouth were speedily beneficial. He was soon so well as to be able to enjoy the open air, and whilst he was out his room was thoroughly aired. This course was attended by increasing benefit for some weeks, and he had almost completely recovered when he one day by staying out too long in severe weather, took cold, and was confined to the house in a febrile state. The precaution of opening the window was omitted, without my being aware of it. His former symptoms now rapidly returned, the ulcers in the throat and on the other parts of the body broke out with increased violence, and even the glans penis was rapidly perforated by deep, rapidly spreading ulcers here and there, but not on the seat of the former chancre. The fever with the night sweats, the pains in the limbs and the salivation returned, and increased daily in violence. I made use of every thing that had previously proved serviceable, but

---

[1] I had also to give the healthy person who slept in the same room the same remedy for salivation and night sweats, that had arisen spontaneously, so saturated was the air of the room with mercurial exhalations.

without success; in the course of a few days he was brought to the verge of the grave. He would take nothing more, had frequent hiccough, recognized his friends no longer, and could not move himself. I now began to suspect that the confined atmosphere of the room might perhaps be loaded with mercurial vapour, which had again penetrated his system, and thus caused a recurrence of these sufferings. I ventured to give the half-dead patient three grains of hepar sulphuris every hour, with such good results, that in the course of twelve hours I observed some traces of amendment, and by continuing this and the former remedies, I gradually restored him to life and health, and I did not neglect to place a solution of hepar sulphuris for some weeks in his room, in order completely to mineralize and to destroy the mercurial vapour in the room, by the evaporation of the sulphuretted hydrogen. I leave every thinking man to draw his own inferences from this striking case.

END OF THE VENEREAL DISEASES.

THE FRIEND OF HEALTH.

BY

SAMUEL HAHNEMANN,

Doctor of Medicine, Member of the Academy of Sciences of Mentz.
and of the Economical Society of Leipzig.

———— •◦•◦•◦◦ ◦◦•◦•◦•◦ ————

PART I.[1]

PREFACE.

WHEN we behold the large family of mankind acting as they
do, when we see with what perseverance they go through their
more or less important spheres of action, which some wretched
passion often traces out for them, when we see how they all
strive after the attainment of some kind of happiness, be it ease,
rank, money, learning, amusement or excitement, scarcely
deigning to cast a single glance towards the real blessings of this
world, wisdom and health, which beckon them back into Eden,
we can scarcely refrain from pitying a race of such noble origin
and high destiny. My mission permits me not to point out the
means of ennobling the mind ; it behoves me only to preach upon
the greatest of corporeal blessings, health, which scarcely any
take the trouble to seek after, and few know how to value until
it is lost. It will scarcely be credited when I assert that nought
is shunned more earnestly, nay is held to be more disgraceful,
than rational care about the health. We indeed hear it occasionally remarked that this or the other article of diet is wholesome
or hurtful, that this or that remedy is a specific for this or that
disease, this or the other habit is injurious ; in the higher and
lower circles of society, people interest themselves with fashionable modes of treatment, marvellous diseases, cases of sudden
death, beautifying remedies, and anecdotes about physicians.
But all this is only vain trifling.

---

[1] Published at Frankfort on the Main, in 1792.

The lover of highly spiced dishes exclaims against the indigestible nature of puddings; the tea-drinker can speak like a book about the evils of spirit-drinking; the lady who has a weakness for coffee talks learnedly on the coarse juices of her who has a liking for beer; and the guzzler of puddings declaims upon the poisonous nature of mushrooms.

Hearken to that gouty fellow how well he can describe the hurtful character of the day-labourer's life; to that young gentleman with his pimpled face, how he depicts the disadvantages of a sedentary life; hear how that lady who sticks close to her tapestry work inveighs against the dangers of dancing; and how the dancing nymph points out that much sewing causes green-sickness. All know something, only not what is wholesome for *themselves*.

To take *ourselves* to task about our pernicious habits, to study our own system, to follow the regimen most appropriate for our own constitution, and heroically to deny ourselves everything that has a tendency to undermine our own health, or that may already have done so, to bestow a thought upon all this, is held to be puerile, old-fashioned, and vulgar. The courtier rebels at the idea of attending to the advice of his physician on dietetic points; the young lady who excels in dancing would think it beneath her to listen to the warning voice of her mother; the romance-reading damsel scorns to be corrected by the sarcasms of her old-fashioned uncle; and the wild student will not be persuaded by his banker to frequent better company.

I readily grant that excessive concern about one's health is an evil; that there is no occasion for an active lad to trouble himself about fur-boots, for a rosy-cheeked lass to interest herself in the various kinds of obstetric forceps, or for the pleasure-seeker to concern himself about hospitals; but everything has its proper bounds; every human being his particular sphere, which he ought to be thoroughly conversant with, and which he should blush to be unacquainted with.

If the minister of state were to possess no thorough knowledge of medical police, the chief municipal magistrate no accurate notion respecting the arrangement of prisons, workhouses and hospitals, if the general officer were to know his hospitals only by plan, if the student who has completed his studies were to bring away with him from the university no knowledge of physiology or anatomy, if the laughing girl were to enter into the married state without ever having heard of a mother's duties, if the governess can do nothing but descant on silly gentilities to her chlorotic pupils, and if the pedantic usher, enveloped in a mist of phrases, elegances and verbiage, were unable to perceive how numbers of hopeful boys entrusted to his care fall victims to the most enervating vices, how unfit for their respective spheres these persons would be. Indeed I should like to know if there is any condition in life, where some medical knowledge and some care for our own and our neighbour's health are not necessary, or if it is ridiculous or degrading, beyond the mere rude routine of our actual business, to devote some time to the finer but often not less important study of the structure and modes of preservation of the human body.

Of course I do not mean to say that the works of Frank, or Howard, or Fritz, or Haller, or Levret, or Whytt, are for such persons as these, and I should commit a most egregious blunder were I to recommend a total reformation in the plan of education to those who have made it their special study. But, jesting apart, for all these there are studies of general utility, springs to which all may resort with profit, for they flow only to supply the wants of all the conditions of life.

Oh! that in the following pages I were so fortunate as to be able to contribute something to the happiness of mankind, if they would listen to the voice of a warm friend of his fellow creatures, as if it were the voice of a friend! In a few years, nay days, and we have reached the termination of our earthly life ; would that I could now and then prolong it were it but for a few hours, would that I could improve it were it only in trivial things!

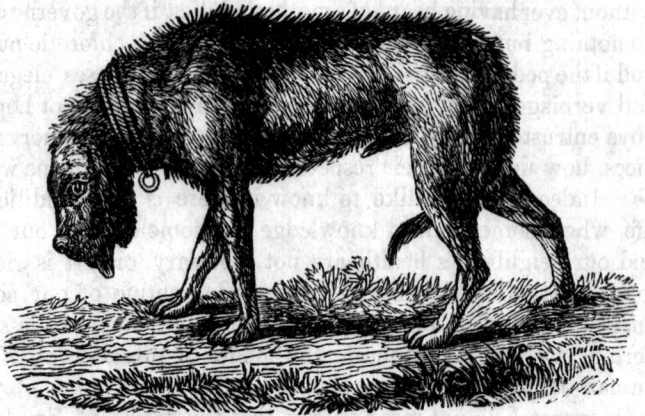

CANINE RABIES.

THE BITE OF MAD DOGS.

THE disease that results from the bite of rabid animals, most frequently of mad dogs, is of such an extraordinary and terrible character, that we are struck with horror on beholding a patient affected by it, and the mere description of his sufferings causes us to shudder. Among a thousand persons affected by real hydrophobia, often not one is saved. The most vigorous constitution, the best physician, the most recondite remedies, and the most implicit obedience of the patient and his friends, are in most cases all of no avail; in the possession of perfect conscious-ness the unfortunate being is usually, amid the most fearful symptoms, hurried off in a few days to an untimely end.

The patient feels an accession of pain in the bitten part, which may either be perfectly healed or still an open wound, it becomes surrounded by a blue border; a creeping sensation proceeds from it up to the throat, which feels as if contracted. The patient has pain in the head and stomach, and sometimes bilious vomiting. His sleep is disturbed by frightful dreams, he becomes restless, the hands, feet and tip of the nose grow cold, the features distorted. He thinks he sees fiery sparks dancing before his eyes. He feels neither hunger nor usually thirst, the tongue is moist but covered with viscid mucus, stools and urine suppressed, or he passes them of natural colour, but with pain. The pulse is weak and jerking, but not inflammatory. He cannot bear the approach of any liquid without trembling all over, with wild, anxious, sad expression. In like manner he cannot bear anything glittering, bright or white, anything approached suddenly towards him, loud talking, a draught of air, &c. In the lucid intervals he speaks rationally, but in a more timid rapid and nervous manner than usual; a hacking cough, sometimes combined with hiccough, interrupts his speech. His face becomes always paler and more distorted, the anxiety that dominates over all his actions is expressed also by the cold clammy sweat on his face and hands, his eyes are tearful and the pupils dilated. He tosses convulsively about in his bed. He seeks to run away. At length he hides his face, becomes quieter and expires.

The *post mortem* examination exhibits usually nothing abnormal.[1] The extreme tension and excessive irritability of the nervous system and the sense of self-preservation shewn in the anxious dread of approaching dissolution, these are the sole characteristics of this fearful disease.

I shall not here enter into a description of the countless remedies that have been proposed for it; their enormous quantity is of itself to a certain extent a proof that no sure mode of cure is yet known, otherwise that would be adhered to. I shall merely endeavour to remove some erroneous notions prevalent on the subject, and thus if possible endeavour to render this disease of less frequent occurrence.

The *first* and most prejudicial of these is the great confidence reposed in certain remedies said to be infallible, among which I allude chiefly to internal remedies. Some persons are bitten by a dog supposed to be mad. They use with all speed the renowned specific, and none of them takes the hydrophobia; all recover from their wounds without any serious consequences following; and in all the country round nothing is talked of but the wondrous curative virtues of, it may be, the may-worm electuary,[2] or whatever else these patients used. It follows, of course, that in similar cases occurring in this district nothing

---

[1] [In two instances, a medical friend of ours has made very thorough and careful dissections of dogs which had died of hydrophobia, but in neither case could any morbid changes be discovered which would in any way account for death. In one of these examples, portions of the brain, spinal-cord and nervous apparatus, were submitted to microscopic examinations, but without throwing any new light upon the subject.]—*Am. P.*

[2] [A nostrum for the hydrophobia purchased at an extravagant price by the Prussian Government.]

more will be done than to give the bitten individuals the may-worm electuary. One of these, however, dies of hydrophobia, but the vaunters of the nostrum can furnish reasons for its inutility in this case, at all events this single unfortunate case is regarded as the exception, against the many successful ones. Should it happen a third time that some one or other in the neighbourhood is inoculated with the poison of a mad dog, so that in the course of nature he must be affected by the hydrophobia, the electuary is at once confidently administered to the unfortunate individual, and it is only by the sad termination of this case that the remedy falls into disrepute.

Had the first cases of reported success been more carefully investigated, it would have been found that these first patients had received no true virus of rabies into their wounds, and that consequently the electuary had no difficulty in curing, as there was nothing to cure. The subsequent unfortunate cases might then have been prevented, had not such implicit confidence been placed in this internal remedy, but the far more trustworthy external preventive remedies been employed.

But what are the best external preventive remedies, and how can we confidently pronounce on the madness of an animal? These questions shall be answered farther on.

Thus much is certain, that the commencement of the malady is at first merely local. The poisonous saliva of the animal lies at first inactive in the bitten wound. The wound heals, and not the slightest inconvenience is experienced, until, after a longer or shorter period, symptoms of irritation of the nervous system, and along with them the fatal hydrophobia make their appearance. Could we at first extract the poisonous saliva from the wound as completely as we can a splinter or a bullet, it would be impossible that rabies could result from such a bite. But if it be already present we know *no* remedy whereby it may be certainly cured. Hence all trusting to such specifics is unsafe and injurious if we have not already frequently tested their efficacy on fully developed hydrophobia.

The second error which may prove injurious, is the belief, that a dog has communicated the poison by its bite if he die within a few days of rabies, and has not communicated it if he continue alive; consequently that a dog that soon dies with the symptoms of this disease, which fear magnifies excessively, was mad, but that one that recovers could not have been mad. In the former case (and who can deny it, as we know as yet so little of the maladies of the domestic animals) it might have been quite a different disease that the dog had which inflicted the bites, and the remedies employed for these bites thus falsely acquire a reputation as specifics for hydrophobia. In the latter case in spite of all the danger, none is apprehended; the only useful remedies for the parts infected by the virus are neglected, and the fatal disease is in all certainty allowed to break out.

We find in the records of medicine many instances [1] in which the severe bite of a dog that afterwards died with all the signs of rabies, infected some persons but not others, without the latter employing anything, and on the other hand there are undeniable instances shewing that dogs of whose bite persons have died of hydrophobia have remained alive.

To refer to but one case of the latter sort, I may mention that Martin Lister, in the 13th vol. of the *Philosophical Transactions*, relates the case of a robust young man, who, six weeks after being bitten, became affected by hydrophobia, of which he died fourteen days thereafter. At the same time, the same dog bit a little dog, which died the day following of rabies; but the large dog itself recovered, and was quite well eight weeks after it had been mad.

A similar instance of a rabid dog which recovered, some children, at the risk of their lives, diligently washing its wounds, is to be found in the 20th volume of this instructive collection, where we also meet with the cases of two young men, related by Dr. Kennedy, *who recovered from the hydrophobia without employing any means.* Had any of the renowned specifics been used in these cases, would not the cure have been infallibly ascribed to it? Can a medicine be extolled as infallible for this disease, or even as very useful, that has not cured at least ten cases of developed hydrophobia?—Where is there such a medicine? [2]

The third error is the delusion entertained even by physicians, that the virus of mad dogs can only cause infection when

---

[1] Vaughan saw from twenty to thirty persons bitten by a mad dog, of whom only one among them, a boy, died of hydrophobia, the rest escaping unaffected.

[2] Unless it be perhaps the root of belladonna. Might not a very strong extract of black henbane, prepared *without heat*, administered in sufficient quantity in the form of pills, be able to cure this disease? A number of *theoretic* reasons lead us to have strong hopes that it might. But the extract must be so strong that two grains of it are sufficient to cause in a healthy individual, troublesome symptoms, stupefaction, &c.

11

introduced into the wound caused by a bite, or some other open wound.

As a proof of the incorrectness of this, cases are not rare where mad dogs have merely licked the external skin, and yet have communicated the disease. Two boys, as we learn from De la Prime, in the 20th vol. of the *Philosophical Transactions*, frequently cleaned with their hands the wounds of a dog that had been bitten by a mad dog; many months afterwards *without ever having been wounded*, they both were attacked simultaneously by hydrophobia, which lasted a week, when the eldest recovered, and said timidly to his father, "I am well." The same happened to the other. They remained well three or four days, then again had violent attacks of hydrophobia for a week, and thereafter recovered without relapsing.[1] Likewise in the 23d vol., we find the history of two servants, who frequently inserted their fingers into the throat of a dog (that had been bitten by another rabid dog, and did not die for three weeks afterwards), in order to feel if there was anything the matter with it. Both were affected by hydrophobia without having been wounded; the stronger of the two recovered without using any medicine, but the younger died of hydrophobia on the third day.

I myself knew a boy whose face was licked by a dog that was going mad, and who died of hydrophobia.[2]

---

[1] [These are probably cases of *sympathetic hydrophobia*. The painful mental impression which continued to prey upon their imaginations for so long a period, finally induced pschychological phenomena, viz., symptoms of the very malady which they had so much dreaded. An instance of this kind occurred in our own knowledge, several years since, in the person of a nervous girl of 16 years. She had been bitten about a year previously by a dog, which was at the time supposed to be rabid, and which was immediately killed. The idea that she should have the hydrophobia continued to torment her, and to wear upon her health and spirits, until, finally, all the symptoms of hydrophobia made their appearance. These symptoms continued at intervals for two days, when the dread of water, the convulsive motions, the anxious and wild expression, &c., disappeared, leaving only a general soreness throughout the body, and a sense of debility.

We fully believe that there is such a disease as genuine hydrophobia, from the absorption into the system of the virus of rabid dogs; yet, it is quite probable that cases not unfrequently occur, and terminate fatally, in which there has been *no absorption of the virus*, but simply a painful and intense action upon the imagination, thus inducing pschychological phenomena, somewhat analogous to those produced by the mesmeric processes. It would not be difficult for a mesmerizer, or a pschychologist, to induce in his subject a temporary condition closely similating hydrophobia.] —*Am. P.*

[2] Cœlius Aurelianus, Palmarius, Van Hilden, Callisen, Odhelius, Gruner, and Morando have recorded similar cases.

It is in general the safest plan to consider the bite of an un-irritated dog as that of a mad dog, and to treat it accordingly. This is the surest way to guard against hydrophobia.

The wound should be immediately washed out with water in which a quantity of potash has been mixed, and this should be repeated frequently, and until the surgeon arrives, who should bring with him a piece of caustic potash, and touch the open wound therewith until a slough the thickness of the back of a knife is formed, whilst the moisture that exudes should be removed by blotting-paper. The pain is not very severe, the slough falls off in a few days and the clean wound soon heals. If this is done first of all and very quickly, we may feel quite at ease, and do all in our power to comfort and console the pa-tient,[1] and tranquilize his circulation. A moderate blood-let-ting in plethoric individuals, or a glass of wine given to per-sons of an opposite constitution, will suffice for this purpose. If this frightful disease can by any means be prevented, it is by such means; but *not by any internal medicine* hitherto known.

The part of the skin which, although not broken, may have been wetted by the saliva of a dog which has become suspicious from having bitten others, must be diligently rubbed with potash, and washed continually for an hour with the solution of the alkali. If a blister be afterwards applied to the spot, then all danger will be more than warded of.

No dog should be trusted that bites people unirritated, and has a gloomy wild expression. It is far better to kill too many of these often useless beasts, than to allow one actually rabid to roam at large; man's life is too precious, and should be held paramount to every other consideration. Merely to shut up for a few days dogs bitten by a mad one, is always dangerous, as examples are not wanting where they only became mad several weeks after being bitten. They must either be killed, or be kept in safe custody for at least four weeks, before they are trusted; the former must absolutely be done in case the dog that inflicted the bite was very suspicious.

A dog may be suspected of commencing rabies when it ceases to be friendly, will scarcely wag its tail on being patted by those it likes best, appears very tired and lazy, is cross and dejected,

---

[1] A clergyman was affected by chronic hydrophobia merely from imagining that a dog that had bitten him was mad. He would have died had not a physician pointed out to him the erroneous nature of his idea. He soon recovered after the physician had succeeded in convincing him, and without taking any medicine.

dreads the light, and creeps into dark corners, where it lies down without sleeping. It never barks, not even when there is the greatest cause for it doing so; it merely growls at any thing approaching it suddenly, and springs out at it. The eyes are dim, the tail and ears hang done. At this stage the bite commences to be dangerous.

This state lasts but half a day, or a whole day, and then the second stage of rabies breaks out. The animal no longer knows its own master, eats and drinks no more, becomes restless, growls with a hoarse whine, without ever barking, goes about threateningly with dependent head, red watery eyes, having a sad expression and directed towards the ground. It involuntarily moves the lower jaw in a mumbling manner; its leaden-coloured tongue, dripping with saliva, hangs out of the mouth; the tail is stuck betwixt the legs; the hairs of the whole body stand out in a disorderly manner. It tries to run away, snaps at every thing before it, and runs along, irrespective of the road, without apparent object, straight and crooked, at a quick, usually unsteady pace. Other dogs run away from it.

The wood-cut at the head of the article represents a dog in this state.

THE VISITER OF THE SICK.

If it be not from want of something better to do or from mere curiosity, which, as the story goes, is among the attributes of the fair sex—if, in a word, it be not from some important object that Mrs. X. visits Mrs. Z. in her serious febrile disease, if she does it out of christian, sisterly, or cousinly affection and friendship, I fear I should be denounced as a bad man were I in this last case to forbid such visits. And yet it must be done; I must forbid them, but I beg to be heard before being condemned.

Malignant fevers that spread among the people have usually, at all events often, a contagious character, notwithstanding that some of my colleagues have endeavoured, most learnedly, to prove the contrary. It is safer to consider them so, as it is in all cases safer to believe in a little too much hell than too little, in order that we may take greater precautions to preserve ourselves from it, whether it be a reality or only a sort of a woodcut *in rerum natura*. It is likewise quite praiseworthy to make our children believe that the brook that flows by is somewhat deeper and more fearful than it actually is.

The very probably contagious nature of prevalent fevers being conceded, it must be highly criminal, at least very imprudent, for the healthy lady to sit beside her deadly-sick gossip for hours at a time without the slightest necessity.

"She would be very much offended if I did not visit her; what would the relations say to my impoliteness? I am told she longed to see me—if she should die without me seeing her once more, I should never forgive myself!" Such excuses might probably be considered as valid by a gallant man; but they have no weight with me, for I am not a gallant man. Admitting she had a real affectionate desire to see her friend once more, this good intention must remain unfulfilled, just as many good things in this world must remain undone because they cannot be done, or at least not without great injury or palpable danger.

If you wish to save your friend from drowning you must be able to swim; if you cannot, do not jump into the water after him—for any sake don't! but run for assistance, and if he is drowned by the time assistance arrives, then help to drag the water for him; help with all your might to bring him back to life, or if all is of no avail, follow his body to the grave. There are in like manner cases where you can do nothing but pray when your neighbour is being burnt to death in the fourth story and your heart is bleeding for him.

Your sick friend most probably knows you no longer in her delirium; but supposing she would know you, you may, when she recovers, make up in many ways for this neglected service of love, as such unnecessary and dangerous visits to the sick are commonly called. (Would that we poor creatures began to testify our friendship more in deed and in truth than in empty compliments and visits; there is already enough of the empty and windy in this world of ours!)

No one requires fewer persons about him than a dangerously sick person, himself nearly related to death, which slumbers in solitude beneath grave-mounds, as we learn from friend Hain.

Who does the patient who is seriously ill prefer having near him? none but the necessary person, at the most a father, a mother or a spouse, but best of all the sick-nurse and the doctor (two persons ordained by God and placed, like Uriah in the battle, in the thickest of the fight—forlorn hopes quite close to the advancing enemy, without any hours of relief from their irksome guard—two very much misunderstood beings, who sacrifice themselves at hard-earned wages for the public weal, and, in order to obtain a civic crown, brave the life-destroying, poisoned atmosphere, deafened by the cries of agony and the groans of death).

Let patients affected with contagious fevers be left to these two, the only necessary, the only useful individuals, and to a beneficent God; they alone can attend to them properly, from their hands must they expect all the good that we can wish for them, *life and health*.

The anxious lady that visits her sick friend can do her no manner of good; all she can do will be to shew her a pocket-handerkchief which she has moistened with her sympathizing tears, irritate her morbid nerves with chattering, help to spoil the air of the close sick-room with her breath, increase the noise that is often so hurtful to patients, disarrange the good order by her officious interference, give well-meant but erroneous advice, and, what is of still greater consequence, carry back the disease with her into her own house.

Let it not be alleged that the sick nurse and the doctor must run the same risk if the doctrine of contagiousness be true. They do so no doubt to a certain degree, as the death of many doctors and nurses shew. But they do not do so much as Madam Gossip, and this is the reason.

The Creator of mankind has so ordained that *habit* shall be a protector against many dangers. Thus the chimney-sweeper gradually accustoms himself to the smoke from wood, which would choke any one else, and he can, if it be not too intense, easily exist in it. The glass-blower, from gradual custom withstands the most intense heat of his furnace, and goes much closer to it than other persons can. The Greenlander, a man like ourselves, laughs and jokes in a degree of cold that would freeze to death those unused to it. The courier who travels many hundred miles in a few days, and the runner who makes a day's journey in a few hours; the fisherman who spends much of his life in the water without taking cold, and the Scotch miner who lives to the age of a hundred years in his unhealthy occupation. are all proofs of this.

In like manner some stout-hearted men can gradually accustom themselves to the exhalations of the most infectious diseases, and their system in course of time becomes quite insensible to them. There are some layers-out of dead bodies in large cities who attain a great age, and have breathed the exhalations from thousands of corpses that have died of infectious diseases. There have also been grave-diggers who in the time of a pestilence have buried the last inhabitant of their district.

But it is only cautious nurses and physicians that can rejoice in this immunity from infection ; they must accustom themselves to it very gradually, continue to habituate themselves and employ various precautions in order not to be destroyed by the murderous exhalation.

A casual visiter cannot pretend to such advantages, she must be totally unused to the insidious miasm, and in all probability she runs the greatest risk to her life.   She may be happy if her imprudence does not make orphans of her children, or even cause the death of all of them, without any fault of theirs.

PROTECTION AGAINST INFECTION IN EPIDEMIC DISEASES.

For every kind of poisonous exhalation there is in all probability a particular antidote, only we do not always know enough about the latter.   It is well known that the air of our atmosphere contains two-thirds of a gas that is immediately fatal to man and beast, and extinguishes flame.   Mixed up along with it is its peculiar corrective; it contains about one third of vital air, whereby its poisonous properties are destroyed; and in that state only does it constitute atmospheric air, wherein all creatures can live, grow and develop themselves.

The suffocative and flame-extinguishing exhalations in cellars in which a quantity of yeast or beer has fermented, is soon removed by throwing in fresh slaked lime.

The vapour developed in manufactories where much quicksilver is employed, together with a high temperature, is very prejudicial to health ; but we can in a great measure protect ourselves against it by placing all about open vessels containing fresh liver of sulphur.

To chemistry we are indebted for all these protective means against poisonous vapours, after we had discovered, by means of chemistry, the exact nature of these exhalations.

But it is quite another thing with the contagious exhalations from dangerous fevers and infectious diseases.   They are so subtle that chemistry has never yet been able to subject them to analysis, and consequently has failed to furnish an antidote for them.   Most of them are not catching at the distance of a few paces in the open air, not even the plague of the East; but in close chambers these vapours exist in a concentrated form and then become injurious, dangerous, fatal, at a considerable distance from the patient.

Now as we know of no specific antidotes for the several kinds of contagious matters, we must content ourselves with general prophylactic means. Some of these means are sometimes in the power of the patient, but most of them are solely available by the nurse, the physician, and the clergyman, who visit the sick.

As regards the former of these, the patient, if not too weak, may change his room and his bed every day, and the room he is to occupy may, before he comes into it in the morning, be well aired by opening the doors and all the windows. If he have curtains to his bed he may draw them to, and let the fresh air circulate once more through his room, before the physician or clergyman comes to visit him.

The hospitals used by an army in a campaign, which are often established in churches, granaries, or airy sheds, are for that reason much less liable to propagate contagion, and also much more beneficial for the patients than the stationary hospitals, which are often built too close, low, and angular. In the latter, the nurses, physicians, and clergymen often run great risks. And what risks do they not constantly run in the half underground damp dwellings of the lowest class of the people, in the dirty cellars of back courts and narrow lanes that the sun's reviving rays never shine in, and the pure morning air never reaches, stuffed full with a crowd of pauper families, where pale care, and whining hunger seem for ever to have established their desolating throne!

During the prevalence of contagious diseases the poisonous qualities of the vitiated air are concentrated in such places, so that the odour of the pest is plainly perceptible, and every time the door is opened, a blast of death and desolation escapes. These are the places fraught with greatest danger to physician and clergyman. Is there any mode whereby they can effectually protect their lungs from the Stygian exhalation, when the crying misery on all sides appeals to them, shocks them, and makes them forgetful of self? And yet they must try to discover some preventive! How are they to do so?

I have said above, that we may gradually accustom ourselves to the most poisonous exhalations, and remain pretty well in the midst of them.

But, as is the case with accustoming ourselves to every thing, *the advance from one extreme to the other must be made with the utmost caution, and by very small degrees*, so it is especially with this.

We become gradually accustomed to the most unwholesome prison cells, and the prisoners themselves with their sighs over the inhuman injustice of their lot, often, by their breathing and the exhalations from their bodies, gradually bring the few cubic feet of their atmosphere into a state of such pestilential malignity, that strangers are not unfrequently struck down by the most dangerous typhoid fevers, or even have suddenly died by venturing near them, whilst the prisoners themselves, having been gradually accustomed to the atmosphere, enjoy a tolerable health.

In like manner we find that physicians who see patients labouring under malignant fevers rarely and only occasionally, and clergymen whose vocation only requires them to pay a visit now and then, are much more frequently infected than those who visit many such cases in a day.

From these facts naturally proceeds the first condition for those who visit such sick-beds for the first time, "that they should in the commencement rather see their patients more frequently, but each time stay beside them as short a time as possible, keep as far away as possible from the bed or chamber utensil, and especially that they should take care that the sick room be thoroughly aired before their visit."

After these preliminary steps have been taken with proper caution and due care, we may then, by degrees, remain somewhat longer, especially beside patients with the slighter form of the disease, and of cleanly habits, we may also approach them sufficiently close to be able to feel their pulse and see their tongue, taking the precaution when so near them, to refrain from breathing. All this can be done without any appearance of affectation, anxiety, or constraint.

I have observed, that it is usually the *most compassionate, young* physicians, who, in epidemics of this sort, are soonest carried off, when they neglect this insufficiently known precaution, perhaps from excessive philanthropy and anxiety about their patients; that on the other hand, the hard hearted sort of every-day doctors who love to make a sensation by the large number of patients they visit daily, and who love to measure the greatness of their medical skill by the agility of their limbs and their rapidity, most certainly escape infection. But there is a wise middle path (which young clergymen who visit the sick are counselled to adopt), whereby they may unite the most sensitive and warmest philanthropy with immunity to their own precious health.

The consideration "that a precipitate self-sacrifice may do them harm but cannot benefit the patient, and that it is better to spare one's life for the preservation of many, than to hazard it in order to gratify a few," will make the above first precaution acceptable, viz.—*by very gradually approaching and accustoming ourselves to the inflammatory material of the contagion, to blunt by degrees our nerves to the impression of the miasm* (morbid exhalation) *otherwise so easily communicable.* We must not neglect to impress the same precautionary measures on the attendants of the sick person.

The second precaution is "that we should, when visiting the patient, endeavour to maintain our mind and body in a good equilibrium." This is as much as to say, that during this occupation we must not permit ourselves to be acted on by debilitating emotions; excesses in venery, in anger, grief and care, as also over-exertion of the mind of all sorts, are great promoters of infection.

Hence to attend either as physician or clergyman a dear friend sick of the prevalent fever is a very dangerous occupation, as I have learnt from dear-bought experience.

We should endeavour moreover to preserve as much as possible our usual mode of living, and whilst our strength is still good we should not forget to take food and drink in the usual manner, and duly apportioned to the amount of hunger and thirst we may have. Unusual abstinence or excess in eating and drinking should be carefully avoided.

But in this respect no absolute dietetic rules can be laid down. It has been said that one should not visit patients when one's stomach is empty, but this is equally erroneous as if it were to be said, one should visit them with an empty stomach. One who like myself is never used to eat anything in the forenoon, would derange his digestion and render himself more susceptible of infection were he, following the old maxim, to eat something for which he had no appetite and visit his patients in this state; and *vice versa.*

On such occasions we should attend more than ordinarily to our desires for particular articles of diet, and procure if possible that for which we have most appetite, but then only eat as much as will satisfy us.

All over fatigue of the body, chills and night-watchings, should be avoided.

Every physician who has previously been engaged in practice, every clergyman and nurse will of course have learned to get over the unnecessary repugnance he may feel.

Thus we become gradually habituated to the occupation of tending patients suffering from malignant fevers, which is fraught with so much danger and cannot be compensated by any amount of pecuniary remuneration, until at length it becomes almost as difficult to be infected at all as to get the small-pox twice. If under all these circumstances we retain our courage, sympathizing compassionate feelings, and a clear head, we become persons of great importance in the state, not to be recompensed by the favour of princes, but conscious of our lofty destiny and rising superior to ourselves, we dedicate ourselves to the welfare of the very lowest as well as the highest among the people, we become as it were angels of God on earth.

Should the medical man experience in himself some commencing signs of the disease, he should immediately leave off visiting the patient, and if he have not committed any dietetic or regiminal error, I would recommend, notwithstanding I have endeavoured in this book to avoid anything like medicinal prescriptions, the employment of a domestic remedy, so to speak, empirically.

In such cases I have taken a drachm of cinchona bark in wine every three quarters of an hour, until all danger of infection (whatever kind of epidemic fever the disease might be) was completely over.

I can recommend this from my own experience, but am far from insisting upon the performance of this innocuous and powerful precaution by those who are of a different opinion. My reasons would be satisfactory if I could adduce them in this place.

But as it is not enough to protect ourselves from infection, but also necessary not to allow others to come in the way of danger through us, those who have been engaged about such patients should certainly not approach others too nearly until they have changed the clothes they had on when beside the patients for others, and the former should be hung up in an airy place where no one should go near them, until we again need them to visit our patients. Next to the sick-room, infection takes place most easily by means of such clothes, although the person who visits the patient may not have undergone any infection.

A highly respectable and orderly individual who for years

had never walked anywhere, but only to his office at the fixed hours, had a female attendant with whom he was on very friendly terms, an old good-natured person, who without his knowledge employed all her leisure hours in making herself useful to a poor family living about a hundred yards from his house, who were lying sick of a putrid fever, the prominent character of which was, a malignant typhoid fever. For a fortnight all went on well; but about this time the gentleman received some intelligence of a very annoying and depressing character, and in a few days, although to my certain knowledge he had seen no one affected with such a disease, he got, in all probability from the clothes of his attendant who was often very close to him, exactly the same kind of malignant fever, only much more malignant. I visited him as a friend with unreserved sympathy as I ought, and I fell sick of the same fever, although I had been already very much accustomed to infection.

This case, together with many other similar ones, taught me that clothes carry far and wide the contagious matter of such fevers, and that depressing mental emotions render persons susceptible to the miasm, even such as are already used to its influence.

It would appear that the lawyer who draws up a will, the notary and the witnesses would, on account of not being habituated to such impressions, run much greater risk of being infected in these cases. I do not deny it; but for them there are modes of escape which are not so accessible to the other persons of whom we have spoken.

Where there is nothing, the sovereign has lost his rights, there is no will to be made. But when wealthy persons wish to make their last will and testament on their sick bed, there are two circumstances in favour of the lawyer and his assistants. As in the formalities of a legal testament, the patient's bed often cannot remain in its usual situation, and as moreover it is essential for such a testament that the testator should be in full possession of his intellectual faculties, it follows that for those patients *who are not absolutely poor* another room and another bed may be got ready, thoroughly aired and free from infectious atmosphere. They do not need to remove thither until all this has been properly performed a short time before.

The weakness of the intellect in such patients generally keeps pace with their corporeal weakness, and a patient who possesses

sufficient strength of intellect to make his will would not allege
that he is too weak to be removed to another bed and room.

How little chance there is of the legal officials catching the
infection under these circumstances (provided they take moderate care not to approach the patient nearer than necessary), I
need not dwell upon.

I should mention that after one has once accustomed himself
to any particular kind of miasm, for example the bloody flux,
the nerves remain for a considerable time, often for years, to
some degree insensible to the same kind of disease, even though
during all that time we may have had no opportunity of seeing
patients affected with that disease, and thus as it were of keeping the nerves actively engaged in keeping up this state of specific unsusceptibility. It gradually goes off, but more slowly
than one would suppose. Hence with moderate precaution a
nurse, a physician, or a clergyman, may attend dysenteric patients this year if they have had to do with similar patients
several years previously. But the safest plan is to employ even
in this case a little blameless precaution.

But as the superstitious amulets and charms of our ancestors'
times did harm, inasmuch as full credit was given to their medicinal virtues, and better remedies were consequently neglected,
so for like reasons the fumigations of the sick room with the vapour of vinegar, juniper-berries and the like, is inadvisable, although the majority of my colleagues highly recommend it,
and assert that the most infectious miasms of all kinds have
thereby been overpowered and driven away, and thus the air
purified.

Being convinced of the contrary, I must directly contradict
them, and rather draw upon myself their disfavour than neglect
an opportunity of rendering a service to my fellow-creatures.
But as the spoiled (phlogisticated, foul, fixed, &c.) air can never
be restored to purity or turned into vital air by means of these
fumes, and as there is not a shadow of a proof that the subtle
contagious exhalations, whose essential nature is quite unknown
to us and not perceptible to our senses, can be weakened, neutralized, or in any other manner rendered innocuous by these
fumes, it would be foolish, I would almost say unjustifiable, by
recommending such fumigations for the supposed purification
of the air, to encourage ordinary people in their natural indolence and indisposition to renew the air of their apartments,
and thereby expose every different person who comes in con-

tact with them to a danger to his life, which shall be all the more obvious and great, the more confident he has been made by the futile representation that, without driving away the disease-spreading miasm by means of repeated draughts of air, the pestilential atmosphere of the sick room has been converted into pure healthy air by means of simple fumigations with vinegar and juniper berries. That is just like the old superstition of hanging an eagle-stone at the hip of the woman in labour, at the very moment when all hopes of saving her, even by the forceps, are over.

When a physician or clergyman enters an unfumigated chamber he can at once tell by his sense of smell whether his needful order to air the room has been obeyed or not. All sick people make a disagreeable smell about them. Therefore the freedom from smell of a chamber is the best proof that it has previously been aired, but if fumigations have been had recourse to, the latter becomes doubtful and suspicious. Neither the physician nor the clergyman, neither the sick-nurse nor the patient, require perfumes when they have to think and speak seriously concerning a matter of life and death. They should never be used!

IN OLD-WOMEN'S PHILOSOPHY THERE IS SOMETHING GOOD, IF WE ONLY KNOW WHERE TO FIND IT.

I hope by this section, at all events by the title of it, to have made my peace for all future times with that, please heaven, small portion of my fair readers who suspect me of heresy from the faith of our grandmothers, and I should be sorry to fall out with these respectable old people, certainly I should.

So let us hasten from the preface to the main point of our matter. I once lived in a place where the midwife, who was there called emphatically the *wise woman*, gave to all newly confined (peasant) women a good large quantity of brandy. Even I had to submit to this inevitable fate, and I did it without a murmur. For who dare say a word against the Parcæ, especially against the the third and last of them?

I was assured that this fiery spirit did great good in many cases. With folded hands I held my peace, as was reasonable, and looked on, and I found that in this locality there were actually many puerperal women who when left to themselves had serious symptoms arising from weakness or excessive irritability of the nervous system, accompanied by impurities of the stomach and bowels, or by plethora—in these the brandy did real service, but these were exactly the cases in which we find opium (a very analagous thing) of use.

Here then the old-woman's philosophy was really right for once. But what became of the other cases in which the brandy was poured into the poor creatures in a useless and hurtful manner? I shall say nothing about that, because at the present time the third fate is still much too intractable, and has even become fearful to the sons of Æsculapius.

"If you are a woman, tie a man's stocking round your swollen neck, and it will subside; say, I said it." This good counsel of the old dame is true in so far as slightly swollen cervical glands in lymphatic constitutions only require a warm covering in order to dissipate the swelling, more especially a covering which (as will readily be done by a woollen cloth on the tender skin of a lady's neck) shall cause friction and produce irritation and redness. Thus far the old women's philosophy is again correct. But why a dirty stocking? might we not use flannel—and how! in true inflammations of the throat what good will a dry, woollen, heating covering do!—Here the old witch holds her tongue, and so do I, for it is advisable to do so in her presence.

Swollen cervical glands are cured by the lucky hand of some wise woman or midwife, who must each time that the moon is on the wane, in silence press thrice upon the swollen glands with her thumb, in a crucial manner. Superstition places much confidence in this semi-magical remedy, which sometimes is actually of great service. Thus much is certain, that glandular swellings in middle-aged individuals of lymphatic constitutions who have not much general scrofulous disposition, not unfrequently disappear rapidly by rubbing and moderate pressure. Thereby is produced an increased circulation of the blood and a greater activity of the lymphatic vessels, and even an incipient inflammation, whereby the swelling is removed. In so far the vaunted petticoat wisdom is right.

But what the period of the wane of the moon has to do with the matter, we, who belong to the inferior class of untranscendental doctors, are too dull to perceive, because, alas, we are not endowed with the super-subtle sixth or perhaps seventh sense; were it otherwise we might see the great importance of the triple and crucial pressure, more especially if the excessively lucky precaution is observed of commencing and carrying out the operation from beginning to end *without speaking a word*, which indeed it were almost too much to expect from an ordinary woman.

THINGS THAT SPOIL THE AIR.

It cannot be indifferent to those of my readers who wish to enjoy a long and healthy life whether the air of their rooms possess the necessary degree of purity or not.

There are many familiar things that render the air that we breathe more or less unsuitable for the maintenance of life, so my readers must listen to the warnings of a friend.

Flowers are an ornament to a room, and if we are content to deck one room with but *a few* of extreme beauty, and *very few*, on account of their perfume, it will not much signify; it is rather praiseworthy than blameworthy. The more we refresh our senses in an innocuous manner the more lively and easy does our power of thinking become, the more capable and disposed for business are we, and the delight of the sight and the smell in flowers, the pride of lovely nature, is especially of this character.

But an excess does harm in all things, so it does likewise here. A large bouquet of lilies, tuberous plants, love-flowers, centifolia, jasmine, lilac, and so forth, makes such a strong perfume in a small room that many sensitive persons have occasionally been made to faint by them. This does not depend so often on the antipathy of the nervous system to such odours as it does on the injurious property of such strong-scented flowers of quickly spoiling the air and rendering it unfit for respiration. Other writers have already called attention to this fact, so that I need not dwell longer on it, and will content myself with having repeated the warning.

People who wish to be very genteel, love to burn in the evening more candles than are necessary; and if they are entertaining company, they light up chandeliers, sconces and all the other receptacles for candles they may possess, in order that the fashionably dressed ladies and gentlemen may see each other well. It is considered a capital holiday spectacle to see so many candles burning at once; it dazzles one's eyes so brilliantly that we scarcely know where we are; it also costs a good round sum.

But if we view all this display of candles in the proper light, we shall find that they spoil the air in a very ugly manner. Considering that they are only lighted for a number of guests who are to be well feasted, who, seated in close rows, pollute the atmosphere for each other by their breathing and exhalations, in one word that they are only lighted for feasts and balls, considering this, I say, I know not what sort of complimentary speech I can make to my entertainer for purposely depriving me of the little bit of pure God's-air, and giving me the very worst sort instead, in which an animal could with difficulty sustain life. Amid how many attacks of faintness will not yon lady express her thanks to him, after having worked away for hours at her toilette, preparing for the festivities, in the endeavour to diminish by one third the capacity of her chest by means of a whalebone apparatus, until, drawn in so tightly as to look like a wasp, she could scarcely take in air enough to support life in a pure atmosphere! Relish it who may—I must say, for my part, that I have no wish to be regaled with so many candles in a room.

He who wishes to act wisely will not tarry in the room where he has dined, and where the vapour from the warm food has deteriorated the air, until it has been thoroughly aired.

It is very unwholesome to sleep in rooms where, as is often the case among the lower classes, there is a store of green fruit. A quantity of phlogiston that exhales from the fruit in the form of their odour soon approximates the pure atmospheric air to the condition of phlogistic and unhealthy air.

Also store-rooms of other kinds, where domestic articles and food from the animal and vegetable kingdoms are kept in quantity, such as oils, candles, lard, raw, boiled, and roasted meat, pastry, &c., are not healthy places for people to dwell in. It should be observed that everything that emits much smell, perceptibly vitiates the atmosphere.

In foul linen the excretions from the skin are present, and no rational person would submit to have them kept or washed in his room for similar reasons, but also for delicacy's sake.

No one who can avoid it should sleep in the room in which he remains during the day. The beds part very gradually with the exhalation they have received from the sleeper during the night, and continue to vitiate all day long the air of the

12

room, even though it had been thoroughly aired in the morning.

Six busy watchmakers do not spoil the air nearly so much as two workmen engaged in sawing wood. I would therefore advise that the workshops in manufactories, especially where much corporeal exercise is employed, should be built rather too high than too low, rather too airy than too close, and be they ever so cleanly and well situated they should be frequently aired. It is incredible in how short a time in such cases the air of the room becomes vitiated and unfit for respiration. The miserable, sick aspect and the great mortality of the workmen of many manufactories renders further proof of my proposition superfluous.

Working with unclean wool, with oil-colours, or with things for which burning charcoal is employed, is for other reasons not innocuous.

But even though the air should not be altered in its composition, it may become hurtful in another way by the mixture of something extraneous. Such is especially *moisture.*

Reservoirs attached to chamber-stoves, wherein the water is kept hot for domestic use, are in this respect injurious. For this reason also, workmen who are engaged in drying wet things in highly heated rooms, cabinet-makers, turners, potters, bookbinders, &c., are very liable to swellings and other affections proceeding from relaxation of the absorbents.

A person who from an idea of extreme convenience should, notwithstanding the vicinity of a water-closet, keep a night-chair in his sleeping apartment, should bear in mind that the disgusting exhalation from it spoils the air uncommonly, and renders the bed-chamber in which we pass a third of our life (if it be not very roomy) a very unwholesome place of abode. There are however many houses so ill-arranged as either to have no water-closet at all, or where it is at such a distance as as not to be very accessible in the night.

If this is the case, and cannot be remedied, we should have a small closet constructed of stone in the corner of some public room near the bed-chamber which has a good opening to the outside of the house, and a well fitting door to enter at. In this place we may, under such circumstances, place the night-chair, and have it carried out afterwards, without having to fear any vitiation of the air or bad smell.

We should not permit large thickly-leaved trees to stand

close to the windows of a house. In addition to their preventing the access of daylight and of the pure air, their exhalations in the evening and at night are not very favourable to health. Trees at a distance of from ten to twelve paces from the house admit the air much more readily, and cannot be sufficiently recommended, as well on account of their beautiful appearance and their pleasant shade, as on account of the wholesomeness of their exhalations by day. If we have the choice we should have the windows of our bed-room to the east, where the view is quite free, uninterrupted by very close trees, and unpoisoned by the febrile exhalation from a marsh.

Poverty has brought many injurious habits into this world, one of the worst of which is that where persons in the lower ranks of life, especially women, sit over a vessel filled with red hot charcoal, in order thereby to save themselves the expense of a stove in winter. The closer the room is shut up in such circumstances, and the more the external air is excluded, the more dangerous and fatal is this habit, for the air inside will thereby soon become a stupifying poison.

We feel a pressive, stupifying headache, that seems to bore throug' oth temples, at the same time we experience an inclination to vomit, which however is soon suppressed by a rapidly increasing comatose state, in which we sink helplessly to the ground and generally die without convulsions.

When the person falls down the clothes are apt to catch fire from the burning charcoal, and indeed fires have often originated in this manner, which are all the more dangerous because it is only when they have fairly burst forth that they will be observed by strangers, seeing that the person who originates it is too stupified to be able to extinguish the first flames.

Not less dangerous to life is it to close the valve in the chimneys of stoves that are heated from within, as long as the stove continues full of glowing cinders. From motives of economy people often like to retain the heat in the room. An economy that is very ill-directed. The more glowing charcoal there is in the stove, and the tighter the valve is closed, the quicker is the air vitiated, just as it is by a brazier full of red hot charcoal standing free in the room, and there ensue accidents just as bad as those above described, and not unfrequently fatal.

The valves in the chimneys of stoves are solely intended to moderate the draught of air into the stove and the violence of the fire, or in the event of the soot in the chimney catching fire to prevent a destructive conflagration by entirely shutting the chimney. If this latter should happen, every sensible person will as soon as he has shut the valve at once open the doors and windows in order to remove the air of the room that has been deteriorated by the confined fire.

We should rather seek to save wood by using well constructed stoves, than, by stopping up every hole and cranny in the doors and windows, exclude every breath of air, as is done by many persons of slender and of moderate means. Such persons must be ignorant of the incalculable value of air, who paste up with paper every chink and hole, and even hang up cloths before their doors, and thus retain all the unwholesome exhalations from the pores of the skin and from the lungs in their small rooms, so as to respire, instead of life and health, disease and death. I have seen melancholy examples of this nature, and I fear that my warning will have some difficulty in penetrating to the miserable cellars they have themselves selected.

Deathly pale and spiritless they feel an unknown poison permeating all their bloodvessels, they feel their health gradually being undermined, just as the water that runs down from their windows rots the window-frames; cachexy, dropsical swellings and pulmonary consumptions carry them off after having seen their children die around them of low, wasting diseases, which they attribute principally to teething or bewitchment, or reduced by rickets to cripples. Where is the compassionate man who will teach them something better?

THERE IS GOOD EVEN IN HURTFUL THINGS.

It is well known that the tailor's trade is not one of the healthiest of occupations. We find in these good folks, if they are diligent workmen, usually emaciated legs, knock-knees, a dragging of the left leg, round shoulders, the head bent forwards, drawn-in abdomen, and so forth. Their complexion shews very plainly the unhealthiness of their occupation; loss of appetite, piles, constipation, weakness of the body, itch, &c., are things quite common among them, and yet there are cases in which this mode of life has been favourable to health.

A young man in England was born with the feet turned inwards. A surgeon whom his mother consulted pronounced the deformity incurable. When he grew up, he could only walk with difficulty upon the outer border of his feet and heels, he always knocked one foot against the other, and frequently fell; the muscles of his thighs and calves were extremely attenuated, and the turned-in feet were so deformed, that shoes of a particular shape and tie had to be made for him.

The poor-house authorities bound him apprentice to a tailor, thinking that this was the only trade that his deformity permitted him to follow.

In this work, whereby one usually sits at the shop-board, as is well known, with the legs crossed, he observed a gradual change in his limbs, which, without the slightest employment of external or internal remedies, continued to turn outwards. In the course of three years they attained their natural position, so that he could wear ordinary shoes, they were indeed directed more than usually outwards. The muscles of his legs grew stout, and his body was so well formed that he enlisted in the marines, and thenceforward remained in the service.

Probably in this case a peculiar stiffness (rigidity) of the muscles that adduct the foot was the cause why the abductor muscles could not maintain the balance of power, and so allowed the foot to be drawn inwards. The strain upon the former, when the legs were crossed at his work, stretched and relaxed them more, and thus the abductor muscles of the leg and foot were enabled gradually to attain their natural opposing power; indeed the latter gained in this way an excess of power, and his feet were turned outwards more than is usual.

Joiners and cabinet-makers usually have the right shoulder higher than the left, because they exert the former most during their work. It might be tried whether individuals whose left shoulder was the highest, would not become straight by following these trades.

In like manner, to give another example of the good effects of hurtful things, there have been cases where by a stab of a sword in the chest, purulent deposits in its cavity that threatened a fatal result, have been opened, and where, after the murderous wound was healed, general health was the result.

So, also, persons who were paralysed on one side of the body, on being struck by lightning, have recovered the perfect use of their limbs.

I knew a melancholic gentleman who in a fit of the spleen wounded the veins in his neck, and after losing several pounds of blood, recovered from his melancholy madness.

Cases have been recorded of patients who, in order to put a period to their sufferings, swallowed large doses of opium, and attained their object in this way—that they did not indeed die, but were completely delivered from their disease.

And how many instances might be cited where persons have become wiser and better by disease, or have grown healthier by calamity, misery and hunger, and have become more useful members of society! I know a physician, to whom the world owes much, who would never have adopted this honourable profession, had not the delicate state of his health when a young man almost compelled him to do so.

He who has made a narrow escape from drowning learns to swim, and by this accomplishment is enabled to save the lives of others.

The police-inspector has his house burnt down, and the fire-engines of the place are put by him into a state of perfection.

Yon prince would not have placed the lands of his subjects in a state of security against inundations, had not some of his own estates been fearfully inundated; and had not his throne been several times shaken by the thunderstorm, he would not have introduced the valuable lightning-conductor into his dominions.

Pfeffel and Euler must lose their sight in order to surpass the most of their fellow-beings in poetical and mathematical talent; and if we had space, we might adduce many other examples of benefits derived from injurious things, to the glory of the Creator.

DIETETIC CONVERSATION WITH MY BROTHER, CHIEFLY ABOUT THE INSTINCT OF THE STOMACH.

He. Are you not ashamed of yourself to be eating pears early in the morning? you will chill your stomach, and then you can't say I did not warn you.

I. Certainly not, for I have no fear of such a catastrophe. But tell me, at what time of day should one eat fruit?

He. After dinner, and as a rule, after having taken something warm into the stomach; such was the opinion of our ancestors, and they were no fools.

I. But we moderns on the contrary are of course? and this I would almost concede to you for the sake of peace, if this verdict only applied to some of us. But tell me, can the stomach of different individuals be regulated by one general rule, even were it as old as the twelve commandments. Is not every one's stomach as peculiar as every person's foot, which the shoe of another will not and cannot fit?

He. Yes, I grant you that; but we can take the measure of the foot, it is something visible and tangible, but who can tell the exact and peculiar condition of the stomach? Would we not act more wisely, by following in its proper place, the general rules for it laid down by wise men; and not attempting to speculate further on such a ticklish subject?

I. Did then the wise men of former generations know every individual stomach, its condition and requirements, so clearly as to enable them to lay down those general rules for their posterity, which were suited for each one of the innumerable varieties of stomachs? Is that possible?

He. Not that exactly! but you moderns have apparently been more lucky in finding a general rule for the stomach (*dietetics* as it is commonly termed), as I guess from your eating fruit in the morning.

I. Just so, I just wished you to tell me that the moderns were diet-mongers. They are but too much so, to reply seriously to your irony. In their law-giving mania they imagine themselves just as wise, and make just as many mistakes, as the ancients.

He. In what horrible uncertainty, brother, would we be groping about in a matter of such importance for preserving the proper standard of health! how unlucky would we be were what you say correct!

I. Neither unlucky, nor yet in horrible uncertainty, I should think.

This article in our vital breviary is of such great importance that it is certain the beneficent Creator could not have founded it upon the shifting standard of the professional dietists; he must have given us an infallible guiding principle to direct us in the selection of food and drink. Could any one seriously attempt to bring up good children according to the literal principles of a pedagogic book? What think you? the good Claudius will cut off his finger if this be true.

He. And what then is your infallible guide to the only saving system of dietetics?

I. Just what you yourself usually follow, without thinking about it?

He. And what is that I demand, you tantalizing fellow?

I. I should suppose, "Moderation and attention to what best suits your individual constitution in every condition." I will allow a finger to be cut off if this be not the natural religion of the stomach and the only infallible dietetic rule for every one.

He. No doubt, if we had the instinct of beasts, you might be right.

I. What mutilater of the rights of man could have told you that our beneficent mother Nature has not endowed us with just as much instinct as we require? Who teaches the infant to prefer its mother's milk to pastry? Who instructs him that is sunk in grief and distress to take a glass of wine? Who tells the patient ill of a bilious fever to avoid meat? the dysenteric patient to pant for grapes? Who tells us when we are hungry, when thirsty? A rotten egg is just as repulsive to us as it would be dangerous to life, and arsenic is as abhorrent to a delicate tongue as it is fatal to the stomach.

But all these are only striking fragmentary reasons for the reality of a beneficial instinctive principle in us. I am incapable of erecting a scholastic system upon it, irrefragable though it be in itself.

Do not retort by referring me to the appetite with which the parched brandy-drinker pours in his murderous liquor; to the ravenous hunger with which the glutton fills the very last cubic line of his stomach with hurtful chef-d'œuvres of the culinary art; to the greediness wherewith the hypochondriac swallows his malt liquor, which has frequently before caused him dangerous colics; to the coffee-drinking woman who will give her last farthing in order to purchase the enervating drink, although she is just about to lose her last pair of black teeth, or must sigh over her unfruitful marriage amid the reproaches of her husband.

To retort in that way would be as if from the innumerable daily examples of want of conscientiousness we should seek to prove that there was no such thing as conscience.

Oh my brother! he who has preserved this delicate, never-deceptive feeling for the good and the noble, in all its simplicity and innocence, and exercises it with the readiness of an unsophisticated child, for his own and his brother's benefit; he asks not if there be human beings so degenerate as to presume to demonstrate away the conscience to a mere shadow, who assert knavery to be a necessary fashion, and a Sybarite's life to be a lawful recreation. In like manner he who, moderately enjoying the gifts of God, has made it his study to discover the reality

of his desires for articles of food, and has by degrees acquired a
facility in being able to determine before he sees it, and from
the mere name alone, whether this or that food, this or that
drink would agree with him at the time,—he does not inquire
if there be men who bid defiance to all nature's wholesome hints,
turn a deaf ear to all her wanings, confound the mere tickling
of the palate with a sufficiency, and repletion with the satisfaction of their wants, and acknowledge no dietetic rule besides the
gratification of their taste, their indolent habits, and the example of their neighbours. He inquires not about them, I repeat,
nor does he imitate them in the crowd of ailments and maladies
that from time to time endeavours harshly enough to call them
back to resolutions of temperance. Do not, however, take up
my observations as though I imagined that the instinct of our
stomach should in all cases indicate even particular varieties of
nutritious articles which we must especially partake of in order
to keep in good health; this would be foreign to the purpose of
the Creator.

In its healthy state the human stomach only needs an instinct
to direct us to certain classes of food, which we should partake
of from time to time if we would continue in right good health.[1]
Thus, for instance, the peasant who has overworked himself,
says to his wife when she is about to set before him cheese and
eggs, " I wish you would make me a little salad ; if you have any
sour milk, give me a little of the whey in place of any food, or
something else sour." Or if, during a couple of holidays, he
has not had an opportunity of working at all, he only asks for
weak soup for supper, or will not eat any thing at all. Or, if
he has been dissipating for several days, he asks her for something strong, something tasty, a bit of bacon, cheese, peas, and
the like. In this case he would feel as if he wanted something
more were he to get nothing but a dish of milk ; he does not
name any article of food in particular that he must absolutely
have, he only wishes something of a very nutritious character.
In like manner many persons of from eighty to ninety years of

---

[1] [This is true, and the reason is quite obvious. When the palate, or, as our Author terms it, the " *instinct of the stomach*," calls for certain articles of food, the salivary glands, the stomach, the pancreas, and the liver all pour out their secretions
abundantly, and thus produce the conditions essential to healthy digestion. If, however, food or drink be taken which is repugnant to the palate, the digestive secretions
are not furnished, and, as a consequence, chylification is imperfectly performed, and
indigestion, with its concomitants obtain. The ideas advanced by our great master
upon this subject are of great importance in a dietetic point of view.]—*Am. P.*

age, commence from mere instinct to live upon honey, sugar and milk. Who informs them that such substances only will keep their fibres in a pliant condition?

But whenever we get into a morbid state, and accustom ourselves to attend dispassionately to the wants of our stomach, then the voice of this true guardian of our life becomes louder and more audible. We perceptibly lose our appetite for certain classes and even varieties of food, and a desire for other classes and varieties is developed, without our knowing why. The pleuritic patient calls for water, cold water, the patient ill of putrid fever demands beer; soups and the like are intolerable to both.

The delicate woman in the family way puts chalk into her mouth, and if we keep it from her she scrapes the lime from the wall and consumes it. She knows not that she has an intolerable acid in her stomach, and still less does she know the chemical property of the chalk of neutralizing and removing acids. What teaches her to swallow greedily this specific for her ailment? What else but the awakened wise instinct implanted by the infinitely wise Creator?

The man who is extremely exhausted from starvation desires a spoonful of wine; what tells him that a supply of meat and bread which an ignorant person would endeavour to force him to swallow, might prove fatal to him?

I saw a lying-in woman, who, after a difficult labour, suffered from intolerable after-pains and a great loss of blood. She cried for coffee, although when she was well she could scarcely endure it. Who told her that her hæmorrhage resulted from atony of the womb, and this from diminished irritability of the fibres, and that the specific remedy for this was coffee? A few cups of very strong coffee were given to her, and hæmorrhage and pains ceased suddenly; opium would have had no effect in such a case.

A person who has contracted a bilious fever from anger and vexation, longs for nothing so much as fruit, who tells him that this is almost the only thing that can do him good?

And so I might give you many more examples of the expression of the instinct of the stomach, did I not fear to weary you. We understand it under the terms appetite and repugnance, two very important but much neglected monitors for our wellbeing!

If we would only study this voice of nature often enough,

and in a perfectly unprejudiced manner, we would obtain a great facility in understanding its feeblest manifestations; we should be enabled thereby to escape a large number of diseases, and in many cases to attain to long life without difficulty.

But we find (as a proof of all I have said) that this small voice of nature is only audible to persons who live upon very simple articles of food, and that they come at last to understand it in a very remarkable manner; almost just as the cattle, which we allow to range at large over the fields, never swallow a plant that would hurt them, but only those that are suitable for them; but when they are ill they often recover, if we drive them out to the meadows where they can instinctively select the food that will do them good.

But how often does it happen that cattle before whom we place hurtful plants, mixed with good hay, are gradually induced to swallow the former along with the latter, and so grow ill? Just as often (let me be permitted to employ this appropriate comparison as regards animal nature in general) as a gentleman gets ill at the richly furnished table by the artistic mixtures of his cook; the taste of the healthy person decoys him into eating unwholesome things without knowing they are so; or the viands become unwholesome by the contradictory mixtures, and the palate is seduced, deceived.

But as the Creator did not wish to limit our appetite when in health specially to one single particular kind of food or drink, and only directed our stomach's instinct to general classes of nutriment, in order that we might remain healthy and useful members of society in every condition, under various relations, in all degrees of latitude, and under all circumstances of fortune, so he sought to avert all injurious consequences that might arise from this instinct of the stomach, that is so much less limited than is the case with the lower animals, by endowing us with an accurate, definite sense of when it is time to leave off or to partake of food and drink.

This sense, which we term *hunger, thirst,* and *satiety,* is in the case of healthy persons who have not much choice of food, almost the only guardian of their health. This feeling, this instinct, as I may term it, is in persons who regard moderation as one of the greatest of virtues, so watchful, so active—they hear this internal voice as distinctly as any animal to which we especially attribute instinct, so distinctly, that they can determine to a mouthful when they have taken enough for their health; that they would deny themselves half a glass of wine or beer beyond what would agree with them. (The sick man, however, whose imagination has got a wrong direction, does not belong to this class.) And it is this last kind of bodily sensation, (hunger, thirst, satiety,) dear brother, that I, as a physician, cannot sufficiently recommend to be kept in an active state.

Moderation, strict moderation, that is not to be bribed by a pampered, corrupt palate, is a sublime corporeal virtue, without which we cannot become healthy nor happy.

This virtue, which is nothing more than faithful obedience to the internal voice of our digestive organs, relative to the proper quantity of nutriment we should take in, has the most perceptible influence even over all other virtues (which, in fact, do also consist mainly in some kind of moderation or another)— and just as certain is it that excess is always accompanied by at least one vice.

We may readily attain sufficient proficiency in this attention to ourselves, but, on the other hand, it is much more difficult to maintain in an active and understandable condition, under the various circumstances of life, that instinct, those secret hints of our digestive organs which beckon us to certain classes or even certain varieties of nutriment that are most wholesome for the particular state of our system for the time being. If you desire it, however, you may acquire even this latter art, but only after having perfected yourself in the former one.

But where is the wise man to be found who is capable of rightly dictating to me in a book once for all what and how much I ought to eat and drink? To me, an isolated individual, with a peculiar constitution, in all the daily varying relations of my life, and the circumstances of my health? I must judge by my own sensations what and how much will suit me; *I* must know it, or no one else can, unless, perhaps, my ordinary medical attendant.

Do not blame me, therefore, brother, if I am somewhat prejudiced against those general dietetic rules for sensible persons; do not blame me if I eat or drink this or that at this or that time, and again pass over whole periods for meals without taking anything, as I do all this only when I am so inclined.

He. But tell me what is meant by depraved appetite, which makes so many people ill? Most derangements of the stomach seem to me to proceed from that cause.

I. Tell me, on the other hand, whence do most of the moral deformities come into the world ? is it not from misguided, perverted feeling for the good and the desirable ? And these erroneous directions of our moral faculty, whence come they, if not from a seared conscience and ignorance of what is good and desirable ?

He. Ignorance you say, and I take you at your word. Consequently in order that your analogy should hold good, we require, in order to carry out a rational system of diet, a historical knowledge of wholesome and unwholesome articles of food ; and hence the dietists should be most acceptable to us.

I. There is not and cannot be any thing which as a general rule is absolutely unwholesome or wholesome. Just as bread is useless to him that has an inflammatory disease, and to him that has his belly full, and as belladonna can in certain cases restore the health, so none of the other general maxims of the dietists can be accounted good—such as, veal is the most wholesome butcher's meat, chervil is a wholesome vegetable, &c.

How can a thing that we can swallow be, under all circumstances and in every condition of the body, universally wholesome healthful, innocent, hurtful, or poisonous? There is a time for every thing, says the king-sage, and to my mind he speaks much more sensibly than most of the dietists.

It is, however, very good and laudable (and in this respect you are right) to have some knowledge of the various articles of food, their nature and properties, before entering on the great world, in order that we may avoid mistaking toad-stools for mushrooms, or swallowing a solution of corrosive sublimate for liqueur. But I should like if our dietists were more careful and exact in respect of these matters, I should like them to enter more into details, and that their maxims in regard to the particular constitution of the body in which this or that article of food makes this or that peculiar impression, were derived more from trustworthy and select authorities and from their own experience, than from mere hear-say. But this is a herculean task, and a useful system of diet of this kind will long remain ideal only. And with this, adieu, dear brother. Think over the subject and tell me on some future occasion where you think I am wrong.

AN OCCASIONAL PURGATIVE, SURELY THAT CAN DO NO HARM.

My dear Doctor,

      I have been advised to apply to you, as you have the

character of always telling people in a pretty straightforward manner what they ought to do. It occurs to me, and my family-surgeon also has often reminded me, that it is surely high time for me, my wife and my children, to take a good dose of purgative physic. " Your honour," he is always saying, " only think what a quantity of dirt must accumulate in the abdomen in the course of half a year, if the refuse be not swept out and cleansed away at least once a month." The like of us, to be sure, do not understand it, but one would think, that of all the food and drink we take, somewhat must occasionally stick in the body, though it may not be so desperately bad as my surgeon alleges. Thinks I to myself, if everything collects in the body in that way, then my shepherd, who is in his seventieth year, and has never taken any medicine in his life, must carry about with him in his belly an accumulation of impurities enough to fill a barrel. But my surgeon ought to know more about the matter than I do. The fellow has, as he assures me, had great experience during the seven years' war; he has amputated a fearful number of arms and legs in the military hospitals, and helped to extract many bits of broken skulls. Do not blame me, doctor, for adopting his views; the chap makes an impression on one with his talk. He looks as fierce as a savage, stammers out horrible Latin and Greek words, gesticulates with his arms, and distorts his features to such an extent that one cannot help being moved when one listens to him. And what he says may be perfectly correct; and is there any greater blessing than health? What a lot of diseases with Greek and Latin names one might get in one's gullet by neglecting the proper precautions! My wife and children are very precious to me; they are all lively and ruddy, and as sound as a nut. May God keep them so! But all my household must lend a hand, and work according to their abilities. After being busy all day in the open air they get a brave appetite for their meals. None of them ail in the least, that is true. If we could but prevent their suffering hereafter! If you should think a good purgative advisable for us, please to send us our portions, and say how we should take them. The chemist will tell you the ages of myself and family. You may send the stuff to us by the brewer's cart.   I am, &c.,

W. von TEUTON,

Retired Capt-in.

Schloss Berghausen,
1st October.

Answer.

My dear Captain,

It is well that you have not given the preference to the idle talk of your Bramarbas of a surgeon over your sound judgment, as so many in your situation do.

You appear to appreciate the truth of that very sensible maxim, "The whole need not the physician, but they that are sick." Who would take medicine if there was nothing the matter with him? Is there any better preventive of diseases than a good robust state of health? That you enjoy, as I perceive from your letter, along with your family; do you wish for anything better?

It is only in cases of excessive over-loading of the stomach in delicate persons, and such as are afflicted with chronic diseases, that the circumstance occurs of nature being too weak to expel the ordure at the right time, and we require to assist her by means of a purgative medicine. But in the healthy state, nature is able of herself to evacuate the useless refuse of the food, and that infinitely better than can be done by our good art.

Therefore, trust me, take no physic, neither you nor your family. Anything else that you have to ask I shall be happy to inform you of. Let your barber-surgeon stick to your beard; the inferior class of these gentry usually only understand the art of making healthy people less healthy, and the sick worse than they were; they bring nothing out of the military hospital with them but disregard for the sufferings of others. Farewell.

ON MAKING THE BODY HARDY.

Modern instructors and other clear-headed men have deeply felt the necessity of making young persons destined for various pursuits and for fighting their way in the great world, hardy, as they term it, and thereby rescuing them from that effeminating and coddling mode of rearing which has for long been the privilege of fashionable people, in which they have been encouraged by the ordinary class of physicians, who are accustomed to reap a golden harvest from the fur-coats, fur-boots, fur-caps, the heated rooms, the intemperance, the warm drinks, and the destructive passions of their clients.

The many unfruitful marriages, the delicacy and bad health of the richer classes have excited attention, and it has been found that these favourites of fortune have been changed into the most wretched specimens of humanity by the habits of life they adopt, that many of their families gradually die out inevitably, and that the delicate members that may still remain of some, encompassed by a host of diseases and pains, joylessly drag out their existence, without any pleasure in life, in the midst of their abundance of the good things of this world, like the fabled Tantalus of heathen mythology.[1]

The open air was never warm enough, it chilled the young ambassador; the comfortable travelling carriage was altered a dozen times in order to exclude every breath of air.

The prince was not allowed to walk, for how easily might he not get his feet wet, and in consequence die suddenly of appoplexy!

The young count, destined to be a general, slept in beds of the softest eider-down, was fed upon sweet cakes, coffee, highly seasoned dishes, two servants must wait on him to assist him to dress, but not before ten o'clock in the morning, because the tender plant might have withered if exposed to the rude morning air. And so he grows up, enters upon his important post, and must now play the iron denizen of camps; only imagine!

In like manner there are king's messengers who would be suffocated in a peasant's heated cot, and rangers of the royal forests who would catch their death if they were forced to wade through the snow.

How many toothaches and diarrhœas has not last night's opera occasioned! what an amount of colics, rheumatisms, sore-throats and erysipelas will not our to-morrow's illumination give rise to!

I said before, that effeminacy is the privilege of the rich fashionable classes; I am wrong! This privilege has been said to belong to the nobility. In order to appear fashionable, the manners of *haut ton* have been assumed by the very lowest classes. A merchant's wife, nay a hair-dresser's lady, would think it a disgrace not to be able to talk about vapours, *perte blanche* and digestive lavements from her own experience. The son of the poor secretary takes his afternoon nap on soft pillows, and the ostler's daughter eats her Swiss biscuits with her sugared coffee; she would blush to wash her own clothes.

These depraved habits have crept in, even among country people: for the farmer's daughter can undoubtedly not consider

---

[1] [We are here reminded of the remark since made by Majendie, "that Paris would become depopulated in two or three generations, were it not for the robust recruits who constantly come in from the country as residents."]—*Am. P.*

herself thoroughly educated until she has acquired the blanched complexion of the French lady. She carries on an affected courtship with the downy-bearded young squire, Fritz, with his false calves, artificially enlarged thighs, and coat padded with feathers; a striking contrast to the shirt of mail of his great-grandfather. Siegwart, Idris, Musarion, Grecourt, and Ecole des Filles! are you not partly to blame for this climax of enervation?

But the philanthropic genius of the last quarter of this century saw all this abomination and destructive degeneracy, and deplored it. It resorted to bathing in cold rivers.

In these the tender sprouts of gentle lineage were immersed; they were forced to tramp over the frosty ground, bare-footed; bare-headed and with uncovered chest, and to rest for but a few hours on a hard bed.

Of thy good intention, dear genius, there could not be a doubt, even though the poor children from these experiments got their hands and feet frostbitten, died of consumption and catarrhal fevers, or in other ways shewed in lamentable manner that a hot-house plant should not be transplanted in November in order to accustom it to the northern climate.

Thy good intention, I repeat, could not be doubted, only the interpreters of thy counsels did not quite enter into thy spirit, and by their imperfect execution of them caused thy name to be reviled among the heathen.

Allow me (if I understand thee better) to translate thy heavenly ideas into the common language of mortals, and if not to inculcate doctrines, at least to throw out hints, as to how the effeminate race may be changed into men bearing at least a distant resemblance to the rock-like bodies of the ancient Germans; how they may, if engaged in business, manfully encounter the dangers of their calling, regardless of all variations in the weather, undergo the labours of life with courage and strength, and see their great grandchildren play like young eagles around their untottering knees.

Father Hippocrates, whose knowledge of mankind was of the most profound, remarks in one part of his writings that changes from one extreme to another cannot be undertaken without danger and caution, and I cannot too strenuously insist upon the truth of this observation. Nature does nothing without preparation; all her operations are performed gradually, and the more complex and artistic the work is that she performs, so much the more cautiously and gradually does she do it.

13

She never goes from summer to winter without interposing the transition period of autumn.

The cherry tree loaded with fruit would immediately wither and die if January followed immediately after June. She knows better how to prepare it for the winter's frost. She first causes the tree to drop its fruit, protects the buds for the next year by means of hard barks and balsamic resins, and during five months diminishes the circulation of its juices so gradually that the sap-tubes contract and the moisture in them is evaporated almost to dryness by January; she sends cold and ever colder nights and days, so that the biting frost, when it arrives, finds the tree prepared to encounter its tyranny. In an equally gradual manner does she put the sap again into circulation, until its activity, fostered by the increased warmth of spring and its rains, is in a condition to bear the full glow of the dog-days.

Let us imitate nature—let us never make January to follow close upon June, nor July upon January, if we do not wish our tender plants to be blasted and withered by both of these extremes.

The hardening of the human creature in respect to heat and cold no doubt is commenced with greatest safety in childhood (with older persons it is more difficult to effect such changes, just as it is more difficult to transplant an old tree to a new soil), but we require to exercise the greatest caution at first with these tender creatures, in order to prevent numbers of them from remaining behind, withering and fading during the transition to a mode of life to which they are unused!

When the sunshiny days commence, the gardener removes the shutters from the windows of his forcing frames; when the air becomes warmer he opens the windows to allow of the entrance of fresh air: he opens them more and more as the warm weather becomes more constant, and only transfers permanently to the open air the tender plants which he has thus accustomed as it were to the atmosphere, when he no longer dreads the occurrence of night-frosts.

The modern hardening methods seem to bear a great resemblance to the incautious transference of hot-house plants to the open air in February.

It is incredible what man can endure if he be gradually habituated to it. The Russian leaps into the ice-covered Neva the instant he creeps out of the stewing-hot sweating bath; the Halle brewer plunges into the Saale after roasting half naked

beside his brewing vat; the negro readily endures the heat of
the equator, and works under it like a horse; the Greenlander
goes forth to hunt the bear by moonlight in a cold of which we
can form no conception, and returns to his lowly hut, which is
filled by the exhalations from the large oil-lamp, and from his
own and other families, with a deteriorated air that would
almost suffocate a stranger; here he is cheerful and gay, and
gratifies his palate with things that disgust would prevent us
bringing near our lips.

If it be supposed that there are peculiar varieties of the
human species, that would be to make a great mistake; they
have come from their mother's womb as delicate and soft as
any of ourselves.

All these people, however, give their children no other education but their own example; they abandon them to their own
will until they have attained a good age.

The young creature at first creeps on all fours after his father
as far as he can, in heat and in cold, and creeps home again
when he can go no farther. This he does day after day, until
he can bear it better and go farther; no one forces him, he turns
back again when he has had enough, but he is always acted on
by that most powerful of all agents in education, the imitative
faculty, the desire to act as like his father as possible; this is a
stimulus that will not easily induce him to do anything that
might endanger his life, because he can unrestrainedly atten
to his sensations of pain, and of his own free-will return to
place of security. The stronger of the children of these people
(their young offspring know not the pleasure of mischief, as ours
do) assist the weaker, pull them out of the snow, fetch them
away from the burning sand-desert, or rescue them by swimming when they fall into the water, and thus the child learns
gradually (but only *gradually*, be it observed) to endure as much
as his father can.

The objection might fairly be made to what I have said that
this kind of gradual accustoming to heat and cold, and so forth
is not applicable to our education and to our mode of living.

This objection is a fair one, I repeat; but only partially so.
True, the father and the mother among us cannot become Samo-
jedes or Ethiopians, but the teacher of the children (be he a
peasant, a schoolmaster or a tutor) must have brought this kind
of hardening process to a certain degree of perfection in his own
person, he ought to have several children at once under his

superintendence, for the purpose of excittng emulation among them. Here it is much worse on the part of the teacher to err on the side of doing *too much* than *too little*. He may leave it to the free-will of the children to inure themselves; he does it before them, they imitate him, each according to his strength, and none must be forced to overstep the latter.

The teacher cannot put himself in the situation of the boy, cannot enter thoroughly into his feelings, consequently the boy must be allowed to draw back when he wishes to do so. He will rather have sometimes to keep him back, for imitation is often too powerful a spur.

It is best that these exercises should be carried on in the presence of the pupils only, without any other spectator, for then all present would be animated by the same mind.

But to send one's children with bare feet, head, chests and arms through the crowded streets of a town, accompanied by a well clothed tutor, amid the jeers of the boys in the street, and the audible expressions of compassion from the windows, would be to turn to ridicule an affair of great seriousness, and to inspire the children with an invincible repugnance to the hardening system generally.

When the children have played long enough in their ordinary clothing in the cold or in the heat, and if they have advanced so far as to be able in such guise to bear both extremes readily, we may proceed to diminish the amount of their clothing somewhat and by degrees, and even allow them to go with sundry parts of their person uncovered when they are alone.

But this should not be done in the severest winters, for the bodies of children will not be able to stand so much cold; there is besides no possible case when their being habituated to it would be necessary. Even beggar-children find rags to put their feet in, when they have no shoes; and we should only seek to prepare our children for the positions in which they may chance to be placed!

Here I must refer to what I should long since have spoken about. The new hardening-system commits the usual fault, of seeking to harden the body only in reference to the endurance of cold. But would it not be just as delicate, to be unable to endure heat? Persons who cannot bear the heat of the sun, or of very warm rooms, are liable to the most serious, even fatal accidents; why are they not accustomed to this also? To be able to endure cold, will not require much effort on the part of the Russian, but the alternations of heat and cold and vice versa (this great promoter of diseases in the delicate denizens of towns), these he endeavours to learn to endure by his alternate sweating and ice-water baths; to these he seeks to become quite indifferent. He attains his object, as we well know, and is the hardiest soldier history makes mention of.

But in the case of children this habituation to heat must also take place only gently and by degrees, and we should take care that they have not too much given them to do at first. They should have for their instructor a wise man, who knows the capabilities of each of his pupils, and he must not urge them on but rather keep them back, if he sees that his example is likely to make them go too far.

Frequent recreation (without witnesses, or among suitable companions) in the open air, in summer, will furnish many opportunities for this.

For pupils of more mature age, there can be no better opportunity for hardening them against the variations of temperature, than little pedestrian excursions. Here under the rational guidance of their master, they have at the same time an opportunity of habituating themselves to other inconveniences and dangers of the world; I allude to fatigue, the various atmospheres of different houses, to draughts, and damp.

One may be able to bear very well the pure, dry, cold air of winter, and the heat of summer, but readily get ill in a damp cellar-like room.

Draughts of wind are something quite different from the open air, and a damp stocking in cold weather may often cause one who is used to swimming to be laid on the bed of sickness. And yet all these are incidents occurring in human life, which can scarcely be escaped by him who mixes with the world, or who does not dread dangerous consequences to his health from such every-day trifles.

In all these exercitations it is necessary to employ caution when accustoming ourselves to them, beginning with the less and going on to the greater, but always only *gradually, interruptedly and by progressive advances.*

Very young children, that is, such as are not above seven years of age, cannot become very habituated to the deteriorated air of rooms. If we carry things too far with them we render them liable to become ricketty.

But since if we wish to render ourselves useful for business, we must also live in unhealthy deteriorated air, and be particularly anxious to preserve our health in it, so we must endeavour to render growing children capable of living not only in pure country air, but also in rooms; in rooms filled with people they must be able to exist at first for half an hour at a time, then for a whole hour, for several hours, and at length for whole days; and the hardening process must put them in a condition to remain well in spite of this, the most pernicious of all situations in which man can be placed. If their habituation be performed gradually, they will be able to do this bravely. Those children, however, should not be under ten or twelve years of age if we do not wish the whole plan to fail.

Pedestrian expeditions afford many opportunities for this also; these the teacher should direct, limit and define with wisdom and forbearance.

A teacher who is acquainted with the habits of life of the lowest class of peasants' children, and has observed how they have to bear all the discomforts of life, and to get a hardy body thereby, will be enabled to employ many of their practices upon his pupils.

When the peasant-lad, for instance, falls through the ice and gets wet up to the knees, he commences to jump about more vigorously than his companions; in order not to be laughed at, he carries on this process of warming himself by moving about until either he becomes quite dry, or until he can bear it no longer; he then goes home and dries his stockings. If he has got himself chilled, he does not much care, he only waits till he is dry and then runs out again to play with his companions.

If he has the care of horses he gains courage, if of oxen he learns patience, if he has to cart dung he learns to overcome his feelings of disgust, if he is engaged in mowing grass he acquires caution in handling sharp instruments, the rigour of the schoolmaster tends to make him docile, listening to a wretched sermon teaches him to be silent—from going barefoot his feet lose their tendency to get corns, gout and dropsy, climbing makes him lose his liability to turn giddy. His black bread needs no layer of butter, and his water requires not the addition of sugar and lemon-juice.

To unite the good that is to be found in this station of life with the cultivation of the mind, such is, in my opinion, the *ne plus ultra* of a rational and suitable education.

Gleaning corn in August, sheep-washing, crab-catching, tending the cattle in all kinds of weather in the open fields, as well when he remains motionless beside them as when he runs after them over the hills, fetching wood from the distant forest in all weathers, the damp school-room, the fair that excites disgust at the excesses committed, the three-hours' sermon in the cellar-like church—all these are excellent exercises and modes of hardening the body, which would be serviceable to a person in after life, whatever position he might occupy.

In the centre of a great and populous city it is utterly impossible to bring up healthy children, and equally so to harden their frames. Should they walk all through the town in order to get into the open country, they would be tired before they could escape from the depraved air of the city. Tired children could not endure any of the exercises we have proposed without getting ill; they would require strength, I might say a superlative degree of strength, to stand heat or cold, wind, damp, &c. Should they drive out of town, there are several difficulties in the way; to endure all sorts of weather seated in an open carriage can only be done by robust, grown-up people. Should they only drive out in good weather, then, during bad weather, confined to the air of the town rooms, they would go back farther than they had gone forward from the few exercises in the country. In shut-up carriages the space is so confined that the depravation of the air by breathing soon attains to a great height. If the carriage windows be let down, a draught is produced which the poor hot-house plants cannot bear.

In small towns of about a couple of thousand of inhabitants, or in the environs of larger towns, it is more possible to rear healthy and hardy children with proper care, provided we withdraw them gradually and as much as possible from the enervating influences of genteel life, and allow them to pass at least one-third of the day in the open air, mindful always of their relative strength and of the necessity of accustoming them gradually to all that is strange and unusual to them.

Children can be brought up healthy and hardy most easily and certainly at a distance from towns, for example on an estate or in a village residence, but the circumstances of all parents do not admit of this, and equally certain is it that we may, even in the most healthy villages, make our children delicate and puny. To do this we need only to deprive them of their freedom, to leave them usually shut up in the low, damp, hot room, to overload their stomachs, and to let them sleep in hot, soft feather beds, to encourage uncleanliness, and so forth.

But on the other hand the propinquity of a town offers so many advantages for the cultivation of the mind of growing children, that we should make the greatest sacrifices in order that, in all the circumstances in which we parents may be placed, we may give or cause to be given to the bodies and minds of our children the development most suitable for their destined situation in life.

PART II.[1]

SOCRATES AND PHYSON.
ON THE WORTH OF OUTWARD SHOW.

Socr. I am pleased that thou comest nearer me, Physon; I have been admiring thy beautiful garment at a distance.

Ph. It cost me a great many drachmas; thrice must the purple shell-fish yield its costly dye to produce this rich colour. Now none can compare with me; the greatest in Athens enviously makes way for me, and, only think! before I inherited my property, nobody cared an iota for me.

Socr. Then I presume thou art now worth infinitely more, art infinitely happier, than formerly, when thou usedst to dig my little garden for a scanty hire.

Ph. I should think so indeed! He that can regale himself for hours together at the most richly furnished table with the most delicious viands, that can set before twenty guests wine from the Cyclades fifty years of age, and complete their intoxication with the music of the lute and the sweet voices of female choristers, that can drive over great estates as the sole possessor, and can issue his commands to a hundred slaves—should such an one not be deemed happy?

Socr. But thou wast formerly a healthy, sensible man before thou inheritedst the property; thou hadst thy house, wast beloved by thy wife, thy children and thy neighbours; thou earnedst thy bread, together with an excellent appetite and robust health.— At what dost thou value thy fortune?

Ph.—At five millions.

Socr. How much richer dost thou esteem a man with a sound reason than that unfortunate maniac Aphron.

Ph. The greater richness of the former is to be measured by no amount of wealth.

---

[1] Published at Leipzig, in 1795.

Socr. At what price woldst thou part with thy five children?

Ph. Certainly not for all my wealth. Physicians would be kings could they make women fruitful or save children from death.

Socr. Thou art right, but in that case thy wife could not have been much less valued?

Ph. By Juno! I would not part with her for millions if she still lived! The charming woman, with whose fidelity and thriftiness and goodness, and excellent manner of bringing up children when I used to live upon boiled beans, all the treasures of the earth were not to be compared.

Socr. But blindness, lameness, a pair of deaf ears, and a lingering fever, thou wouldst suffer for an inconsiderable sum?

Ph. Zeus forbid! Dost thou imagine that this prospect of the sun gilding the mountain tops as in the morning it issues forth from the misty ocean, diffusing life and joy over all the habitable globe, that the melting song of Apollo's rival, the nightingale, that my warm blood, the healthy breath of my lungs, my strong stomach and my refreshing sleep, could be bartered by me for any amount of gold?

Socr. Hygieia preserve them to thee! But it seems from thy calculation that thou hast not become richer by thine inheritance than the sea-shore would become by the addition of a spoonful of sand. What are thy boasted five millions when compared with the innumerable millions of thy former blessings! Of a truth, when thou commencest to esteem thyself happy only after thou hast got this little addition, when thou lookest down so contemptuously on thy former apparently poor condition, I must pity thee; thou shewest thereby that thou hast never rendered the thanks due from thee to the immortal gods! I am sorry for thee, thou that was formerly so brave a man! Did they formerly regard less beneficially thy well-meant offering of salt and roasted flour, than they do now thy proud sacrifice of a bull? I am sorry for thee!

Go into the dark at midnight and feel the costliness of thy purple garment; thou seest nought, thou feelest nought but that thy nakedness is covered, and was not this also the case when thou performedst thy hard manual labour for a few oboli. Are the flatteries of thy fawning guests dearer to thee than formerly was the pressure of thy master's hand when he was pleased with thee? Dost thou really walk softer on thy gold-embroidered carpets than thou usedst to do on the unpaid-for green turf?

Perhaps the dark Persian wine now quenches thy thirst better than the spring that formerly trickled forth beside thy moss-grown cottage; perhaps thou risest now more refreshed from thy soft bed at noon, to which time a splendid supper causes thy sleep to be prolonged, than thou didst formerly from thy not very soft straw matrass, which the fatigues of the day's work made welcome to thee? Probably flamingoes' tongues served on gold plate, though from repeated repletion thou hast but little hunger left, are much more relished than milk and bread after hard work! Perhaps the thousand forced and artificial endearments of the hired girls that hover round thee now afford a purer, more permanent enjoyment to thy senses, nearly worn down to obtuseness, than did formerly the artless, trusting embrace of thy true and hearty wife in rare moments of happiness, when the unadorned black hair fell artlessly upon her neck browned by the sun, her constant heart throbbed for thee alone, and love for thee alone streamed forth from her dark eyes. Perhaps we live more secure from diseases, lightning and thieves, in marble pillared palaces, filled with numbers of dear-bought slaves, in beds inlaid with ivory, and beside bags filled with the precious metals, than in the lowly cottage covered with ivy, provided with the necessaries of life for several days to come, among honest neighbours and friends? Physon! Physon! mistake not the destiny of man, forget not the happiness of thy former days which the gods granted to thee, and which were dear to thee. Only ask thyself, if ever thou hast an hour to spare for this purpose, whether thou hast not more cause to envy thy former lot, than others have to envy thee thy present life!

Knowest thou the man that has just passed us clad in a coarse woollen garment? In his venerable aged form beams universal philanthropy. That is Eumenes, the physician. The many thousands that he yearly makes by the practice of his art, he does not spend on fine country houses and on the other vain trifles of the luxurious. His happiness consists in doing good! About the tenth part of his large income he uses for his limited wants, the rest he puts out to interest in the state. And how? thou askest me. To the poor he gives his aid, his medical skill. With his stores he supports the convalescent families until they can again help themselves, and with the costliest of his wines he revives the dying. He seeks out the miserable in their dirty hovels, and appears to them as a beneficent divinity; yes, when

the all-vivifying sun, the image of the unknown God, refrains
from shewing the dying its life-bestowing face, and even at midnight, he appears in the huts of the miserable to assist them,
and lavishes on them consolation, advice and aid.   They worship him as our ancestors worshipped the beneficent demi-gods,
Osiris, Ceres and Æsculapius.   Wilt thou soon commence to
envy him?   Go, Physon, and engage in some better pursuits,
and then count on my esteem.

PLANS FOR ERADICATING A MALIGNANT FEVER.

IN A LETTER TO THE MINISTER OF POLICE.

Sir,

You will, no doubt, yourself, see the results that the
infection that was brought to   *   *   *   four weeks ago might
produce if its farther spread be not arrested, still I consider it to
be a duty, as I have, here and there, had considerable experience
in extensive epidemics, to offer my mite at the altar of fatherland, in the form of some unpretending propositions.

Taking into account the malignancy of this fever, if the epidemic be left to itself, it may, in the course of half-a-year, at this
season, and in the present condition of the town, sweep away
about 250 individuals, a considerable human capital, seeing that
it is especially adults, the most useful class, that will first and
most certainly be cut off by it.   Should it, as soon will happen,
once penetrate into the damp dirty houses of the poor, who are
already often rendered liable speedily to catch the disease, by unhealthy miserable fare, by sorrow and depression, it is difficult,
very difficult, to extinguish it in these situations.   In addition to
this, there is the carelessness of the common people, who incline
to Turkish fatalism, as the most convenient of all creeds respecting Providence, and their want of reflection in only considering
as dangerous what they can see with their eyes, such as a flood
or a conflagration.   From these they will flee, but they are indifferent to a murderous pestilential vapour, because it does not
fall within the recognizance of their coarse senses.   So the ignorant person fearlessly approaches a charged electric battery, and
smilingly enters the pit filled with poisonous gases, though his
predecessor may just have been brought out of it dead.   Every
one thinks he possesses enough strength to resist the enemy of

life. But vain are his expectations; the giant himself if breathed on by the breath of death sinks down, and the wisest loses his consciousness. Resistance is not to be thought of. In flight, in flight alone, is safety.

The *only* means on which we can rely for checking epidemics in their birth, is the separation of the diseased from the healthy. But if it be left to the public to preserve themselves from infection, every one for himself, even with the help of published advice, experience teaches us that all such recommendations do little good—and often, in spite of the best intentions, cannot be carried out.

But just as the police, when a conflagration breaks out in the town, does not leave it to the caprice of the possessor of the house, to extinguish the fire in the way he thinks fit, but makes itself the necessary arrangements, and erects the fire-stations to be employed without delay, if necessary in opposition to the will, and even in spite of the resistance of the owner of the tenement,—acting upon the just principle, that the security of the community ought to weigh infinitely more than the property of an individual—in like manner, I assert it ought not be left to the individual's caprice to nurse his relatives affected with infectious disorders, in his house, since it is not to be presumed that he has either sufficient power, or judgment, or opportunity, to prevent the spread of the disease, and no amount of wealth on his part, no damages expressible in figures, can compensate for the life of one, not to speak of many families, fathers, mothers, husbands, wives, children, endangered by him.

Of a truth if ever the better part of the public ought anxiously to look to the authorities and to the police for protection, it is in the case of the invasion of epidemics, if the protecting divinities of fatherland do not stretch forth their powerful hands on that occasion, where else can we look for deliverance from the danger?

I could easily exhibit a picture of the most frightful scenes, that still haunt me from similar epidemics, whereby the most uncosmopolitan soul must be deeply moved—but to you, sir, such things are not unfamiliar, and you require not such reasons to induce you to put your hand to the work.

Taking for granted, then, that you concede the above premises, I make bold to make the following preliminary proposals, for whose efficacy experience is my warranty, and thereon I stake my honour.

They may all be set in action in the course of a few days; in this case speed saves expense and human life.

1. Let a hospital or other public building without the gates of the town be prepared, solely for the reception of such patients; the court-yard must be surrounded by a stone or wooden fence, as high as a man.

2. From twenty to thirty cheap bedsteads are requisite, provided with straw matrasses and frieze coverings.

3. The male and female nurses—of whom there should be one for every four or five patients—must always remain in the house with their patients, and should never go outside the door. The food and medicines they require should be brought to them daily in the open court by persons who should immediately afterwards retire, so that the two parties shall not approach within three paces of each other, and nothing should be brought from the house into the town.

4. In order to enforce this regulation, place a guard of two soldiers before the outer door, which they only are to open, and command them to let none but these persons and the physician and surgeon in and out.

5. A small sentry-box formed of boards will protect them from the weather, outside of which should hang a linen (or, still better, an oil-cloth) cloak for the physician and surgeon, which they should put on when they enter the house and lay aside on leaving it.

6. The medical officers should get a written notice of the mode in which it is desirable that they should protect themselves and others from infection, and the attendants of the sick should get instructions of a similar character.

7. All who fall ill of this malignant nervous fever in the town (the police officers should get a gratuity for all they detect) should be removed to the hospital by their friends in a covered sedan chair, kept for this purpose in the court-yard of the hospital, and there they should be taken care of and cured—(at the expense of their friends?).

Persons so dangerous to the community cease to belong to their friends; from the nature of their malady they come under the surveillance and care of the state, like a highwayman, a madman, a murdering quack-doctor, an incendiary, a robber, a poisoning courtesan, &c. They belong to the state until they are rendered innocuous. *Salus publica periclitatur* is the simple standard for determining all the wholesome regulations of a philanthropic police in such cases. To forbear pulling down neighbouring houses during a spreading conflagration, in consequence of the unreasonable request of their owners, this is a fault that no police now-a-days would commit. In the case we allude to, however, there is no pulling down, but on the contrary, building up. Men's lives, not houses, are to be saved.

Should my patriotic general propositions meet with your approbation, I shall not fail, if no one else does it, to treat of the subject in greater detail, and to furnish, in writing, the additional plans for the general weal, as circumstances prevent me taking a personal share in them.

If I could thereby prevent some misfortune, I should feel myself richly rewarded. But the reason why I, a private individual, occupying no official post, and not intimately connected with this country, wish to lend my aid in this matter, is owing to this, that I think that in such public calamities the motto should be *sauve qui peut!* and hence I am wont to exert myself to the utmost, and to save what can be saved, be it friend or foe.

I am, &c.

DR. H.

More particular directions.

The police officials ought to ascertain where any person has been suddenly taken ill in the town, or has suddenly complained of headache, rigour, stupefaction, or has rapidly become very weak and delirious; they should report what they learn to the appointed physician, who, after a rapid but careful examination, during which he attends to the directions below for avoiding infection, sees that the patient is conveyed to the hospital. At the same time the police officer receives his fixed remuneration.[1]

The large hall of the hospital should be divided longitudinally by means of a partition of boards; the one part so divided to form the patient's ward, whilst the other and much narrower division forms a kind of passage, into which the bedstead of each patient, which should be placed on castors, may be pushed through a trap-door in the partition, in such a manner as that only the patient in the bed shall come into the passage, where

---

[1] If this remuneration be considerable (about a thaler [3s. 6d.] for the discovery of every case of this kind), the progress of the epidemic will be speedily checked, there will soon be no more sick to be separated from the healthy. The sick will be discovered in time, before they can (easily) communicate the infection. Again in human life and in the smaller sum required, will be the manifest result.

on the trap-door falls to again. Here the physician examines the external and internal condition of the patient, in the presence of the surgeon, then he causes him to be pushed back into the ward, and the next patient to be brought forward, and so on.

But before performing this examination, and indeed before the arrival of the physician, all the windows of the passage should be opened in order to air it. Before the patients are brought in they must be closed.

The physician, accompanied by the surgeon, both covered with the oil cloth cloak,[1] visits the patients twice a day, and questions them at a distance of three paces. If he require to feel their pulse, he must do this with averted head, and immediately afterwards wash his hand in a basin containing water and vinegar. If the patient's face be directed towards the light, it is not difficult to observe the state of the tongue at a distance of three paces. At a less distance it is scarcely possible to avoid the danger of inhaling the patient's breath,[2] whence the contagious principle spreads farthest and most powerfully.

When the patient has a clean tongue,[3] as is found in those who are most dangerously ill, it is often advisable to give him large quantities of bark and wine, in place of any other medicine; and as it is to be apprehended that the nurse might make away with the wine, it is better to prescribe the bark and wine mixed, or for the physician to mix it himself. After every visit the medical officers should wash their hands and faces in vinegar and water.

The nurses must also be warned not to hold their faces near the patient's mouth, and after every time they raise up, turn or touch the patient, they should immediately wash their hands and faces. It is advisable to use a mixture of vinegar and water for the purposes of ablution.

Each bed should be provided with a linen matrass, well stuffed with straw,[4] over which is spread a linen sheet, and on

[1] When the disease is particularly malignant in its character, it is advisable to have a hood attached to the cloak, which the medical officer may draw over his head when he makes his visit, for it has been observed that the contagious matters attach themselves most readily to wool and hair.

[2] The odour of the contagious miasm of malignant typhus fever is a kind of earthy, mouldy smell, like that from old graves newly opened. It has little or no resemblance to the odour of putrid flesh.

[3] This disease was chiefly a goal-fever without anything in the first passages.

[4] Matrasses equally, smoothly and firmly stuffed with some vegetable substance,

this a piece of oil-cloth[1] about three feet in length, whereon the nates and back of the patient lie.

There should be two frieze-coverlets for each bed, in order that the one may hang all day long in the open air, whilst the other is covering the patient. They should be washed once a week by the nurses, together with the rest of the patient's linen, either in the open court yard, or beneath a shed only covered at top. They should first be washed clean in merely tepid water with soap, and subsequently scalded with boiling water, care being taken to avoid the steam that rises, and they should not be washed a second time until the whole is almost quite cooled down.[2]

The oil-cloth should also be frequently wiped with a wet cloth.

Every day at noon all the windows of the sick-room should be opened, and a draught of air kept up for an hour, during which the patients' beds should be pushed through into the ante-room, and remain there all the time.

In the centre of the ward should stand a stove, heated from within.[3]

The most trustworthy of the nurses must be responsible for the accurate carrying-out of these directions, as well as those of the physician.

---

as barley-straw, hay or moss, are for this object preferable to feather beds. The former allow the exhalations to pass through, do not retain the miasm so long, and as they are not so yielding form no wrinkles, and are cooler : they prevent the formation of those often fatal bed sores (*spacelus a decubitu*) so often met with in malignant fevers.

[1] By its smoothness it prevents the formation of bed-sores, and catches the fæces that often pass involuntarily in patients seriously ill. They may be easily removed without soiling the bed linen or matrass, which has a very bad effect on the purity of the air.

[2] A washerwoman in America had to wash some dirty clothes that had been brought over by a ship from England (among them were some that had been worn by a person who had recently recovered from small-pox in London), and she was immediately thereafter infected with malignant small-pox, from the hot steam that arose from the wash-tub. Boerhaave has brought forward abundant proof of the frequency and facility with which washerwomen are infected. He recommended soap not to be used in washing, probably because he thought that the miasmatic matter was more apt to be volatilized by it; but this danger is only to be apprehended from the employment of hot water.

[3] Stoves heated by a fire in their interior, and still more open fire-places, renew the air of the room very effectually as long as the fire burns (and also to a certain extent at other times), because the flame must always have fresh nourishment from the air which it draws through the vent-hole of the stove in large quantity. At the same time pure fresh air penetrates through the chinks of the windows, or through the the air-holes above them, into the room.

Those nurses who have already attended patients affected with the complaint, are more secure from infection than those who have not. To the former should be assigned the duty of the more immediate attendance on the patients. A new nurse should during the first days only be employed in work at some distance from the patients, such as scrubbing, sweeping, &c., until she is gradually habituated to the miasm.

The state of the health of the whole household should be every day carefully investigated by the physician, even though they consider themselves to be quite well. They should each day be reminded of the directions for their own preservation.

The excrements of the patients should be carried in well-covered night-stools to the most distant part of the court or garden, and there emptied in such a way that the wind shall blow the exhalations from them away from the bearer. This should be done by those of the nurses who are most habituated to the contagious virus (not by the new-comers), upon a thick layer of saw-dust, and the ordure immediately covered with one or several bundles of lighted faggots or straw, whereupon the nurse should withdraw, and allow the excrement to be consumed by the fire.

Two of the attendants who have been longest in the service should be appointed the bearers of the sedan-chairs, for the purpose of fetching new patients from the town. For this purpose they should each time put on clean clothes, and apply to the sentry, who will give them from a chest in the sentry-box a clean linen cloak, which they are to put on, leaving their house cloak hanging up on the outside of the sentry-box; they fetch the patient in the chair, and whenever they have brought him within the inner door (whence he is removed by others into the sick ward), they take off their clean cloak and return it into the custody of the sentry.

All the attendants, male and female, should wear a linen cloak in the house, reaching down to the feet; this should be washed at least once a fortnight.

The attendants cook the meals for themselves and the convalescents, but they ought to be supplied daily with fresh meat and vegetables; half a pound of the former should be reckoned as the daily allowance of each person. The male attendants should get about three pints of good beer a-piece, the females somewhat less.

They should get double the amount of the daily wages usual

14

in the town. It would be well to promise them additional re-muneration in the event of the happy termination of the epi-demic. It is inconceivable the power to prevent infection pos-sessed by the beneficent emotions, hope, content, comfort, &c., as also by the strengthening qualities of good living, and of that liquor that is so refreshing to such people, beer!

They should, moreover, have no lack of wood, soap, vinegar, lights, tobacco, snuff, &c.

If a clergyman is wanted for any of the patients, his visit must be paid in the presence of a physician, and the same for-malities must be gone through as when the latter makes his visit, namely, the passage must be well aired before the bed containing the patient is pushed through the trap-door. The physician instructs him how near and in what manner he may approach the patient.[1]

When a patient dies he must be immediately pushed through on his bed into the passage, and left there until the physician has convinced himself of his decease. The corpse is then to be covered with straw, and carried out on his bed into the court-yard or dead-house, where he is to be put, along with the clothes in which he died, into a coffin well stuffed with straw; the corpse should be covered with straw, and in the presence of the physi-cian and clergyman, conveyed to the churchyard in silence. The grave should be four feet in depth, and the coffin should rest upon a layer of faggots, and straw piled upon the top of it up to the level of the top of the grave. After the lapse of three days in this manner, the grave should either be covered over with earth, or, still better, the straw ignited and the miasmatic virus consumed along with the corpse, or at least dried till it is render-ed innocuous. This is a precautionary measure that cannot be too forcibly recommended.

When a patient recovers so as to be able to be restored to his friends, he should be taken into a clean room, the key of which should be kept by the physician alone, and there put into a bath and well washed over all the body, not excepting the hair, at first with clean warm water, and then sprinkled all over with vinegar before being finally dried. He is then to put on the clean clothes which his friends have sent him; and all his old clothes, without exception, are to be burnt in the court-yard, in

---

[1] By incautiously approaching the beds of such patients, I have frequently seen the most promising young clergymen infected and die.

the presence of the physician,[1] and finally he is to be accompanied home by the physician and surgeon.

Whenever a patient has recovered or died, the wooden close-stool he has used must be burnt in the open air, and the pot-de-chambre broken and the fragments thrown into the fire.

After the epidemic has been subdued, the male attendants should not be dismissed until they have whitewashed the whole of the interior walls of the house, not only the sick ward, but every other room, and the females not until they have thoroughly scrubbed all the floors, all the wood-work and all the utensils.

The sick-ward should then be heated in the early morning as much as possible, at least up to 100° Reaum., and after this heat has been kept up for two hours, all the windows should be opened and kept so till night.

Before they quit the house, both male and female attendants should bathe themselves, each sex in seperate apartments, and all their articles of clothing and the linen they have used during their residence in the hospital should be placed in an oven of about the temperature of a baker's oven after the bread has been removed (about 120° Reaum.), and kept there for at least a quarter of an hour,[2] the vent-hole being duly regulated the time.

After this is done, all the other linen or woolen articles which have been used by the patients, the straw matrasses (after taking out the straw), the towels, sheets, &c., should also be exposed for fully an hour to the same heat in the oven, and thereafter the bedsteads, after they have been well scoured, should be put in the oven and left there till it cools.

The straw out of the matrasses, the accumulated sweepings, rags, bandages, scrubbing cloths, brooms, and other articles of small value, should be burnt in the court-yard in the doctor's presence.

---

[1] Too much care cannot be taken to secure the destruction of such things, as the paltry love of gain of the nurses induces them to keep them for themselves, in spite of the danger to themselves and others of doing so.

[2] The pestiferous miasmata which have become attached to clothes, linen, beds, &c., can according to my observations be expelled from such things and *destroyed* by no means more certainly than by a heat of upwards of 100° Reaum., the higher the temperature the better, even should the articles suffer a little from its effects. The celebrated Cook expelled in this manner the morbific vapours that had become attached to the cabins of his ships and infected the walls; the efficacy of this measure is well known. The earliest physicians discovered the wholesome effect of fire and heat in destroying the plague virus, and their excellence is corroborated in our infectious epidenics by Howard, Lind and Campbell. It is moreover remarkable that all the infection of typhus fever ceases when ships are under the line.

In his presence the attendants should leave the house all together and the sentinels should be withdrawn.

The house may be allowed to stand empty, and reserved for similar purposes on a future occasion, one of the best-deserving male attendants, with his wife, being allowed to live in it gratuitously as housekeeper. Their business would be to see that the building is kept in good repair (in case it is required for another epidemic).

A house of this description and so arranged might subsequently be used with the greatest advantage, with some slight modifications, in epidemics of small-pox, measles, dysentery, and other infectious maladies dangerous to the population, and might be the means of preserving many useful citizens to the state.

There might be a few beds kept there permanently for the reception of all sick journeymen, beggars and trampers from the inns and lodging houses (a fine being imposed for the concealment of such cases), whereby a source of epidemics of no small importance, but one that is *frequently overlooked*, might be effectually checked at its origin.

This should be the duty imposed upon the housekeeper in return for his free dwelling, but at the same time he should receive an adequate (not paltry[1]) remuneration for each patient who recovers, whenever he leaves the house.

———

SUGGESTIONS FOR THE PREVENTION OF EPIDEMICS IN GENERAL, ESPECIALLY IN TOWNS.

A well-ordered police should take care that *rag-gatherers* are not allowed to live anywhere but in isolated houses near the paper mills,[2] nor should they be permitted to have in any house in the town a place where they may deposit the rags by little and little, only to remove them when they have collected a large quantity. The regulations prevalent in Electoral Saxony should be adopted, viz.: that the rag-gatherer should keep in the open street with his barrow or cart, by some signal summon

---

[1] If the remuneration be not very small, he and his friends take good care to be ever on the watch for any such patients that may have slipped into the town, and he will do his utmost to obtain it as speedily as possible by the rapid recovery of the patient, to the great advantage of the state (and of the patients).

[2] Which should never be built close to towns and villages.

around him those who have rags to sell, and not remain in the town with his collection of rags, but go into the country, and when he puts up at a country inn, leave his cart in the open court-yard, or before the door of the inn ; in a word, leave it in the open air.   He should be forbidden, under penalty of imprisonment, to pick out from his heap of rags and sell to others for their use any articles of clothing that may be still fit for wear.

They should also be forbidden to wear such articles themselves or put them on their children, which they will often do, to the great detriment of their health, as I have often observed. I have seen a malignant epidemic of small-pox spread over the country from so doing.

The *paper-mills* should be so arranged that the supply of the crude rags should be kept in well ventilated buildings far away from the dwelling houses, and the reception of the rags from the gatherer, and the weighing of them, in order to determine the sum he is to receive, should be carried on in a shed only covered at top.

The *dealers in old clothes* should only be allowed to carry on their trade in open shops, and should not be permitted to sell them in their houses under penalty of imprisonment.   All the linen and articles of clothing they have for sale in their shops should be previously washed, not excepting even the coloured and woollen articles ; and a police officer should be charged to examine if they be washed, who should overhaul the whole contents of the shop on undetermined days.   Every article that he finds still dirty should become his property after having shewn it to the inspector of police in the presence of the dealer.[1]

It should only be permitted to the burghers of the town to deal in old clothes.   Jews engaging in this trade should be deprived of their letters of protection.   Women found carrying it on should be put in the House of Correction.

The civic-crown merited by him who improves the *prisons* has been gained from us Germans by an Englishman—Howard. Wagnitz follows in his steps.   It is inconceivable how often the most destructive vapours are concentrated in these dens of

---

[1] Should it be feared that such an article of clothing, probably worn by a sick person, might prove dangerous to the policeman, it should be considered that the poor broker, in order to avoid such a loss, will most certainly take care to have none but clean washed things in his shop, and thus the police agent will have little or nothing to confiscate.

misery, fraught with death to those that enter them; how often their visiters are prematurely sent to the grave by fatal typhus. Destructive epidemic diseases often have their origin in these death-laden walls.

There are several kinds of prisons. I shall here allude only to those where the imprisonment is for life and to those gaols where prisoners guilty of capital crimes are kept until the termination of their trial, often for several years, the visitation or inspection of which is not unfrequently the cause of infectious diseases. Even when the prisoners themselves have not been ill of such fevers, their exhalations, their breath, and the miasm lurking about their dirty clothes, have often occasioned malignant fatal fevers. Heysham, Pringle, Zimmermann, Sarcone and Lettsom adduce a number of cases of this kind.

Now as in the true spirit of laws that are free from all barbarity, even the punishment of death should have (and can have) no other aim than to render an incorrigible criminal innocuous, and to remove him from human society, what else can both these kinds of imprisonment be than rendering the prisoner harmless, in the former case for life, in the latter for a certain time pending the duration of the trial. None but Syracusan tyrants could dream of uniting a more inhuman object with such prisons.

If then the gaol even for capital offenders can and ought to be nothing but a means of depriving them of all opportunity of injuring society, in that case every torture that is unnecessarily inflicted on them when thus in custody *is a crime on the part of the police.* I only allude here to the pain inflicted on them by unhealthy (disease-producing) prisons. In order to avoid this, prisons should never be raised less than four feet above the ground, and the openings of the windows, while they are sufficiently narrow, should be always so long as to allow the free access of fresh air. Where two windows opposite each other cannot be obtained (which is the best plan), there ought to be at least three windows for each small cell. The floor should either be paved with slabs of stone or better, with rounded stones, so that it may be deluged and scrubbed, once a week, with boiling water. The walls and roofs should be lined with wooden boards, like the peasants' houses, in order to allow of their being also washed with hot water,[1] as is customary with

---

[1] The exhalation from these wretched creatures, that constantly tends to decomposition, and the animal poison developed from their breath, whereby the air of their

the country people. By these means these dismal habitations are at all events rendered dry residences, and the cachexias and tumours so frequently met with in such as have undergone a long imprisonment are in a great measure prevented. If it were possible to construct an air-hole for the purpose of carrying off the deteriorated vapours into the open air, gaols would thereby lose much of their dangerous aptitude to generate pests. The prisoner should have at least once a week a bundle of fresh straw for his bed. His bed-cover, together with his clothes and linen, should be washed at least once a week in hot water. He himself should be forced, before putting on his clean clothes, to wash his body all over. His chamber utensil should be emptied daily, and rinsed out with boiling water. He should be allowed to walk about in the open air at least once a week, for at least an hour at a time.

When he is removed from prison, his cell must be prepared for the reception of future prisoners by washing anew the floor, the walls and the roof with hot water, and by placing a small stove in it, the funnel of which goes out at the window. With this the cell is to be heated very highly, so that the heat shall almost take away one's breath (up to 120° Reaum.), and then the stove should be again removed, supposing it is not allowed to have one in the cell.

If not, an iron tube communicating with the open air should open in the floor of the cell, passing in winter through a heated stove, in order to conduct in a supply of fresh warm air.

It is great cruelty to shut up many prisoners together without allowing at least 500 cubic feet of space and air for each. If this be not allowed, the better ones among the prisoners are exposed to much annoyance by the bad behaviour of the worse ones; and it is incredible the rapidity with which that most destructive of all animal poisons, the virus of the most fatal pestilence, is generated. Police authorities, be humane!

I scarcely need to remark, that the (often long-continued) imprisonment of debtors who are frequently deserving of compassion, ought to be made at least as innocuous for the health of the prisoners, of the turnkeys, and of those who visit them, &c., as that of criminals.

When *foreign prisoners* or *field-hospitals* are introduced into a

---

narrow cells is deteriorated, attaches itself in great quantity to the walls of gaols, and in course of time degenerates into a pestilential miasm; by the process above described it is removed and washed away by the boiling water.

healthy country in time of war, whether temporarily or permanently, the authorities, if they have it in their power to act, should take care that an epidemic is not thereby brought into the country.

Prisoners of war, who are not unfrequently suffering from typhus and putrid fevers, in their transit through a country, are generally, when remaining for the night in towns, lodged in the town-halls, apparently in order that they may be kept more securely. But how often has this practice given rise to the spread of epidemics!

It would be safer to quarter them in large coach-houses, stables, barns, &c., outside the town, to make them lie undressed on straw matrasses, keeping them warmly covered in winter, and in this manner retaining them until their march can be renewed.[1] If the season of the year admit of it, they must be compelled to wash each other's clothes and linen with hot water, and to dry them in the open air.

The most destructive pestilences are most easily engendered by *military-hospitals*. It would be the most disgraceful barbarity even in an enemy, to erect them in the middle of towns.

But if, nevertheless, this is done, there remain for the poor town's-man, if they bring pestilence along with them, as they usually do, very few means of preserving the life and health of himself and family, and these he should carefully attend to.

If he will not or cannot leave the town, he must at all events avoid all intercourse and communication with the sick, with infected houses, and even with those who frequent such houses. If they bring him any thing he should take it from them at his house-door or in the open court. Should it be articles of clothing or linen, he should not make use of them before he has plunged them into hot water mingled with vinegar, in the open court, or thoroughly fumigated them with sulphur. Should it be articles of food,[2] let him not partake of them before preparing them on the fire, or otherwise heating them.

---

[1] On the march they have plenty of air and exercise; in this way they get rest and warmth, and are incapacitated from making their escape.

[2] A person who is exposed to the danger of infection, should not allow his courage to sink, should not leave off any of his accustomed comforts, rest, exercise, food, or drink; but he should also carefully avoid all excess in any of these things, as also in passions, venereal excitement, &c. The other prophylactic measures that should be adopted will be found in the first part of the "Friend of Health." A slight increase of stimulants, such as wine, tobacco and snuff, is said to be a powerful prophylactic against infectious disorders.

Infectious diseases have even been communicated by money and letters; the former may be washed in boiling water, the latter fumigated with sulphur.

Although the animal poisons called infectious miasmata are not infectious at the distance of several paces in still open air, so that we may (with the exercise of great care) preserve our house free from infection in the midst of houses where the malady is raging, we should remember that a draught of air can carry the miasm arising from a sick person to a distance of many paces, and then occasion infection.

On that account we should avoid traversing narrow lanes where we should have to pass close by a sick person, and for a similar reason we should shun narrow passages through houses. Above all we should refrain from looking into an open window and conversing with people in whose house or room cases of infectious disease may exist.

Acquaintances kiss each other or shake hands; this ceremony should be omitted when the danger is so iminent, as also drinking out of another's glass. We should particularly avoid making use of a stranger's water-closet, or allowing a stranger to use ours.

At such times we should never bring second-hand furniture[1] into our premises.

Domestic animals that are given to rove, such as dogs and cats, often carry about with them in their hair the virus of infectious diseases. For security's sake it is advisable to get rid of them at such times, and not to allow strange dogs or cats to approach us.

The drying up of *marshes* and *old ditches* close to human dwellings has frequently been the occasion of the most murderous pestilences.[2]

If the fosse surrounding the town is to be cleared out or dried

---

[1] I have seen putrid fevers occur periodically for many years in the country, merely by old furniture, which had belonged to persons who had died of such affections, coming into other families by purchase.

[2] I saw the fortieth part of the inhabitants of a large town die of typhus, in consequence of the incautious draining of the town fosse.

Whenever the slime of such a town fosse, which may have been accumulating for many, perhaps hundreds of years, is deprived of the fresh water covering it, the half putrified animal matters contained in it immediately pass into the last stage of decomposition. This last stage of decomposition of animal substances is infinitely more poisonous than all the previous ones, as we may see in the rapid fatality of the exhalations from cess-pools which have not been cleared out for thirty years or more. Of this more hereafter.

up, as is highly desirable for the health of the inhabitants of all towns, this work should only be undertaken in the depth of winter. The water should be carried off in the form of ice-layers, and the ice that forms again in a few nights should next be taken away, and so on till no more water remains.

But as the removal of the mud from town-ditches is much preferable to letting it gradually dry up, seeing that throughout the whole time required for the latter, noxious vapours are constantly exhaling, there is no better time for removing it than in severe cold. The mud which is always in a state of putrefaction is always warm, and never freezes so much as to prevent its being easily dug out in winter. We can also more readily dispense with draught-cattle on account of the excellent condition of the roads in severe frosty weather.

After great *inundations* on flat land, the spontaneous drying up of which cannot be expected to take place in a short time, it is requisite that all should lend a hand to cut ditches through and round about the inundated country ; but if it is impossible to drain off the water into the river on account of its low level, a number of small wind-mills must be erected in order to pump off the water as quickly as possible and dry the land; for if this be not done the water readily takes on the putrefactive process, giving rise from spring to autumn to dysenteries and putrid fevers.

The *low-lying houses that have been inundated* by the water are a fertile source of epidemic diseases (see Klöckhoff). The police authorities must see that every householder digs a deep ditch round his premises, and especially round his dwelling-house; that he has all his windows and doors open for the greater part of the day; that he occasionally lights fires even in summer; and that in winter, at all events before he rises in the morning, all the doors and windows are left open for an hour at a time.

There are places that are destitute of the (often unacknowledged benefit of a sufficient supply of *fresh* flowing *water*, in place of which the inhabitants are obliged to make use of spring or rain-water brought from a distance, or to put up with rain-water only. In all such cases they collect their supply of water for a long time in large reservoirs, in which it becomes stale in a few days and furnishes a very unwholesome drink, the source of many diseases. Soon, it again becomes clear and inodorous; but in a short time the putrefaction recommences, and so it goes on until the water is all consumed, the greater part of it in a very bad state. I shall not here attempt to determine whether these disadvantages might not be obviated by the construction of artificial aqueducts on no very expensive scale, or of (very deep) wells; but I am convinced that in flat localities on firm soil it is possible to resort to one or other of these plans, whatever may be alleged against it by the paltry parsimony of many corporations, who look on unmoved whilst many such communities gradually die out. In the absence of such a radical cure, I would advise every householder to keep his supply of water in casks, in which for every 400 pounds of water one pound of powdered wood charcoal should be thrown, which, according to the discovery of Lowitz, possesses the power of preserving water from putrefaction and of making stale water sweet. The clear fluid may be drawn off when required through a tap provided with a tight linen bag.

A similar precaution against the production of disease is adopted in large *ships* that go to sea, which are often reduced to great straits on account of a deficient supply of fresh water. But many causes conspire in ships to produce destructive[1] diseases. Among these are the mode of feeding the crew so much in vogue, with often half-decayed, dried and salted meat, with unwholesome fatty substances of various kinds; the want of fresh air when during continued storms they have to pass many days together below deck with the port-holes closed, when the exhalations from their bodies increase to a pestilential fetor; the exhaustion of the sailors when kept at work too long, during which their wet clothes check the perspiration. These causes engender and keep up scurvy, dysentery, and other maladies.

The risk of such disorders may be avoided by the following measures: supplying vegetable food, and in the absence of green herbs, dried legumes that so easily ferment; sour-crout; sometimes brown sugar in place of oil; brandy for strengthening; meat-soups boiled down and dried, in place of kept meat; malt-liquor to drink in addition to water; the division of labour into eight-hours' work; care that the crew have always dry clothes to put on, and that their habits are cleanly; frequent pumping out of the necessary; and the purification of the air between decks by means of large braziers of burning charcoal according to

---

[1] Major Nante observed during the war betwixt England and North America a pestilential gaol-fever break out on board the fleet lying off the Havana, of such severity that numbers of men who seemed to be in perfect health died after an illness of not more than from three to four hours.

Cook's method. The frequent washing with sea-water of the various utensils, the floor, the walls and the decks, must not be neglected. If powdered charcoal be mingled with the sea-water used in scrubbing, the stench of the walls will be effectually got rid of. In addition to all this care should be taken not to take on board sick persons, or such as have scarcely recovered from illness; and all the utensils and furniture should be frequently exposed to the air on deck when the weather is good.

By the employment of Sutton's method of conducting leaden pipes into all parts of the ship which all terminate in the kitchen fire-place, the deteriorated air will most certainly be drawn off by the fire. But Cook's braziers do much more, for they heat the walls, and thus destroy the contagious matter much more effectually. Hale's ventilator (a kind of wooden bellows) are little used in ships. Would not the so-called garden-cress (*lepidium sativum*) be a valuable vegetable, or at all events be useful on board ship as a medicine, in order to diminish the noxious matters in the first passages? The facility with which its seed grows is well known. We only need to strew it upon a piece of old wet sail cloth, and cover it with unravelled pieces of old moistened tow.

In towns where no rapid stream of water can be conducted through even the small streets wherein the animal excrements, the washing-water, the urine and other impurities of men and animals can be carried off without doing any harm, covered *cess pools* cannot be dispensed with.

These cess-pools are always a bad thing for the health of man, from their aptitude to engender, or at least to promote, pestilence.

In order to render them as innocuous as possible, they should be built up with masonry, not only on the roof and walls, but they should also be paved on the floor with stones cemented together, in order that the putrefying impurities may not sink into the ground, but be capable of being taken clean away. They must be frequently cleansed out, and the odour removed quickly.

The time selected for cleansing them should be during the prevalence of a strong wind, more especially one from the north, north-east, east or south-east, and those days should be avoided when a long period of warm rain, calm and foggy weather, with a low state of the barometer prevails.

Though we are not able to adduce any instances in which the exhalations from *old privies* have spread a pestilence of any duration, yet no good police which attends to the health of the community should permit them; and moreover, cases have occurred where workmen suffocated in such places have spread such a virulent exhalation from their clothes, that many of those approaching them have been cut off by typhus fever.

In order to avoid the pestilential poison proceeding from animal substances in the last stage of putrefaction, the most destructive of all poisons, the removal of such murderous pits should be advised, and no sensible person will object to this.

But when they are already in existence and require to be cleared out, we must not go to work incautiously. The simplest method of freeing such pits from their poisonous exhalations is always the lowering into them of small loose bundles of ignited straw attached to a wire, since there is rarely in them any inflammable gas that might endanger the house by its ignition. These bundles are to be let down to the depth at which they will almost be extinguished by the vapour, and then they should be allowed to burn out. This process is to be repeated with larger and larger ignited bundless until the stratum of gas is removed to the very floor of the pit, and atmospheric air occupies the place of the fire-extinguishing gas. But our precautionary measures should not cease here: for it is not only want of atmospheric air that kills the workmen in such situations, but still more the vapour that rises, though not to any great height in consequence of its weight, from stirring up the human excrement that has entered on the last stage of putrefaction. In order to render this as harmless as possible, a quantity of dry faggots ignited should be thrown into the pit, sufficient to cover all the bottom of it, and there they should be left till they are totally consumed. The heat thus generated will, after the lapse of an hour, have rendered the odour innocuous to at least a foot in depth. This quantity should then be removed by the workmen; faggots are then to be burnt as before on what is beneath, whereupon the next layer is removed, and so on until it is all cleared away.

Should it really prove true, that the most of our police authorities have abolished burials in churches, we should not be thereby set quite at our ease. *The old graves* still exist in our churches, in which the last and most poisonous stage of decomposition of the dead bodies has not yet ceased to emit its destructive emanations.[1] Hence alterations and building operations in the

---

[1] It should be borne in mind that the most fatal gas generated by the last stage of putrefaction does not readily rise, but is heavy, and not unfrequently reposes in a

floors of such churches are fraught with manifest danger to the life of the workmen and the congregations in the churches, whence diseases may spread over a considerable portion of the population.

In June, 1773, a grave was opened in the church of Saulieu, Burgundy, and church-service performed soon afterwards, in consequence of which, 40 children and 200 grown-up people, together with the clergyman and sexton, were assailed by the exhalation that arose, and carried off by a malignant disorder. Moreover, it has not yet been perfectly ascertained how many years the contagious principle may remain attached in undiminished virulence to the buried corpses of those who have died of malignant diseases.

In many countries, *the lying in state of all bodies* is very properly forbidden. But in others where not so much enlightenment prevails, infectious diseases are often propagated by the exposure of such poisonous bodies, of which I could adduce many examples from Saxony.

In 1780 a girl brought a putrid fever with her to Quenstädt from Aschersleben. All her numerous brothers and sisters and her parents took ill of it, one after the other, but they all gradually recovered except one grown-up daughter, who died of bed-sores. I took the greatest pains to prevent the disease being propagated to others from this house. I succeeded in this for five months until this girl had to be buried. The young men of the village bore the body in a coffin nailed up according to my directions, to the grave. Here, from their attachment to the deceased, they disobeyed the strict orders given by my friend, the clergyman; they forced open the lid of the coffin, in order to see the corpse once more before it was let down into the grave. Others, moved by curiosity, approached. The third and fourth day thereafter, all those that had been guilty of this excess, lay mortally sick of this fever, as also all those who had come near the grave (some of them from neighbouring villages,) to the number of eighteen, of whom only a few escaped death. The epidemic of putrid fever spread around at the same time.

It is not desirable that those important personages in the state called *inspectors of the dead* and *corpse washers*, whose business it originally was to form a silent judgment respecting the kind

_____

low stratum above the corrupting matter, until it is stirred up, and is thus rendered dangerous to life.

of death that had occurred, and to verify the decease, should receive from the juridical medical officer accurate instructions on this by no means easy point, before undertaking such an important, such an exceedingly important duty ? How many lives of those apparently dead might they not be instrumental in restoring, how many cases of murder might they not detect, and, what interests us peculiarly in this place, how often might they not discover that some who have died without having been seen by any physician, might have laboured under contagious diseases?

We should not be too rash with bodies brought to the *dissecting rooms*, not receive such as we may suspect to have died of contagious diseases, nor keep the subjects until they are in the last stage of putrefaction, nor, for the sake of bravado, have too much to do with macerated parts in a state of extreme decomposition, and often melting away under our touch, which can no longer teach us anything. Examples are not wanting of the students who were merely looking, on being rendered dangerously ill thereby.

But chiefly are the contagious pestilences in towns harboured, renewed, promoted, and rendered more contagious and more murderous, in the small low, *old houses*, situated close to the town-walls, huddled together in narrow *damp lanes*, or otherwise deprived of the access of fresh air, where poverty dwells, the mother of dirt, hunger and despondency. In order to save firing and the expensive rent, several miserable families are often packed close together, often all in one room, and they avoid opening a window or door to admit fresh air, because the cold would enter along with it. He alone whose business takes him into these abodes of misery, can know how the animal matters of the exhalations and of the breath are there concentrated, stagnant and putrefying; how the lungs of one are struggling to snatch from those of another the small quantity of vital air in the place, in order to render it back laden with the effete matters of the blood; how the dim, melancholy light from their small darkened windows is conjoined with the relaxing humidity and the mouldy stench of old rags and decayed straw; and how grief, envy, quarrelsomeness and other passions strive to rob the inmates completely of their little bit of health. In such places it is where infectious pestilences not only smoulder on easily and almost constantly, when a spark falls upon them, but where they take their rise, burst forth and even become fatal to the wealthy citizens.

It is the province of the authorities and the fathers of the country, to change these birth-places of pestilence into healthy, happy, human dwellings. Nothing is left for me but to turn my face away from them, and to keep my compassion to myself.

If, however, the inmates of them be not without employment, their systems, accustomed to meagre fare and hard work, resist infections tolerably well; but when they are out of work, when *dearness* of the first necessaries of life and *famine* prevail among them, then, from these dirty sources of misery and woe, diseases of malignant character and pestilences perpetually issue. It is only since the fearful years 1771, 1772 and 1773, that some rulers have learned, from the dangers to which they themselves were exposed, to provide for the safety of their many thousand subjects, by establishing corn-granaries and flour-magazines against seasons of scarcity.

I must make the general observation belonging to this place, that most of our towns are not adapted, not calculated, to promote health. High town-walls and ramparts are now generally acknowledged to be useless for towns that are not fortified. That they are injurious by preventing the access of fresh air, will also be readily conceded. But that the masses of houses of most towns are too closely huddled together is not yet generally seen, and when it is, it is attempted, but without success, to be excused, by the greater facilities offered for business and trade by having everything within a small circle.

In towns about to be built, it should not be allowed to build houses higher than two stories, every street should be at least twenty paces in width, and built quite straight, in order that the air may permeate it unimpeded, and behind every house, (the corner houses perhaps excepted,) there should be a court-yard and a garden, as broad and twice as long as the house. In this way the air may be readily renovated, behind the houses in the considerable space formed by the adjoining gardens, and in front in the broad and straight streets. This arrangement would be so effectual for suppressing infectious diseases and for preserving the general health,[1] that if it were adopted most of the

---

[1] The deteriorated air in closely built towns with high houses is especially injurious to children and gives rise to those deformites of the beautiful human figure denominated rachitis, which consists of a softening of the bones, combined with laxness of muscles, inactivity of the lymphatic system, and a high degree of irritability. The non-medical observer does not readily notice the large number of these pitiable little monstrosities in closely built towns, partly because a great many of them sink into the grave in the first years of their life, partly because the cripples who escape conceal themselves for shame from the public gaze.

precautionary measures against pestilence I have inculcated above would be rendered to a great degree superfluous. What advantages in this respect do not Neuwied, Dessau, &c., possess!

The handsome, roomy, high and airy *bucthers' shops* we meet with in some towns, (*e. g.* Dresden) are not so good as the open butchers' stalls standing in market places, and only covered by a roof. A putrid stench is always concentrated in the shops built for the sale of meat.

The shops for the sale of stock-fish and herrings should be situated in the open air, at the outside of the city-gates; the disgusting stench that proceeds from them is sufficient evidence of their unwholesomeness.

Were it possible to banish entirely from the interior of towns all the manufactories and warehouses of the butchers, soap-boilers, parchment-makers, catgut-spinners, glue-boilers, and all other trades that are engaged with animal substances that become readily decomposed, and to transfer them to special buildings outside the town-gates, this would be a great advantage as regards infectious diseases. I have seen many butchers' houses in narrow lanes completely cleared of their inmates in epidemics, whilst the houses in the neighborhood suffered much less severely.

It is astonishing how the indolence of that class of men who cherish their prejudices, inspires them with such deep respect for some things that appear horrible to them, so that there is with them but little difference[1] betwixt them and things that are holy. It can only be attributable to this unaccountable prejudice that the *bodies of dead domestic animals,* as also those persons who have to do with them, have been considered as not to be meddled with and as exempt from the regulations of a good police. Owing to this, great confusion and injuries to the health of the community have resulted. In this place I shall only complain of the custom of leaving the bodies of dead domestic animals in the open air, on greens and commons not far removed from the dwellings of man, a custom so opposed to all ideas of the preservation of health.[2] If, as is assuredly the case, all putrefying animal sub-

---

[1] It is curious that in almost all languages the same expressions are applied to the most horrible as well as to the most revered things—*schaudervoll, sacer, awful,* are instances in point.

[2] Does this custom originate in the vanity of man, who thinks to vindicate his right to the title of sole lord of creation by assuming to be alone worthy of the high honour of being buried beneath the ground, and to shew his supreme contempt for animals (even of such as are most useful and most valuable to us), gives them the vilest names and leaves them unburied in the open air, in defiance of nature which seeks to conceal all putrefying processes from the public gaze?

15

stances make a horrible impression on our senses, if, moreover, all contagious diseases are hatched in corruption, how can we imagine that such large masses of putrefying flesh of horses and horned cattle, particularly during periods of great mortality among cattle, can be a matter of indifference as far as human health is concerned. The thing speaks for itself!

It is in large well-regulated towns only that I have met with some (although seldom sufficient) attention directed to the *sale of spoilt-food*, especially animal food. In districts where fish abound, many kind, especially smaller ones, are brought to market with all the signs of putrefaction upon them. They are chiefly purchased by poor people, because they are cheap— nobody gives himself any concern about the matter, and the labourer when he is taken ill throws the blame of his sickness on any cause but the right one. Nobody concerns himself; the seller of this pernicious food returns home after having pursued his avocation unimpeded. The authorities who may perchance hear of it, say to themselves : Where there is no complainant, there is no judge. Can such be called Fathers of the town? Other kinds of spoilt food can also produce infectious typhus fever.

In large *manufactories* and *workhouses* where the workpeople live in the house, those who fall ill should, whenever they commence to complain, be immediately separated from the healthy workmen, and kept apart until they have completely recovered their health. And even where the workmen reside out of the house but come to work together in large workrooms, it is the duty of the master manufacturer, especially at the time of the prevalence of epidemics, to send home immediately such of the workmen as begin to complain of illness. Great care should be taken always, but especially when disease is about, to have the workrooms and warerooms well aired and clean.

Public schools are generally places for the diffusion of contagious diseases, such as small-pox, measles, scarlet fever, malignant sore throat, miliary fever, (hooping cough?) and many skin diseases. If schoolmasters in general were given to attend more to the physical and moral training of their pupils than to cramming their memories, much mischief of this character might be prevented. It should be impressed upon them not to admit any sick child to the classes, whose altered appearance betrays the commencement of a disease. Besides, a sick child can learn nothing.

In times of prevailing sickness the clergymen should publicly warn the members of their congregations, not to come to church when they are feeling indisposed, and thereby expose their neighbours to danger.

I cannot here enter into details regarding the power of bad arrangements in *poor houses, houses of correction, orphan asylums* and *invalid hospitals,* as also of *ordinary hospitals* and *infirmaries,* in producing and promoting infectious diseases, and still less can I describe the best plans for such institutions designed for the relief of the most miserable classes of society. The subject is too important, and in many respects much too vast to be dismissed here with a few words.

ON THE SATISFACTION OF OUR ANIMAL REQUIREMENTS, IN ANOTHER THAN A MEDICAL POINT OF VIEW.

Man seems manifestly created for enjoyment. This is the language of the infant when it cries for its mother's breast; this is the language of the shivering old man as he pokes the fire; this is the language spoken by the child playing with its doll, of the girl eager for the dance, of the youth disporting himself in the bath, of the matron preparing for the domestic festival, of the delighted look of the father returning home from his daily work, as old and young run out to meet him.

All creation around him is happy and rejoices; why should man, endowed as he is with finer sensibilities, not do so likewise?

Certainly he ought to do so. But in his choice of enjoyments and in the quantity of them he indulges in, he alone transgresses the bounds of moderation; he alone of all living beings. No animal living in a state of a freedom partakes of any food except what is suitable for its nature and health; it consumes no more than what it requires for its well-being; it drinks not after its thirst is quenched; rests itself only when it is weary; and indulges in sexual pleasures only when the period for the propagation of its species has arrived, and when its matured irresistible instinct attracts it to the delightful object of its desires.

The satisfaction of our animal requirements has no other object than the preservation of our life, our health, our species; the pleasure accompanying it is lively and great in proportion to the strength and completeness of the requirement, but in the happiest class of human beings (those who live in conformity with nature) it instantly assumes a shade of indifference as soon as the requirement has received the appropriate degree of satisfaction.

When we pass the boundary line beyond this moderation, as is so frequently the case among the higher and middle ranks of society, luxury, gluttony and depraved sensuality commence. Persons in easy circumstances are apt to imagine that the excessively multiplied indulgence in excitement of the senses of all kinds is *to live* in the true sense of the word. "*I have lived much,*" says the enervated voluptuary; to me it seems that he has lived *little*.

To every human being only a certain amount of corporeal enjoyments has been allotted, which his nervous system is capable of partaking of and of indulging in only to that amount without prejudice to the health. The temperate man easily discovers these limits assigned to his organization by experience uninfluenced by partiality, and in the observance of the laws he has discovered he is happy, happier than the intemperate man can have any idea of.

But if, seduced by bad example or by the flattering advantages of fortune, I should exceed the measure of indulgence consistent with my health, I shall find that this excess is at first repugnant to my senses. There occur satiety, disgust—the warnings of nature in her wisdom! But if I go on undeterred, making it my business to force more indulgencies upon my body than is consistent with its well-being; if I employ ingenious methods, by means of stimulants of various kinds, to coax the nerves fatigued by the excess, to the reception of new and immoderate enjoyments, I shall doubtless at length be enabled to indulge in debauchery, that is, to burden my nerves with an unnatural number of impressions, which the temperate man could not bear; but this is only a semblance of greater enjoyment. There is no reality in it.

In proportion as we seek to increase to multiply our animal enjoyments by unnatural means, our other senses become blunted, and commence to derive less and less pleasure from a number of enjoyments.

By spices, condiments, and fiery wines, the gourmand must seek to keep the nerves of his tongue up to the mark to enable them to allow still more food to pass down his throat, and at length he comes to such a state that even his highly seasoned dishes are relished no more, and he must stir up his respected *chef de cuisina* to invent something new to tickle the languid palate of his poor master, and so to over-stimulate the cardiac orifice of his stomach that it shall forget its office to reject what is superfluous. If his honour have fully satisfied his appetite with the first two dishes, the omnipotent genius of his cook must follow these up by one or more dozen dishes, which by their elegant appearance, their enticing odour, the dissimilarity of their taste, and their stronger seasoning, shall deceive, ever anew, ever more powerfully, the sister senses, and particularly the sense of taste.

But this is only a vain artifice, an imaginary greater enjoyment, not a real enjoyment, accompanied by inward entire gratification. It is all vain, vain pitiable imagination.

The thresher regales himself with his black rye-porridge, with his potatoes and salt, much more than his worshipful lord and master, though his meal may not perhaps have cost a thousandth part of the latter's sumptuous repast. The former is gay and happy over his frugal fare, and sleeps soundly until the cheerful morn wakes him up refreshed and vigorous; whilst the latter in his satiety finds the world too small for him, and his dull, dream-beset slumber scantily fills up the long hours of night, until he rises unrefreshed from his soft down bed, with confused head, foul tongue, and spasmodic yawning.

Whose repast was worth most? which of the two had the higher, the more genuine enjoyment, the greater sensuous pleasure?

The ploughman who only drinks his pot of beer in an alehouse on a Sunday after church, has in the few hours he spends over it perhaps twice as much enjoyment for his few half-pence as my Lord Mayor who can boast perhaps of having swallowed during the week a thousand times as much money in luscious Constantia wine. The former quenched his thirst on working-days at a spring behind his cottage, and was refreshed whilst the latter was made hot, sleepy and stupid, by the excessive quantity of his costly liquor.

Which of the two best enjoys life? which has the higher enjoyment?

In vain does the libertine imagine that the disgusting dissipation of his faculties that were created for higher objects can procure him great pleasure and real enjoyments. Not to speak of the enervation and the innumerable sufferings that must result from his head-strong folly? not to speak of how incapable he is rendering himself for future paternal joys, or of the deep lamentable furrows ? he is ploughing in his youthful brow ; not to mention these and a thousand other considerations (which I purposely avoid touching upon) ; he is the unhappy slave of a habit which from the falsely dazzling, inebriating goblet confers on him far more pains than pleasures. Poor fellow ! he knows not the ecstatic feeling of a rare, an ardent embrace of the faithful wife, whose virtue and modesty inspire the deepest respect, and can conjure love of the real sort into her enraptured husband.

But he who has a fancy for the dregs of beastly lust may drink them to satiety in the shameless intercourse with mercenary courtesans. Soon will all his fine feelings be blunted in such laudable society ; true love, that daughter of heaven, is to this deluded being a ridiculous absurdity. Soon does his sexual passion become deadened to such a degree, that, in order to excite it, he must resort to a number of coarse stimulants and aphrodisiacal arts, revolting to every chaste imagination. Exhaustion of body and mind, self-contempt, disgust for life, and a wretched and premature death, such are the natural results of this destructive intemperance.

The wealthy classes in other respects seek to distinguish themselves by the refinement of their manners, of their appearance, and of all the things wherewith they are surrounded ; why do they in the gratification of their animal requirements sink so far beneath the poorest classes of the people, and I might say still lower ? Apparently for this simple reason, that they are bent on having much enjoyment here below, and this they might have, if they knew the proper, the true, the sole means of attaining it it ? that genuine mother of ecstatic, inexhaustible enjoyments, that rich awarder of pleasure—*moderation !*

A NURSERY.

I lately paid a visit to one of my relations. Our conversation soon turned upon my favourite subject, children. My fair cousin (her husband very properly left her to speak) talked like a book about physical education, and made me very desirous to see her young family.

She led me to the corridor at the back of the house that abutted on the court-yard, and opened the door of a dark, low receptacle full of disgusting smells, which she informed me was her nursery.

A steaming tub in which dirty linen was soaking stood in the front of the room, surrounded by some low washerwomen, whose unmannerly chattering polluted the ear, as the vapour from the dirty hot water did the lungs. The steam condensed into drops ran down the window panes.

I expressed to my fair cousin my incredulity as to the utility of this arrangement, and hinted how much the emanations from the clothes that were being washed must deteriorate the air the little ones had to breathe, how the excessive humidity thereby engendered relaxed all the fibres of our bodies, and must consequently be doubly injurious to children of a tender age.

" Do you really mean to say," cried she, "that washing causes any pollution? I'm sure I see no dirt made by it, and a little moisture can't do much harm."

" I allude to the invisible, but very injurious, deterioration of the air, the bad effects of which on such delicate creatures as children are, you must have heard of."

" Oh," she replied, " I fumigate occasionally 'with juniper berries, and they soon remove all impurities."

I now perceived that a learned demonstration of the difference betwixt the properties of azotic gas and pure oxygen, although they differ but slightly in odour, and not at all in appearance, would have been quite incomprehensible to my dear cousin, nor could I hope to make her understand how a prolonged sojourn in impure air acted as a slow poison on animal life, especially at a tender age, and how impossible it was that children could enjoy even tolerable health in such an atmosphere, and so forth. Neither did I venture to speak of the quantity of humidity that was imperceptibly taken up by the warm air of the room from the scalding water, and equally imperceptibly absorbed by the open mouths of the absorbent vessels in the child's soft body, whereby the natural exhalations were obstructed. Nor did I attempt to prove to her by the syllogysm in *Barbara*, though I had it on my scholastic tongue, that fumigation with juniper berries and such-like things would rather tend to plogisticate and deteriorate the air, but could never transform the impure air into vital gas.—However, as I have said, I luckily suppressed my spirit of logical refutation that was about to burst forth, and endeavoured to bring forward some *argumentum ad hominem*.

" It is possible," I said, "that I may be mistaken, and that you, my esteemed cousin, contrary to all expectation, are in the right in supposing that the frequent repetition of a washing festival in a nursery, together with the exhalations that arise from the blankets hung to dry near the stove there, may be without any unfavourable influence on the health of children, and I shall give up my point at once when you produce me your dear little children, who doubtless are very lively and stout."

"Produce them," she replied, "I cannot, but you may see them yourself back there. I don't know what ails my poor Freddy, yonder; he is nine years old, but cannot walk well without his crutches."

At these words a little miserable looking figure crawled towards us with difficulty. His knees were bent inwards, and his legs completely destitute of muscle. His head drawn backwards, stuck betwixt his shoulders; his face was pale and withered; his eyes dull, but projecting beyond the prominent forehead. His large ears stuck out; his nostrils were expanded; his broad tongue always hung partially out of his half-open mouth. His emaciated arms could scarcely support him on his crutches.

He soon returned panting to his little arm-chair, to rest himself after this slight exertion.

I involuntarily shrugged my shoulders, and heaved a deep sigh

A mixed feeling of gratitude to God and profound pity took possession of me, as I called my own rosy cheeked Fritz to my side and bade him shake hands with this innocent victim of a false and injurious method of bringing up children. My little urchin kissed this poor object affectionately, and asked him what was it he drank out of the large jug beside him. "My afternoon coffee"—was his reply, and at the same time he poured out a cup for my boy, who, however, refused it, as he was not in the habit of drinking things he was not acquainted with.

"You do not seem to approve of that," said my cousin, "but what else can the child drink, it is the only thing that seems to do him good; he cannot enjoy any thing else."

"Do him good?" I hastily asked, in a paroxysm of half-suppressed, but extreme anger—and I turned away from the odious sight.

Oh! what an inclination I felt to give this unhappy mother a severe lecture, and to shew her that a drink which sets our blood in agitation, whilst it exalts the irritability of our muscular fibre to such a degree as in course of time to render it quite lax, and to weaken it so that it trembles - which gradually exhausts our vital heat—which, possessing no nutritive properties in itself, unnaturally stifles hunger and thirst, and which communicates a false overstrained liveliness to its votaries, who are often reduced to the last stage of weakness, that like a transient intoxication leaves behind it an opposite state of the nervous system,—how injurious such a drink must be for the delicate child, endowed as it is with great irritability, and how impossible it is that such a badly treated creature can become any thing but rachitic and cachectic in the last degree—a shrivelled diminutive of a human being, for whom death were the most desirable lot.

With all these evident truths I should have wished to fan the smouldering spark of a mother's love in her breast, but I refrained from so doing because it occurred to me that coffee was the favourite beverage of mamma herself, so suppressing my feelings, I mildly gave her to understand that in my opinion coffee should only be an occasional beverage of persons above forty years of age, or employed in certain cases as a medicine."

"I suppose, my censorious cousin," was her reply, "you would be for depriving the little creature yonder at the table of her favourite food?"

It was some kind of confectionery which the girl three years old, who could not stand on her legs and could not be taught to walk, was swallowing with a degree of greediness that excited my disgust and horror. This pale, bloated creature had a rattling at the chest, slavered at the mouth, had a dull look, a projecting abdomen, and, as I learned, little sleep, and a perpetual diarrhœa, whereby, my cousin assured me, all impurities of the body were discharged.

I begged her to try whether she herself would remain in good health if she were constantly eating sweet things, and if she would not get sour eructations, worms, deficient or excessive appetite and diarrhœa, and if so, how much more the delicate stomach of a child who was incapable of taking exercise, and in whom there was a natural tendency to acidity.

This seemed to make some impression on her, especially when I begged her to try the strength of my home-made vinegar, which was made of sugar and yeast alone.

"I wish you would advise me what to do for the miserable skeleton yonder in the cradle at the side of the stove; it has constant cold sweats, it does not sleep, and is always crying as if it were on the rack. It has fits occasionally. I wish God would mercifully take it to himself, its sufferings are so heart-rending to witness. I have already buried three boys, peace be with them! they all died teething. The little fellow has been about his teeth these three months; he is always putting his little hands to his mouth. I only trust he has not got into this state from the evil eye of some bad people, as my mother-in-law confidently asserts must be the case; it was she tied the scarlet rags round its little hands. They are said to be good for bewitchment. She also often fumigates with nine kinds of wood."

"What harm," I replied, "could the poor innocent child have done to the bad people? where are these bad people that possess the power to make ill by a few words a healthy child fed moderately on wholesome food and strengthened by exercise in the open air and cleanliness? I am perfectly convinced," I continued, with some bitterness, caused by the sight of so much misery, "I am convinced that if you left off letting the poor child suck such a quantity of chewed bread from that bag, whereby its stomach is made sour and overloaded, if you would clean and dry it often enough so that all the stench I observe about its cradle were removed, if you would not cover it up so warm, would wash it all over every day with cold water and take it away from the unnatural heat of the stove, if you would send it, or, better, take it yourself frequently into the open air, would never give it unwholesome food, nor overload its stomach with the most wholesome—the little creature might still be able to enjoy life, it would not have to whine so much at all the misery you heap upon it and which you attribute to teething and witchcraft; it would become healthy and lively, in a word it would be to you a source of joy, and not as now, one of sorrow. Believe me, teething diseases are almost impossible, almost unheard of among quite healthy children; this name is a mere invention of ignorant persons, and is applied by them to children's diseases which they know nothing about, and the blame of which they lay upon nature, whereas they are in reality the fault of the mothers, the nurses and the doctors! None of my six children have manifested any serious illness when cutting their teeth; when I looked into their mouths I usually found their teeth as I expected, planted along their gums in an even row. Why do we hear those everlasting complaints about the pretended teething diseases of children, for which we have ourselves to blame?"

I went on in my overflowing zeal to give her to understand, in the most decided manner, what a poisonous atmosphere the air of this low, dark, hot room was, filled as it was with exhalations of all kinds, and so often with the emanations from the dirty clothes washed in it—how well children were worth the trouble of giving them a roomy, high, bright, frequently aired and extremely clean room to stay in during those hours of the day which they do not spend in the open air, which is quite indispensable for little children.

"Come, Fritz," I added, "let us quit this wretched children's hospital and clear our lungs in the autumnal breeze outside from this bad air. God will provide for these helpless children in the cold earth, including the poor cripple whose sad state causes your tears to flow. Come away!"

My cousin was much affected, wished to have more advice from me, wished to thank me, and so forth. But I hastily took my leave, exclaiming that she had got quite enough to do for the present if she made those changes which my compassionate zeal had induced me to suggest, and away I went with my stout and healthy little Fritz.[1]

---

[1] [Respecting the fate of this same Fritz or Frederick Hahnemann, the only son of the founder of Homœopathy, nothing is known for certain. To those conversant with Hahnemann's Materia Medica his name is very familiar, as it constantly appears among the early proved medicines, and indeed he seems to have been one of the most devoted and daring among those who were the pioneers of our pathogenetic knowledge. In 1811 he wrote an admirable reply to Hecker's attack upon the Organon, which may still be read with interest and profit.* After taking his degree in Leipzig, he contracted a matrimonial alliance with a widow, who I believe still lives in Dresden with a daughter, but who, according to what I have heard, was not well qualified to make his married life happy. This marriage gave great offence to his father, and led to an estrangement between them which was never removed. Frederick left the paternal roof and set up in practice in Wolkenstein, a small town in the Saxon Erzebirge where his success obtained him great celebrity, so much so that it is said his house was beset with crowds of patients. The jealousy of his professional brethren was aroused, and by some intrigue a letter was obtained from the Medical College of Saxony forbidding him to practice. Young Hahnemann on this was obliged to remove, but before doing so he wrote a most contemptuous letter to the College, which gave great offence, as it was intended it should. What became of him for a long time after that is not known. I find it stated in the Augsburg *Allg. Ztg. f. Hom.* that he went to Edinburgh and staid there several years, but I am unable to ascertain the truth of this statement. In the same journal it is mentioned that some years previous to 1830 a traveller calling himself Frederick Hahnemann had visited the interior of Pennsylvania and cured many people by means of small powders. Since that time no authentic traces of him have been met with, and I was last year assured by his sister, who cherished his memory with a sister's love, that she knew not whether he was dead or alive, never having heard any tidings of him since he quitted his native country.]

* This work is entitled " *Friedrich Hahnemann's des Sohnes Widerlegung der Anfælle Hecker's auf das Organon der rationellen Heilkunde.*" Dresden, 1811.

ON THE CHOICE OF A FAMILY PHYSICIAN.

Dear Doctor,

Since I left your neighbourhood I have felt a want, to supply which I am sure you are able, and I now write to request you to do so. When anything happens to me I know not what doctor to apply to; and yet you have repeatedly and urgently recommended me to pay more than ordinary attention to my health. We have here many doctors whom you know, and also some with whom I presume you are not acquainted. Some of them have pressed their services upon me, have got themselves recommended to me in various ways, and some have even recommended themselves. Now I know very well what recommendations are, especially to a person of my rank. It is the most forward, the most insolent, I might say the most impudent, that gets the best recommendation, though he may be the most ignorant and most immoral of the lot. Either monstrous vanity (and you know full well that this is *always* allied to ignorance) trumpets forth that its important possessor is the mighty hero he thinks himself to be, who can boldly offer himself for the most important posts without fear of a repulse; or a mixture of self-satisfaction and avarice makes him fertile in all kinds of devices in order to enlist in his interest those whose recommendation may be serviceable, whilst the latter are weak enough to bring all their influence to bear in his favour.

Such is the character of most recommendations, and he who trusts to them will have to put up with sorry trash; I have no faith in them, and must be perfectly satisfied in my own mind before I can make my choice.

But tell me, dear Doctor, how can I become satisfied in my case? On what principles must I choose a physician in order to avoid the bait of the ordinary run of recommendations, in which we are not always sharp enough to perceive the point of the hook? Pray give me your advice.

Yours, &c.

Prince of * * *

My dear Prince,

You are right in supposing that I am not well acquainted with the medical men of your capital; I know none of them sufficiently well, and I perceive with pleasure that you have a decided objection to receive the recommendations of those who are unknown to you.

Without being oneself a very great physician, it is impossible to form an immediate judgment respecting the scientific attainments of another physician; therefore you as a non-medical person must, in order to be able to select a really good man of this profession, have recourse to some circuitous methods, which shall guide you to your object with not less certainty than the knowledge attained by school learning can bestow. Certain trivial things in their outward appearance, a certain mode of conducting themselves when professionally engaged, and some other accessaries characterize the different classes of medical men.

Look how A. walks into the assemblage that reverentially expects him, with carefully measured steps, with expanded chest and elevated head; how he announces the dignity of his great person by a gracious, slow inclination of his body, and how he decides the most important questions with a few short words and a disdainful air. He only honours the great people in the company with his notice, he flatters them in high sounding phrases, in order to be entertained by them in return, and he talks about the highest personages in the land and the greatest savants, as he would about the most ordinary trifles which may be estimated with the fifth part of a glance. Merit rewarded or neglected, heart-breaking domestic occurrences, danger and delivery, life and death, are all the same to him; nothing produces any change in his frigid manner, or at the most they elicit from him a witty remark, which the crowd of his admirers do not omit to acknowledge with their plaudits. He talks the modern languages with the most refined accent; his house is the model of fashion and the furniture in the best taste.

You surely would never be so foolish, Prince, as to seek to make a display by selecting such a Khan among Doctors. Such an eccentric part must engage the whole mind of the best actor; it has to be learned, rehearsed, played. Who can be surprised that the details of a case of disease are tiresome to him, and that he defers till to-morrow doing anything for the urgent symptoms of some poor man, the sole support of a wretched family, because he must go and leave his card on some lord who is passing through the town. His medical wisdom must, in the face of all these fashionable accessaries, be but a thin coating which he has enough to do to keep well polished, so that all uninvited inquiring glances may be arrested by its mirror-like gloss, and be repelled without having penetrated its shallow depth.

Should I advise you to select B. I felt half inclined to do so! See : by half-past four in the morning he is in his carriage, for this morning he has thirty visits to pay to patients. His horses foam with the rapidity of the pace, and have to be changed for fresh ones in a few hours. Whilst he drives along he is seen to bend in deep meditation over a long clearly written list, wherein the names and abodes of the patients who are sighing for him, and the minute at which he believes he will be at each of them, are carefully marked. He looks at his watch which indicates the seconds, he calls to the coachman who instantly draws up. Out he jumps, says a few words to his servant and runs up the stairs. Doors fly open at his approach, three steps bring him to his patient's side. He feels his pulse, asks him a couple of questions, and without waiting a reply he calls for pen, ink and paper : and after deep reflection for two seconds in his chair he suddenly dashes off the complex prescription, politely hands it to the patient for his uninterrupted use with a few solemn words, rubs his hands together, makes his bow and disappears, in order to be with another patient six seconds afterwards, on whom also he bestows his two minutes of advice ; for his presence is in such great request that he is perfectly unable to devote a longer period to each patient. He wipes the perspiration from his brow, complains of having too much to do, makes his servant call him half a dozen times out from a party where he stays altogether only half an hour ; beckons to him every surgeon he meets, in order to whisper a few important words in his ear, pointing at the same time to some houses or streets. At his consultation hour his ante-room teems with the friends of patients, sick-nurses, midwives, surgeons, and patients. There he dispenses in profusion, prescriptions, recommendations, advice— like tickets for the theatre.

Do you still hesitate, prince, to select this the most renowned practitioner in the town, whose residence every child knows, who according to the unanimous opinion of the whole public owes his great and wide-spread reputation to his indefatigable industry, his enormous experience and knowledge of disease, which must of necessity procure him such an extensive practice ? Methinks I hear you insinuate that with such a superabundant practice the man cannot attend to any of his patients properly, cannot in a few minutes maturely reflect upon all the circumstances of each case, and still less find the proper remedies for it, seeing that the greatest and best physicians sometimes require half and whole hours for the consideration of similar cases. You will doubtless consider him to be some delusive, fleeting phantom, whose charlatanism consists in having too much to do, and whose only recommendations are a light hand, agile legs, and fleet horses. Well, I presume you will be inclined to look out for some one else.

Possibly your approbation may be bestowed on the next most celebrated practitioner, Dr. C., late surgeon in the army. He unites in his person to perfection all the arts that can enhance his superiority as a physician. His very appearance gives an aristocratic dignity to our science. His dress is in the last style of fashion. The cloth of his coat—which by the way is not yet paid for—could not have cost less than thirty shillings the yard, and the pattern of his gold-embroidered waistcoat excites the admiration of every lady. Those ambrosial curls on his hair, which are dressed thrice a day, are the work of the greatest artist in town. Look how elegantly he sticks out the little finger of his left hand, and how neatly he advances his foot—calumny asserts that he does so in order to show off his diamond rings and sparkling buckles. See with what grace he kisses the lily hands of dames and damsels, how charmingly he seats himself beside them on the sofa in order to feel their pulse in his inimitable manner, with what sweet words he commences the conversation, how fascinatingly he carries it on, and how artfully his philanthropic spirit revives it when it commences to flag, with scandalous half-invented anecdotes about other families, who had unfortunately made him their confidant. In order to charm the ears of his curious auditors he never forgets to tell them about all the false teeth, stuffed backs, and *pertes blanches*, of all their friends and neighbours; but all this he does in mysterious whispers and under the solemn promise of inviolable secresy, which he had not omitted to swear to observe in all the other houses. If he is ever at a loss for something else to talk about, he delights to pass his colleagues in malicious review. This one has no knowledge of the world, that one is deficient in anatomical knowledge, the other has a repulsive appearance; a third wants genius, a fourth has got a bad pronunciation, a fifth has no skill in dancing, a sixth has little practical talent; and so he goes on to a seventh and a tenth, ascribing to them all, heaven knows what faults. Every unsuccessful case of his colleagues is retailed from house to house, and he takes care at the same time, by delicate insinuations, to extol the wonderful powers of his own far superior genius. To the wife who complains of her husband he gives ingenious reasons to confirm her suspicions; and on the other hand, he expresses to the husband by a few dexterous shrugs of his shoulders the honest sympathy he feels for him on account of the unhappiness the conduct of his wife must occasion him. Those who employ him must prefer him to all his colleagues, for he launches out into praise of every-thing about them. Thus any ordinary looking children are darling angels, the new furniture of the room is in the best pos-sible taste, the pattern of the knitted purse has not its equal for ingenuity of invention, the cut of the new gown forms an epoch in fashion, the favourite daughter's wretched strumming on the piano is the music of the spheres, her stupid remarks are sparks of the most brilliant genius. He has the conplaisance to allow his patients to drink their favourite mineral waters, and to take their favourite medicines as often as they choose, and deferen-tially conforms to their fancies with regard to having their me-dicine in the form of powders, pills, draughts, or electuaries. He can also give it them as liqueur, lozenges, or confections. He whispers many a sly word in the chamber-maid's ear; and no one gives more in christmas-boxes to the servants who bring him his annual presents. He is perfectly conscious of his own talents; before ladies he parades his profound knowledge of the Greek and Hebrew languages, and his nocturnal studies of the Latin author Hippocrates; to the police magistrate he exhibits his botanicol lore; to the clergyman his anatomical acquire-ments; and to the mayor his skill in writing prescriptions.

"In a calumnious mind no love for mankind can dwell," me-thinks I hear you say "and he whose head is occupied in trying to ingratiate hinself by the elegancies of the toilette, by indirect self-praise, and all sorts of dishonourable practices, cannot possess any real merit."

The fear of wearying you, my prince, prevents me pursuing further the disagreeable occupation of displaying more of these caricatures composed of fragments, and which are by all means to be shunned. Thank God! their number is daily diminishing and it cannot be a matter of much difficulty for you to find a good physician if you will only be guided by your own feelings.

Search for some plain man of sound common sense, who takes great pains to ascertain the truth of all he hears and says, and does not merely look to its passing muster, who knows how to give clear and condensed information respecting everything that belongs to his art, and never obtrudes his opinion unasked or at an improper time, and who is no stranger to everything else important for man as a citizen of the world to know. More especially let the man you choose be one who does not shew temper nor get angry, except when he beholds injustice, who never turns away unmoved from any except flatterers, who has but few friends but these men of sterling principle, who listens attentively to the complaints of those who seek his aid, and does not pronounce an opinion without mature reflection, who prescribes but few, generally single, medicines in their natural state, who keeps out of the way until he is sought for, who is not silent respecting the merits of his colleagues, but does not praise himself; a friend to order, quiet and beneficence.

And when, my prince, you have found such a person, as is not so very difficult now-a-days, no one will rejoice more than

Yours, &c.,
S. H.

P. S. One word more! Before you finally fix on him, see how he behaves to the poor, and if he occupies himself at home unseen with some useful work!

CONTENTS OF THE FRIEND OF HEALTH.

PART I.

PART II.

DESCRIPTION OF KLOCKENBRING

DURING HIS INSANITY.[1]

AFTER having been for several years much occupied with the treatment of diseases of the most tedious and desperate character in general, and with all sorts of venereal maladies, cachexiæ, hypochondriasis and insanity in particular, with the assistance of the excellent reigning duke, I established three years ago a convalescent asylum for patients affected with such disorders, in Georgenthal, near Gotha. Hither the privy secretary of the chancery, Klockenbring, of Hanover, who lately died from the effects of a surgical operation in the 53d year of his age, was brought and placed under my care. He was a man who in his days of health attracted the admiration of a large portion of Germany by his practical talents for business and his profound sagacity, as also by his knowledge of ancient and modern lore, and his acquirements in various branches of science.

His almost superhuman labours in the department of state police, for which he had a great talent, his constant sedentary life, the continued strain upon his mind, together with a too nutritious diet, had, five years before the mental alienation occurred, brought on a deranged state of the system, which gradually assumed the form of offensive whimsicality and intolerable ill-humour; I am unable to say how much his copious indulgence in strong wines contributed to bring on this state.

His hypochondriasis had already attained a considerable height when that most disgusting satire of a petulent and degenerate wit, *Barth mit der eisernen Stirne*, appeared, wherein he found himself held up to ridicule in a manner that would have set even the coldest philosopher on fire. His mird, that was almost too sensitive to honour and fair fame, sank deep into the dust beneath this hail-storm of abusive accusations, which were, for the most part, without foundation, and left it to his disordered nervous system to complete the sad catastrophe.

In the winter of 1791-2, the most fearful furious madness burst forth, that for half a year completely baffled all the most

[1] From the *Deutsche Monatsschrift*, February, 1796.

assiduous treatment of one of the greatest physicians of our age, Dr. Wichmann, physician to the Hanoverian court.

He was brought to me towards the end of June, in a very melancholy state accompanied by the strong keepers.

His bloated body, which in his days of health was somewhat unwieldy, now exhibited a wondrous agility, quickness and flexibility in all its movements. His face was covered with large reddish-blue elevated spots, was dirty, and bore an expression of the greatest mental aberration. Smiles and grinding of the teeth, inconsiderateness and insolence, cowardice and defiance, childish folly and unlimited pride, desires without want—such was the admixture of traits displayed by the patient.

For the first fortnight I only observed him without treating him medicinally.

Incessantly, day and night, he kept on raving, and was never composed for a quarter of an hour at a time. When he sank down exhausted on his bed, he rose to his feet again in a few minutes. He either pronounced with the most threatening gestures capital sentences on criminals, which he often declared his former superiors to be; or he lost himself in declamations of a heroic character, and spouted, as Agamemnon and Hector, entire passages from the Iliad; then he would whistle a popular song, roll about on the grass, and sometimes vary his amusements by singing a stanza from Pergolese's *Stabat mater*. Anon it would occur to him to relate to his honest keeper, Jacob, the bargain made by ancient Jacob with Esau, about the birth-right, in the exact words of the Hebrew text; but he finished nothing that he began, for some new idea constantly led him into a different region; thus he would sing an ode of Anacreon, or of the Anthologia, to what he imagined to be an ancient Greek melody, or he would burst forth in an agony of weeping and sobbing, often throwing himself at the feet of the amazed attendant. But all at once he would often suddenly arise and with the most extraordinary hideous roars, hurl imprecations at his enemies, mingled with passages from Milton's *Paradise Lost* and Dante's *Inferno;* or he would mutter a form of exorcism for evil spirits in the Vandal tongue, point with any stick he could lay his hands on to the four quarters of heaven, write magical characters on the sand at his feet, make the sign of the cross, &c., and then he would burst out into immoderate fits of laughter, or recite an amorous rhapsody from some play, and, in the fire of his deluded imagination, he would warmly embrace one of his cold keepers, taking him for his beloved Daphne.

The most wonderful thing was the correctness with which he delivered all the passages from writings in all languages that occurred to his memory, especially all that he had learnt in his youth. The farrago he uttered was certainly a proof of his great acquirements in languages, but was at the same time a kind of ostentatious display of learning, which shone through all his extraordinary actions.

But nothing equalled the confidential friendship in which he pretended he had lived with emperors and queens, the love affairs he had had with princesses, his relationship to the highest personages in the world, &c., of which he often talked under the seal of the strictest confidence to his keepers, with laughably important gestures and half-whispered words.

In his worst period he called every one *thou*, and would not allow any one to address him otherwise.

When he was awake and alone he always kept talking to himself.

If his conversation was disordered, his other behaviour was not less so.

In spite of all remonstrances he tore and hacked to pieces his attire and his bed, generally when unobserved, with his fingers or with fragments of glass and the like.

Every instant he had some urgent desire, he wanted to eat or to drink, or he wished for some article of dress, or some piece of furniture, or a musical instrument, or some one of his private friends, or tobacco, or something else, although at first all food was rejected, laid aside, thrown out or dirtied, and in spite of his rapid pulse and white tongue, all drink was put aside,[1] spilt, mixed with all sorts of impurities, and at length poured out. He never waited till he got one thing before ordering another.

By taking his piano to pieces and setting it together again in an absurd manner, he endeavoured in the midst of the most tremendous noise and the most absurd tricks, to discover the ancient complementary tone of harmony, the προσλαμβανόμενον, he drew up algebraic formulas for it, explained them and his important projects to his keepers, and day and night he was always exceedingly busy.

At first he ran about and bellowed, mostly at night.

He exhibited a great inclination to dress himself up, so as to

---

[1] At the worst period his nervous system was so powerfully influenced by the irritation of his disordered imagination, that 25 grains of tartar emetic only caused him usually to vomit moderately three times, sometimes even less frequently.

give himself an amazingly majestic or half heroic, half Merry-Andrew-like appearance. He painted his face with variously coloured dirt, fat and such-like things, curled his hair, drew up his shirt collar and pulled down the ruffles of his shirt, scarcely ever went without a wreath of hay, straw, flowers, or something similar on his brow, never without a kind of girdle over his hips, a pathognomonic sign that he felt some disorder in the organs seated there[1] that required attention; but what kind of attention? his instinctive somnambulic sensibility did not teach him so much.

But he once put my metaphysical learning fairly at fault, when one evening, in the midst of the most extravagant paroxysm of folly, he hastily called for pen, ink and paper, and though on other occasions he would not listen to anything about corporeal diseases, he now wrote a prescription[2] which he wished to be made up immediately. The extraordinary ingredients of this were so extremely well arranged and so admirably adapted to the cure of an insanity of this sort, that for the moment I was almost tempted to consider him a very well instructed physician, had not the ridiculous direction he gave as to how it should be used—namely, with a few bottles of burgundy as a vehicle, to be followed up by lard—given another turn to my thoughts. But how was it[3] that in the midst of the very hurricane of its most extravagant passion, his mastless and helmless mind lighted on a remedy so excellent for insanity and unknown to many physicians? How came he to prescribe it for himself in the most appropriate form and dose?

Scarcely less remarkable was the circumstance that in the very worst period of his insanity he would, when asked, tell not only the exact day of the month (that one could understand, though he had not an almanac), but even the true hour by day or by night with astonishing accuracy.

As he began to improve, this faculty of divination became always more and more vague and uncertain, until at last, when his reason was completely restored, he knew neither more nor less about the matter than other people.

When he had completely recovered I begged him, in a friendly manner, to explain this enigma to me, or at least to describe the sensation that used to teach him this knowledge.

---

[1] He never forgot this appendage, even when he ran or rolled about naked, which sometimes could not be prevented.

[2] The commencement was: R. *Sem. Daturæ*, gr. ij. &c.

[3] He had no access to books or writings of any sort.

"I shudder, and a cold chill comes all over me," he replied, "when I think about it; I must beg of you not to remind me of this subject." And yet at that time he was able to talk with perfect sang-froid about his whole previous madness.

The first and worst period of his insanity he described as a death-like state, and indicated the day on which he felt as if he awoke.

From time to time, especially when he commenced to improve, he used to give me things that he had written, among which I often found some subjects which must have cost him much profound meditation. The chief part of these consisted of sonnets and elegies in various languages upon his present state, or addressed to his friends, odes to God, to his king, to me, to my family, &c. The language of these was usually correct, and they were interspersed with quotations from the ancient poets and philosophers, or the Bible, of which book, chapter and verse were given with great accuracy, although, as I before remarked, he had not a single book at his command.

Whilst he was still very ill he wrote his autobiography in classical Latin, composing a portion each day, and although he kept no copy he always resumed the thread of his tale exactly where he had left off.

But all these prose essays, odes, romances, ballads, elegies, &c., though in themselves often irreproachable, always betrayed their origin by something ludicrous about them. They were either written on pieces of paper torn into a triangular form, or if on square pieces they were written so that the lines ran obliquely across the sheet, the writing commencing in one of the corners. Or he drew various kinds of geometrical figures, in which he childishly wrote in a small hand these compositions, which sometimes consisted of the most sublime dithyrambics.

His whim was to apply the triangular figure and the number three wherever he could; thus he folded his bed-clothes and laid his pillow in a triangular manner, he disenchanted his drink, his food and his clothes by spitting thrice, by making the sign of the cross thrice, &c., and this folly he kept up partially until very near the period when he had almost recovered his full reason, and in every other respect could be perfectly well trusted by himself.

His propensity to compose verses[1] was remarkable, and this

---

[1] He played very well on the flute, but even after his reason had been considerably restored I could not allow him to do so, nor yet to play the organ, which he did in a most masterly style, as both of these instruments threw him into paroxysms of

was especially the case when his reason was somewhat restored; these chiefly consisted of popular songs conveying a moral lesson, combating popular prejudices, &c., illustrated by examples, many of which were excellent, in the style of ancient times. He set them them to simple appropriate melodies, in the same style, and often sang them, accompanying himself on the piano, which he played with great skill.[1]

In the midst of all these sometimes very pleasing performances, to which I did not in the least incite him, the rest of his behaviour, especially when one noticed him unseen, was very foolish, adventurous, grotesque.

But I must do him the justice to say, that in all his oral and written communications, and even when he was not observed, both during the periods of his greatest insanity and afterwards, he never shewed the slightest traces of any unbecoming behaviour in regard to sexual morality, but very frequently the very reverse. On this point he was certainly no saint in the strict meaning of the word, still he was much better than most men of the world. His body in this respect was in the most untainted and healthy condition; he must have therefore felt all the more deeply the calumnies that had been spread concerning him, and especially the satire alluded to above.

Loyalty to his sovereign and affection for his family and for some of his deceased friends, was perceptible through all the stages of his malady.

Much as he loved[2] and esteemed me, even in the height of his madness, as also after his complete recovery, and though he

madness. Even during the height of his mania he was uncommonly sensitive to certain things. Although my presence was always very agreeable and consolatory to him, yet he often begged me, especially when he was still considerably insane, not to put my hand on his arm or to touch his bare hand; it went through his marrow and bones, so he expressed himself, like an electric shock.

[1] I repeatedly requested him, when he was completely restored, to compose me a small poem by way of a souvenir. He tried to do so, but was unable to produce any thing tolerable, just as previous to his malady he had but little talent for making rhymes.

[2] I never allow any insane person to be punished by blows or other painful corporeal inflictions, since there can be no punishment where there is no sense of responsibility, and since such patients only deserve our pity and cannot be improved, but must be rendered worse by such rough treatment. He often however shewed me with tears in his eyes the marks of the blows and stripes his former keepers had employed to keep him in order. The physician of such unfortunate creatures ought to behave so as to inspire them with respect and at the same time with confidence; he should never feel offended at what they do, for an irrational person can give no offence. The exhibition of their unreasonable anger should only excite his sympathy and stimulate his philanthropy to relieve their sad condition.

was obliging and pleasant to every one after his recovery, yet he became malicious, deceitful and offensive as he was passing from the first state into the last, I mean when his reason was just beginning to dawn, when he was able to entertain himself with visitors for half-hours at a time, and when he could behave himself quite well as long as he was noticed. A most puzzling phenomenon! This perverted state of the disposition, in which head and heart seemed, so to speak, to have mutually lost their equilibrium, was accompanied in a corresponding degree by an astonishing canine hunger, or to speak more correctly, insatiableness.[1] They both went away together gradually, when, under the medicines used, health and reason were completely restored.

His friendship, which I enjoyed for two years after his complete restoration, has richly repaid me for these and thousands of other sad moments I passed on his account.

Before he quitted my establishment he shewed to the public, by his translation of a statistical work of Arthur Young, his regenerated intelligence in a very advantageous manner, and after he quitted me, the government of his native land bestowed on him, in place of his former too toilsome office, the direction of the lottery, which he continued to hold till his death, which was caused by a retention of urine.[2]

Peace be with his ashes!

ESSAY ON A NEW PRINCIPLE FOR ASCERTAINING THE CURATIVE POWERS OF DRUGS,

WITH A FEW GLANCES AT THOSE HITHERTO EMPLOYED.[3]

AT the commencement of this century, the unmerited honour was conferred on chemistry, more especially by the Academy of Sciences of Paris, of tempting it to come forward as the discoverer of the medicinal virtues of drugs, particularly of plants. They were subjected to the action of fire in retorts, generally

---

[1] He was not satisfied with ten pounds of bread daily, besides other food. When he had recovered his health he ate very moderately, I might almost say extremely little.

[2] [Where among modern authors, can be found so clear and masterly a description of a case as this of Klockenbring? Surely not in any of the medical records of the 19th century.]—*Am. P.*

[3] From *Hufeland's Journal der praktischen Arzneykunde.* Vol. ii, Part iii. 1796.

without water, and by this process there were obtained, from the most deadly as from the most innocent, very much the same products, water, acids, resinous matters, charcoal, and from this last, alkali; always the same kind. Large sums of money were thus wasted on the destruction of plants, before it was perceived that none of the important component parts of vegetables could be extracted by this fiery ordeal, far less that any conclusion respecting their curative powers could be come to. This folly, which was, with divers variations, perpetrated for nearly half a century, gradually produced an unfavourable impression on the minds of modern physicians, which had been in the mean time more enlightened respecting the chemical art and its limits, so that they now almost unanimously adopted an opposite view, and denied all value to chemistry in the search for the medicinal powers of drugs, and in the discovery of remedial agents for the diseases to which humanity is liable.

In this they palpably went too far. Although I am far from conceding to the chemical art a universal influence on the materia medica, I cannot refrain from alluding to some notable discoveries in this respect which we have to thank it for, and to what it may hereafter effect for therapeutics.

Chemistry informed the physician who sought a palliative remedy for the evils occasioned by morbid acids in the stomach, that the alkalis and some earths were their remedies. If it was desired to destroy in the stomach poisonous matters which had been swallowed, the physician applied to chemistry for the antidotes that should speedily neutralize them, before they should injure the alimentary canal and the whole organism. Chemistry alone could tell him that the alkalis and soap were the antidotes of acid poisons, of vitriol, of aquafortis, of arsenic, as well as of the poisonous metallic salts; that the acids were the counter-poisons of the alkalis, of quicklime, &c., and that for speedily counteracting the effects of all metallic poisons, sulphur, liver of sulphur, but especially sulphuretted hydrogen, were effectual.

It taught him to remove lead and tin from a cavity of the body by living quicksilver, to dissolve iron that had been swallowed by acids, and ingested glass and flint by fluoric and phosphoric acids, in the way it is seen to take place, with respect to the last substance, in the stomach of fowls.

Chemistry produced vital air in its purity, and when the physiologist and clinical observer perceived its peculiar power of maintaining and increasing the vital energy, chemistry showed that a part of this power lay in the great specific caloric of this air, and furnished a supply of it, which neither the therapeutic materia medica nor clinical experience could do, from many different sources, in greater and greater purity.

Chemistry alone could supply a remedy for those suffocated by fixed air, in the vapour of caustic ammonia.

What would the Galenic school have done in cases of suffocation from charcoal vapour, had chemistry not pointed out vital air, the second component of atmospheric, as the proper thing wherewith to inflate the lungs?

Chemistry discovered a means of destroying the remains of poisons which had penetrated the system, by administering sulphuretted hydrogen in drinks and baths.

What but chemistry taught us (with nitrous ether and acetate of potash) how to dissolve those gall stones that often give rise to so many most troublesome diseases?

For centuries, chemistry has been applied to by medicine for a remedy for stone in the bladder, and with what result? Those that applied to it know best. It has at all events done something, since it has brought soda saturated with fixed air into repute. A still better remedy will be found in the employment of phosphoric acid.

Were not all sorts of medicinal agents applied to mammæ in which the milk had curdled and caused pain? This was a hopeless, fruitless way. Chemistry showed a true remedy in fomentations of hartshorn, which renders curdled milk once more fluid.

Chemical experimentation with colombo root and morbid bile, showed that that vegetable substance must be a remedy in deranged biliary secretion in the human body, and medical experience has confirmed the accuracy of chemical induction.

Does the practitioner seek to know if a new remedy is of a heating description? Distillation with water, by showing the presence or absence of an ethereal oil, will with few exceptions suffice to solve the problem.

Practice cannot always tell by sensible signs if a vegetable substance possess astringent properties. Chemistry discovers that astringent principle, sometimes of no small use in practice, and even its degree, by means of sulphate of iron.

The science of dietetics alone cannot tell if a newly-discovered plant possess anything nourishing in its composition. Chemistry shows this, by separating its gluten and its starch, and can, from the quantity of these ingredients, determine the degree of its nutritive quality.

Although chemistry cannot directly point out medicinal powers, yet it can do this indirectly, by demonstrating the powerlessness of medicines, in themselves powerful, from being mixed; or the noxious properties of mixtures of medicines, in themselves innocuous. It forbids us, when we seek to produce vomiting by means of tartar emetic, to add to it substances containing gallic acid, by which it is decomposed; it forbids us to drink lime water when we seek to obtain benefit from the astringent principle of cinchona bark, by which it is destroyed; it forbids us, if we do not wish to produce ink, to mix bark and iron in the same potion; it forbids us to make the Goulard lotion powerless by adding alum; it forbids the mixture of an acid with those laxative neutral salts having cream of tartar for their bases, which remove acids from the primæ viæ; it forbids us to render poisonous, by admixture, those otherwise innocuous substances, diaphoretic antimony and cream of tartar; it prohibits the use of vegetable acids during a milk diet, (whereby an insoluble curd would be formed,) and when acids are required for digestion, it points to the vitriolic acid.

It furnishes the tests for detecting the adulteration of remedies, extracts the deadly corrosive sublimate from calomel, and teaches the difference betwixt the latter and the poisonous white precipitate which it so closely resembles.

These few examples may suffice to show that chemistry cannot be excluded from a share in the discovery of the medicinal powers of drugs. But that chemistry should not be consulted with respect to those medicinal powers which relate, not to hurtful substances to be acted on immediately in the human body, but to changes wherein the functions of the animal organism are first concerned, is proved, *inter alia*, by the experiments with antiseptic substances, respecting which, it was imagined that they would exhibit exactly the same antiputrefactive power in the fluids of the body, as they did in the chemical phial. But experience showed that saltpetre, for instance, which out of the body is so highly antiseptic, shows exactly opposite qualities in putrid fever and in tendency to gangrene; the reason of which, I may mention, though out of place here, is, that it weakens the vital powers. Or shall we seek to correct the putrefaction of matters in the stomach with saltpetre? An emetic will remove them at once.

Still worse for the materia medica was the advice of those who sought to ascertain the medicinal powers of its various agents, *by mixing the unknown drug with newly-drawn blood*, in order to see whether the blood grew darker or lighter, thinner or thicker; just as if we could bring the drug into the same immediate contact with the blood in the artery, as we can in the test-tube; just as if the drug must not first undergo an infinity of changes in the digestive canal, before it can get (and that only by a most circuitous method) into the blood. What a variety of appearances does not the blood itself present when drawn from the vein, according as it is taken from a heated or a cool body, by a smaller or larger opening, in a full stream or by drops, in a cold or warm room, in a flat or a narrow vessel.

But such paltry modes of ascertaining the powers of medicines bear on their face the stamp of their worthlessness.

Even the *injection of drugs into the bloodvessels of animals* is for the same reason a very heterogeneous and uncertain method. To mention only one circumstance,—a teaspoon full of concentrated cherrylaurel-water will most certainly kill a rabbit, when taken into the stomach, whereas, if injected into the jugular vein, it causes no change, the animal remains lively and well.

But at all events, some will say, *the administration of drugs to animals by the mouth* will furnish some certain results respecting their medicinal action. By no means! How greatly do their bodies differ from ours! A pig can swallow a large quantity of nux vomica without injury, and yet men have been killed with fifteen grains. A dog bore an ounce of the fresh leaves, flowers, and seeds of monkshood; what man would not have died of such a dose? Horses eat it, when dried, without injury. Yew leaves, though so fatal to man, fatten some of our domestic animals. And how can we draw conclusions relative to the action of medicines on man, from their effects on the lower animals, when even among the latter they often vary so much? The stomach of a wolf poisoned with monkshood was found inflamed, but not that of a large and a small cat, poisoned by the same substance. What can we infer from this? Certainly, not much, if I may not say, nothing. Thus much, at least, is certain, that the fine internal changes and sensations, which a man can express by words, must be totally wanting in the lower animals.

In order to try if a substance can develope very violent or dangerous effects, this may in general be readily ascertained by experiments on several animals at once, as likewise any general manifest action on the motions of the limbs, variations of temperature, evacuations upwards and downwards, and the like, but never anything connected or decisive, that may influence our conclusions with regard to the proper curative virtues of the agent on the human subject. For this, such experiments are too obscure, too rude. and if I be allowed the expression, too awkward.

As the above-mentioned sources for ascertaining the medicinal virtues of drugs were so soon exhausted, the systematizer of the materia medica bethought himself of others, which he deemed of a more certain character. He sought for them in the drugs themselves; he imagined he would find in them hints for his guidance. He did not observe, however, that their *sensible external signs* are often very deceptive, as deceptive as the physiognomy is in indicating the thoughts of the heart.

Lurid-coloured plants are by no means always poisonous; and on the other hand, an agreeable colour of the flowers is far from being any proof of the harmlessness of the plant. The special qualities of drugs, which may be ascertained by the smell and the taste, will not allow us to form any trustworthy conclusions respecting untried substances. I am far from denying utility to both these senses in corroborating the probable properties of drugs which have been ascertained in other ways, but I would counsel, on the other hand, great caution to those who would form their judgment from them alone. If the bitter principle strengthens the stomach, why does squill weaken it? If bitter aromatic substances are heating, why does marsh rosemary diminish the vital temperature in such a marked manner? If those plants only are astringent that make ink with sulphate of iron, how is it that the highly astringent principle in quinces, medlars, &c., cannot furnish ink?

If the astringent taste gives evidence of a strengthening substance, why does sulphate of zinc excite vomiting? If the acids are antiseptic, why does arsenious acid produce such rapid putrefaction in the body of one poisoned by it? Is the sweet taste of sugar of lead a sign of its nutritive properties? If the volatile oils, and everything that tastes fiery on the tongue, are heating for the blood, why are either, camphor, cajeput oil, oil of peppermint, and the volatile oil of bitter almonds and cherry-laurel, the very reverse? If we are to expect a disagreeable odour in poisonous plants, how is it so incosiderable in monks-hood, deadly nightshade, and foxglove? why so imperceptible in nux vomica and gamboge? If we are to look for a disagreeable taste in poisonous plants, why is the most deadly juice of the root of *jatropha manihot* merely sweetish, and not the least acrid? If the expressed fatty oils are often emollient, does it follow that they are *all* so, even the inflammatory oil expressed from the seeds of the *jatropha curcas*? Are substances which have little or no smell or taste destitute of medicinal powers? How is that ipecacuan, tartar emetic, the poison of vipers, nitrogen, and lopez-root, are not so? Who would use bryony-root as an article of diet, on the ground that it contains much starch?

Perhaps, however, *botanical affinity* may allow us to infer a similarity of action? This is far from being the case, as there are many examples of opposite, or at least very different powers, in one and the same family of plants, and that in most of them. We shall take as a basis the most perfect *natural system*, that of Murray.

In the family of the *coniferæ*, the inner bark of the fir-tree (*pinus sylvestris*) gives to the inhabitants of northern regions a kind of bread, whereas the bark of the yew-tree (*taxus baccifera*) gives—death. How come the feverfew (*anthemis pyrethrum*), with its burning root, the poisonous cooling lettuce *lactuca virosa*), the emetic groundsel (*senecio vulgaris*), the mild scorzonera, the innocuous cudweed (*gnaphalium arenarium*), the heroic arnica (*a. montana*), all together in the one family of the *compositæ*? Has the purging *globularia alypum* anything in common with the powerless *statice*, both being in the family of the *aggregatæ*? Is there any similarity to be expected betwixt the action of the skirret root (*sium sisarum*) and that of the poisonous water-dropwort (*œnanthe crocata*), or of the water-hemlock (*cicuta virosa*), because they are in the same family of the *umbelliferæ*? Has the not harmless ivy (*hedera helix*), in the family *hederaceæ*, any other resemblance to the vine (*vitus vinifera*), except in the outward growth? How comes the harmless butcher's-broom (*ruscus*) in the same family of the *sarmentaceæ* with the stupifying cocculus (*menispermum cocculus*), the heating *aristolochia*, and the *asarum europæum*? Do we expect any similarity of effect from the goose-grass (*galium aparine*) and the often deadly *spigelia marylandica*, because they both belong to the *stallatæ*? What resemblance can we find betwixt the action of the melon (*cucumis melo*) and the elaterium (*momordica elaterium*), in the same family of the *cucurbitaceæ*? And again, in the family *solanaceæ*, how comes the tasteless great mullein (*verbascum thapsus*), along with the burning Cayenne pepper (*capsicum annuum*); or tobacco, which has such a powerful spasm-exciting action on the primæ viæ, with nux vomica, which impedes the natural motions of the intestines? Who would compare the unmedicinal perriwinkle (*vinca pervinca*) with the stupifying oleander (*nerium oleander*), in the family *contortæ*? Does the watery moneywort (*lysimachia nummularia*) act similarly to the marsh trefoil (*menyanthes trifoliata*), or the powerless cow-slip (*primula veris*), to the drastic sowbread (*cyclamen europæum*), in the family of the *rutaceæ*? From the strengthening effects of the bear-berry (*arbutus uva ursi*) on the urinary apparatus, can we infer the heating, stupifying action of the *rhododendron chrysanthum*, in the family *bicornes*? Among the *verticillatæ*, can any comparison be made betwixt the scarcely astringent self-heal (*prunella vulgaris*) or the innocent bugle (*ajuga pyramidalis*), and the volatile germander (*teucrium marum*), or the fiery majoram (*origanum creticum*)? How can the powers of the verbena (*v. officinalis*) be said to resemble those of the active hyssop (*gratiola officinalis*) in the family *personatæ*? How different are the actions of the *glycyrrhiza* and *geoffroya*, although in the same family of the *papilionaceæ!* In the family of the *lomentaceæ*, what parallel exists betwixt the properties of the *ceratonia silliqua* and those of the fumatory (*fumaria officinalis*), of the *polygala senega* and the Peruvian balsam (*myroxylon peruiferum*)? Or is there any likeness in properties amongst the *nigella sativa*, the garden rue (*ruta graveolens*), the peony (*pœonia officinalis*), and the cellery-leaved crowfoot (*ranunculus sceleratus*), although one and all are in the family of the *multisiliquæ?* The dropwort (*spiræa filipendula*) and the tormentil (*tormentilla erecta*) are united in the family *senticosæ*, and yet how different in properties! The red currant (*ribes rubrum*), and the cherry-laurel (*prunus laurocerasus*), the rowan (*sorbus aucuparia*), and the peach (*amygdalus pirsica*), how different in powers, and yet in the same family of the *pomaceæ!* The family *succulentæ* unites the wall-pepper (*sedum acre*) and the *portulaca oleracea*, certainly not because they resemble each other in effects! How is it that the stork's-bill and the purging-flax (*linum catharticum*), the sorrel (*oxalis acetosella*), and the quassia (*q. amara*), are in the same family? Certainly not because their powers are similar! How various are the medicinal properties of all the members of the family *ascyroideæ!* and of those of the *dumosæ!* and

of those of the *trihilatæ!* In the family *tricoccæ,* what has the
corrosive spurge (*euphorbia officinalis*) in common with the box
(*buxus sempervirens*), which has such a decided influence on the
nervous system? The tasteless rupture-wort (*herniaria glabra*),
the acrid *phytolacca decandra,* the refreshing goosefoot (*chenopo-
dium ambrosioides*), and the biting persicaria (*polygonum hydro-
piper*), what a motley company in the family *oleraceæ!* How
dissimilar in action are the *scabridæ!* What business has the
mild, slimy, white lily (*lilium candidum*) beside the garlic (*allium
sativum*), or the squill (*scilla maritima*); what the asparagus (*a.
officinalis*) beside the poisonous white hellebore (*veratrum album*),
in the family *liliaceæ?*

I am far from denying, however, the many important hints
the natural system may afford to the philosophical student of
the materia medica and to him who feels it his duty to discover
new medicinal agents; but these hints can only help to confirm
and serve as a commentary to facts already known, or in the
case of untried plants they may give rise to hypothetical conjectures, which are, however, far from approaching even to
probability.

But how can a perfect similarity of action be expected
amongst groups of plants, which are only arranged in the so-
called natural system, on account of often slight external similarity, when even plants that are much more nearly connected,
plants of one and the same genus, are sometimes so different in
their medicinal effects. Examples of this are seen in the species of the genera *impatiens, serapias, cystisus, ranunculus, calamus, hibiscus, prunus, sedum, cassia, polygonum, convallaria,
linum, rhus, seseli, coriandrum, æthusa, sium, angelica, cheno-
podium, asclepias, solanum, lolium, allium, rhamnus, amygdalus,
rubus, delphinium, sisymbrium, polygala, teucrium, vaccinium,
cucumis, apium, pimpinella, anethum, seandia, valeriana, anthemis, artemisia, centaurea, juniperus, brassica.* What a difference betwixt the tasteless tinder amadou (*boletus igniarius*) and
the bitter, drastic *boletus laricis;* betwixt the mushroom (*agaricus deliciosus*) and the agaric (*agaricus muscarius*); betwixt the
woody stone moss (*lichen saxatilis*) and the powerful Iceland
moss (*lichen Islandicus!*)

Though I readily admit that, in general, similarity of action
will be much oftener met with betwixt species of one genus,
than betwixt whole groups of families in the natural system,
and that an inference drawn from the former will have a much

17

greater degree of probability attaching to it, than one from the latter; yet my conviction compels me to give this warning, that, be the number of genera ever so many whose species resemble each other very much in their effects, the lesser number of very differently acting species should make us distrustful of this mode of drawing inferences, since we have not here to do with mechanical experiments, but that most important and difficult concern of mankind—health.[1]

As regards this method also, therefore, we come to the conclusion, that it cannot be considered as a sure principle to guide us to the knowledge of the medicinal powers of plants.

Nothing remains for us but *experiment* on the human body. But what kind of experiment? *Accidental* or *methodical?*

The humiliating confession must be made, that most of the virtues of medicinal bodies were discovered by *accidental, empirical* experience, by *chance;* often first observed by non-medical persons. Bold, often over-bold, physicians, then gradually made trial of them.

I have no intention of denying the high value of this mode of discovering medicinal powers—it speaks for itself. But in it there is nothing for us to do; chance excludes all method, all voluntary action. Sad is the thought, that the noblest, the most indispensable of arts, is built upon accident, which always pre-supposes the endangering of many human lives. Will the chance of such discoveries suffice to perfect the healing art, to supply its numerous desiderata? From year to year we become acquainted with new diseases, with new phases and new complications of diseases, with new morbid conditions; if, then, we possess no better method of discovering the remedial agents around us than chance allows, nought remains for us to do but to treat these diseases with general (I might often wish with *no*) remedies, or with such as have seemed to be of service, in what we imagine, or what appear to us to be, similar diseased states. But how often shall we fail in accomplishing our object, for if there be any difference, the disease cannot be the same! Sadly

---

[1] Conclusions relative to similarity of action betwixt species of a genus become still more hazardous, when we consider that one and the same species, one and the same plant, frequently shows very various medicinal powers in its different parts. How different the poppy head from the poppy seed; the manna that distils from the leaves of the larch from the turpentine of the same tree; the cooling camphor in the root of the cinnamon laurel, from the burning cinnamon oil; the astringent juice in the fruit of several of the mimosæ, from the tasteless gum that exudes from their stem; the corrosive stalk of the ranunculus from its mild root!

we look forward into future ages, when a peculiar remedy for this particular form of disease, for this particular circumstance, may, *perhaps,* be·discovered by chance, as was bark for pure intermittent fever, or mercury for syphilitic disorders.

Such a precarious construction of the most important science —resembling the concourse of Epicurian atoms to make a world—could never be the will of the wise and most bountiful Preserver of mankind. How humiliating for proud humanity, did his very preservation depend on chance alone. No! it is exhilarating to believe that for each particular disease, for each peculiar morbid variety, there are peculiar directly-acting remedies, and that there is also a way in which these may be *methodically* discovered.

When I talk of the *methodical discovery of the medicinal powers still required by us,* I do not refer to those empirical trials usually made in hospitals, where in a difficult, often not accurately noted case, in which those already known do no good, recourse is had to some drug, hitherto either untried altogether, or untried in this particular affection, which drug is fixed upon either from caprice and blind fancy, or from some obscure notion, for which the experimenter can give no plausible reason, either to himself or to others. Such empirical chance trials are, to call them by the mildest appellation, but foolish risks, if not something worse.

I speak not here, either, of the somewhat more rational trials, made occasionally in private and hospital practice, with remedies casually recommended in this or that disease, but not further tested. These, also, are performed, unless under the guidance of some scientific principle, to a certain degree at the peril of the health and life of the patient; but the caution and practical skill of the physician will often avail to smooth much that is uneven in his half-empirical undertakings.

As we already possess a large number of medicines, which are evidently powerful, but concerning which we do not rightly know what diseases they are capable of curing, and moreover, others which have sometimes proved serviceable, sometimes not, in given diseases, and concerning which we have no accurate knowledge of the exact circumstances under which they are applicable, it may not at first sight appear very necessary to increase the number of our medicinal agents. Very probably all (or nearly all) the aid we seek lies in those we already possess.

Before I explain myself further, I must, in order to prevent misapprehension, distinctly declare that I do not expect, and do not believe, there can be a thoroughly specific remedy for any disease, of such and such a name, burdened with all the ramifications, concomitant affections and variations, which, in pathological works, are so often inconsiderately detailed as essential to its character, as invariably pertaining to it. It is only the very great simplicity and constancy of ague and syphilis that permitted remedies to be found for them, which appeared to many physicians to have specific qualities; for the variations in these diseases occur much more seldom, and are usually much less important than in others, consequently bark and mercury must be much more often serviceable than not so. But neither is bark specific in ague, in the most extended sense of the term,[1] nor mercury in syphilis, in its most extended sense; they are, however, probably specific in both diseases, when they occur simple, pure, and free from all complication. Our great and intelligent observers of disease have seen the truth of this too well, to require that I should dwell longer on this subject.

Now, when I entirely deny that there are any absolute specifics for individual diseases, in their full extent, as they are described in ordinary works on pathology,[2] I am, on the other

---

[1] Pity it is, that it was not observed *why*, for example, of the seven-fifteenths of all the so-called agues in which bark was useless, three-fifteenths required nux vomica or bitter almonds, another fifteenth opium, another fifteenth blood-letting, and still another fifteenth small doses of ipecacuan, for their cure! It was thought sufficient to say, "Bark was of no use, but ignatia cured;" the *why* was never satisfactorily answered. Were it a case of pure ague, bark must be of service; where there were complications, with excessive irritability, especially of the primæ viæ, however, it was no longer a pure case of ague, and it could not do good; here were now *reasons* for choosing as a remedy, or as an auxiliary means, ignatia, nux vomica, or bitter almonds, according to the different conditions of the system; and it could not and should not have been wondered at, that bark was not useful.

[2] The history of diseases is not yet advanced so far that we have been at pains to separate the essential from the accidental, the peculiar from the adventitious, the foreign admixture, owing to idiosyncrasy, mode of life, passions, epidemic constitutions, and many other circumstances. When reading the description of one disease, we might often imagine it was a compound admixture of many histories of cases. with suppression of the name, place, time, &c., and not true, abstractedly pure, isolated characteristics of a disease separated from the accidental (which might be afterwards appended to it, as it were). The more recent nosologists have attempted to do this: their genera should be what I call the peculiar characteristics of each disease, their species the accidental circumstances.

Before all things, we have to attend to the chief disease; its divergencies and concomitant circumstances only demand particular aid when they are serious, or offer

hand, convinced that there are as many specifics as there are
different states of individual diseases, *i. e.*, that there are peculiar
specifics for the pure disease, and others for its varieties, and
for other abnormal states of the system.

If I mistake not, practical medicine has devised three ways
of applying remedies for the relief of the disorders of the human body.

The *first way, to remove or destroy the fundamental cause of the
disease*, was the most elevated it could follow. All the imagin-
ings and aspirations of the best physicians in all ages were
directed to this object, the most worthy of the dignity of our art.
But, to use a Spagyrian expression, they did not advance beyond particulars; the great philosopher's stone, the knowledge
of the fundamental cause of all diseases, they never attained to.
And as regards most diseases, it will remain for ever concealed
from human weakness. In the mean time, what could be ascertained respecting this point, from the experience of all ages,
was united in a general system of therapeutics. Thus, in cases
of chronic spasms of the stomach, the general weakness of
the system was first removed; the convulsions arising from tape-
worm were conquered by killing that animal; the fever arising
from noxious matters in the stomach was dissipated by powerful emetics; in diseases caused by a chill the suppressed perspiration was restored; and the ball was extracted that gave rise to
traumatic fever. This object is above all criticism, though the
means employed were not always the fittest for attaining it. I
shall now take leave of this royal road, and examine the other
two ways for applying medicines.

By the *second way*, the symptoms present were sought to be
removed by medicines *which produced an opposite condition;* for
example, constipation by purgatives; inflamed blood by venesection, cold and nitre; acidity in the stomach by alkalis: pains
by opium. In acute diseases, which, if we remove the obstacles to recovery for but a few days, nature will herself generally
conquer, or, if we cannot do so, succumb; in acute diseases, I
repeat, this application of remedies is proper, to the purpose,
and sufficient, as long as we do not possess the above-mentioned
philosopher's stone (the knowledge of the fundamental cause of

---

obstacles to recovery; they demand our chief attention, and the primary disease
may be less regarded, when the latter, by passing into the chronic state, has become
of less importance, and is less urgent, whilst the former has gradually become the
chief disease.

each disease, and the means of its removal,) or as long as we have no rapidly-acting specific, which would extinguish the variolous infection, for instance, at its very commencement. In this case, I would call such remedies *temporary*.

But if the fundamental cause of the disease, and its direct means of removal are known, and we, disregarding these, combat the symptoms only by remedies of this second kind, or employ them seriously in chronic diseases, then this method of treatment (to oppose diseases by remedies that produce an opposite state) gets the name of *palliative*, and is to be reprobated. In chronic diseases it only gives relief at first; subsequently, stronger doses of such remedies become necessary, which cannot remove the primary disease, and thus they do more harm the longer they are employed, for reasons to be specified hereafter.

I know very well that habitual constipation is still attempted to be cured by aloetic purgatives and laxative salts, but with what melancholy results! I know well that efforts are still made to subdue the chronic determination of blood of hysterical, cachetic, and hypochondriacal individuals, by repeated, although small venesections, nitre, and the like; but with what untoward consequences! Persons living a sedentary life, with chronic stomachic ailments, accompanied by sour eructations, are still advised to take repeatedly Glauber salts; but with what disastrous effects! Chronic pains of all kinds are still sought to be removed by the continued use of opium; but again, with what sad results! And although the great majority of my medical brethren still adhere to this method, I do not fear to call it palliative, injurious, and destructive.

I beseech my colleagues to abandon this method (*contraria contrariis*) in chronic diseases, and in such acute diseases as take on a chronic character; it is the deceitful by-path in the dark forest that leads to the fatal swamp. The vain empiric imagines it to be the beaten highway, and plumes himself on the wretched power of giving a few hours' ease, unconcerned if, during this specious calm, the disease plants its roots still deeper.

But I am not singular in warning against this fatal practice. The better, more discerning, and conscientious physicians, have from time to time sought for remedies (the *third way*) for chronic diseases, and acute diseases tending to chronic, which should not cloak the symptoms, but which should remove the disease radically, in one word, for *specific* remedies; the most desirable, most praiseworthy undertaking that can be imagined. Thus, for instance, they tried arnica in dysentery, and in some instances found it a useful specific.

But what guided them, what principle induced them to try such remedies? Alas! only a precedent from the empirical game of hazard from domestic practice, chance cases, in which these substances were accidentally found useful in this or that disease, often only in peculiar unmentioned combinations, which might perhaps never again occur; sometimes in pure, simple diseases.

It were deplorable, indeed, if only chance and empirical *apropos* could be considered as our guides in the discovery and application of the proper, the true remedies for chronic diseases, which certainly constitute the major portion of human ills.

In order to ascertain the actions of remedial agents, for the purpose of applying them to the relief of human suffering, we should trust as little as possible to chance; but go to work as rationally and as methodically as possible. We have seen, that for this object the aid of chemistry is still imperfect, and must only be resorted to with caution; that the similarity of genera of plants in the natural system, as also the similarity of species of one genus, give but obscure hints; that the sensible properties of drugs teach us mere generalities, and these invalidated by many exceptions; that the changes that take place in the blood from the admixture of medicines teach nothing; and that the injection of the latter into the bloodvessels of animals, as also the effects on animals to which medicines have been administered, is much too rude a mode of proceeding, to enable us therefrom to judge of the finer actions of remedies.

Nothing then remains but to test the medicines we wish to investigate on the human body itself. The necessity of this has been perceived in all ages, but a false way was generally followed, inasmuch as they were, as above stated, only employed empirically and capriciously in diseases. The reaction of the diseased organism, however, to an untested or imperfectly tested remedy, gives such intricate results, that their appreciation is impossible for the most acute physician. Either nothing happens, or there occur aggravations, changes, amelioration, recovery, death—without the possibility of the greatest practical genius being able to divine what part the diseased organism, and what the remedy (in a dose, perchance, too great, moderate, or too small) played in effecting the result. They teach nothing, and only lead to false conclusions. The everyday physicians held their tongues about any harm that ensued, they indicated with one word only the name of the disease, which they often confounded with another, in which this or that remedy appeared to do good, and thus were composed the useless and dangerous works of Schröder, Rutty, Zorn, Chomel, Pomet, &c., in whose thick books are to be found a monstrous number of mostly powerless medicines, each of which is said to have cured radically this and at least ten or twenty other diseases.[1]

The true physician, whose sole aim is to perfect his art, can avail himself of no other information respecting medicines, than—

First—*What is the pure action of each by itself on the human body?*

Second—*What do observations of its action in this or that simple or complex disease teach us?*

The last object is partly obtained in the practical writings of the best observers of all ages, but more especially of later times. Throughout these, the, as yet, only source of the real knowledge of the powers of drugs in diseases is scattered: there we find it faithfully related, how the simplest drugs were employed in accurately described cases, how far they proved serviceable, and how far they were hurtful or less beneficial. Would to God such relations were more numerous!

But even among them contradictions so often occur, one condemning in a certain case what another found of use in a similar case, that one cannot but remark that we still require some natural normal standard, whereby we may be enabled to judge of the value and degree of truth of their observations.

This standard, methinks, can only be derived from the effects that a given medicinal substance has, by i self in this and that dose developed in the healthy human body.

To this belong the histories of designedly or accidentally swallowed medicines and poisons, and such as have been purposely taken by persons, in order to test them; or which have been given to healthy individuals, to criminals, &c.; probably,

---

[1] To me, the strangest circumstance connected with these speculations upon the virtues of single drugs is, that in the days of these men, the habit that still obtains in medicine, of joining together several different medicines in one prescription, was carried to such an extent, that I defy Œdipus himself to tell what was the exact action of a single ingredient of the hotch potch; the prescription of a single remedy at a time was in those days *almost* rarer than it is now-a-days. How was it possible in such a complicated practice, to distinguish the powers of individual medicines?

also, those cases in which an improper powerfully acting substance has been employed as a household remedy or medicine, in slight or easily determined diseases.

A complete collection of such observations, with remarks on the degree of reliance to be placed on their reporters, would, if I mistake not, be the foundation stone of a materia medica, the sacred book of its revelation.

In them alone can the true nature, the real action of medicinal substances be *methodically* discovered; from them alone can we learn in what cases of disease they may be employed with success and certainty.

But as the key for this is still wanting, perhaps I am so fortunate as to be able to point out the principle, under the guidance of which the lacunæ in medicine may be filled up, and the science perfected by the gradual discovery and application, *on rational principles*, of a suitable specific[1] remedy for each, more especially for each chronic disease, among the hitherto known (and among still unknown) medicines. It is contained, I may say, in the following axioms.

Every powerful medicinal substance produces in the human body a kind of peculiar disease; the more powerful the medicine, the more peculiar, marked, and violent the disease.[2]

We should imitate nature, which sometimes cures a chronic disease by superadding another, *and employ in the* (especially chronic) *disease we wish to cure, that medicine which is able to produce another very similar artificial disease*, and the former will be cured; *similia similibus.*

We only require to know, on the one hand, the diseases of the human frame accurately in their essential characteristics, and their accidental complications; and on the other hand, the pure effects of drugs, that is, the essential characteristics of the specific artificial disease they usually excite, together with the accidental symptoms caused by difference of dose, form, &c., and by choosing a remedy for a given natural disease that is capable of producing a very similar artificial disease, we shall be able to cure the most obstinate diseases.[3]

---

[1] In this Essay my chief object is to discover a permanently acting specific remedy for (especially) chronic diseases. Those remedies which remove the fundamental cause, and the temporary acting remedies for acute diseases which in some cases receive the name of palliative medicines, I shall not touch on at present.

[2] Non-medical people call those medicines which produce the most powerful specific diseases, and which therefore are actually the most serviceable *poisons*.

[3] The cautious physician, who will go gradually to work, gives the ordinary

This axiom has, I confess, so much the appearance of a barren, analytical, general formula, that I must hasten to illustrate it synthetically. But first let me call to mind a few points.

I. Most medicines have more than one action; the first a *direct* action, which gradually changes into the second (which I call the indirect secondary action). The latter is generally a state exactly the opposite of the former.[1] In this way most vegetable substances act.

II. But few medicines are exceptions to this rule, continuing their primary action uninterruptedly, of the same kind, though always diminishing in degree, until after some time no trace of their action can be detected, and the natural condition of the organism is restored. Of this kind are the metallic (and other mineral?) medicines, *e. g.* arsenic, mercury, lead.

III. If, in a case of chronic disease, a medicine be given, whose direct primary action corresponds to the disease, the indirect secondary action is sometimes exactly the state of body sought to be brought about; but sometimes, (especially when a wrong dose has been given) there occurs in the secondary action a derangement for some hours, seldom days. A somewhat too large dose of henbane is apt to cause, in its secondary action, great fearfulness; a derangement that sometimes lasts several hours. If it is troublesome, and we wish to diminish its duration, a small dose of opium affords specifically almost immediate relief; the fear goes off. Opium, indeed, in this case, acts only antagonistically, and as a palliative; but only a palliative and temporary remedy is required, in order to suppress effectually a transitory affection, as is also the case in acute diseases.

---

remedy only in such a dose as will scarcely perceptibly develope the expected artificial disease, (for it acts by virtue of its power to produce such an artificial disease,) and gradually increases the dose, so that he may be sure that the intended internal changes in the organism are produced with sufficient force, although with phenomena vastly inferior in intensity to the symptoms of the natural disease; thus a mild and certain cure will be effected. But if it is sought to go rapidly to work, with the otherwise fit and properly chosen remedy, the object may be certainly attained in this way too, though with some danger to life, as is often done in a rude manner by quacks among the peasants, and which they call miraculous, or horse cures, a disease of many years' standing being thereby cured in a few days; a proceeding that testifies to the truth of my principle, while at the same time it shows the hazardous nature of this mode of effecting it.

[1] Opium may serve as an example. A fearless elevation of spirit, a sensation of strength and high courage, an imaginative gaiety, are part of the direct primary action of a moderate dose on the system: but after the lapse of eight or twelve hours an opposite state sets in, the indirect secondary action; there ensue relaxation, dejection, diffidence, peevishness, loss of memory, discomfort, fear.

IV. Palliative remedies do so much harm in chronic diseases, and render them more obstinate, probably because after their first antagonistic action they are followed by a secondary action, which is similar to the disease itself.

V. The more numerous the morbid symptoms the medicine produces in its direct action, corresponding to the symptoms of the disease to be cured, the nearer the artificial disease resembles that sought to be removed, so much more certain to be favourable will the result of its administration be.

VI. As it may be almost considered an axiom, that the symptoms of the secondary action are the exact opposite of those of the direct action, it is allowable for a *mas er of the art*, when the knowledge of the symptoms of the direct action is imperfect, to supply in imagination the lacunæ by induction, *i. e.* the opposite of the symptoms of the secondary action; the result, however, must only be considered as an addition to, not as the basis of, his conclusions.

After these preliminary observations, I now proceed to *illustrate by examples* my maxim, *that in order to discover the true remedial powers of a medicine for chronic diseases, we must look to the specific artificial disease it can develope in the human body, and employ it in a very similar morbid condition of the organism which it is wished to remove.*

The analogous maxim, *that in order to cure radically certain chronic diseases, we must search for medicines that can excite a similar disease (the more similar the better) in the human body—* will thereby almost become evident.

In my additions to Cullen's Materia Medica, I have already observed that *bark*, given in large doses to sensitive, yet healthy individuals, produces a true attack of fever, very similar to the intermittent fever, and for this reason, *probably*, it overpowers, and thus cures the latter. Now after mature experience, I add, not only *probably*, but *quite certainly*.

I saw a healthy, sensitive person, of firm fibre, and half way through with her pregnancy, take five drops of the volatile oil of chamomile (*matricaria chamomilla*) for cramp in the calf of the leg. The dose was much too strong for her. First there was the loss of consciousness, the cramp increased, there occurred transient convulsions in the limbs, in the eyelids, &c. A kind of hysterical movement above the navel, not unlike labour pains, but more annoying, lasted for several days. This explains how chamomile has been found so serviceable in after-pains, in excessive mobility of the fibre, and in hysteria, when employed in doses in which it could not perceptibly develope the same phenomena, that is, in much smaller doses than the above.

A man who had been long troubled with constipation, but was otherwise healthy, had from time to time attacks of giddiness that lasted for weeks and months. Purgatives did no good. I gave him *arnica root* (*arnica montana*) for a week, for I knew that it causes vertigo, in increasing doses, with the desired result. As it has laxative properties, it kept the bowels open during its employment, by antagonistic action, as a palliative; wherefore the constipation returned after leaving off the medicine; the giddiness, however, was effectually cured. This root excites, as I and others have ascertained, besides other symptoms, nausea, uneasiness, anxiety, peevishness, headache, oppression of the stomach, empty eructation, cutting in the abdomen, and frequent scanty evacuations, with straining. These effects, not Stollen's example, induced me to employ it in an epidemic of simple (bilious) dysentery. The symptoms of it were uneasiness, anxiety, excessive peevishness, head-ache, nausea, perfect tastelessness of all food, rancid bitter taste on the (clean) tongue, frequent empty eructation, oppression of the stomach, constant cuttings in the abdomen, complete absence of fæcal evacuations, and instead, passage of pure grey or transparent sometimes hard, white, flocculent mucus, occasionally intimately mixed with blood, or with streaks of blood, or without blood, once or twice a day, accompanied with the most painful constant straining and forcing. Though the evacuations were so rare, the strength sank rapidly, much more quickly, however (and without amelioration, but rather aggravation of the original affection), when purgatives were employed. Those affected were generally children, some even under one year old, but also some adults. The diet and regimen were proper. On comparing the morbid symptoms arnica root produces with those developed by this simple dysentery, I could confidently oppose to the totality of the symptoms of the latter, the collective action of the former. The most remarkable good effects followed, without it being necessary to use any other remedy. Before the employment of the root, I gave a powerful emetic,[1] which I had occasion to repeat in scarcely two cases, for arnica sets to right

---

[1] Without using the arnica root, the emetics took away the rancid bitter taste for but one or two days; all the other symptoms remained, though they were ever so often repeated.

the disordered bile (also out of the body,) and prevent its derangement. The only inconvenience resulting from its use in this dysentery was, that it acted as an antagonistic remedy in regard to the suppression of fæces, and produced frequent, though scanty evacuations of excrement; it was consequently a palliative; the effect of this was, when I discontinued the root, continued constipation.[1]

In another less simple dysentery, accompanied by frequent diarrhœa, the arnica root might be more useful and suitable, on account of this latter circumstance; its property of producing frequent fæcal evacuations in its primary direct action would constitute it a similarly acting, consequently, permanent remedy, and in its secondary indirect action it would effectually cure the diarrhœa.

This has already been proved by experience; it has been found excellent in the worst diarrhœas. It subdues them, because, *without weakening the body*, it is capable of causing frequent evacuations. In order to prove serviceable in diarrhœas without fœcal matter, it must be given in such small doses as not to produce perceptible purgation; or in diarrhœas with acrid matters, in larger purgative doses; and thus the object will be attained.

I saw glandular swellings occur from the misuse of an infusion of flowers of arnica; I am much mistaken if, in moderate doses, it will not remove such affections.

We should endeavour to find out if the *millefoil* (*achillea millefolium*) cannot itself produce hæmorrhages in *large* doses, as it is so efficacious in moderate doses in chronic hemorrhages.

It is not to be wondered at that *valerian* (*valeriana officinalis*) in *moderate* doses cures chronic diseases with excess of irritability, since in large doses, as I have ascertained, it can exalt so remarkably the irritability of the whole system.

The dispute as to whether the *brooklime* (*anagallis arvensis*) and the bark of the *misletoe* (*viscum album*) possess great curative virtues or none at all, would immediately be settled, if it were tried on the healthy whether large doses produces bad effects, and

---

[1] I had to increase the dose daily, more rapidly than is necessary with any other powerful medicine. A child of four years of age got at first four grains daily, then seven, eight, and nine grains. Children of six or seven years of age could at first only bear six grains, afterwards twelve and fourteen grains were requisite. A child three quarters of a year old, which had taken nothing previously, could at first bear but two grains (mixed with warm water) in an enema; latterly six grains were necessary.

an artificial disease similar to that in which they have been hitherto empirically used.

The specific artificial disease and the peculiar affections that the *spotted hemlock* (*conium maculatum*) causes, are not nearly so well described as they deserve ; but whole books are filled with the empirical praise and the equally empirical abuse of this plant. It is true that it can produce ptyalism, it may therefore possess an excitant action on the lymphatic system, and be of permanent advantage in cases where it is requisite to restrain the excessive action of the absorbent vessels.[1] Now as it, besides this, produces pains (in *large* doses violent pains) in the glands, it may easily be conceived that in painful induration of the glands, in cancer, and in the painful nodes that the abuse of mercury leaves, it may be the best remedy, in *moderate* doses, not only for curing almost specifically this peculiar kind of chronic pains, in a more effectual and durable manner than the palliative opium and all other narcoctic remedies which act in a different manner, but also for dispersing the glandular swellings them-selves, when they either have their origin, as above described, in excessive local or general activity of the lymphatic vessels, or occur in an otherwise robust frame, so that the removal of the pains is all that is required in order to enable nature to cure the complaint herself. Painful glandular swellings from external injuries are of this description.[2]

In true cancer of the breast, where an opposite state of the glandular system, a sluggishness of it, seems to predominate, it must certainly do harm on the whole (it may at first soothe the pains), and especially must it aggravate the disease when the system, as is often the case, is weakened by long-continued suf-fering ; and it will do harm all the more rapidly, because its continued use produces, as a secondary action, weakness of the stomach and of the whole body. From the very reason that it,

---

[1] If employed in inactivity of these vessels, it will first act as a palliative ; after-wards do little one way or other ; and lastly, prove injurious, by the production of the opposite condition to that wished for.

[2] A healthy peasant child got, from a violent fall, a painful swelling of the under lip, which increased very much in the course of four weeks in hardness, size, and painfulness. The juice of the spotted hemlock applied to it, effected a cure without any relapse in fourteen days. A hitherto uncommonly healthy, robust girl, had severely bruised the right breast, whilst carrying a heavy burden, with the strap of the basket. A small tumour arose, which for six months increased in violence of pain, in size, and hardness, at each monthly period. The external application of spotted hemlock juice cured it within five weeks. This it would have done sooner, had it not affected the skin, and produced there painful pustules, in consequence of which it had frequently to be discontinued for several days.

like other umbelliferous plants, specifically excites the glandular
system, it may, as the older physicians remarked, cure an excessive secretion of milk. As it shows a tendency to paralyse
the nerves of sight in large doses, it is comprehensible why it
has proved of service in amaurosis. It has removed spasmodic
complaints, hooping cough, and epilepsy, because it has a tendency to produce convulsions. It will still more certainly be of
use in convulsions of the eyes and trembling of the limbs, because
in large doses it developes exactly the same phenomena The
same with respect to giddiness.

The fact that *fool's parsley* (*œthusa cynapium*), besides other
affections, as vomiting, diarrhœa, colicky pains, cholera, and others
for the truth of which I cannot vouch (general swelling, &c.),
produces so specifically imbecility, also imbecility alternately
with madness, should be of use to the careful physician in this
disease, otherwise so difficult of cure. I had a good extract of
it prepared by myself, and once, when I found myself, from much
mental work of various kinds coming upon me in rapid succession, distracted and incapable of reading any more, I took a grain
of it. The effect was an uncommon disposition for mental labour,
which lasted for several hours, until bed-time. The next day,
however, I was less disposed for mental exertion.

The *water hemlock* (*cicuta virosa*) causes, among other symptoms,
violent burning in the throat and stomach, tetanus, tonic cramp
of the bladder, lockjaw, erysipelas of the face, head-ache, and
true epilepsy; all diseases for which we require efficient remedies,
one of which, it may be hoped, will be found in this powerfully,
acting root, in the hands of the cautious but bold physician.

Amatus the Portuguese observed that *cocculus seeds* (*menispermum cocculus*), in the dose of four grains, produced nausea,
hiccough, and anxiety in an adult man. In animals they produced a rapid, violent, but when the dose was not fatal, a transitory stupefaction. Our successors will find in them a very
powerful medicine, when the morbid phenomena these seeds
produce shall be more accurately known. The Indians use the
root of this tree, among other things, in malignant typhus (that
accompanied by stupefaction).

The *fox-grape* (*paris quadrifolia*) has been found efficacious in
cramps. The leaves cause, in large doses at all events, cramp
in the stomach, according to the still imperfect experience we
possess of the morbid phenomena they are capable of developing.

Coffee produces, in large doses, head-aches; it therefore cures,

in moderate doses, head-aches that do not proceed from derangement of the stomach or acidity in the primæ viæ. It favours
the peristaltic motion of the bowels in large doses, and therefore
cures in smaller doses chronic diarrhœas, and in like manner
the other abnormal effects it occasions might be employed against
similar affections of the human body, were we not in the habit
of misusing it. The effects of opium in stupifying the senses,
and irritating the tone of the fibres, are removed by this berry
in its character of an antagonistic palliative remedy, and that
properly and effectually, for here there is no persistent state of
the organism, but only transitory symptoms to be combated.
Intermittent fevers, too, where there is a want of irritability and
inordinate tension of the fibres, precluding the employment of
otherwise specific bark, it apparently suppresses in large doses,
merely as an palliative remedy; its direct action, however, in
such large doses, lasts for two days.

The *bitter-sweet* (*solanum dulcamara*) produces, in large doses,
among other symptoms, great swelling of the affected parts and
acute pains, or insensibility of them, also paralysis of the tongue
and of the optic nerves?). In virtue of the last powerful action,
it is not to be wondered at that it has cured paralytic affections,
amaurosis, and deafness, and that it will render still more specific service in paralysis of the tongue, in moderate doses. In
virtue of the two first properties, it is a main remedy in chronic
rheumatism, and in the nocturnal pains from the abuse of mercury. In consequence of its power of causing strangury, it has
been useful in obstinate gonorrhœa, and from its tendency to
bring about itching and shooting in the skin, it shows its utility
in many cutaneous eruptions and old ulcers, even such as arise
from abuse of mercury. As it causes, in large doses, spasms of
the hands, lips and eyelids, as also shaking of the limbs, we may
easily understand how it has been useful also in spasmodic affections. In nymphomania it will probably be of use, as it acts so
specifically on the female genital organs, and has the power of
causing (in large doses) itching and pains in these parts.

The berries of the *black nightshade* (*solanum nigrum*) have caused
extraordinary convulsions of the limbs, and also delirious raving.
It is, therefore, probable that this plant will do good in what are
called possessed persons (madness, with extraordinary, emphatic,
often unintelligible talking, formerly considered prophesying and
the gift of unknown tongues, accompanied by convulsions of the
limbs), especially where there are at the same time pains in the

region of the stomach, which these berries also produce in large doses. As this plant causes erisypelas of the face, it will be useful in that disease, as has already been ascertained from its external employment. As it causes, to a still greater degree than bitter-sweet, by being used internally, external swellings, that is, a transient obstruction in the absorbent system, its great diuretic power is only the indirect secondary result; and hence its great virtue in dropsy, *from similarity of action*, is plainly perceptible; a medicinal quality of so much the greater value, as most of the remedies we possess for this disease are merely antagonistically acting (exciting the lymphatic system in a merely transitory manner), and consequently palliative remedies, incapable of effecting a permanent cure. As, moreover, in large doses it causes not only swelling, but general inflammatory swelling, with itching, and intolerable burning pains, stiffness of the limbs, pustular eruptions, desquamation of the skin, ulcers, and sphacelus, where is the wonder that its external application has cured divers pains and inflammations? Taking all the morbid symptoms together that the black nightshade produces, we cannot mistake their striking resemblance to raphania, for which it will, *most probably*, be found to be a specific remedy.

It is probable that the *deadly nightshade (atropa belladonna)* will be useful, if not in tetanus, at least in trismus (as it produces a kind of lockjaw), and in spasmodic dysphagia (as it specifically causes a difficulty of swallowing); both these actions belong to its direct action. Whether its power over hydrophobia, if it do possess any, depends on the latter property alone, or also on its power of suppressing palliatively, for several hours, the irritability and excessive sensitiveness that are present in so great a degree in hydrophobia, I am unable to determine. Its power of soothing and dispersing hardened, painful and suppurating glands, is owing, undeniably, to its property of exciting, in its direct action, boring, gnawing pains in these glandular swellings. Yet I conceive that it acts antagonistically, that is, in a palliative and merely temporary manner, in those which proceed from excessive irritation of the absorbent system (with subsequent aggravation, as is the case with all palliatives in chronic diseases); but, by virtue of similarity, that is, permanently and radically, in those arising from torpor of the lymphatic system. (Then it would be serviceable in those glandular swellings in which the *spotted hemlock (conium maculatum)* cannot be used, and the latter will be useful where the former does injury.) As, however, its con-

18

tinued employment (by reason of its indirect secondary action) exhausts the whole body, and when given in too large, or too often repeated doses, has a tendency to produce a gangrenous fever, its good effects will sometimes be destroyed by these secondary bad consequences, and fatal results may ensue (especially in the case of cancerous patients, whose vital powers have been exhausted by the sufferings of many years), if it be not cautiously employed. It produces directly mania, (as also, as above described, a kind of tonic cramp); but clonic cramps (convulsions) it only produces as a secondary action, by reason of the state of the organism that remains after the direct action of belladonna (obstruction of the animal and natural functions.) Hence its power in epilepsy with furor is always most conspicuous upon the latter symptom, whilst the former is generally only changed by the antagonistic (palliative) action of belladonna, into trembling, and such-like spasmodic affections peculiar to weakened irritable systems. All the spasmodic symptoms that belladonna produces in its direct primary action are of a tonic character; true, the muscles are in a state of paralytic relaxation: but their deficient irritability causes a kind of immobility, and a feeling of health, as if contraction were present. As the mania it excites is of a wild character, so it soothes manias of this sort, or at least deprives them of their stormy nature. As it extinguishes memory in its direct action,[1] nostalgia (home sickness) is aggravated, and, as I have seen, is even produced by it.

Moreover, the increased discharge of urine, sweat, menses, fæces, and saliva, which have been observed, are merely consequences of the antagonistic state of the body, remaining after an excessive exaltation of the irritability, or else sensitiveness during the indirect secondary action, when the direct primary action of the drug is exhausted, during which, as I have several times observed, all these excretions are often completely suppressed by large doses for ten hours and more. Therefore, in cases where these excretions are discharged with difficulty, and excite some serious disease, belladonna removes this difficulty permanently and completely, as a similarly-acting remedy, if it be owing to tension of the fibres, and want of irritability and sensibility. I say purposely, *serious disease*, for only in such cases is it allowable to employ one of the most violent of medicines, which demands such caution in its use. Some kinds of dropsy, green sickness, &c., are of this nature. The great ten-

---

[1] It will, therefore, be useful in weakness of memory.

dency of belladonna to paralyse the optic nerve, makes it important, as a similarly-acting remedy, in amaurosis.[1] In its direct action it prevents sleep, and the deep sleep which subsequently ensues is only in consequence of the opposite state produced by the cessation of this action. By virtue, therefore, of this artificial disease, belladonna will cure chronic sleeplessness (from want of irritability) more permanently than any palliative remedy.

It is said to have been found beneficial in dysentery; probably, as in its direct action it retards the stool, in the most simple cases of diarrhœa, with suppressed fæcal evacuations, and rare motions, but not in dysentery with lienteric diarrhœa, where it must do positive harm. Whether, however, it is appropriate for dysentery, by reason of its other actions, I am unable to say.

It produces apoplexy; and if it have, as we are told, been found serviceable in serous apoplexy, it is owing to this property. Besides this, its direct action causes an internal burning, with coldness of the external parts.

Its direct action lasts twelve, twenty-four, and forty-eight hours. Hence, a dose should not be repeated sooner than after two days. A more rapid repetition of ever so small a dose must resemble in its (dangerous) effects the administration of a large dose. Experience teaches this.

The fact that *henbane* (*hyoscyamus niger*) in large doses diminishes remarkably the heat of the body and relaxes its tone for a short time in its direct action, and therefore is an efficacious palliative remedy when given in moderate doses inwardly and outwardly in sudden attacks of tension of the fibres and inflammation, does not fall to be considered in this place. This is not the case, however, with the observation, that this property only enables it to palliate very imperfectly, in any dose, chronic affections with tension of the fibre; in the end, however, it rather increases than diminishes them by its indirect secondary action, which is exactly the opposite of its primary action. On the other hand, it will help to assist the power of the strengthening remedy in chronic relaxation of the fibres, as in its primary action it relaxes, and in its secondary action it tends all the more to elevate the tone, and that in a durable manner. In *large* doses it likewise possesses the power of producing hæmorrhage, especially bleeding of the nose, and frequently recurring cata-

---

[1] I have myself seen the good effects of it in this disease.

menial flux, as I and others have ascertained. For this reason it cures chronic hæmorrhages, in small doses, in an extremely effectual and lasting manner. The most remarkable thing is the artificial disease it produces in *very large* doses, suspicious, quarrelsome, spitefully-calumnious, revengeful, destructive, fearless,[1] mania (hence, henbane was termed by the ancients *altercum*), and this is the kind of mania it specifically cures, only that in such cases a tenseness of fibre sometimes hinders it effects from being permanent. Difficulty of moving, and insensibility of the limbs, and the apoplectic symptoms it produces, it may also very probably be capable of curing. In large doses, it produces, in its direct primary action, convulsions, and is consequently useful in epilepsy, probably also in the loss of memory usually accompanying it, as it has the power of producing want of recollection.

Its power of causing in its direct action sleeplessness with constant tendency to slumber, makes it in chronic sleeplessness a much more permanent remedy than the frequently merely palliative opium, especially as it at the same time keeps the bowels open, although only by the indirect secondary action of each dose, consequently in a palliative way. It causes dry cough, dryness of the mouth and nose, in its direct action; it is, therefore, very useful in tickling cough, probably also in dry coryza. The flow of mucus from the nose, and the flow of saliva observed from its use, only belong to its indirect secondary action. The seeds cause convulsions in the facial and ocular muscles, and by their action on the head, cause vertigo, and a dull pain in the membranes lying under the skull. The practical physician will be able to take advantage of this. Its direct action lasts scarcely twelve hours.

The *thorn-apple* (*datura stramonium*) causes extraordinary waking dreams, unconsciousness of what is going on, loud delirious talking, like a person speaking in sleep, with mistakes respecting personal identity. A similar kind of mania it cures specifically. It excites very specific convulsions, and has thus often proved useful in epilepsy. Both properties render it serviceable in the case of persons possessed. Its power of extinguishing recollection should induce us to try it in cases of weak memory. It is most useful where there is great mobility of the fibre, because its direct action in large doses is increased fibrous mobility. It

---

[1] The subsequent indirect secondary action is a kind of faint-heartedness and fearfulness.

causes (in its direct action?) heat and dilatation of the pupil, a kind of dread of water, swollen, red face, twitching in the ocular muscles, retarded stool, difficult breathing; in its secondary action, slow, soft pulse, perspiration, sleep.

The direct action of large doses lasts about twenty-four hours; of small doses, only three hours. Vegetable acids, and apparently citric acid in particular, suddenly put a stop to its whole action.[1] The other species of datura seem to act in a similar manner.

The specific properties of *Virginia tobacco* (*nicotiana tabacum*) consist, among other things, in diminishing the external senses, and obscuring the intellect; it may therefore be useful in weakness of mind. Even in a very small dose, it excites the muscular action of the primæ viæ violently; a property which is valuable as a temporary oppositely-acting remedy (as is well known, though it does not fall to be considered here); and as a similarly-acting remedy it is probably serviceable in chronic disposition to vomiting and to colics, and spasmodic constriction of the œsophagus, as indeed experience partially corroborates. It diminishes the sensibility of the primæ viæ ; hence its palliative power of lessening hunger (and thirst?) In larger doses, it deprives of their irritability the muscles of voluntary motion, and temporarily removes from them the influence of the cerebral power. This property may give it as a similarly-acting remedy, curative powers in catalepsy : but this very property makes its constant employment in large quantities (as with tobacco-smokers and snuff-takers) so injurious to the tranquil state of the muscles belonging to the animal functions, that a tendency to epilepsy, hypochondriasis, and hysteria, are in course of time developed. The remarkable fact, that the employment of tobacco is so agreeable to insane persons, arises from the instinct of those unfortunates to produce a palliative obtuseness in the sensibility of their hypochondria[2] and brain (the two usual seats of their complaints). But as it is here an oppositely-acting remedy, it gives them but temporary relief; their desire for it increases, but the end for which it is taken is not attained,—on the whole

---

[1] A patient, who was always violently affected by two grains of the extract of the plant, once experienced not the slightest effects from this dose. I learned that he had partaken of the juice of a large number of red currants ; a considerable dose of pulverized oyster-shells at once restored the full efficacy of the thorn apple.

[2] To this belongs the feeling of insatiable hunger, which many insane persons suffer from, and for which they generally appear to use tobacco; at least, I have seen some, who had no desire for tobacco, especially such as were affected with melancholia, who had very little hunger.

the complaint is thereby increased, as it renders no permanent service. Its direct action is limited to a few hours, except in the case of very large doses, which extend to twenty-four hours (at the farthest).

The seeds of the *poison tree* (*strychnos nux vomica*) are very powerful; but the morbid symptoms it produces are not yet accurately known. The most I know concerning them is derived from my own observation. They produce vertigo, anxiety, febrile rigour, and in their secondary action a certain immobility of all parts, at least of the limbs, and a spasmodic stretching, according to the size of the dose. Hence they are useful, not only, as is already known, in intermittent fever, but in cases of apoplexy. In their first direct action, the muscular fibre has a peculiar mobility imparted to it, the sensitive system is morbidly exalted to a species of intoxication, accompanied by fearfulness and horror. Convulsions ensue. The irritability seems to exhaust itself during this continued action on the muscular fibre, first in the animal, then in the vital functions. On passing into the indirect secondary action, there occurs a diminution of the irritability, first, in the vital functions (general perspiration), then in the animal, and lastly in the natural functions. In the latter, especially, this secondary action lasts several days. During the secondary action, there is a diminution of sensibility. Whether in the primary direct action the tonicity of the muscle is diminished, to be proportionately increased in the secondary action, cannot be accurately determined; this much, however, is certain, that the contractility of the fibre is as much diminished in the secondary action, as it was increased in the direct action.

If this be true, nux vomica produces attacks similar to hysterical and hypochondriacal paroxysms, and this explains why it is so often useful in these complaints.

Its tendency to excite, in its primary direct action, the contractility of the muscles, and cause convulsions, and then again in its secondary action to diminish to an excessive degree the contractility of the muscles, shows such a resemblance to epilepsy, that from this very circumstance we must have inferred that it would heal this disease, had not experience already demonstrated it.

As it excites, besides vertigo, anxiety and febrile rigour, a kind of delirium consisting in vivid, sometimes frightful visions, and tension in the stomach, so it once quickly subdued a fever in a laborious reflective mechanic in the country, which began with tension in the stomach, followed by a sudden attack of vertigo, so as to make him fall, that left behind it a kind of confusion of the understanding, with frightful, hypochondriacal ideas, anxiety, and exhaustion. In the morning he was pretty lively and not exhausted, but in the afternoon, about two o'clock, the attack commenced. He got nux vomica, in increasing doses, one daily, and improved. At the fourth dose, which contained seventeen grains, there occurred great anxiety, immobility and stiffness of the limbs, ending in a profuse perspiration. The fever and all the nervous symptoms disappeared, and never returned, although for many years previously he had from time to time been subject to such attacks suddenly occurring, yet unaccompanied by fever.

Its tendency to cause cramps in the abdomen, anxiety and pain in the stomach, I availed myself of in a dysenteric fever (without purgings), in persons living in the same house with dysenteric patients. In these cases it diminished the feeling of discomfort in the limbs, the feverishness, the anxiety, and the pressure in the stomach; it produced the same good results in some of the patients, but as they had simple dysentery without diarrhœa, it made the evacuations still rarer, from its tendency to cause constipation. The signs of deranged biliary secretion showed themselves, and the dysenteric evacuations, though rarer, were accompanied by just as great tenesmus as before, and were of as bad a character. The symptom of loss of taste, or perverted taste, remained. Its tendency to diminish the peristaltic movements was therefore disadvantageous in the true simple dysentery. In diarrhœas, even such as are of a dysenteric character, it will be more serviceable, at least as a palliative remedy. During its employment, I witnessed twitching movements under the skin, as if caused by live animals, in the limbs, and especially in the abdominal muscles.

St. Ignatius' bean (*ignatia amara*) has been observed to produce trembling of several hours' duration, twitchings, cramps, irascibility, sardonic laughter, giddiness, cold perspiration. In similar cases it will show its efficacy, as experience has partly demonstrated. It produces febrile rigour, and (in its secondary action?) stiffness of the limbs, and thus it has cured, by similarity of action, intermittent fever. which would not yield to bark; probably it was that less simple form of intermittent in which the complication consisted of excessive sensitiveness and increased irritability (especially of the primæ viæ). But the other symptoms it can produce must be more accurately observed, before we can employ it in those cases for which it is exactly suited from similarity of symptoms.

The *purple foxglove* (*digitalis purpurea*) causes the most excessive disgust at food; during its continued use, therefore, ravenous hunger not unfrequently ensues. It causes a kind of mental derangement, which is not easily recognisable, as it only shows itself in unmeaning words, refractory disposition, obstinacy, cunning, disobedience, inclination to run away, &c., which its continued use frequently prevents. Now as, in addition to these, it produces in its direct action violent headaches, giddiness, pain in the stomach, great diminution of the vital powers, sense of dissolution and the near approach of death, a diminution of the rapidity of the heart's beats by one half, and reduction of the vital temperature, it may easily be guessed in what kind of madness it will be of service; and that it has in fact been useful in some kinds of this disease, many observations testify, only their particular symptoms have not been recorded. In the glands it creates an itching and painful sensation, which accounts for its efficacy in glandular swellings.

It produces, as I have seen, inflammation of the Meibomian glands, and is a certain cure for such inflammations. Moreover, as it appears to depress the circulation, so does it seem to excite the absorbent vessels, and to be most serviceable where both are too torpid. The former it assists by virtue of similarity, the latter by virtue of antagonism of action. But as the direct action of foxglove persists so long (there are examples of its lasting five or six days), it may, as an antagonistically acting remedy, take the place of a permanent curative agent. The last observation is in reference to its diuretic property in dropsy; it is antagonistic and palliative, but nevertheless enduring, and valuable on that account merely.

In its secondary action it causes a small, hard, rapid pulse; it is not therefore so suitable for patients who have a similar (febrile) pulse, but rather for such as have a pulse like what foxglove produces in its direct action—slow, soft. The convulsions it causes in large doses, assign it a place among the anti-epileptic remedies; probably it is only useful in epilepsy under certain conditions, to be determined by the other morbid symptoms it produces. During its use, objects not unfrequently appear of various colours, and the sight becomes obscured; it will remove similar affections of the retina. (Its tendency to produce diarrhœa, sometimes so adverse to the cure, is counteracted, as I have have ascertained, by the addition of potash.

As the direct action of foxglove lasts occasionally several days (the longer its use is continued, the longer lasts the direct action of each dose; a very remarkable fact, not to be lost sight of in practice), it is evident how erroneously those act, who, with the best intentions, prescribe it in small but frequently repeated doses, (the action of the first not having expired before they have already given the sixth or eighth), and thus in fact they give, although unwittingly, an enormous quantity, which not unfrequently causes death.[1] A dose is necessary only every three, or at most every two days, but the more rarely the longer it has been used. (During the continuance of its direct action, cinchona bark must not be prescribed; it increases the anxiety caused by foxglove, as I have found, to an almost mortal agony.)

The *pansy violet* (*viola tricolor*) at first increases cutaneous eruptions, and thus shows its power to produce skin diseases, and consequently to cure the same effectually and permanently.

Ipecacuanha is used with advantage in affections against which nature herself makes some efforts, but is too powerless to effect the desired object. In these ipecacuanha presents to the nerves of the upper orifice of the stomach, the most sensitive part of the organ of vitality, a substance that produces a most uncongenial disgust, nausea, anxiety, thus acting in a similar manner to the morbid material that is to be removed. Against this double attack, nature exerts antagonistically her powers with still greater energy, and thus, by means of this increased exertion, the morbid matter is the more easily removed. Thus fevers are brought to the crisis, stoppages in the viscera of the abdomen and of the chest, and in the womb, put in motion, miasmata of contagious diseases expelled by the skin, cramp relieved by the cramp that ipecacuanha itself produces, their tension and freedom restored to vessels disposed to hemorrhage from relaxation, or from the irritation of an acrid substance deposited in them, &c. But most distinctly does it act as a similarly acting remedy to the disease sought to be cured, in cases of chronic disposition to vomit without bringing anything away. Here it should be given in very small doses, in order to excite frequent nausea, and the tendency to vomit goes off more and more permanently at each dose, than it would with any palliative remedy.

Some benefit may be anticipated in some kinds of chronic palpitation of the heart, &c., from the administration of the *rose-bay*

---

[1] A woman in Edinburgh got for three successive days, each day, three doses, each dose consisting of only two grains of the pulverized leaves of foxglove, and it was a matter of surprise that she died from such small doses, after vomiting for six days. It must be remembered, however, that it was the same as if she had taken eighteen grains at one dose.

(*nerium oleander*), which has the power of causing palpitation, anxiety, and fainting. It causes swellings of the abdomen and diminution of the vital temperature, and seems to be a most powerful vegetable.

The morbid symptoms produced by the *nerium antidysentericum* are not sufficiently known to enable us to ascertain the cause of its real remedial powers; but as it primarily increases the stools, it apparently subdues diarrhœas as a similarly acting remedy.

The *bear's berry* (*arbutus uva ursi*) has actually, without possessing any acridity perceptible to the senses, not unfrequently increased the difficulty of passing water, and the involuntary flow of urine, by some power peculiar to itself; thereby showing that it has a tendency to produce such affections, and hence, as experience also testifies, it is capable of curing similar disorders in a permanent manner.

The *golden-flowered rhododendron* (*rhododendron chrysanthum*) shows, by the burning, formicating, and shooting pains it produces in the parts affected, that it is certainly fitted to relieve, by similarity of action, pains in the joints of various kinds, as experience also teaches. It causes difficulty of breathing and cutaneous eruptions, and thus it will prove useful in similar disorders, as also in inflammation of the eyes, because it produces lacrymation and itching of the eyes.

The *marsh-tea* (*ledum palustre*) causes, as I have ascertained, among other effects, difficult, painful respiration; this accounts for its efficacy in hooping cough, probably also in morbid asthma. Will it not be useful in pleurisy, as its power of so greatly diminishing the temperature of the blood (in its secondary action) will hasten recovery? It causes a painful shooting sensation in all parts of the throat, as I have observed, and hence its uncommon virtues in malignant and inflammatory sore throat. Equally specific is, as I have noticed, its power of causing troublesome itching in the skin, and hence its great efficacy in chronic skin diseases.

The anxiety and the faintings it occasions may prove of use in similar cases. As a transitory and antagonistically acting powerful diuretic and diaphoretic remedy, it may cure dropsies; more certainly however, acute, than chronic.

On some of these properties depends its reputation in dysentery. But were they real cases of dysentery, or some of those painful diarrhœas so often taken for it? In the latter case it may, as a palliative remedy, certainly hasten the cure, and even help to complete it; but in true uncomplicated dysentery, I have never seen it of any use. The long-continued weakness it occasions was against its being used for a length of time, and it ameliorated neither the tenesmus nor the character of the excretions, though these became more rare. The symptoms of deranged biliary secretion were rather worse during its use, than when the patients were left without medicine. It causes a peculiar ill-humour, headache, and mental confusion; the lower extremities totter, and the pupils dilate. (Do both the latter symptoms, or merely the last, belong to the secondary action only?) An infusion of ten grains once a day was a sufficient dose for a child six years old.

The primary direct action of *opium* (*papaver somniferum*) consists in transitory elevation of the vital powers, and strengthening the tone of the blood-vessels and muscles, especially of those belonging to the animal and vital functions, as also in excitation of the mental organs—the memory, the imagination, and the organ of the passions;—thus, moderate doses are followed by a disposition to work, sprightliness in conversation, wit, remembrance of former times, amorousness, &c.; large doses by boldness, courage, revenge, inordinate hiliarity, lasciviousness; still larger doses by furious madness, convulsions. The greater the dose, the more do the individuality, the freedom, and the voluntary power of the mind suffer in sensations, and in power of judgment and of action. Hence, inattention to external disagreeable circumstances, to pain, &c. This condition, however, does not last long. It is gradually followed by loss of ideas, the pictures of fancy fade by degrees, there supervene relaxation of the fibre, sleep. If the use of elevated doses is continued, the consequences (indirect secondary action) are, weakness, sleepliness, listlessness, grumbling, discomfort, sadness, loss of memory (insensibility, imbecility), until a new excitation by opium, or something similar, is produced. In the direct action, the irritability of the fibre seems to be diminished in the same proportion as its tone is increased; in the secondary action, the latter is diminished, the former increased.[1] The direct action, still more than the secondary action, prevents the mind from

---

[1] There occurs a marked sensitiveness, especially for things that produce disagreeable effects, for fright, grief, fear, for inclement weather, &c. If the mobility of the fibre which occurs secondarily is called increased irritability, I have nothing to object to the term; its sphere of action, however, is but small: it is either that the fibre is too relaxed, and cannot contract much, or that it is in a too contracted condition, and

taking cognizance of sensations (pain, sorrow, &c.), and hence its great pain subduing power.

(In cases where only the direct action as a cordial is necessary, it will be requisite to repeat the administration of it every three or four hours, that is, each time before the relaxing secondary action, which so much increases the irritability, ensues. In all such cases it acts merely antagonistically, as a palliative remedy.

Permanent strengthening powers are not to be expected from it used in this manner, least of all in chronic weakness. This, however, is a digression.)

But if it is wished to depress permanently the tone of the fibre, (I give this name to the power of the fibre to contract and relax completely), to diminish permanently the deficiency of irritability, as is the case in some cases of mania, in such circumstances we may employ opium with success, as a similarly acting remedy, given in elevated doses, and making use of its indirect secondary action. We must consider the treatment which consists in giving opium in true inflammatory diseases, e. g. pleurisy, to be according to this principle.

In such cases, a dose is necessary every twelve or twenty-four hours.

It appears that this indirect secondary action has been made use of on the principle of a similarly acting remedy; which, as far as I am aware, is not the case with any other medicine. Opium has, for instance, been given with the greatest success, (not in true venereal diseases, for that would be a delusion,) but in the disastrous effects that so often arise from the abuse of mercury in syphilis, which are sometimes much worse than the syphilis itself.

Before illustrating this employment of opium, I must say something appropriate to the subject, concerning the nature of syphilis, and introduce here what I have to say concerning mercury.

Syphilis depends upon a virus, which, besides other peculiarities that it developes in the human body, has an especial tendency to produce inflammatory and suppurating swellings of the glands (to weaken the tone?), to make the mechanical connexion of the fibres so disposed to separation, that numerous spreading ulcers arise, whose incurable character may be known

---

is relaxed easily indeed, but not sufficiently, consequently is incapable of making any powerful effort. In this condition of the fibre, the tendency to chronic inflammation is unmistakable.

by their round figure; and lastly, to increase the irritability. Now, as such a chronic disease can only be cured by a remedy capable of developing a disease of similar character, no more efficacious remedy could be conceived than mercury.

The most remarkable power of mercury consists in this, that in its direct action it irritates the glandular system, (and leaves behind its glandular indurations as its secondary indirect action,) weakens the tone of the fibres and their connexion, and disposes them to separation in such a manner, that a number of spreading ulcers arise, whose incurable nature is shown by their round form; and lastly, increases uncommonly the irritability (and sensibility). Experience has confirmed it as a specific; but as there does not exist any remedy similar to the disease, so the mercurial disease (the changes and symptoms it usually produces in the body) is still very different from the nature of syphilis. The syphilitic ulcers are confined to the most superficial parts, especially the deuteropathic ones, (the protopathic ulcers increase slowly in extent,) they secrete a viscid fluid in place of pus, their borders are almost level with the skin (except the protopathic ones), and are almost quite painless (excepting the protopathic ulcer, that arising from the primary infection, and the suppurating inguinal gland). The mercurial ulcers burrow deeper, (rapidly increase in size,) are excessively painful, and secrete sometimes an acrid thin ichor; sometimes they are covered with a dirty cheesy coating, their borders also become everted. The glandular swellings of syphilis remain but for a few days; they are either rapidly resolved, or the gland suppurates. The glands attacked by mercury are stimulated to increased action by the direct action of this metal, (and thus glandular swellings from other causes disappear rapidly under its use,) or they are left in the state of cold indurations during the indirect secondary action. The syphiltic virus produces induration of the periosteum of those bones which are nearest the surface and least covered with flesh; they are the seat of excessive pains. In our days this virus, however, never produces caries, notwithstanding all my researches to discover the contrary. Mercury destroys the connexion of the solid parts, not of the soft parts only, but also of the bones; it first corrodes the most spongy and concealed bones, and this caries is only aggravated the more rapidly by the continued use of the metal. Wounds which have arisen from external violence are changed by the use of mercury into old ulcers, difficult of cure; a circumstance that does not occur with syphilis. The trembling, so remarkable in the mercurial disease, does not occur in syphilis. From the use of mercury there ensues a slow, very debilitating fever, with thirst, and great and rapid emaciation. The emaciation and weakness from syphilis come on slowly, and remain within moderate limits. Excessive sensitiveness and sleeplessness are peculiar to the mercurial disease, but not to syphilis. The most of these symptoms seem to be owing rather to the indirect secondary action, than to the direct action of the mercury.

I have been so circumstantial on this subject, because it is often very difficult[1] for the practitioner to distinguish the chronic mercurial disease from the symptoms of syphilis; and thus he will be apt to consider symptoms as belonging to that disorder, whilst they are only mercurial, and go on treating them with mercury, whereby so many patients are destroyed; chiefly, however, because my object is to depict the mercurial disease, in order to show how opium can cure it, by virtue of similarity of action.

Opium raises the sinking forces of patients suffering from the mercurial disease, and allays their irritability, when its direct action is kept up, that is, when it is given at least every eight hours; and this it does as an antagonistically-acting remedy. This happens, however, only when it is given in large doses, proportioned to the degree of weakness and irritability, just as it is serviceable only in large and oft-repeated doses in the excessive irritability of hysterical and hypochondriacal patients and in the excessive sensibility of exhausted individuals. The normal condition of the body seems thereby to be restored; a secret metamorphosis seems to take place in the organism, and the mercurial disease is geadually conquered. The convalescent patient can only bear smaller and smaller doses. Thus the mercurial disease seems to be vanquished by the palliative antagonistic power of the opium; but any one who is aware of the almost uneradicable nature of the mercurial disease, the irresistible manner in which it destroys and dissolves the animal frame when it is at its height, will be convinced that a mere palliative could never master this excessively chronic malady, were it not that the secondary effects of opium were very analogous to the mercurial disease, and that these tended to overcome the latter.

---

[1] Stoll (Rat. Med. Part iii, p. 442,) doubts if there are certain signs of a perfectly cured syphilitic disease, i. e., he himself knew not the signs whereby this disease is distinguishable from the mercurial disease.

The secondary effects of the continued use of opium in large doses, increased irritability, weakness of the tone, easy separation of the solids, and difficult curability of wounds, trembling, emaciation of the body, drowsy sleeplessness, are very similar to the symptoms of the mercurial disease; and only in this do they differ, that those of mercury, when they are severe, last for years, often for a lifetime whilst those of opium last but hours or days. Opium must be used for a long time, and in enormous doses, for the symptoms of its secondary action to last for weeks or longer. These brief secondary effects of opium, whose duration is limited to a short time, are thus the true antidote of the mercurial secondary effects in their greatest degree. which are almost unlimited in their duration; from them alone, almost, can one expect a permanent, true recovery. These secondary actions can develope their curative power during the whole treatment, in the interval betwixt the repetition of the doses of opium, as soon as the first direct action of each dose is passed, and when its use is discontinued.

Lead produces, in its primary action on the denuded nerves (belonging to muscular action?) a violent tearing pain, and (thereby?) relaxes the muscular fibre to actual paralysis; it becomes pale and withered, as dissection shows, but its external sensibility still remains, though in a diminished degree. Not only is the power of contraction of the affected fibres diminished, but the motion that still remains is more difficult than in other similar relaxations, from almost total loss of the irritability.[1] This, however, is observed only in the muscles belonging to the natural and animal functions, but in those belonging to the vital functions this effect occurs without pain and in a less degree. As the reciprocal play of the vascular system becomes slower, (a hard, slow pulse,) this satisfactorily explains the diminished temperature of the blood attending the action of lead.

Mercury also diminishes the mutual attraction of the various parts of the muscular fibres, but increases their susceptibility for the stimulus, so as to impart to them an excessive mobility. Whether this effect be the direct or the indirect secondary action it suffices that it is very enduring; and hence, even if of the latter character, it would be very efficacious, as an oppositely-

---

[1] The convulsive vomiting and dysenteric diarrhœa which sometimes follow the ingestion of large quantities of lead, must be explained on other principles, and do not fall to be considered here; neither does the vomiting that ensues from large doses of opium.

acting remedy in the lead disease; if of the first character, however, it will act as a similarly-acting remedy. Rubbed in externally, as well as given internally, mercury has an almost specific influence over the lead disease. Opium increases in its direct action the contraction of the muscular fibre, and diminishes its irritability. By virtue of the former property, it acts as a palliative in the lead disease; by the latter, however, permanently, as a similarly-acting remedy.

From the above idea of the nature of the lead disease, it will be seen that the service this metal (lead has afforded, when cautiously used in diseases, depends entirely on its antagonistic, though uncommonly long-lasting, action, the consideration of which does not belong to this Essay.

The true nature of the action of *arsenic* has not yet been accurately investigated. Thus much I have myself ascertained, that it has a great tendency to excite that spasm in the blood-vessels, and the shock in the nervous system, called febrile rigour. If it be given in a pretty large dose (one-sixth or one fifth of a grain) to an adult, this rigour becomes very evident. This tendency makes it a very powerful remedy as a similarly-acting medicine in intermittent fever, and this all the more, as it possesses the power, observed by me, of exciting a daily-recurring, although always weaker, paroxysm, even although its use be discontinued. In typical diseases of all kinds (periodical head-ache, &c.), this type-exciting property of arsenic in small doses (one-tenth to at most one-sixth of a grain in solution) becomes valuable, and will, I venture to guess, become invaluable to our perhaps bolder, more observant, and more cautious successors. As its action lasts several days, so, frequently-repeated doses, be they ever so small, accumulate in the body to an enormous, a dangerous dose. If, then, it be found necessary to give a dose daily, each successive dose should be at least a third smaller than the previous one. A better procedure is, when we have to treat short typical diseases with, say, two days' interval, always to prescribe a dose only for one fit two hours before it is expected, pass over the following fit without giving any arsenic, and another dose only about two hours before the third fit. It will be best to act so even in the case of quartan fever, and only commence to treat the series of the intermediate paroxysms when we have attained our object with regard to the first series of paroxysms. (In the case of longer intervals, as seven, nine, eleven, and fourteen days, a dose may be prescribed before each fit.)

The continued use of arsenic in large doses gradually causes an almost constant febrile state ; it will thus, as indeed experience has, to a certain degree, taught us, prove useful in hectic and and remittent fever, as a similarly-acting remedy ; in small doses, (about one-twelfth of a grain). Such a continued employment of arsenic, however, will always remain a masterpiece of art, as it possesses a great disposition to diminish the vital heat and the tone of the muscular fibre. (Hence the paralyses from a strong dose, or a long-continued and incautious employment of it.) These latter properties will enable it to prove of service as an antagonistic remedy in pure inflammatory diseases.) It diminishes the tone of the muscular fibre, by diminishing the proportion and cohesion of coagulable lymph in the blood, as I have convinced myself, by drawing blood from persons suffering from the effects of arsenic, more especially such as had a too inspissated blood before the use of this metallic acid. But not only does it diminish the vital heat, and the tone of the muscular fibre, but also, as I think I have fairly proved to myself, the sensibility of the nerves. (Thus, in cases of maniacs, with tense fibre, and inspissated blood, a small dose of it procures quiet sleep, in its character of an antagonistically-acting substance, where all other remedies fail. Persons poisoned by arsenic are more composed about their state, than might be expected. Thus it generally seems to kill more by extinguishing the vital power and sensibility, than by its corrosive and inflammatory power, which is only local and circumscribed. This being borne in mind, the rapid decomposition of the bodies of those poisoned by arsenic, like cases of death by mortification, will be readily comprehended.) It weakens the absorbent system, a circumstance whence, perhaps, we may one day derive some curative power (as a similarly or as an antagonistically-acting remedy?), but which must be always a powerful objection to its long continued use. I would direct attention to its peculiar power of increasing the irritability of the fibre, especially of the system of the vital functions. Hence cough, and hence the above-mentioned chronic febrile actions.

When arsenic is used for a length of time, and in pretty large doses, it seldom fails, especially if diaphoretics and a heating diet be used simultaneously, to cause some chronic cutaneous disease (at least desquamation of the skin). This tendency renders it an efficacious remedy in the hands of the Indian physician, in that frightful skin disease, elephantiasis. Would it not also be serviceable in pellagra? If it be truly (as is confidently

19

affirmed) of service in hydrophobia, it must act by virtue of its power to diminish (the influence of the nerves on) the attraction of the parts of the muscular fibre and its tone, as also the sensibility of the nerves, therefore antagonistically. It produces acute, continued pains in the joints, as I have seen. I shall not attempt to determine how we may avail ourselves of this property in a curative point of view.

What influence the arsenic disease, the lead disease, and the mercurial disease, may have over each other, and if the one may be destroyed by means of the other, future observations can alone decide.

Should the accidents produced by a long-continued use of arsenic become threatening (besides the employment of sulphuretted hydrogen in drinks and baths to extirpate what still remains of the substance of the metal), the free use of opium in the same manner as in the mercurial disease (see above) will be of service.

I revert again to vegetable substances; and first, I shall mention a plant, which in violence and duration of action, deserves to be placed alongside the mineral poisons; I allude to the *yew* (*taxus baccata*). Great circumspection must be employed in the use of its various parts, more particularly of the bark of the tree when in flower; the cutaneous eruptions, with signs of gangrenous decomposition of the fibre, which sometimes occur several weeks after the last dose, the fatal catastrophe that sometimes takes place suddenly, sometimes several weeks, after the last dose, with symptoms of mortification, &c., teach us this. It produces, it appears, a certain acridity in all the fluids, and an inspissation of the lymph; the vessels and fibres are irritated, and yet their functions are more impeded than facilitated. The scanty evacuations, accompanied by tenesmus, the dysuria, the viscid, salt, acrid saliva, the viscid fœtid sweat, the cough, the flying acute pains in the limbs after perspiration, the podagra, the inflammatory erysipelas, the pustules on the skin, the itching and redness of the skin, underneath which the glands lie, the artificial jaundice, the horripilation, the continued fever, &c., it produces, are all proofs of this. But the observations are not accurate enough to enable us to determine which is the primary, which the secondary action. The direct action seems to continue for a considerable time. A lax, unexcitable state of the fibres and vessels, especially of those belonging to the absorbent system, which seem partly deprived of vital power, appears to be its secondary action. Hence the perspiration, the flow of saliva, the frequent discharge of watery urine, the hæmorrhages (a dissolved state of the red parts of the blood); and after large doses, or too long-continued employment, the dropsy, the obstinate jaundice, the petechiæ, the gangrenous decomposition of the fluids. Employed cautiously in gradually-increased doses, it may, as indeed experience has partly shown, be employed with lasting advantage in a similar derangement of the fluids, and in a similar state of the solids; in a word, in similar morbid states to those it is capable of producing. In induration of the liver, jaundice, and glandular swellings, with tense fibre, in chronic catarrh, catarrh of the bladder (in dysentery, dysuria, tumours, with tense fibre?), in amenorrhœa with tense fibre. (On account of its long-enduring, direct action, it may sometimes be of permanent service as an antagonistically-acting remedy in rachitis, in amenorrhœa with relaxation, &c. But this does not belong to our subject.)

The *monkshood* (*aconitum napellus*) excites formicating, also acute tearing pains in the limbs, in the chest, in the jaws; it is a prime remedy in pains of the limbs of all kinds (?); it will be serviceable in chronic tooth-ache of a rheumatic character, in pleurodynia, in face-ache, and in the consequences of the implantation of human teeth. It causes chilling pressure in the stomach, occipital head-ache, shootings in the kidneys, excessively painful ophthalmia, cutting pains in the tongue; the practitioner will be able to employ these artificial diseases in similar natural diseases. It has a peculiar tendency to produce giddiness, faintings, debility, apoplexy, and transient paralysis, general and partial paralysis, hemiplegia, paralysis of particular limbs,—of the tongue, of the anus, of the bladder, obscuration of vision and temporary blindness, and singing in the ears. It is also just as serviceable in general and partial paralysis of the parts just mentioned, as experience has in a great measure proved;—as a similarly-acting remedy, it has in several cases cured incontinence of urine, paralysis of the tongue, and amaurosis, as also paralysis of the limbs. In curable marasmus, and partial atrophies, as a remedy capable of producing similar morbid symptoms, it will certainly do more than all other known remedies. Successful cases of this kind are on record. Almost as specifically does it produce convulsions, general as well as partial, of the facial muscles, of the muscles of the lips on one side, of the muscles of the throat on one side of the ocular muscles. In all these last affections it will prove useful, as it has also cured epilepsies. It causes asthma; how, then, can it be wondered at, that it has several times cured different sorts of asthma? It produces itching, formication in the skin, desquamation, reddish eruption, and is hence so useful in bad cutaneous affections and ulcers. Its pretended efficacy in the most obstinate venereal sufferings, was probably only founded on its power over the symptoms of the mercury that had been previously employed in that disease; and this conclusion is justified by what we know of its action. It is valuable to know that monkshood, as an exciter of pain, cutaneous affections, swellings, and irritability,—in a word, as a similarly-acting remedy, is powerful in subduing the similar mercurial disease, and is even preferable to opium, as it leaves behind it no debility. Sometimes it causes a sensation about the navel, as if a ball rose up thence, and spread a cold feeling over the upper and back part of the head; this would lead us to use it in similar cases of hysteria. In the secondary action, the primary coldness in the head seems to change into a burning sensation. In its primary action are observed general coldness, slow pulse, retention of urine, mania; in its secondary action, however, an intermitting, small, rapid pulse, general perspiration, flow of urine, diarrhœa, involuntary fæcal evacuation, sleepy intoxication: (Like several other plants that produce a cooling effect in their primary action, it resolves glandular swellings.) The mania it causes is a gay humour alternating with despair. As a similarly-acting remedy, it will subdue manias of that sort. The usual duration of its efficacy is from seven to eight hours, excepting in cases of serious effects from very large doses.

The *black hellebore* (*helleborus niger*) causes, if used for a long time, severe head-aches, (hence, probably, its power in some mental affections, also in chronic head-aches,) and a fever; hence its power in quartan fever, and hence also, partly, its efficacy in dropsies, the worst kinds of which are always accompanied by remitting fever, and wherein it is so useful, aided by its diuretic power. (Who can tell whether this belongs to its primary, or, as I am inclined to think, its secondary action? This power is allied to its property of exciting to activity the blood-vessels of the abdomen, rectum, and uterus.) Its power of causing a constrictive, suffocating sensation in the nose, would lead us to prescribe it in similar cases (as I once did in a kind of mental disease). The frequency with which it is confounded with other roots is the reason why we are only in possession of these few true data of its effects.

The boring, cutting pain that the internal use of the *meadow anemone* (*anemone pratensis*) causes in weak eyes, led to its successful employment in amaurosis, cataract, and opacity of the cornea. The cutting headache caused by the internal employment of the inflammable crystalline salt obtained by distillation with water, would lead us to employ this plant in a similar case. Most likely it is on this account that it once cured a case of melancholia.

The *clove gilliflower* (*geum urbanum*), besides its aromatic qualities, possesses a nausea-exciting power, which always causes a febrile state of body, and hence its service in intermittent fever, when used as an aromatic along with ipecacuanha.

The principle that constitutes the medicinal power of the kernel of the *cherry* (*prunus cerasus*), of the *sour cherry* (*prunus padus*), of the *peach* (*amygdalus persica*), of the bitter variety of the *almond* (*amygdalus communis*) and more especially of the leaves of the *cherry-laurel* (*prunus laurocerasus*), possesses the peculiar property of increasing the vital power and contractility of the muscular fibre in its direct action, as notably as it depresses both in its secondary action. Moderately large doses are followed by anxiety, a peculiar cramp of the stomach, trismus, rigidity of the tongue, opisthotonos, alternately with clonic cramps of various kinds and degrees, as its direct action;[1] the irritability is gra-

---

[1] If it is sought to deny the primary action of the principle of bitter almond, which I have represented as producing the phenomena of increased power of contraction in the muscular fibre and exaltation of the vital power, on this ground, that in some cases of monstrous doses, death occurs almost instantaneously without any perceptible reaction of the vital power or pain, as great a mistake would be made, as if all pain should be denied to death by the sword, and it should be affirmed that the stroke of the sword did not produce a peculiar condition different from the death that followed it. This pain will be just as intense, although perhaps less than momentary, as the sensation of anxiety and torment will be indescribable, which may and must follow a fatal dose of cherry-laurel water, though its action lasts scarce a minute. This is proved by the case recorded by Madden, of excessive anxiety in the region of the stomach (the probable region of the chief organ of the vital power) of a person killed in a few minutes by a large dose of cherry-laurel water. That in this brief space of time, the whole series of phenomena that follow a not fatal dose, cannot make their appearance, is easily understood; yet it is probable that changes and impressions, similar to those of the direct action I have described from nature, do actually take place in the animal organism, in this short time (until a few instants before death, i, e., the few instants that the indirect secondary action lasts.) Thus, electrical phenomena may be seen, when they can be gradually passed before the eyes; but in the lightning rapidly flashing before us, we scarce can tell what we see or hear.

dually exhausted,[1] and in the secondary action the contractility
of the muscular fibre and the vital power sink in the same degree
that they had previously been exalted.   There follow cold, relaxation, paralysis,—which also, however, soon pass off.

(Cherry-laurel water has now and then been used as a domestic
analeptic, in debility of the stomach and body, that is, as an
oppositely-acting palliative, and, as might have been guessed,
with bad effect.   The result was paralysis and apoplexy.)

More remarkable, and peculiarly belonging to our subject, is
the curative power of its direct action (which consists in a kind
of febrile paroxysm) in intermittent fever, especially, if I mistake
not, in that kind of intermittent depending on a too great contractility of the muscular fibre, which is incurable by bark alone.
Equally efficacious has black cherry water proved in the convulsions of children. As a similarly-acting remedy, cherry-laurel
water will prove efficacious in diseases from too tense fibre, or
generally where the contractility of the muscular fibre far exceeds its relaxing power; in hydrophobia, in tetanus, in the
spasmodic closure of the biliary excretory ducts and similar tonic
spasmodic affections, in some manias, &c.,[2] as several observations
have shown.   In proper inflammatory diseases it also deserves
attention, where it would, to some extent, operate as a similarly-
acting remedy. If the diuretic property observed from the bitter-
almond principle lies in its indirect secondary action, we may
hope much from it in dropsy, with a chronic inflammatory condition of the blood.

The power of the bark of the *sour cluster-cherry* (*prunus padus*)
over intermittent fever lies likewise in the bitter-almond principle it contains, by means of which it comports itself as a similarly-acting remedy.

Of the *sundew* (*drosera rotundifolia*) we know nothing certain,
except that it excites cough, and hence it has been of use in most
catarrhal coughs, as also in the influenza.

The curative principle in the flowers and other parts of the

---

[1] A small lizard (*lacerta agilis*), that had moved about pretty rapidly for a minute
in diluted cherry-laurel-water, I placed in concentrated cherry-laurel water. The
motions became instantly so excessively rapid, that the eye could scarcely follow
them for some seconds; then there occurred one or two slow convulsions, and then
total loss of motion: it was dead.

[2] Tonic (and clonic) spasms without an inflammatory state of the blood, and when
the consciousness is little affected, appear to be the peculiar sphere of action of the
principle of bitter almonds, as it, as far as I know, does not elevate the vital
temperature even in its direct action, and leaves the sensitive system unaffected.

elder (*sambucus niger*), appears to lie in its primary direct action of exalting the contractive power of the muscular fibres belonging chiefly to the natural and vital functions, and of raising the temperature of the blood, whilst, in its indirect secondary action, it brings down the strength of the muscular fibre, lowers the temperature, relaxes the vital activity, and diminishes sensation itself. If this be the case, as I think it is, the good that it does in the true spasm of the finest extremities of the arteries, in diseases from a chill, catarrhs, erysipelas, is in virtue of its similarity of action. Have not the elder species the power of producing transitory erysipelatous inflammation?

Various kinds of *sumach*, considered to be poisonous, *e. g., rhus radicans*, appear to possess a specific tendency to produce erysipelatous inflammation of the skin and cutaneous eruptions. May it not be useful in chronic erysipelas, and the worst kinds of skin diseases? When its action is too violent, it is checked by elder, (a similarly-acting remedy?)

Camphor in large doses diminishes the sensibility of the whole nervous system; the influence of the, as it were, benumbed vital spirits (if I may be allowed to use a coarse expression), on the senses and motion is suspended. There occurs a congestion in the brain, an obscuration, a vertigo, an inability to bring the muscles under the dominion of the will, an incapacity for thought, for sensation, for memory. The contractile power of the muscular fibres, especially of those belonging to the natural and vital functions, seems to sink to actual paralysis; the irritability is depressed in a like degree, especially that of the extreme ends of the blood-vessels,[1] that of the larger arteries less, and still less that of the heart. There occur coldness of the external parts, small, hard, gradually diminishing pulse, and on account of the different state of the heart from that of the extreme ends of the bloodvessels, anxiety, cold sweat. The above condition of the fibre causes an immobility of the muscles, *e. g.*, of the jaws, of the anus, of the neck, that resembles a tonic spasm. There ensue deep slow breathing, fainting.[2] During the transition to the secondary action, there occur convulsions, madness, vomiting, trembling. In the indirect secondary action itself, the awaken-

[1] The nervous power and its condition seems to have most influence on these, —less on the larger vessels, least of all on the heart.

[2] A proof, according to Carminati, that Camphor, far from extinguishing the irritability, only suspends it so long as the muscles are in connexion with the benumbed state of the nerves—is, that when all sensation is extinguished by means of camphor, the heart, if cut out, continues to beat all the more strongly for hours afterwards.

ing of the sensibility; and if I may be allowed the expression, the mobility of the previously benumbed nervous spirit first commence; the almost extinguished mobility of the extremities of the arteries is restored, the heart triumphs over the previous resistance. The previous slow pulsations increase in velocity and in fulness, the play of the circulating system attains, or in some cases (from larger doses of camphor, from plethora, &c.) surpasses, its former state,—the pulse becomes more rapid, and more full. The more motionless the bloodvessels were previously, the more active do they now become; the temperature of the whole body becomes increased, with redness, and uniform, sometimes profuse, perspiration. The whole process is ended in six, eight, ten, twelve, or at most twenty-four hours. Of all the muscular fibres, the mobility of the intestinal canal returns latest. In every case where the contractile power of the muscular fibres greatly preponderates over their power of relaxation, camphor, as an antagonistically-acting remedy, procures rapid but only palliative relief; in some manias, in local and general inflammations, of a pure, of a rheumatic, and of an erysipelatous character, and in diseases arising from a chill.

As in pure malignant typhus, the system of the muscular fibre, the sensitive system, and the depressed vital power, presents something analogous to the direct primary action of camphor, it operates as a similarly-acting remedy, that is, permanently and beneficially. The doses must, however, be sufficiently large to produce the appearance of a still greater insensibility and depression, but given seldom, only about every thirty-six or forty-eight hours.

If camphor actually removes the strangury caused by cantharides, it does this as a similarly-acting remedy, for it also causes strangury. The bad effects of drastic purgatives it removes, chiefly as a suspender of sensation, and a relaxer of the fibre (consequently an antagonistic, palliative, but here, admirable remedy). In the bad secondary effects of squill, when they are chronic—a too easily excitable action of the contractile and relaxing power of the muscular fibre—it acts only as a palliative, and less efficaciously, unless the doses be frequently repeated. The same may be said with regard to its effects in the chronic symptoms caused by the abuse of mercury. As a similarly-acting remedy, it is eminently serviceable in the long-continued rigour of degenerated (comatose) intermittent fevers, as an adjunct to bark. Epilepsy and convulsions dependent on relaxed fibre deprived of its irritability, are rapidly cured by the similar action of camphor. It is an approved antidote to large doses of opium, in which it is chiefly an antagonistic palliative, but efficacious in consequence of the symptoms being but tran·sitory. In like manner, opium is, as I have ascertained, an excellent antidote to large doses of camphor. The former raises the sunken vital power and diminished vital temperature caused by the latter, antagonistically, but in this case effectually. A curious phenomenon is the action of coffee in relation to the direct action of large doses of camphor; it makes the stomach, whose irritability was suspended spasmodically mobile; there occur convulsions, vomiting, or when given in clysters, rapid evacuation; but neither does the vital power become raised, nor do the nerves become relieved from their stupified state, they rather become more stupified, as I think I have observed. As the most striking effect of camphor on the nerves consists in this, that all the passions are lulled, and a perfect indifference to external things, even of the most interesting character, occurs, as I have ascertained, it will accordingly be of service as a similarly-acting remedy in manias, whose chief symptom is apathy, with slow, suppressed pulse, and contracted pupil,—also, according to Auenbrugger, retracted testicles. It is by no means advisable to use it in manias of every description. Used internally, camphor removes acute general and local inflammations, and also such as are chronic, in a few hours; but in the former case, the doses must be very often repeated to admit of anything efficacious being performed, *i. e.*, always a new dose before the secondary action comes on. For in its secondary action, camphor does but the more strengthen the tendency to renewed inflammation, makes it chronic, and predisposes the organism chiefly to catarrhal diseases, and the bad effects of a chill. Used externally for a length of time, it can do more good, and its bad effects may be easily remedied in another manner.

The patrons of new medicines generally commit the error of carefully but injudiciously concealing the disagreeable effects of the medicines they take under their protection.[1] Were it not for this suppression of the truth, we might, for instance, from the morbific effects the bark of the *horse-chesnut* (*aesculus hip-*

---

[1] Thus we often read, that this or that powerful medicine has cured so many hundred cases of the worst diseases, without causing the slightest bad effects. If this last be correct, we may certainly infer the perfect inefficacy of the drug. The more serious the symptoms it causes, the more important is it for the practitioner.

poscastanum) is able to produce, form a just estimate of its medicinal powers, and determine if, for instance, it is suitable for pure intermittent fever, or some of its varieties; and if so, which. The sole phenomenon we know belonging to it is, that it produces a constrictive feeling in the chest. It will accordingly be found useful in (periodical) spasmodic asthma.

The symptoms produced on man by the *phytolacca decandra* deserve to be particularly described. It is certainly a very medicinal plant. In animals it causes cough, trembling, convulsions.

As the bark of the *elm* (*ulmus campestris*), when exhibited internally, produces at the commencement[1] an increase of cutaneous eruptions, it is more than probable that it has a tendency to produce such affections of itself, consequently, that it will be serviceable in them, which is amply proved by experience.

The juice of *hemp leaves* (*cannabis sativa*) is, it would seem, a narcotic, similar in action to opium. This is only in appearance, however, and owing to the imperfect accounts we have of its pathogenetic action. I am much mistaken if it do not possess differences indicative of peculiar medicinal powers, if we but knew it sufficiently. It produces dimness of vision; and in the madness caused by it there occur many phenomena, generally of an agreeable character.

It appears as if *saffron* (*crocus sativus*), in its direct action, brought down the circulation and vital heat. Slow pulse, pale face, vertigo, exhaustion, have been observed. In this stage most probably occur the melancholy and headache that have been observed from its action, and in the second stage (the indirect secondary action), occur the senseless, extravagant gaiety, the stupefaction of the senses, the increased action in the arteries and heart, and lastly, the hæmorrhage which have been observed from its use. For this reason it may be useful in restoring flows of blood that have been checked, as a similarly-acting remedy, as its power of increasing the circulation occurs first in the secondary action; consequently, the opposite must take place in its direct action. It has been found useful as a similarly-acting remedy in vertigo and headache, with slow pulse. In

---

[1] In order to draw a favourable induction from the aggravating action of a drug in a disease, this aggravation must occur at the commencement of its use, that is, in its direct action; in such cases only can it be considered a similarly-acting efficacious remedy. The morbid aggravations occurring so often subsequently (in the indirect secondary action) prove the contrary in ill-chosen remedies.

some cases of melancholia with slow pulse, and in amenorrhœa, it appears also to be of service as a similarly-acting remedy. It has (in its direct action) produced death by appoplexy, and is said to have proved efficacious in similar affections (probably in relaxed organisms). The phenomena of its secondary action point to much increased irritability of the fibre, hence probably the cause of its so readily producing hysteria.

The *darnel* (*lolium temulentum*) is such a powerful plant, that he who knows its pathogenetic action must congratulate the age when, for the benefit of humanity, its application shall be known. The chief phenomena of the direct action of the seeds are cramps, apparently of a tonic character (a kind of immobility), with relaxation of the fibre and suspension of the vital spirits, great anxiety, exhaustion, coldness, contraction of the stomach, dyspnœa, difficult deglutition, rigidity of the tongue pressive headache and vertigo (both continue longer than is known from any other drug, in the greatest degree, for several days), noises in the ears, sleeplessness, insensibility, or weakness of the external senses, red face, staring eyes, sparks before the eyes. In the transition to the secondary action, the cramps become clonic, there occur stammering, trembling, vomiting, diuresis, and (cold) perspiration (cutaneous eruptions, ulcers on the skin?) yawning (another kind of cramp), weak sight, long sleep. In practice, cases of obstinate vertigo and cephalalgia present themselves, which we are inclined to avoid treating, from their incurability. The darnel appears to be made expressly for the worst of such cases, probably also for imbecility, the opprobium of medicine. In deafness and amaurosis something may be hoped from its use.

Squill (*scilla maritima*) appears to possess an acrid principle that remains long in the body ; the mode of operation of which, from want of accurate observation, cannot be very well separated into primary and secondary action. This acrid principle possesses a tendency to diminish for a long period the capacity of the blood for caloric, and hence to establish in the organism a disposition to chronic inflammation. Whether this power can be applied to useful purposes, instead of being, as hitherto, a stumbling-block to the use of the drug itself, I am unable, on account of the obscurity of the subject, to determine. As, however, this power must certainly have its limits, at least in the commencement, it has only an acute inflammatory action, and afterwards, especially after long-continued use, leaves behind it the slow chronic inflammatory action ; so it seems to me to be rather indicated in pure inflammations with tense fibre, when its use is otherwise required, than in a cold or hectic inflammatory condition of the fluids and mobility of the fibre. The incomparable aid derived from squill in inflammation of the lungs, and the extraordinary injury inflicted by its *continued* employment in chronic purulent consumption of the lungs, as also in pituitous consumption, prove this satisfactorily ; there is no question here of palliative relief. This acrid principle puts the mucous glands in a condition to secrete a thin, instead of a viscid mucus, as is the case in every moderately inflammatory diathesis. Squill causes a great degree of strangury, shewing thereby that it must be very useful in restoring the secretion in the suppression of the urine accompanying several kinds of dropsy, as daily experience confirms. Rapid, acute dropsical swellings appear to be its chief sphere of action. It has cured some kinds of tickling cough, because it can of itself cause cough.

That most incomparable remedy, *white hellebore (veratrum album)*, produces the most poisonous effects, which should inspire the physician who aspires to perfection with caution, and the hope of curing some of the most troublesome diseases that have hitherto usually been beyond medical aid. It produces in its direct action a kind of mania, amounting from larger doses to hopelessness and despair; small doses make indifferent things appear repulsive to the imagination, although they are not so in reality. It causes in its direct action, *a.* heat of the whole body ; *b.* burning in different external parts, *e. g.*, the shoulder-blades, the face, the head ; *c.* inflammation and swelling of the skin of the face, sometimes (from larger doses) of the whole body ; *d.* cutaneous eruptions, desquamation of the skin ; *e.* a formicating sensation in the hands and fingers, tonic cramps ; *f.* constriction of the gullet, of the larynx, sense of suffocation ; *g.* rigidity of the tongue, tough mucus in the mouth ; *h.* constriction of the chest ; *i.* pleuritic symptoms ; *k.* cramp in the calves ; *l.* an anxious, (gnawing ?) sensation in the stomach, nausea ; *m.* gripes, and cutting pains here and there in the bowels ; *n.* great general anxiety ; *o.* vertigo ; *p.* head-ache (confusion of the head) ; *q.* violent thirst. On passing into the indirect secondary action, the tonic cramps resolve themselves into clonic cramps ; there occur, *r.* trembling ; *s.* stammering ; *t.* convulsions of the eyes ; *u.* hiccough ; *v.* sneezing (from the internal use) ; *w.* vomiting (when at its height, black, bloody vomiting) ; *x.* painful, scanty evacuations, with tenesmus ; *y.* local, or (from large doses) general convulsions: *z*. cold (from large doses, bloody) sweat; *aa*. watery diuresis; *bb*. ptyalism; *cc*. expectoration; *dd*. general coldness; *ee*. marked weakness; *ff*. fainting; *gg*. long profound sleep.—Some of the symptoms of its direct action, *l. m. n. p. q.*, would lead us to use it in dysenteric fever, if not in dysentery. The mania it causes, together with some symptoms of its direct action, *e. f. g. g. h. n. q.*, would lead us to employ it in hydrophobia, with hopes of a good result. A dog to which it was given had true rabies, lasting eight minutes. The ancients speak of it with approbation in hydrophobia. (In tetanus?) in spasmodic constriction of the gullet, and in spasmodic asthma, it will be found specific on account of *f.* and *h.* It will prove of permanent advantage in chronic cutaneous diseases, on account of *c.* and *d.* as experience has already shown with regard to herpes. In so-called nervous diseases, when they are dependent on tense fibre or inflammatory symptoms, (*a. q.*) and the symptoms in other respects resemble the veratrum disease, it will be of benefit; so also in manias of like character.—The landlord of a country inn, a man of firm fibre, robust make, red blooming countenance, and somewhat prominent eyes, had almost every morning, soon after waking, an anxious feeling in the stomachic region, which in the course of a few hours involved the chest, producing constriction there, sometimes amounting to complete loss of breath; in the course of a few hours the affection attacked the region of the larynx, and suffocation became imminent (swallowing solids or fluids being impossible); and as the sun declined it left these parts, and became confined to the head, with timorous, despairing, hopeless suicidal thoughts, until about ten o'clock, when he fell asleep, and all the morbid symptoms disappeared. The mania resembling that peculiar to veratrum, the firm fibre of the patient, and the symptoms *f. g. h. l. n.*, induced me to prescribe three grains of it every morning, which he continued for four weeks, with the gradual cessation of all his sufferings; his malady had lasted four years or more.—A woman, thirty-five years of age, after having had many epileptic attacks during her pregnancies, was affected a few days after her last delivery, with furious delirium and general convulsions of the limbs. She had been treated for ten days with emetics and purgatives, without effect. At midnight every night she was attacked by fever, with great restlessness, during which she tore all the clothes off her body, especially what she had about her neck. Cinchona bark always made the fever a few hours later, and increased the thirst and anxiety; the expressed juice of stramonium, used according to Bergius' method, soon quelled the convulsions, and produced some rational hours, in which it was ascertained that her worst symptom (except the fever) was the suffocating feeling in the throat and chest, besides pain in all her limbs. More, however, it could not do; on the contrary, its continued use seemed rather to increase the last mentioned serious symptoms; the face was swollen, the anxiety infinite, the fever greater. Emetics did no good; opium caused sleeplessness, increased the restlessness; the urine was dark-brown, the bowels much constipated. Blood-letting, which was evidently not adapted to this case, was, moreover, contra-indicated by the excessive weakness. The deliria returned, notwithstanding the extract of stramonium, with increased convulsions and swelling of the feet. I gave her in the forenoon half a grain of veratrum powder, and a similar dose in the afternoon at two o'clock. Deliria of another kind made their appearance, along with viscid mucus in the mouth, but no fever returned, the patient slept, and in the morning passed white cloudy urine. She was well, quiet and rational, except that the great weakness continued. The suffocating sensation in the throat was gone, the swelling of the face fell, as also that of the feet, but the following evening, without her having taken any medicine, there occurred a constrictive sensation in the chest. She therefore got another half grain of veratrum the following afternoon; this was followed by scarcely perceptible delirium, tranquil sleep, in the morning copious discharge of urine and a few small evacuations. For two more days she got half a grain of veratrum in the afternoon. All her symptoms disappeared, the fever vanished, and the weakness yielded to a good regimen.

I shall on a subsequent occasion[1] record a case of spasmodic colic still more rapidly cured by it. As a producer of mania and spasms it has shown itself useful in cases of persons possessed. In hysterical and hypochondriacal attacks, dependent on tense fibre, it will be useful, as it has been practically proved. Inflammation of the lungs will find in it a powerful remedy. The duration of its action is short; limited to about five, at most eight or ten hours, inclusive of the secondary action; except in the case of serious effects from large doses.

Sabadilla seed causes confusion of the intellect and convulsions, which it can also cure; the peculiarities of its action, however,

---

[1] See next article.

are not yet known. It also causes a creeping sensation through all the limbs, as I have experienced, and is said to produce pain in the stomach and nausea.

The *agaric* (*agaricus muscarius*) produces, as far as I can ascertain, a furious and drunken mania (combined with revengeful, bold resolves, disposition to make verses, to prophesy, &c.), exaltation of the strength, trembling and convulsions, in its primary direct action; and weariness, sleep, in its secondary action. It has therefore been employed with benefit in epilepsy (caused by fright), combined with trembling. It will remove mental affections and possession, similar to those it causes. Its direct action lasts from twelve to sixteen hours.

The *nutmeg* (*myristica aromatica*) diminishes the irritability of the whole body, but especially that of the primæ viæ, for a considerable time. (Does it not increase the contractile power of the muscular fibre, especially of the primæ viæ, and diminish its capability of relaxing?) In large doses it causes an absolute insensibility of the nervous system, obtuseness, immobility, loss of reason, for its direct action; headache and sleep for its secondary action. It possesses heating properties. May it not be useful in imbecility, combined with laxness and irritability of the primæ viæ?—against the first as a similarly, against the second as an antagonistically-acting remedy? It is said to have done good in paralysis of the gullet, probably as a similarly-acting remedy.

Rhubarb is useful in diarrhœas without fæcal evacuations, even in the smallest doses, more in consequence of its tendency to promote the action of the bowels, than on account of its astringent power

The topical pain-producing applications, as catharides, mustard plasters, grated horse-radish, spurge-laurel bark, crushed ranunculus acris, the moxa, allay pain often permanently, by producing artificially pain of another kind.

CASE OF RAPIDLY CURED COLICODYNIA.[1]

L——IE, a compositor, 24 years of age, lean, of a pale and earthy complexion, had worked at the printing-press a year and

---

[1] From Hufeland's *Journal der practischen Arzneykunde.* Vol. iii. 1797.

a half before he came to me, and then for the first time suddenly felt great pain in the left side which obliged him to keep his bed, and which after several days went away under the use of ordinary medicines. Ever since that, however, he had experienced a dull disagreeable sensation in the left hypochondrium. Some months afterwards, when he had overloaded his stomach with sweet beer-soup flavoured with caraway, he was attacked with a severe colic, the violence of which he could not express, but at the same time could not say whether it corresponded with the colicodynia which succeeded it.

The attack passed off this time, I don't know how, but he observed, that after it he could not bear certain kinds of food. The mischief increased unobserved, and the colicodynia with its distinctive symptoms took firm root.

The worst kinds of food for him were carrots, all sorts of cabbage, especially white cabbage and sour-crout, and every species of fruit, but pears in particular.

If he were so incautious as to eat any of these things within eight days after an attack which had been brought on by them, the liability was so increased that he could not eat even a morsel of a pear, for example, one or two weeks after without bringing on another severe attack.

The course of a severe attack was as follows. Four hours or four hours and a half after eating of such food—having previously felt quite well—a certain movement was felt about the umbilical region; then there took place suddenly, always at the same place, a pinching as if by pincers, but attended with the most intolerable pain which lasted half or a whole minute, and each time suddenly went away with borborygmus extending to the right groin—about the region of the cœcum. When the attack was very bad the pinching came back, and the subsequent borborygmus more and more frequently, until in the worst attacks they were almost constant. There occurred also the sensation of a constriction above and below, so that flatus could pass neither upwards nor downwards. The uneasiness and pains increased from hour to hour, the abdomen swelled and became painful to the touch. Along with all this suffering, which resembled a fever, there came an inclination to vomit, with sense of constriction of the chest, the breathing was shorter and attended with more and more difficulty, cold sweat broke out, and there came on a sort of stupefaction with total exhaustion. At this period it was impossible for him to swallow a drop of liquid, much less any solid food. Thus he lay stupified and unconscious, with swollen face and protruded eyes, and without sleep for many hours; the attack of spasmodic colic gradually subsided by diminution of the pain, then followed some escape of flatus either upwards or downwards, and so the attack went off, (sometimes only after sixteen or twenty-four hours from its commencement). The strength only returned after three or four days, and thus he was again like a person in health, without any other uneasiness except the dull fixed pain before described, and general weakness and sickly appearance. He could not positively say whether this dull pain went off during the severe attacks or not, but he thought it did.

In these circumstances he could not retain his situation at the printing-press; he became a compositor. The attacks always recurred under the condition described, and had continued to do so for more than a year when he put himself under my care.

It might easily be supposed that the attacks arose from flatulence; this however was not the case. He could take, without the least inconvenience, a good meal of dry peas, lentils, beans or potatoes, and he was obliged to do so moreover, as his position did not allow him the opportunity of getting much else.

Or it might be supposed to arise from some kind of fermentation in the primæ viæ, or from some idiosyncrasy in respect to sweet things. But nothing was further from the case. He could take cakes baked with yeast, and sugar and milk as much as he pleased, even to satiety, without the slightest threatening of colic, although the first attack, *seemed*, as I have said, to be occasioned by the beer soup.

Or could an injurious acidity have occurred within the four hours (for the attack *never* occurred sooner, after partaking of the above things)? This was not the cause. Lemon-juice and vinegar were both innocuous. Neither did he ever vomit sour matter, either during the retching that occurred with the attack or when ordered an emetic. None of the absorbent earths or alkalis were of any use to him, whether taken during or before the attack.

A physician had suspected tape-worm, and subjected him to Herrnschwand's treatment,[1] without any result. Neither before nor after he had passed anything which had the smallest

---

[1] [Herrnschwand's method consisted chiefly in the employment of the powder of male-fern root, followed by purgatives, principally castor-oil.]

resemblance to a tape-worm or indeed to any kind of worm at all.

When he came to me the idea of tape-worm had taken so firm a hold of his mind that I was obliged to order him all that was peculiar in the methods of Nuffer[1] and of Clossius.[2] He used all the medicines with patience, and pressed me to try every means with this view. Tartrate of antimony, gamboge, scammony, male-fern (four ounces daily for four hours together) charcoal, artemesia in large quantities, colocynth with oils, castor oil, tin, iron, sabadilla, sulphur, petroleum, camphor, assafœtida, and laxative salts—nothing was left untried; but they were given, as I have said, rather on account of his urgent request than to satisfy my own conviction, for besides the fact that no worms were ever seen, the two symptoms which I have so often observed to attend worms were absent, viz., the deeply wrinkled countenance and the sensation of a cold stream winding itself towards the back immediately after a meal.

Immediately after the sabadilla, which produced a creeping sensation like ants upon the skin (formication) and a heat in the stomach and over the whole body, I let him try the test of eating a piece of pear. It appeared indeed as if the attack had returned quite mildly, but after I had left him without medicine for eight days and again tried him with a small piece of pear, the colic came on just as bad as ever.

I have forgotten to mention that I had already previously tried all sorts of powerful so-called antispasmodic remedies at the commencement of the paroxysm. Small doses of ipecacuanha taken dry, lukewarm foot-baths and larger baths, opium and cajeput oil, without any result, even without any palliative effect. I only sought to palliate the symptoms at that time in order that he might continue without molestation to use cinchona bark and to wash with cold water, to get the better of his weakness.

As his condition required immediate help, inasmuch as the colicodynia began to appear even upon the use of the smallest quantity of vegetable food, and as all I have done at his entreaty

---

[1] [Madame Nuffer's method, which was purchased by the French Government for 18,000 livres, consisted mainly of the adminstration of the powder of the male-fern root, accompanied by a number of complex directions which were to be implicitly followed to ensure success.]

[2] [Clossius' method was to feed the patient during four weeks on salted meat cheese, and a good allowance of wine, and thereafter to give drastic purgatives consisting chiefly of gamboge.]

had been of no service whatever, I determined to give him a medicine which produced very similar morbid symptoms. The similarity of the griping pain, anxiety, constriction of the chest, fever, loss of strength, &c., produced by *veratrum album* appeared to me calculated to give permanent relief.

I gave him four powders, each containing four grains, and told him to take one powder daily, but to let me know at once if any violent symptoms appeared. This he did not do. He did not return until five days thereafter. His unlimited confidence in my aid had nearly played him an awkward trick. The benefit I had promised from the powders had induced him to take two instead of one daily. After the second powder, without his having eaten anything injurious, there began an attack which he could not otherwise describe than as his spasmodic colic, or something very like it. This did not prevent him, however, from taking the third and fourth powder the following day (taking thus sixteen grains in rather less than two days), upon which, this artificial colic, if I may so speak, increased to such a dreadful extent, that, to use his own expression, he wrestled with death, covered with cold sweat and almost suffocated. He had required the remaining three days to recruit, and had returned for further directions. I reprimanded him for his imprudence, but could not avoid notwithstanding comforting him with the prospect of a good issue. The result confirmed it; under the use of tolerably good diet he regained his strength, and he has not had for half a year even a threatening of an attack, although from time to time he has eaten of the food which before was so injurious to him, but in moderation, as I impressed upon him he should. Since this event he has taken no more medicine, and no tapeworm was passed after the use of the veratrum.

The dull pain in the left hypochondrium likewise went at the same time.

ARE THE OBSTACLES TO CERTAINTY AND SIMPLICITY IN PRACTICAL MEDICINE INSURMOUNTABLE?[1]

Dr. Herz's essay " *On the Medicinal uses of the Phellandrium aquaticum,*" &c., in the first part of the second volume of the *Journal der practischen Arzneykunde*, plunged me into a sort of

[1] From *Hufeland's Journal der practischen Arzneykunde*, Vol. iv., Part iv., page 106. 1797.

melancholy, which only by dint of long continued reflection has given place to a remote but lively hope.

Here one of the most thoughtful physicians of our time, after twenty years of active practice, finds himself obliged repeatedly to make the open, but most melancholy acknowledgment: (p. 40.)

"That we can lay no claim to the attainment of the ideal of simplicity in medical treatment."

"That the hope of ever arriving at perfect simplicity in medical practice, cannot be otherwise than very feeble" (p. 47).

The obstacles to pure observation of the effects of medicines in the various diseases, he enumerates with most overwhelming fulness of detail, and there he leaves us alone in the old well-worn path of uncertainty, almost without a cheering glance at a better futurity, a simpler, surer method of cure; unless we are to reckon his very complaints as foreshadowing coming improvements, just as the impassioned warmth of the sceptical casuist has always appeared to me a proof of that immortality he would deny.

I myself felt the external hindrances to our art more than I could have wished; they continually beset my sphere of action; and I, too, long considered them insurmountable, and had almost made up my mind to despair, and to esteem my profession as but the sport of inevitable accident and insuperable obstacles, when the thought arose within me, " *are not we physicians partly to blame for the complexity and the uncertainty of our art ?* "

OBEDIENCE OF PATIENTS.

I have seen medical men take under their care *patients who had only half confidence*, and from whose demeanour any one might perceive that they put themselves under the physician whom they had chosen, not from any enthusiastic regard for him, nor from a strong desire to be relieved from their sufferings. How could implicit obedience be expected from such persons? And even when they spoke of, and commended in commonplace terms, strict attention to the physician's orders, could he trust them, and with confidence ascribe the issue to his prescriptions, his medicines? By no means!

DIET AND REGIMEN.

It is a constant complaint of physicians that patients will not observe the *prescribed* diet. " Who shall give them assurance of such compliance? and how impossible, then, is it to determine the issue of a disease, or the effect of the remedies employed, since on this point in no case can any certainty be attained? "

Pardon me! We may be perfectly sure of such as with implicit confidence entrust themselves to the care of their almost worshipped physician. Of course, others are less to be relied upon.

Methinks, however, that medical men when thus complaining, do not draw a sufficient distinction between, 1st, the *errors of diet* which produced and kept up the patient's disease; 2d, their ordinary *indifferent diet;* and, 3d, the *new dietetic regulations* laid down by the physician.

If, with respect to the first of these (the correction of the errors of diet), the physician thinks that he does not possess sufficient authority with his patient, who will not pay strict attention to rules, rather let him dismiss such fickle-minded persons; better no patients at all than such!

Who, for example, would undertake to cure a drunkard of induration of the liver, who merely consulted the physician *en passant,* because, perhaps, he met him in the street; or had some business-matters to arrange with him; or, because the physician has come to reside in the neighbourhood; or has become a connexion of his; or for some other trifling reason, but not from having implicit confidence in his skill? What immense influence the medical man must have with such a confirmed debauchee, to feel assured that he will pay attention to his orders, and daily diminish his allowance of the poisonous liquor!

A patient with such bad habits, must show by some considerable sacrifice, that he intends to submit himself entirely to the will of the physician. The physician would do well to try to dissuade him from submitting to treatment; to represent to him, in strong terms, the difficulties which his ruinous vice throws in the way, and the magnitude of the disease. If he return repeatedly, and express his willingness to make any sacrifices, then, what should prevent the physician trusting him, so long as he sees indubitable proofs of his resolution? If he cannot withstand temptation, then let him go his way; he will, at any rate, not bring discredit on the art, nor disappoint the hopes of the much-deceived physician.

Are there not enough of patients, who, when solicitously advised by a universally esteemed physician, will, for example, scrupulously abstain from eating pork during a quartan fever, and for months afterwards; who will carefully avoid potatoes, if they are asthmatic or leucophlegmatic; sedentary occupations, if they are gouty; and sour wine, if suffering from the wasting diseases of youth brought on by venereal excesses?

In the case of a woman affected with a nervous disorder, should not a good physician be able to effect a gradual diminution in the quantity of coffee taken; or, if otherwise, will he not be able to perceive that she will not follow his advice? From my own experience I can say, that it is no uncommon circumstance to meet with both these cases; and in each the physician may reckon with certainty on his observation.

If we go to work in this manner, we shall attain to a high degree of empirical certainty. Is this not certainty? Or does the statesman, the teacher, the lawyer, the merchant, the general, possess any other than empirical certainties? Or is there any other positive rule to guide us, in any imaginable profession in which the free-will of man is involved?

But is the *ordinary diet* of those classes of the community who are not altogether corrupted, of such an objectionable nature, that we are compelled, in every disease, to prescribe a new one? This is one of the rocks on which so many physicians split. In every acute or chronic disease that comes under their notice, they earnestly insist on a very complicated *artificial system of diet*, withholding many things, and ordering a host of others.

Do we physicians, however, know with such extreme precision, the effects of all kinds of food, as to be able with certainty to say, in this case such and such an article of diet is to be taken, and this and that other to be avoided! How does experience refute our fancied omniscience!

For what a length of time did our forefathers insist in their so-called acute (putrid) fevers with diminished vital power, on watery drinks, tea, &c.; and exclaimed against beer and wine as little better than poison—which, however, the patients long for so much, and which is now the main support of our practice! How long did we forbid fresh meat in cases of hæmorrhage from passive plethora, in wasting pulmonary complaints, in scurvy, and in most other chronic non-gastric diseases, where it is now reckoned, if not a perfect panacea, at any rate indispensable! A universal diet, like a universal medicine, is an idle dream; but speaking generally, nothing is more wholesome than fruit in abundance, and green vegetables *ad libitum;* and yet they frequently oppress the stomach of those who have poverty of the blood, of exhausted persons, and those suffering from the effects of a sedentary life, and increase in them the disposition to acidity, flatulence and diarrhœa! Roast beef and raw ham are considered more difficult of digestion for a relaxed stomach than veal boiled to rags. Coffee has the reputation of strengthening and assisting digestion, and yet it only hastens the expulsion of half-digested food from the bowels. I have seen children deprived of the breast-milk, crammed to death with wafer-biscuits, and perishing in numbers of jaundice. My expostulations on the indigestible nature of this unleavened and hard-baked mass of dough, were of no avail against the plausible folly of my colleagues—"it is impossible to imagine any thing lighter (in weight), or more delicate (to the touch)!"

I once knew an ignorant over-officious practitioner prescribe such a severe diet to a healthy young woman after a favourable first-labour, that she was on the eve of starvation. She held up for some days under this water-gruel diet—all meat, beer, wine, coffee, bread, butter, nourishing vegetables, &c., were denied her; but at last she grew excessively weak, complained of agonising after-pains, was sleepless, costive, and, in short, dangerously ill. The medical attendant attributed all this to some infraction of his dietetic rules. She begged to be allowed some coffee, or broth, or something similar. The practitioner, strong in his principles, was inflexible: Not a drop! Driven to desperation by his severity and her hunger, she gave way to her innocent longings, drank coffee, and ate in moderation whatever she fancied. The practitioner found her, on his next visit, much to his surpirse, not only out of danger, but lively and refreshed; so he complacently noted down in his memorandum-book the excellent effects of slop-diet in the treatment of lying-in-women. The convalescent took good care not to hint to him her natural transgression. This is the history of many, even published observations! Thus the disobedience of the patient not unfrequently saves the credit of the physician.

Is the *error calculi*, in such a case, the fault of the art or the patient, or is it not rather the fault of the physician?

The artificial diet prescribed by the physician, is frequently much more objectionable than the accustomed diet of his patient; or, at least, he frequently does wrong in rejecting the latter all at once.

As the physician would do well, in order to observe more distinctly and simply the course of the disease and the effects of his medicines, not to give any orders at all about the diet, except with regard to articles of which he possesses a positive knowledge, and these will be but few; he would also be consulting the good of his patient by not depriving him of any thing which long habit had rendered innocuous, or perhaps indispensable.

A country midwife fell sick of a gastric fever. I purged her. I ordered her for drink, water and weak beer, and extreme moderation in eating. At first, things went on very well; but, after a few days, a new continued fever, with thirst, wakefulness, weariness, confusion of ideas, came on to such an extent as to render her state dangerous. I left none of the ordinary remedies untried. All in vain. I now left off every thing, from the sulphuric acid to the soup (at the time I was not sufficiently acquainted with the properties of opium), and promised to prescribe something on my return. I informed the relations of the danger I apprehended. The following day I was told that the patient was recovering, and that I need not give myself any further trouble. To my astonishment, I saw her pass my window, a few days afterwards, perfectly recovered, I subsequently learned, that when I had discontinued the medicine, a quack had been called in, who had given her a large bottle of essence of wood, his universal medicine, and told her to take so many drops of it. No sooner had she tasted the brandy in it than she gained, as it were, new life. She took the drops by *table-spoonfuls*, and, after a good sleep, she rose completely cured.

This happened when I first began practice, else I should have ascertained at the commencement that, when in health, she could not live without her daily dram, consequently could not recover without it.

It is far less frequently necessary than most physicians think, to make a material alteration in the diet of patients suffering from chronic complaints, at least in ordinary cases; in acute diseases, the awakened instinct of the patient is often considerably wiser than the physician who does not consult nature in his prescriptions.

I do not now allude to cures effected by dietetic rules alone, which, if simple, are not to be despised, and which are very serviceable in many cases. What I particularly call attention to is, the frequently useless change of diet, when treating a case with medicine, whereby the simplest method of treatment is rendered complex, and a composite result is produced, of which I would defy Œdipus himself to guess what part was owing to the new diet, and what to the medicine.

We must certainly prohibit what we know to be hurtful in this or that complaint; but this can at the most be but two or three articles of diet in chronic diseases; the *gradual* disuse of which (for sudden suppression is always dangerous in such affections), cannot produce any great revolution in the system; cannot, therefore, have much effect in deranging the pure action of the medicine we are using.

If it be necessary to make *considerable changes in the diet and regimen*, the ingenious physician will do well to mark what effect such changes will have on the disease, before he prescribes the mildest medicine.

A deeply rooted scurvy can often be cured by the united action of warm clothing, dry country air, moderate exercise, change of the old salted meat for that freshly killed, along with sour-crout, cresses, and such like vegetables, and brisk beer for drink. What would be the use of medicine in such a case? To mask the good effects produced by the change of diet! Scurvy is produced by a system of diet opposite to this, therefore it may be cured by a dietetic course—the reverse of that which produced it; at any rate, we may wait to see the result of this method, before we begin with our medicines.

Why should we render the syphilitic patient, for example, worse than he is by a change of diet, generally of a debilitating nature? We cannot cure him by any system of diet, for his disease is not produced by any errors of the sort. Why then, should we, in this case, make any change?

Since this occurred to my mind, I have cured all venereal diseases (excepting gonorrhœa), without any dietetic restrictions, merely with mercury (and, when necessary, opium); the metal has not a debilitated constitution to act upon, and my patients recovered more rapidly than those of my colleagues. I also knew for certain, that every change that took place, either for the better or the worse, was owing to the medicine.

An old colonel, with "fair round belly," and apparently fond of the pleasures of the table, had suffered for the last forty years from ulcers almost all over the legs, and issues on the thighs. His food consisted of the strongest and most nutritive materials —he drank a good deal of spirits, and, for several years past, he had been in the habit of taking a monthly purge. Otherwise, he was vigorous. I allowed the issues to heal up, made him keep his legs rolled up in a narrow flannel bandage, and immerse them daily a few minutes in cold water, and afterwards dress them with a weak solution of corrosive sublimate. *I made not the slightest alteration in his diet;* I even did not forbid the monthly purge, as he was so constantly in the habit of taking it. In the course of a year his legs gradually healed, and his vigour rather increased than diminished in this his seventy-third year. I watched him for two years, during which he remained perfectly well, and I have since had good accounts of his health. The legs have always continued completely healed. Can I suppose that he would have recovered more rapidly or permanently had I deprived him of his eight or ten dishes, and his daily allowance of liquors? Had I changed his diet, and had he grown worse, would I have known whether this unfavourable turn proceeded from the food so much lauded in works on dietetics, but so different to what he had been accustomed to, or from my external applications, for I gave nothing internally? It would have been easy for me to conform to the schools, and sacrifice my patient methodically to the ordinary dietetic regulations; but how could I at the same time abide by my conviction, my conscience, and that prime guiding principle of the physician, *simplicity!*

I have no intention of exalting myself at the expense of my brethren, when I acknowledge that I have cured the most difficult chronic diseases, without any particular change of diet.

I consider that I do quite enough if I advise moderation in all things, or diminish or forbid altogether particular articles of diet, which would be prejudicial to the object I wish to accomplish; as, for example, acids, when I am employing stramonium, belladonna, foxglove, monkshood, or henbane (the effects of these medicines being entirely counteracted by vegetable acids); or *salted meats*, when I prescribe oxyde of mercury; or *coffee*, when I am giving opium.

Thus, if my treatment fail, I know that I have done no harm by an artificial system of diet (how much that is dangerous and hypothetical is there not in our dietetic regulations!), I know it is owing to the medicine used that the case grew worse, or, at least, did not improve.

If amendment ensue, then I know that the medicine produced it, as it certainly was not owing to any change in the diet.

Hippocrates, himself, if I recollect right, hints at something similar in his aphorisms, when he says, that medicine and the *vis naturæ* produce much more considerable and profound changes in diseases than any small irregularity in diet.

How near was this great man to the philosopher's stone of physicians—*simplicity!* and to think that after more than two thousand years, we should not have advanced one single step nearer the mark! on the contrary, have rather receded from it!

Did he only write books? or did he write much less than he actually cured? Did he do this so circuitously as we?

It was owing to the simplicity of his treatment of diseases alone, that he saw all that he did see, and whereat we marvel.

CLIMATE, WEATHER, STATE OF THE BAROMETER, ETC.

Should we abandon ourselves to despair, because we do not know, to a nicety, what is the exact influence which a slight change in geographical position, a small variation of the hygrometer, the barometer, the anemometer, the thermometer, &c., exercises upon the action of our medicines or our patients?

According to many observations of the first medical men, it is not so very difficult to arrive at a pretty accurate general knowledge of the differences produced by a warmer or colder climate on the nature and treatment of ordinary diseases. They are, for the most part, merely differences in degree. The most opposite climates never produce a completely opposite code of medical laws. Is not bark as efficacious for the cure of pure intermittent fever in Mexico as in Norway; in Batavia and Bengal (the only difference being in quantity), as in Scotland? The venereal disease is cured in China by mercury, just as it is in the Antilles. In our country, we have inflammations and suppurations of the liver of the same nature as in the tropics; although, in the latter regions, they are twenty times as numerous as here, that makes not the slightest difference in the treatment, as in both situations mercury and opium (or something better still) are serviceable. Typhus, and similar fevers, are here as there fatal, if treated by bloodletting and nitre (not, indeed, so rapidly here as there)! They must also be treated in our country with bark and opium (not, indeed, in such large doses as there), in order to increase the strength. These varieties of climate do not change the treatment in nature, but only in degree, and such differences are determinable.

But that the powers given by nature to man and habit will triumph over all variations of climate, to the preservation of life and health, is proved by there being inhabitants in the island of Terra del Fuego, as well as on the banks of the Ganges, in Lapland, as well as Ethiopia, in the seventieth as well as the third degree of latitude.

And are we so ignorant of the other influences which the nature of the soil and country have upon diseases; so very ignorant that we cannot reckon the influence they would have on our practice? Do we know nothing of the different effects produced by a residence in a hilly country and on the sea-coast, on hæmoptysis and phthisis; nothing of the action of the effluvia from marshes and seething intramural grave-yards in the production of intermittent fever, and diseases of the liver and lymphatic system; nothing of the power of pure air on those affected with rickets and those debilitated by sedentary occupations; nothing of the advantages of a level country over confined Alpine valleys, the cradle of cretinism, goitre, and idiocy; nothing of the peculiar power of certain winds and seasons in the production of inflammatory, or asthenic diseases, or of the effect of a low state of the barometer on the apoplectic; nothing of the influence of the air of hospitals in the production of gangrene and typhus?

And it is only these, and similar great and important differences, which exercise a marked influence on health and life itself, which it is necessary for us to know in our treatment of diseases. We do know them, and can calculate their influence.

The influence of the finer shades of these differences is too insignificant to prevent us treating successfully the ordinary diseases. The vital power and the proper medicine generally obtain the victory over any influence which such very fine shades of differences could exert.

What might be said of the Creator, who, having afflicted the inhabitants of this earth with a vast host of diseases, should at the same time have placed an inconceivable number of obstacles in the way of their cure; to discover the influence of each of which would defy the greatest efforts of the physician—a knowledge of which in their full extent (if they were of such great importance) could not be attained by the greatest genius?

We cure diseases in pestilential dungeons, although we cannot, at the same time, impart to the patient the vigour of the mountaineer. Who would desire us to transform the delicate city lady into the buxom peasant girl? We remove, however, most of the ailments of the former. The sedentary man of business seeks at our hands only tolerable health, for the nature of things denies us the power of giving him the strength of the blacksmith, or the ravenous appetite of the porter.

"But," objects some one, "look what a perceptible influence a slight variation of the temperature, moisture, or relative proportion of oxygen and nitrogen in the atmosphere, a slight change in the wind, a higher or lower state of the barometer, a greater or less quantity of atmospherical electricity, and a thousand other physical powers, small though they may be, which are perhaps, as yet unknown to us, sometimes have upon diseases, at least upon the nervous, hysterical, hypochondriacal. and asthmatic!"

Shall I speak out what I think? It appears to me much less profitable to endeavour to ascertain (which is moreover impossible) all the degrees and varieties of the influence of those physical impressions, when they approach the minute, than to do our endeavour to fortify the sufferers against all these innumerable impressions, by implanting in them a certain degree of strength, whereby their system will be enabled to resist these, and many other still unknown physical impressions; just as I consider it much more practicable to dispel the morose ideas of the melancholic by medicine, than to abolish for him the countless evils of the physical and moral world, or to argue him out of his fancies.

Or could all the physical and moral adverse circumstances of the atmosphere, and of human life, be more effectually prevented exercising their pernicious influence on the gossamer nervous system of yon nervous, spasmodic, chlorotic girl, did we, with angels' understanding, completely investigate and maturely weigh, in quality and quantity, all these impulses in their full extent, than if we should restore her monthly periods?

I do not believe that it is the smallness of our knowledge, but only the faulty application of it, that hinders us from approaching, in medical science, nearer to certainty and simplicity.

A young man twenty years of age, the son of an oil manufacturer, thin and weakly, had been from his childhood subject to a spasmodic asthma, which used always to increase from the commencement of autumn until the depth of winter, and gradually decline from that period until the mild weather in spring. Every year he had grown worse, and this autumn he hoped might be his last. Already (I saw him first at Michaelmas) the attack commenced more violently than the last year at this time. The probable issue was evident. Last year, and for years past, every fall of the barometer, every south-west, and more particularly north wind, every approaching fall of snow, every storm of wind, had brought on an asthmatical fit of hours and days in duration, when he not unfrequently passed the night with both hands grasping the table, exerting all his strength to draw the smallest quantity of breath, and every moment in dread of suffocation. The intervals between such fits were occupied by slighter attacks, brought on by a draught of air, the vapour from the heated oil-cakes, dust, a cold room, or smoke. He told me of these symptoms with the utmost difficulty of utterance, elevating his shoulders to draw a scanty breath, and this at a season of the year when his condition was as yet pretty tolerable.

I could expect no good effects from a change of place. So I allowed him to remain in his father's house, exposed, as it was to every wind, and all the inclemencies of the weather; I let him take his usual diet; I only advised that his fare should be, if anything, more nutritious than otherwise; I let him occupy the same sleeping apartment, and continue his work in the oil manufactory, and, as far as his strength allowed, engage in agricultural employments.

The first medicine I administered was ipecacuhan, in the smallest doses; they produced no nausea, neither did doses of five grains; the latter quantity caused purgation and relaxation of the system. The submuriate of antimony and the sulphate of copper, in quarter of a grain doses, produced no better results. Both of these substances, as well as asarum root, each used singly, caused the same bad effects.

I shall refrain from stating what other medicines, celebrated in asthma, did *not* effect; and shall only mention that squills and bark, each employed separately, did—what they often do—they increased the difficulty of breathing, and made the cough more frequent, shorter and drier.

A medicine was procured which could produce anxiety, and diminish the easy action of the bowels. The choice fell naturally on *nux vomica.* Four grains, given twice daily, removed gradually, but perceptibly, the constriction of the chest; he remained free from the spasmodic asthmatic attacks, even in the worst autumn weather—even in winter, in all winds, all storms, all states of the barometer, all humidity of the atmosphere, during his now increased domestic, manufacturing, and travelling business, in the midst of the oil vapour, and that without any important change in his diet, or any in his place of abode. He had been in the habit, when there was but small prospect of cure, of rubbing his whole body every night with a woollen cloth. Although it did not seem to do any good, I did not let him discontinue it while taking the last medicine, as he had been so long accustomed to it.

He now slept comfortably at night, whereas formerly he had passed the whole night in an arm-chair, bent forwards, or lean- ing against the wall, or coughing without intermission. During this season, which had threatened to be so dangerous to him, he gained strength, agility, cheerfulness, and capacity of resisting inclement weather. It was only severe attacks of cold that could cause the slightest return of asthma, and these he speedily got rid of.

Besides this medicine, nothing at all was employed.

Should I, instead of adopting this treatment, have observed attentively all the meteoric changes, and scrupulously calculated their effects on his most susceptible frame? And had I been able to do this, could I have added weight to the diminished atmos- pheric pressure, supplied the loss of atmospherical electricity, maintained an equilibrium between day and night, dried up the moisture in the air, changed the north into the south wind, reined in the storms, and warded off the attraction of the moon? And had I been able to do all this, should I have better attained my object?

MEDICINES.

Here the question arises, *Is it well to mingle many kinds of medicines together in one prescription; to order baths, clysters, ve- nesections, blisters, fomentations and inunctions all at once, or one after the other in rapid succession, if we wish to bring the science of medicine to perfection, to make cures, and to ascertain for certain in every case what effect the medicines employed produced, in order to be able to use them with like, or even greater success in similar cases?*

The human mind is incapable of grasping more than one subject at a time—it can almost never assign to each of two powers acting at the same time on one object its due proportion of influence in bringing about the result; how, then, can we ever expect to bring medical science to a greater degree of cer- tainty, if we deliberately combine a large number of different powers to act against a morbid condidition of the system, while we are often ill acquainted with the nature of the latter, and are but indifferently conversant with the separate action of the component parts of the former, much less with their combined action?

Who can say for certain, that the adjuvant or the corrective in the complex prescription does not act as the base, or that the excipient does not change the whole character of the mixture? Does the principal ingredient, if it be the right one, stand in need of an adjuvant? Does it say much for its fitness if it require a corrective? or why does it require the aid of a director? "I thought I would complete the motley list, and thereby satisfy the requirements of the school!" exclaims the Doctor.

Does opium mingled with ipecacuan cause sleep, because the excipient in the recipe has been invested with the dignity of the principal ingredient? Does the ipecacuan here perform the part of base, adjuvant, corrective, director, or excipient? Does it cause vomiting because the prescriber wills it?

I have no hesitation in asserting that whenever two medicines are mingled together, they almost never produce each its own action on the system, but one almost always different from the action of both separately—an intermediate action, a neutral action,—if I may be allowed to borrow the expression from chemical language.

The more complex our receipts, the more obscure will it be in medicine.

That our prescriptions are composed of a smaller number of ingredients than those of Amatus Lusitanus, avails us just as little as it availed him that Andromachus framed still more complex prescriptions than he. Because the mixtures of both these worthies are more complicated than our own, does that render ours simple?

Why should we complain that our science is obscure and intricate, when we ourselves are the producers of this obscurity and intricacy? Formerly I was infected with this fever; the schools had infected me. The virus clung more obstinately to me before it came to a critical expulsion, than ever did the virus of any other mental disease.

Are we in earnest with our art?

Then let us make a brotherly compact, and all agree to give but one single, simple remedy at a time, for every single disease, without making much alteration in the mode of life of our patients, and then let us use our eyes to see what effect this or that medicine has, how it does good, or how it fails.—Is not this as simple a way of getting over the difficulty as that of Columbus with the egg?

Is it really more learned to prescribe from the chemist's shop a number of complicated combinations of medicines for one disease (often in one day), than with Hippocrates to treat the whole course of a disease with one or two clysters, perhaps a little oxymel and nothing else? Methinks to give the right, not the many-mixed, were the stroke of art!

Hippocrates sought the simplest from out an entire genus of diseases; this he carefully observed and accurately described. In these simplest diseases he gave single simple remedies from the then scanty store. Thus he was enabled to see what he saw—to do what he did.

I hope it will not be considered unfashionable to go to work with diseases as simply as did this truly great man.

Any one who should see me give one medicine yesterday, another to-day, and a third different from either to-morrow, would observe that I was irresolute in my practice (for I am but a weak mortal); but should he see me combine two or three substances in one prescription (and ere now this has sometimes been done), he would at once say, " The man is at a loss, he does not rightly know what he will be at"—" He is wavering"—" Did he know which one of these was the proper remedy, he would not add to it the second, and still less the third!"

What could I rejoin? Nothing.[1]

Should any one ask me what is the mode of action of bark in in all known diseases, I would confess that I know but little concerning it, notwithstanding the number of times I have used it alone and uncombined. Should any one ask me, however, what bark would do if combined with saltpetre, or still more with some third substance, I would at once acknowledge my benighted ignorance, and would bow before any one as before a very divinity who would enlighten me on the subject.

Dare I confess, that for many years I have never prescribed anything but a single medicine at once, and have never repeated the dose until the action of the former one had ceased; a venesection alone—a purgative alone—and always a simple, never

---

[1] The reason which has been frequently given, that we require, by pleasant additions to the medicine, to render it more agreeable to the patient, or to give it a more convenient form for administration, and conceal the disagreeable taste, smell, and colour, is entirely without weight. Grown up patients, whose confidence is ready in one scale of the balance to kick the beam when a bitter, nauseous powder is placed in the other scale, have too scanty a supply of that quantity for my taste. I would abandon them to those needy traders, who, for the miserable fee will prescribe the most dainty sweetmeats, and are willing to submit to all the airs and disobedience of their patients. We all know how to manage children in such case without hurting them.

21

a compound remedy, and never a second until I had got a clear notion of the operation of the first? Dare I confess, that, in this manner, I have been very successful, and given satisfaction to my patients, and seen things which otherwise I never would have seen?

Did I not know that around me there are some of the worthiest men, who in simple earnestness are striving after the noblest of aims, and who by a similar method of treatment have corroborated my maxims, assuredly I had not dared to confess this heresy. Had I been in Galileo's place, who can tell but that I might have abjured the idea of the earth revolving round the sun!

But the dawn begins to glimmer in the horizon!—who can fail to perceive a feeble ray of it in our Herz's commentary on his two cases, to which we alluded above?

What would he not now give that in both instances he had prescribed nothing but the phellandrium, and had met with the same success he did! I, for my part, would willingly give the best, the most satisfactory of all my observations that he had done this.

ANTIDOTES TO SOME HEROIC VEGETABLE SUBSTANCES.[1]

Cases of poisoning often put the practitioner in great straits. It is necessary to administer the specific antidote without delay. But where are the particular antidotes to be met with?

From the time of Nicander to the 16th century, when, if I mistake not, Paré first set his face against them, grand plans were formed by medical men for discovering nothing less than an universal specific for every thing they called poison; and they included under the denomination of poison, even the plague, philtres, bewitchment, and the bites of venomous animals. This extravagant object they sought to obtain by equally extravagant mixtures, such as their mithridate, theriac, philonium, diascordium, &c., and then again, there was a time when all these unimportant compounds were thought to be surpassed by the powerless bezoar and the electuary of jewels. We now know how ridiculous all these efforts were.

---

[1] From *Hufeland's Journal der pract. Arzneykunde.* Vol. v, p. 1, 1798.

The more rational spirit of modern times did not, however, completely abandon this illusory idea of the possibility an universal antidote[1] for all poisons. Among other things, it was sought for in vinegar. But in place of giving us a faithful detail of the cases in which it was truly useful and those in which it did no good, they endeavoured to persuade us that it was specific against everything that bore the name of poison, and yet it is, *e. g.*, of no use in poisoning by opium, and of little or none in that by camphor.

Others saw in milk and fatty substances a supposed universal antidote for all kinds of poisons, but no good can be effected by them, except in cases where inflammatory and mechanically irritating substances have been swallowed.

Emetics seemed to be more generally useful in cases where poisons had been swallowed; but they are by no means so in all cases. They are only serviceable when the quantity of injurious matter, that has been swallowed and is to be evacuated, is considerable in amount. Besides their unadvisableness in cases of poisoning by arsenic, as I have elsewhere[2] shewn, the following cases will suffice to dispel the illusion of their being universal antidotes.

The efforts of our age to discover a peculiar antidote for each individual poison, or at least for particular classes of poisons, are not to be mistaken, and I give in my adhesion to them.

Powerful, heroic, medicinal substances, without which the medical art would be as completely paralysed as the mechanical arts would be without steel and fire, are apt to give rise to violent effects, even in a very small excess of dose, in certain states of the body, as also in idiosyncratic or otherwise very irritable subjects, and these effects the physician must know how to remove in order that the cause he advocates may not suffer.

Antidote to camphor—opium. Antidote to opium—camphor.

1. A girl, five years of age, had swallowed a quantity of

---

[1] There are at least four kinds of antidotes by means of which the hurtful substance may be—

I. *Removed:*

    1. By *evacuation* (vomiting, purging, excising the poisonous bite).

    2. By *enveloping* (giving suet for pieces of glass that have been swallowed)

II. *Altered:*

    1. *Chemically* (liver of sulphur for corrosive sublimate).

    2. *Dynamically* (*i. e.* their potential influence on the living fibre removed) (Coffee for opium).

[2] [*Ueber die Arsenikvergiftung.* 1786.]

camphor, calculated at from eight to ten grains. About ten minutes afterwards she grew pale, became cold, her look fixed; then she became faint, speechless, and senseless. In a short time the head became drawn to the right shoulder, and remained in that position; the rest of the body was limp; the senses extinguished. Occasionally the arms were moved involuntarily. The eyes were turned upwards. There was foam at the mouth. The breathing was scarcely perceptible.

Placed in a warm bed, she occasionally seemed to recover herself a little. Strong coffee was given her; but thereupon the senselessness obviously increased. Violent vomiting set in, (the camphor was in part ejected) but no relief ensued therefrom, the death-agony seemed to increase always more and more.

I poured four drops of tincture of opium into her mouth, but could not observe if they were swallowed, but as I imagined I perceived some signs of amendment after watching carefully for some minutes, I continued to ply her with opium by the mouth, and also (as much seemed to flow out of the mouth again, on account of the inactivity of the œsophagus) by clysters of water mixed with some drops of thebaic tincture.

As far as I could reckon, she might have taken by both methods nearly two grains of opium, (a quantity that under other circumstances would certainly have killed a child of that age) when she recovered perfectly without the employment of any other remedy.

A tranquil sleep of some hours, accompanied by general perspiration, restored all her former liveliness.

In this case it was remarkable how greatly the coffee increased the too powerful action of the camphor.

In other cases I have observed that these two substances taken soon after one another, or together, caused a great and rapid tendency to vomit, a circumstance that might perhaps be turned to account in practice.

The great specific power of opium in removing so speedily the dangerous effects of too large doses of camphor, seems to justify me in regarding *camphor*, on the other hand, as one of the most powerful *antidotes of opium*, as Halle also observed in some degree. And, if we examine the affair accurately, did not the enormous dose of opium that I gave in the above case become innocuous in consequence of the camphor previously swallowed.

Camphor is known, from the observations of others, as an antidote to *cantharides* and *squills*.

Antidote to arnica—vinegar.

2. A man of an irritable system, in the prime of his life and otherwise healthy, during the prevalence of the influenza in April of this year, took, for a headache of several days duration, occasioned probably by this epidemic, six grains of arnica root, a dose that he deemed inconsiderable, as he had previously taken with the greatest benefit, for autumnal fevers, from 15 to 17 grains daily and even twice a day. After the lapse of about eight minutes, he was attacked by frightful palpitation of the heart, which at length became so violent that he could only utter a few words with great difficulty. His look was staring and anxious. A general coldness pervaded his frame, and vertigo almost deprived him of hearing and sight. The open air seemed to revive him, but the effect was not lasting. He tried to promote vomiting, but the efforts to vomit only increased his stupefaction, his anxiety, and his vertigo. His lower jaw fell.

He was scarcely able to indicate his desire for *vinegar* (by this time three quarters of an hour had elapsed). Strong wine-vinegar was brought him, and he felt revived. He drank several ounces at once, but soon perceived that he experienced most relief when he did not drink a draught but only took a little every instant. In the course of half an hour after commencing to use the vinegar he was restored without further traces of these accidents.

If there be any remedy that we require to regulate carefully by the actual constitution of the subject whom we are treating, it is that tremendous irritant arnica, which may be given in the leucophlegmatic cachexies of children of ten years, especially in autumnal diseases and when the pulse is soft, in doses of twelve grains without the slightest bad results; and on the other hand, in certain states of the body where there is already present a general and exalted irritability, eight grains of it in a dose will kill the strongest man in a few hours, as I have known to occur in some instances.

The pathognomonic discrimination of the cases, and when it is at hand, vinegar, will in future prevent such accidents.

Antidote to cocculus indicus—camphor.

3. A druggist, of fine sensibility and otherwise healthy, although but recently convalescent from an acute disease, some years ago wished to ascertain the taste of the cocculus seed, and as he considered it a powerful substance he weighed out a single grain of it, but did not take quite the half of this into his mouth, rolled it about with his tongue over his palate, and he had not

swallowed it two seconds when he was seized with the most dreadful apprehensiveness. This anxiety increased every moment; he became cold all over; his limbs became stiff, as if paralyzed, with drawing pains in their bones and in the back. The symptoms increased from hour to hour, until, after the lapse of six hours, the anxiety, the stupefaction, the senseless stupidity, and the immobility had risen to the greatest height, with fixed, sullen look, ice-cold sweat on the forehead and the hands, and great repugnance to all food and drink. At the slightest increase or decrease of the temperature of the air (75° Fahr.) he expressed his displeasure; every loud word put him in a passion. All that he could still say was that his brain felt as if constricted by a ligature, and that he expected speedy dissolution. He gave no indication of inclination to vomit, of thirst, or of any other want in the world. He wished to sleep, as he felt a great inclination to do so, but when he closed his eyes he immediately started up again, so frightful, he asserted, was the sensation he felt in his brain on going to sleep, like the most hideous dream. The pulse was very small, but its frequency was not altered.

In these frightful circumstances I was called in. A few drops of thebaic tincture appeared not to agree with him. This led me to fix upon a strong camphor emulsion, which I administered to him, a tablespoonful about every minute. I soon observed a happy change in his expression, and after he had thus taken fifteen grains of camphor, his consciousness was restored, the anxiety gone, the heat natural—in something less than an hour. He perspired a little during the night, slept pretty well, but the following day he was still uncommonly weak, and all the parts, which during the direct action of the cocculus were yesterday painful internally, were to-day uncommonly painful externally to the slightest touch. The bowels remained constipated for several days. It is very probable that all these after-sufferings could have been prevented if, in place of giving fifteen grains of camphor, I had at once given thirty.

During the increase of the symptoms from the cocculus, he attempted to smoke tobacco with considerable aggravation; they also increased from taking coffee, though not so strikingly as from the other.

Antidote to gamboge (and other drastic gum-resins)—*salt of tartar*.

4. I saw a child of three years old take a tincture containing two grains of gamboge, prepared with dissolved salt of tartar,

without the slightest sickness or evacuation, with the exception of an uncommonly profuse flow of urine.

Alkalies probably destroy the drastic property of other purgative gum-resins, especially if the latter are still present in the stomach, but not as in the other cases I have adduced, dynamically, by an opposite influence upon the sensitive and irritable fibre, but chemically, by decomposing the resin.

Antidote to datura stramonium—vinegar (and citric acid).

5. In a woman rather advanced in life, there occurred from two grains of the *extract of stramonium*, taken in two doses within eight hours, stupefaction, anxiety, convulsions of the limbs and involuntary weeping; symptoms that were frightfully increased by partaking of coffee. They rapidly disappeared after taking a few ounces of strong *vinegar*.

Besides vinegar, *citric acid* is also a specific antidote to stramonium, as I have shewn in another place, from the use of currants, which contain the latter, and I am very much mistaken if the true antidote of all the *solanaceæ* be not *vinegar, citric* and *malic acid*.

Antidote to ignatia—vinegar.

6. A paralytic stiffness in the lower limbs, with involuntary twitchings in them, great anxiety, coldness of the whole body, with dilatability of the pupil, &c., were the symptoms produced in a youth of 20 years, by an over-dose of *ignatia.* His head was free, his consciousness perfect; but on account of the anxiety, he could not express himself properly. Intelligence of a somewhat unpleasant nature aggravated his condition; the same was the case with coffee and smoking tobacco.

For this unpleasant state I gave some camphor, but no good was thereby effected. But on letting him drink very strong vinegar, eight ounces in the course of half an hour, he was restored so completely that the same afternoon he was able to make one of a party of pleasure.

In poisoning with nux vomica I would also advise vinegar, as it is nearly allied in the natural order of botany to the former.

Antidote to veratrum album—coffee.

7. I had the greatest difficulty in restoring two children, the one a year and three quarters old, the other five years old, who had both taken *white hellebore* by mistake, the former four grains, the latter seven grains. Those conversant with such matters will consider both to be *of themselves* fatal doses, and as long as no antidote is known, *absolutely* fatal.

But few minutes elapsed before the greatest changes were observable in both children. They became quite cold, they fell down, their eyes projecting like a suffocating person's, the saliva ran continually from their mouths, and they seemed devoid of consciousness, when I saw them half an hour after the accident.

It had already been tried to incite them to vomit by means of a feather, without success, indeed with an aggravation of their symptoms, as I was told. Milk administered by clyster and poured down the throat in large quantities had had no effect, except the production of scanty vomiting, which did no good, but only increased the faintness.

When I arrived both seemed to be at the point of death. Distorted, projecting eyes, disfigured, cold countenance, lax muscles, closed jaws, imperceptible respiration. The infant was the worst.

The impending death by apoplexy, the failing irritability, at once induced me to combat the symptoms if possible with strong coffee. I introduced, as far as the clenched jaws would allow me, the warm coffee into the mouth, but I chiefly sought to give it in large quantity by means of the enema. It was successful. In the course of an hour all the danger was gone. The heat, the consciousness, the respiration returned. A sleep of several hours, during which the breathing was slower than usual, refreshed them. All the operations of the animal economy were again almost in good order. But the children remained weak, emaciated, and every night before midnight were attacked with a kind of fever, that threatened to prove fatal in a chronic manner. Peruvian bark given for a fortnight, however, removed this sequela, and as I am informed, they are still (a year and a half have since elapsed) in the enjoyment of good health.

I may here observe, that in the case of severe poisonings we have not unfrequently to combat a remnant of chronic affections, because the antidote of the noxious substance even though it be specific, only *acts in a contrary sense,* consequently, belongs to the class of palliatives which are unable to remove the secondary effects of the poison that has been swallowed, especially if it has had time to make some inroads on the system. Moreover, we must not imagine that an antidote can be such a perfect counterpoison of the poison as that all the symptoms of the latter shall be covered by it, as two triangles with equal sides and angles cover one another; nor can it, consistently with all analogy, be denied, that the noxious substance, in combination with an antidote ever so appropriate, must develope a new action, which could not have been anticipated from each singly, and which will play its part in the body for a longer or shorter time. Thus after poisoning by opium, which has been removed by giving a considerable quantity of coffee, we perceive an extraordinary secretion of urine, even in persons in whom the accustomed coffee did not produce this effect of itself; and a grain of opium in an infusion of from one to one a half ounce[1] of coffee, taken once or several times a day, gives perhaps the most sure and powerful diuretic that the medical art possesses.

Antidote to mezereum—camphor.

8. An otherwise robust man took mezereum internally for some complaints that he had. But as he continued the use of this drug even after the disappearance of these complaints, he became affected with intolerable itching over the whole body, which did not allow him an hour's sleep. He discontinued the medicine, came to me thirty-six hours afterwards, and assured me that he could no longer endure the itching, which increased every hour—the first direct action of mezereum lasts very long. I gave him thirty grains of camphor, six grains to be taken every six hours, and before he had taken it all, his itching had disappeared.

SOME KINDS OF CONTINUED AND REMITTENT FEVERS.[2]

The actual number of genera and species of sporadic and epidemic fevers is probably much greater than is laid down in the works on pathology and nosology. Indeed the morbific agencies that act on the human body are so numerous, their intensity and duration of action so various, that the diseases they give rise to must present a great variety of character.

Although the great epidemics have been more frequently described than the small ones, the sporadic diseases, still these diseases, which present such very different characters, have been confounded under the same name, so that I may be permitted to inquire if they are not quite distinct.

Sporadic fevers are still more diverse and still less known, and it is just from this latter cause, and in consequence of their

---

[1] According as the patient was more or less accustomed to the use of coffee.
[2] From Hufeland's *Journal der practischen Arzneykunde.* Vol. v. 1798.

frequency, that they in general make as many victims as epidemic fevers. Sporadic fevers are no doubt more difficult to describe than the latter, for the fewer the number of observations, the more difficult is it to deduce from them a specific character.

The following facts, imperfect though they be, may however serve as a contribution to the history of these fevers.

I. In January of this year, a kind of sporadic fever, apparently more of a continued than a remittent character, at least in its first stages, prevailed among children. In spite of the heat of skin, the patients experienced continual rigours and great lassitude; the memory was impaired. The respiration was excessively short and spasmodic; some of them had a troublesome cough; the urine was high-coloured, and sometimes deposited a red sediment; there was scarcely any trace of gastro-intestinal derangement; there was an evacuation of the bowels every day. almost quite regularly; the brow was often covered with cold sweat.

Evacuant remedies weakened the patients without producing any amelioration; cinchona bark also produced an injurious effect. The younger the children the worse was the disease. Many sunk beneath it, chiefly those in whom the continued fever no longer presented, towards the last, marked intermissions.

A few grains of *arnica root* produced a rapid change. Although there was in general no amelioration, the fever which till then had appeared to assume a continued character changed into an uninterrupted series of paroxysms of intermittent fever, the rigour of which lasted an hour, and the heat (with very short respiration) a little longer, terminating in general perspiration. On the cessation of the perspiration the rigour presented itself anew, so that this state continued day and night.

On the one hand the shortness of the stages, and on the other the congested state of the chest, the dyspnœa and suffocating cough, contra-indicated the employment of cinchona. *St. Ignatius' bean* on the contrary produced effects that were truly surprising. I gave it in large doses, every twelve hours; to children from nine months to three years of age, from $\frac{1}{2}$ to $\frac{2}{3}$ of a grain; to those between four and six years, from one grain to $1\frac{1}{2}$ grain; to those between seven and twelve years, from 2 to 3 grains. In general this remedy appears to be more suitable than cinchona in intermittent fevers characterised chiefly by a longer duration of the heat. The fever terminated at the end of two or three days without leaving any traces or any weakness.

Ignatia also removed completely, or nearly so, the dyspnœa and suffocating cough in those that presented these symptoms.

II. In the commencement of March of the same year, many children, my own among the rest, were attacked by a fever which also affected adults, though to a much less extent. In addition to the actual paroxysms I noticed the following symptoms : tension and pressure in the forehead just above the orbit on one side, extending in severe cases to below the parietal region ; pressure at the stomach as from weight ; tension at the scrobiculus cordis and violent tensive pains (colic) round the navel, accompanied by clay-coloured diarrhœ, the stools being very fetid, or by consumption alternating with fetid flatus : constant coldness of the limbs without rigour ; humour very bad (morose, disagreeable); rapid emaciation without great debility ; absence of signs of derangement of the bile or of other impurities in the first passages, at least in the stomach ; tongue clean, moist, rarely covered with a somewhat whitish fur ; taste in the mouth natural, sometimes sour ; feeling of tension throughout the body, pupils slightly contracted, not dilating in the dark.

At noon precisely the paroxysms were always renewed with a very distinct rigour, lassitude, somnolence, sopor, and lastly the cheeks burning, but without thirst. Even when the fits were not very severe the patients felt an unconquerable aversion for all kinds of food.

Exactly at midnight a slight attack of a similar character made its appearance : the patient cried out, tossed about in bed ; the limbs were cold. There was rarely at night general perspiration, after which all the symptoms disappeared until the following day ; but in that case the fever reappeared the third day, and so it went on.

The greatest freedom from fever was found in the morning. When the patient rose, the headache, the tension throughout the body, and the abdominal pains reappeared, but the appetite continued good ; the same was the case in the evening.

During this apparent remission the patients expressed a great desire to eat pork. On satisfying this desire to satiety, there occurred more relief than aggravation.

The essential nature of this fever appeared to consist in a diminution of the sensibility and a kind of clonic spasm of the fibre.

The fever shewed itself in the greatest intensity when the wind blew a long time from the east.

It was not dangerous, but it was obstinate and troublesome.

Emetics scarcely produced amelioration for one day; notwithstanding their employment, the following day the fever continued its usual course. Laxatives and the remedies usually employed for acridities completely failed.

Cinchona and ignatia, given in small or large doses, aggravated the patient's state. Arnica, though it palliated the bad humour, the headache, &c., had only an antisymptomatic effect, it did not produce permanent amelioration.

The immobility of the pupil, the pressive, tensive pain in the scrobiculus and around the umbilicus, together with the general sensation of tension throughout the body; the sopor, the apparently insignificant diminution of the strength, and the relief afforded by the occasional perspirations, the benefit produced by the ingestion of pork, which exercises a great influence on the contractility of the fibre, and finally the aggravation occasioned by the east wind, all these symptoms led me to regard *opium* as the remedy indicated. The fetid stools and flatus, whilst the stomach continued in a normal state, contra-indicated its employment all the less as the clay-colour of the evacuations betrayed a spasmodic state of the excretory biliary ducts. I accordingly give this remedy in the morning before the fit, in the dose of $^1|_5$th of a grain to an infant of five years, $^3|_{10}$ths of a grain to one of seven and another of eight years, $^7|_{20}$ths of a grain to one of ten years. I took myself half a grain. The symptoms disappeared completely in the course of the day. Twelve hours afterwards, in the evening, I gave a still weaker dose, and the fever did not return either the following day or on any subsequent day: the constipation likewise ceased. The patients were cured.

III. In the month of April there prevailed an influenza essentially different from that which had been observed five years previously. I know not if the studies that were made of it at that time were correct, or if I am mistaken in my appreciation of the disease. I shall therefore only draw attention to one single point of dissimilarity and leave to my readers the trouble of comparing the others.

In the epidemic of 1782 there was scarcely a third or even a fourth of the inhabitants who were not attacked by a fever presenting all the symptoms of a catarrho-rheumatic fever, though it only lasted seven days. In general they were all affected in the same degree; though there was not danger except to debilitated subjects, to old people, and those suffering from pulmonary consumption. In the influenza of the present year, on the contrary, nine-tenths scarcely had anything more than slight traces of the malady, without fever; the other tenth, on the contrary. were attacked by fever, and danger was imminent.

Patients who had none of the febrile symptoms did not usually seek advice, and were not considered to be affected by the epidemic. It was difficult to observe them, and their symptoms were not perceived by unobservant medical men. All their functions went on regularly ; the only characteristic symptoms they presented were drawing and paralytic pains in some part of the body—some had them in the nape, others only in the external parts of the neck, or only in one half of the chest, in others they were confined to the back, one arm, a thigh, or a few fingers. These fixed pains troubled the patients for weeks, and all the resources of domestic medicine, as the infusion of elder-flowers, the juice of elder-berries, fumigations and emetics. were of no use. When, on the contrary, recourse was had to the appropriate remedy for influenza, the pains ceased quickly in the course of two days or even less.

Other patients had pains in several limbs at once, accompanied by fever.

Those who had at the same time febrile symptoms experienced. before the hot stage, for several hours, and even for some days, a rigour that recurred from time to time, that was *aggravated by every movement*, and was accompanied by ill-humour, *pusillanimity* and *despair*. The patients complained at the same time of weight in the head and dulness, symptoms which they did not consider as headaches, and a difficulty of swallowing, which soon shewed itself on the external parts of the neck and on the nape, or which changed into insufferable tension that did not permit of the slightest motion of the neck, and was aggravated by the touch. In the back they experienced a disagreeable drawing; on the chest a similar very painful sensation, and throughout the body, especially in the thighs, a well marked paralytic stiffness. The patients felt the sensation of laziness and lassitude most when seate d.

After another and more violent rigour (sometimes accompanied by very great anxiety at the heart) which generally appeared in the evening, and in bad cases sooner, the most violent tensive and pressive headache came on just above the orbits and, in many of the patients, in the occiput also. The anxiety increased.

the face became swollen, the eyes red; added to these was a violent heat which lasted six, twelve or more hours, and in some cases till death, which occurred on the fourth, seventh or fifteenth day.

In the mild cases, when the heat diminished, it passed every day (for the paroxysms were usually quotidian, towards the evening, although latterly without rigour) after midnight into general diaphoresis, often characterized by an excessive fetor, and which, in the most favourable cases, only lasted till six o'clock in the morning, but beyond that time in the bad cases. When the perspiration was not very copious, and when it ceased at the time first mentioned, there ensued, throughout the day, a great amelioration of all the pains and the headache; if, on the contrary, it lasted longer and was more abundant, there occurred more disagreeable affections; the head again became confused, and was from time to time affected by pains; the pains on the external parts became twice or even four times more severe during the perspirations that occurred by day, and there was reason to dread the supervention of a continued, a deadly fever.

During the first days there was obstinate constipation; in the most severe cases there was suppression of the urinary secretion that continued sometimes even till death ensued; in these cases there was no perspiration during the greatest severity of the heat of body, and there occurred delirium and tossing about, premonitory symptoms of approaching death. In the most favourable circumstances, the day following the first febrile heat, the *urine*, small in quantity, was of a *greenish-black colour, opaque*, passing the following days, until the recovery was complete, into green and light green.

In the worst cases the tongue was dry and brown to its very point, or when it was slightly moist it was brown or covered by a black coating, and it was yellow in the less serious cases. Notwithstanding the dryness of the tongue, the thirst was not great, and the patients generally expressed a wish for acidulated drinks, rarely for pure water. When amendment ensued they asked for beer. In the mildest cases they felt a bitter taste on the tongue; in less favourable circumstances this taste was very disagreeable; it was not present at all in those cases that presented the most dangerous character. All alleged that they perceived the natural taste of solid and liquid food, though it excited the greatest repugnance in them. The first *stools were black, fetid;* afterwards they became of a greenish-brown colour.

After a constipated state of the bowels had lasted several days, there generally occurred a diarrhœa, similar to that attending colic, with aggravation of the symptoms.

In the bad cases, there was sleeplessness that lasted until death took place; nothing approaching to sleep was observed except a sort of drowsiness, that lasted a few minutes, with delirium and tossing. As the disease diminished, the patient got some sleep before midnight; but even in the most favourable circumstances it only lasted until three o'clock.

The most troublesome symptoms were: dejection and despair, paralytic stiffness, drawing and tensive pains in the external parts, especially in the tendinous and membranous aponeuroses, as it seemed, and in the periosteum of the affected parts; weight in the head, alternating with tensive, drawing and pressive head-ache, and loss of memory.

The character of the affection seemed to betray pain and irritation of the sensitive fibre. Coryza, properly so called, never occurred. In some cases, stitches in the side with expectoration of blood were added to the array of symptoms, but these stitches in the side were not attributable to inflammation.

Sometimes the fever was accompanied at night by attacks of suffocation.

There was never either swelling or redness in the part, even in cases where the pain was excessive, with the exception of some cases where the fingers were sensitive, swollen and red; in one single case the hepatic region was tumefied.

The most annoying drawing headache was often accompanied by nausea that lasted several hours, by faintness and rigours. The catamenia were generally premature and degenerated into metrorrhagia.

The most powerful emetics did not cause vomiting, but sometimes nausea, that lasted for whole days, alternating with syncope; sometimes a single abundant stool occurred, with aggravation of all the symptoms; or again, very small doses of these emetics brought on excessive vomiting for several hours, as often as twenty times, and in severe cases even thirty-six times, always succeeded by obvious aggravation. (Sometimes spontaneous vomiting occurred for twenty-four consecutive hours, and the disease went off entirely.) If, as very seldom happened, the emetics occasioned moderate vomiting, the matter vomited usually consisted of a black, fetid substance, resembling in appearance the grounds of coffee; and, when that was the case, all the other symptoms became speedily aggravated. All attempts made to provoke vomiting by tickling the fauces with a feather only produced loss of strength and increase of the pains.

A similar effect was produced by every kind of laxative, even the mildest kinds, especially when there was present a predisposition to diarrhœa. Thus I saw four grains of rhubarb produce, in the case of a boy of eleven years of age, more than forty stools in the course of two days, and increase the intensity of the symptoms. Many patients sank beneath the constant diarrhœa.

When diaphoretics, which were employed by the poorer classes, sometimes produced the desired effect, excessive perspiration came on, causing an aggravation of all the symptoms. In some patients an abundant uniform transpiration manifested itself until death.

Vegetable acids, which were employed by the medical practitioners in great quantities, occasioned vomiting and diarrhœa, followed by aggravation. Taken by the patients according as their feelings dictated, they seemed to refresh them, but they could only take a very small quantity at a time. In the most violent attacks, they only desired to moisten their lips, and found themselves refreshed thereby.

Mineral acids seemed not to be useful.

Venesection was hurtful in every stage of the disease, but especially when the fever was severe; death then often ensued about the fourth day. Even when the fever seemed slight at the commencement, bleeding[1] was instantly followed by fainting, prostration of strength, increase of the pain, and aggravation of the disease.

Opium subdued the heat and the excessive perspiration, also the delirium and the somnolence; but it increased the constipation; in general, it did not seem to remove the malady radically.

Camphor, on the contrary, surpassed all the expectations that could have been formed of it; it was efficacious, and I may say, specific, in all the stages of the disease, accompanied or not by

---

[1] The local practitioners constantly had recourse to bleeding; they thus caused the death of many patients. If, by chance, a vigorous subject survived after a hard struggle, they raised shouts of triumph, and pretended they had saved him by means of a well-timed bleeding, or by their resolvents and evacuants. One of themselves sank under a similar treatment too exactly followed out, though every effort had been made to dissuade him from it.

fever, especially when it was given as early as possible and in large doses. A large number of patients recovered by its use in the space of four days, in spite of the gravity of their symptoms.

At the commencement I was very cautious in its use, and did not give to adults above from fifteen to sixteen grains per diem, in almond-milk; but I soon perceived that in order to produce a speedy recovery, it was necessary to give, even to weak subjects, thirty grains, and to more robust individuals, forty grains in the twenty-four hours. The favourable result was never long delayed; the constipation ceased; the bad, or at least the bilious taste, rapidly went off, together with the nausea and discomfort; the weight and pain in the head diminished from hour to hour; the febrile rigour was smothered in its birth; the heat diminished, and in those cases where there had been no perspiration, or where it had been abundant, there occurred a general mild diaphoresis, with diminution of all the drawing tensive pains in the external parts. The strength soon returned, along with appetite and sleep; the despondency changed into strength and hope, and the patient recovered his health without a drawback.

I am afraid that this rapid disappearance of the symptoms, the yellow, brown, or black coating of the tongue, the nauseous and bitter taste, the constipation, and the sickness, removed often within the twenty-four hours by the use of camphor alone, given in large doses, will not please the orthodox partisans of the saburral school. Nature, to be sure, often refuses to conform to the requirements of systems: the more's the pity for the dogmatic physician who attempts to fight against her!

When I had been summoned in time, and the disease, in spite of the gravity of its commencement, had radically disappeared at the end of four days, or six at the most, there did not remain a single morbid symptom, not even lassitude.

A nervous lady of great spirit, could not be consoled during the first days for the loss of her betrothed, whom she loved tenderly; he had died of the disease, and she it was who had tended him. She lost her appetite and refused all food. I was advised to prescribe an emetic for her, in order to restore the appetite, but I refused to do so; she was threatened with an attack of influenza, and I merely ordered a glass of wine and sought to raise her spirits.

Her numerous avocations, and still more, her intelligent

22

mind and the consolations of her friends, assuaged her grief; the next week she was more calm, felt her appetite returning, and obtained a little rest in sleep. She only felt some vague pains in the bones, for which she neglected to consult me. Fifteen days after the death of her friend she was seized with a febrile rigour that lasted two hours, and with all the signs of the most violent form of the prevailing epidemic. As regarded her disposition, she was a prey to the most profound despair; day and night she only spoke of her lover, calling him by name, and promising that she would soon join him. Her restlessness was excessive, the tongue was covered with a black coating, she had disagreeable eructations, with bitter taste in the mouth. The heat, the pains in the neck and limbs, the violent headache, filled me with well-grounded apprehensions as to the result. I prescribed from fifteen to eighteen grains of *camphor* the first two days, and an emetic, in consequence of the persistence of the eructations and the bitter taste. The only effect the emetic had was to cause nausea, which lasted several hours; a fresh dose of camphor was given to remove the spasm, and then she had slight vomiting of mucus. Still she felt no relief, and every thing seemed to prognosticate a fatal termination. She spoke of nothing but her lover; her whole body was burning, the face puffed, the pulse 130. Thirty grains of camphor within the twenty-four hours produced a slight moisture of the skin, and diminished the heat and bitter taste of the mouth. The following day she got thirty-six grains, and the day after forty; she slept quietly, spoke no more about the deceased, felt consoled, and regained her courage. She got up and asserted that she felt nothing now except little or no pain in the head and limbs, and she asked for something to eat. Thirty more grains of camphor given on the two following days, re-established her health completely, and from that time she was able to resume her usual occupations.

I only know one case out of more than a hundred where the camphor failed. A lady of rank, very hysterical, subject to hysteria from her youth, had been attacked by influenza. She had taken with good effects twenty grains of camphor in the twenty-four hours, and I prescribed for her fifteen more, to be taken in the space of twenty hours, against some inconveniences that remained. She immediately experienced profuse perspiration, which, in the course of sixteen hours, increased to a very violent degree, with intense heat, faintness and anxiety. The state of the patient was very serious, but half a grain of opium allayed the anxiety, heat and sweat, in less than an hour. I prescribed it anew in much larger doses with much success, and the cure was complete.

The nature of the influenza which generally goes on to copious evacuations (and on the other hand, sometimes to an excessive suppression of the evacuations,) in this case resisted its own specific, probably in consequence of having undergone a modification from the hysterical constitution of the patient.

Before I had ascertained all the efficacy of camphor in this extraordinary disease, I was forced to content myself with opium and cinchona; the first during the hot and sweating stages, and second during the remission. Troublesome and difficult as were these cases, nevertheless the employment of these substances sufficed to remove (although only after several days) the coating of the tongue and bitter taste, and by degrees all the affection. But after it had been subdued, the convalescents could no longer bear the bark; no sooner was it taken than it was ejected. In the epidemic of 1782, I find among the large number of remedies employed by physicians, camphor mentioned incidentally, but no effect superior to that of the other therapeutic agents is attributed to it.

What induces me to believe that on that occasion these various medicaments were employed in a blind and arbitrary manner, is, that among many other remedies arnica[1] is equally recommended for this affection. This substance, though efficacious in many other diseases, is very dangerous in this one. I have seen a robust man affected with influenza, and already convalescent, die in the space of twenty-four hours and a half with all the signs of poisoning, after having taken eight grains of arnica-root, the fatal effects of which shewed themselves by coldness, vertigo, palpitations, anxiety, and loss of voice. Had I at that period known the specific remedy for this kind of poisoning, viz., vinegar, I might have saved this patient's life. The extract of aconite[2] employed in the same way in this epidemic, is equally prejudicial.

This last influenza, in common with all others, as I have had opportunities of convincing myself, presents as a characteristic feature the power of affecting indiscriminately all persons, whatever their constitution may be, a power which the plague of the

---

[1] Languth. *Diss. histor. catarrh. epidem.*, 1782, Helmstadt, p. 157.

[2] *Op. cit.* p. 144.

Levant scarcely possesses in such a high degree. Most epidemic diseases attack chiefly persons in good health; but there are persons affected with chronic diseases, among which I may merely mention severe nervous affections and mental alienation, who are not affected by them; or if so, the old affection is suspended in its course and the new one takes possession of the system; or finally, and this happens tolerably often, the first is cured by the second. It is not so with influenza. Not only does it attack indiscriminately all individuals affected with chronic maladies, but it complicates itself with them and aggravates them. It is when it remains latent itself, that it stirs up and aggravates any ancient disease which may perhaps have slumbered for a long time, and the chronic symptoms thus aggravated no longer yield to the remedies formerly employed with success against them, but only to the specific for the influenza. It reproduces deafness, ophthalmia, cough, asthma, pains in various parts, especially in the chest, head, viscera or limbs, ancient spasms, hypochondriasis, melancholia, all those sufferings that had long been cured; the epidemic constitution and the presence of a few of the symptoms of influenza alone lead us to recognise the existence of influenza, masked by these chronic maladies. Sometimes it has occasioned paralysis, either by metastasis, or in parts previously painful.

A child of twelve years of age, in a district where this epidemic was raging, was seized with characteristic tearing pains in all the limbs, with tensive headache and intolerable pains in the eyes. Having taken a chill, all the signs of the disease disappeared, but the child lost its sight. The pupils were much dilated and unaffected by the strongest light. The employment of fifteen grains of camphor daily, continued for a fortnight, rapidly restored vision without the employment of any other remedy.

About the same time in the mother of this child there was reproduced a melancholia with despair and tendency to suicide, a disease which had disappeared several years previously. Besides tensive pains in the head and anxiety in the precordial region, she complained of drawing pains in the limbs. Of all the remedies given, camphor chiefly contributed to her cure.

A month after the termination of the epidemic there was observed a chronic remission of this fever having a sporadic character. It had this peculiarity, that the pains experienced by individuals in whom convalescence had set in after the influenza, recurred either without fever, or accompanied by a kind of intermittent fever, with quotidian or tertian type. The great lassitude, the prostration, the faintness and the sweat, characteristic of influenza, were entirely wanting. The heat was moderate, the cold all the more obstinate, though not inducing much shivering.

Cinchona, but still better, ignatia, removed the febrile symptoms, but the pains became constant. Camphor failed completely; the *ledum palustre*, on the contrary, in doses of from six to seven grains, three times a day for adults, produced permanent relief.

In some obstinate cases I was forced to have recourse to aconite, which cured them rapidly. I am sorry that I only had an opportunity of treating a small number of those cases that presented themselves at the end of the epidemic, so that I am unable to judge if this plant, whose medicinal properties are much greater than those of ledum, would not have enabled me to attain my object much more rapidly in all the cases that presented themselves to my notice.

SOME PERIODICAL AND HEBDOMADAL DISEASES.[1]

I. A young man, recently recovered from a spasmodic asthma, having drunk some wine, contrary to the dietetic rules I had laid down for him, was heated by it and began to quarrel and fight with his companions. After violent muscular exertion he was seized with an attack of asthma, which became worse and worse, and towards the end of the night reached its greatest intensity. The following day and some days afterwards he felt great lassitude. A week afterwards, without appreciable cause, a similar attack came on, also followed by lassitude. From that time the fits, together with the consequent weakness, came on regularly every Monday afternoon. Eight grains of St. Ignatius' bean once diminished the attack in a marked manner and the weakness did not occur; but strangely enough, the following Monday this attack came on again with renewed force. Cinchona-bark given the following Monday, in the dose of half a drachm in the morning and a drachm after dinner, completely suppressed the fit, and after two more doses all traces of the affection had disappeared.

A circumstance worth mentioning is, that previously the cinchona had always failed in the same person against his asthma when it was continued and not periodical.

II. A lying-in woman, aged 40, one Sunday met with a severe mortification, when confined of her fifth child. Besides other disagreeable symptoms, there came on a sensation of formication that gradually extended from the sacrum up to betwixt the scapulæ, so that by Friday it reached the nape. A sudden stiffness occurred at that spot. The patient experienced at the same time a violent febrile rigour which lasted several hours, followed by diaphoresis which continued till late at night and terminated in profuse sweat. The following day she complained of nothing but lassitude, and on taking the least repose, even if seated, she had general sweat, somewhat cold, during the whole day. A disagreeable sensation of formication, extending from the nape to above the occiput, came on every afternoon and lasted till bedtime. There was no bad taste in the mouth, the tongue was clean, but the appetite almost absent. From that period the same fit of intermittent fever, characterized by the same symptoms and by the same termination, occurred on the Thursday and the following Thursdays for several weeks.

When the patient came to consult me she concealed the exciting cause of her disease, viz., the mortification. The normal taste and the cleanness of the tongue contra-indicated the use of an emetic.

There was evidently in this case an intermittent fever with a quotidian type, and another with a hebdomadal type. The employment of ignatia continued for a week, until the Thursday, entirely removed the febrile symptoms affecting the head. Given also on the Thursday the hebdomadal attack far from diminishing, reappeared, on the contrary, with more violence, but was not followed by lassitude. I discontinued the treatment during the subsequent week; indeed all the corporeal functions were performed regularly, the febrile commotion in the evening and the perspirations by day had disappeared, gaiety, appetite and sleep were restored. From that time I administered every Thursday, with great success, a suitable dose of cinchona. The hebdomadal fever did not return and the patient was cured.

III. A very hypochondriacal man suffered in the spring of last year from a periodical hematuria, the type of which he could not remember. There was at the same time fever, great debility and sleeplessness. He had a relapse of his disease in the month of May of this year. I combatted the accessory febrile symptoms with remedies adapted at the same time for the hæmorrhage, to wit, ipecacuanaha given on an empty stc-mach in the morning, so as to occasion nausea for four hours, and in the evening sulphuric acid. The accessory febrile symptoms sensibly diminished, but the hematuria reappeared the fourth day at seven o'clock in the morning, immediately after awaking, as on the first occasion, and twice on the seventh day thereafter at the same hour. Notwithstanding all the prejudices against the employment of cinchona-bark in hæmorrhages I gave a suitable dose of it every evening before going to bed, fearing to miss the hour in the morning when it ought to be given.

Not knowing if the fit, in place of offering a hebdomadal type, would not recur every three days and a half, as frequently happens, and if an attack might not be expected on the afternoon of Thursday, I prescribed a dose of cinchona for that day at noon, at the same time continuing the evening dose. But before the patient could take it, an attack of hematuria, though not a very severe one, occurred on the Thursday morning about eight o'clock.

I had thus learned: 1st, that the curative power of the evening dose did not last till the following day; 2d, that the semi-hebdomadal type was not bound to precisely the first hour of the second half of the fourth day, but that it could also occur at the regular hour of the hebdomadal paroxysm. I consequently altered my treatment: I thereafter gave every morning a dose of cinchona, taking care to have the patient awakened an hour before his usual time of waking, at six o'clock, permitting him either to go asleep again, which he generally did, or to get up. In the course of a fortnight the hematuria was quite cured.

The hebdomadal type which diseases smoetimes observe, recurring towards the middle of the fourth day, (the fourth day?) the seventh, fourteenth, twenty-first, thirty-first days (the middle of the fourth week), &c., appears to differ essentially from the daily aggravation of most diseases which we observe to take place in the evening, and from the types of quotidian, tertian and quartan intermittent fevers. Experience has taught us that St. Ignatius' bean does not suit the first of these types, which seems peculiar to hysterical, hypochondriacal and spasmodic diseases.

A PREFACE.

I have translated the book entitled " *Thesaurus Medicaminum, a new collection of medical prescriptions, distributed into twelve classes, and accompanied with pharmaceutical and practical remarks exhibiting a view of the present state of the materia medica and practice of physic, both at home and abroad. The second edition, with an appendix and other additions. By a member of the London College of Physicians. London: F. Baldwin, 1794, 8vo.,*" introducing into the body of the work formulas derived from the London and Edinburgh Pharmacopœias and from Lewis, and adding some notes, under the signature of Y., which to some of my readers may facilitate if it do not altogether enable them to dispense with the journey to Anticyra.

If, as the preface to the original informs me, even in London, medical frankness requires the ægis of anonymousness, in order to escape being chid; I need not say a word as to its expediency for some time past in our own dear fatherland! If I, the German editor, would not be less frank, what other course was there for me to pursue? However, as truth can neither be more true nor less true, whether it be said by a man with an imposing array of titles or by one perfectly unknown to fame, the indulgent reader will please to regard merely what is said.

It will be perceived that the original is one of the most recondite collections of selected, at least of elegant prescriptions; but it will also be observed that the writer of the notes is no friend to compound medicines. But how, it will be asked, did he come to edit this work? To which I answer, solely for that very reason! I wished to shew to my countrymen *that the very best prescriptions have a hitch somewhere, are unnatural, contradictory, and opposed to the object for which they are designed.* This is a

---

[1] The work to which this is prefixed was translated by Hahnemann, and published anonymously in the year 1800, under the title of *Arzneischatz oder Sammlung gewählter Rezepte,* aus dem Englischen; Leipzig, bei G. Fleischer.

truth that should be proclaimed from the housetops in our prescription-loving times. When will the time come when I shall see this folly eradicated? When will the physician learn that the cure of his cases requires few, quite simple, but proper, perfectly suitable remedies? Will they for ever deserve the ridicule of such as Arcesilas? Will they never cease to mingle together a heap of remedies in one prescription, each of which (for in the general use of compounds it is impossible to investigate the nature of the several ingredients) remains to the greatest physician often but an imperfectly known, often a whole un-known, thing? If Jones, in London, uses every year *three hundred* pounds of cinchona-bark, what accurate, what perfect knowledge do we obtain of the peculiar mode of action of this powerful remedy? Very little indeed! What do we know of the pure special mode of action of that powerful substance, mer-cury, the monstrous consumption of which in medical practice would seem to imply a thorough knowledge of its relation to our bodies? *Very little!* Little besides the empirical apo-thegm that was enunciated 300 years ago: "it cures the venereal disease," all else are untrustworthy fragments. What certain knowledge do we possess respecting opium that could lead us to such a frantic abuse of it? *Little* or nothing of a sure character! What of Camphor? *Scarcely anything!*

Would that Arcesilas were still alive to know that physicians are still at variance as to whether mercury is capable of produ-cing a change in the strength, mobility and sensibility of the fibres (and in the pulse), in a word, can cause a peculiar kind of fever or no, whether bark is antipyretic, merely by virtue of its being a bitter astringent substance like a mixture of gentian and polygonum, or by some peculiar inherent principle—whe-ther opium strengthens or weakens—whether camphor is cooling or heating, and that those who contend for the one opinion as well as those who defend the other, have both forgotten to state the special conditions of their conclusions. But if the power of these substances of every-day use be so undetermined, how much less known must not those of rarer use be!

If such remarkable obscurity prevail respecting *single* medi-cines, to what a zero in point of value must the phenomena sink, which result from the ordinary tumultuous employment of *seve-ral* of such *unknown* drugs *mixed together*, in diseases—in diseases, those abnormal states of the human body—the most intricate of all organized beings—that are in truth not easily cognizable in individual cases! It is as though one should throw blindfold a handful of balls of various sizes upon an unknown billiard table with cushions of various angles, and should pretend to decide beforehand what effect they would all conjointly produce, what direction each would take, and what position they would finally occupy after their many deflections and their unforeseen mutual concussions! And yet the results of all mechanical forces are much more easily determined than those of dynamic forces.

"In a mixed prescription the case is far otherwise," methinks I hear it contended, "for there the prescribing physician determines for each ingredient the part it shall play in the human body : this one shall be the *base*, this other the *adjuvant*, a third the *corrective*, that one the *director* and this one the *excipient!* It is my sovereign command that none of these ingredients venture to quit the post assigned it in the human body! I command that the corrective be not backward in concealing the blunders of the base, that it cover all the delinquencies of this principal ingredient and of the adjuvant, and direct them for the best; but to go out of its rank and situation and to take upon itself a part of its own contrary to the base, I hereby positively forbid it! Now, adjuvant! to thee I assign the office of Mentor to my base, support it in its difficult task; but mind, thou art only to take it by the arm, but not to do anything else of thine own accord, or dare to act contrary to the order which I have given to the base to cause a certain amount of vomiting; but thou must by no means presume in thine ignorance to undertake any expeditions on thine own account, or to do anything different from the intention of the base ; thou must, though thou art something quite different, act entirely in concert with it; that I command thee! I assign to you all conjointly the highly important business of the whole expedition : see that you expel the impure humours from the blood, without touching in the slightest degree the good ones; alter, transform, what you discover to be in improper combination, in a morbid state. Remember that the commission to alter and to transform gives you unlimited authority to change, God knows or knows not what (just as in warlike tactics it is usual for the general to possess more knowledge than his sovereign lord). You are to diminish the irritability of the muscular fibre, to lessen the sensibility of the nerves, to procure sleep and rest. Do you see the convulsions in yonder arm? I wish them to be quieted, and

the spasm in the sphincter muscle of the bladder to be removed!
That fellow there has the jaundice; I command you to bleach
him and to deobstruate his biliary ducts, whether their imper-
meable condition be owing to spasm or to a mechanical obstacle,
or to some degeneration of the liver. In that hysterical woman,
and in those old skin diseases, all my long years of treatment
and my employment of extracts of spring herbs have proved
useless, from which I infer that there are obstructions in the capillary vessels of the abdomen—my favourite way of accounting for
morbid affections. Now you, most worthy base! were, only a few
days since (and that is a great thing in my estimation), accredited
to me in one of the latest pamphlets as a sure deobstruent. I
therefore give you a commission to resolve those indurations
(though I myself am unacquainted with the invisible indurations
and know not what menstruum can *dissolve* them, what liquifier
can *melt* them, or whatever else the comfortable expressions of
our school may be)—enough, you will know quite well what is
to be done when you yourself get upon the spot. Sömmering,
to be sure, says that hard, swollen glands do not consist of constricted vessels, but on the contrary of unnaturally dilated vessels. But what care we for what that dreamer says. We physicians have been in the habit of deobstruating for so many centuries. Suffice it to say, I command you, base! to deobstruate
for me. See yonder typhus patient, my dear base salpetre! I
pray you to advance and check the putrefactive process, as you
did a year ago to my pork ham. Do not attempt to excuse yourself by alleging that hitherto you have always been unfortunate
in all your expeditions: I give you for ally the sulphuric acid,
to support you in all your attacks, although those fantastic
chemists would try to persuade us that you do not agree with it,
that neither of you remain what you were, that you mutually
change into nitric acid and sulphate of potash. What nonsense!
just as if such a thing were possible without the permission of
the physician who presides over prescriptions! Enough that I
command you to extinguish the putrid fever; for that purpose
you have received from me your diploma of base. Moreover, I
put at your service a troop of auxiliary, corrective and directing
substances.—My dear base, opium! here I have an obstinate,
painful cough to combat. You, who have received from the
Asclepiades the office of subduing all spasms and pains, be they
ever so different in character, just as the seven planets were
commissioned in the almanacs a century ago to preside over

this and that part of our body—to you I give the commission
sanctioned by tradition. But I have been informed that you
have often a bad propensity to constipate the bowels. But in
order that this may not happen I give you as auxiliaries this
and that laxative ingredient, and that your action may not be
disturbed by these, is your own look out; why else should I
constitute you the base! Moreover as you sometimes occasion
heat, and are given to check exhalation, I give you camphor as
a corrective, in order to counteract this bad habit of yours.
Some one lately asserted that you lost all your properties when
camphor was given along with you. But do not let that lead
you astray. How can the saddle-horse allow himself to be obstructed by the draught horse? Each of you must do your duty
as it is indicated for you in the authorized Materia Medica,
whence our opinion is derived. It has also been told me that
the stomach is deranged by you, but to prevent you playing this
trick I have included in the prescription along with you several
stomachic remedies, and will allow a cup of coffee to be drunk
after you are taken, which assists digestion, as the writings of
practitioners allege—regardless of those newfangled persons who
assert of it that it destroys your power: but you must not allow
yourself to be rendered powerless; for that reason I have appointed you the base."

And thus, as though they were independent beings endowed
with free volition, each ingredient in a complete prescription
has its task allotted to it, *vel invitissima Minerva Hygeiaque*, in
many other respects also. For there are many learned considerations in a regular classical prescription. This indication
and that one must be fulfilled; three, four and more symptoms
must be met by as many different remedies. Consider, Arcesilas! how many remedies must be artistically combined in order
to make the attack at once from all points. Something for the
tendency to vomit, something else for the diarrhœa, something
else for the evening fever and night-sweats, and as the patient is
so weak, tonic medicines must be added, and not one alone, but
several, in order that what the one cannot do (which we don't
know) the other may.

But what *if all the symptoms proceeded from one cause, as is almost always the case, and there were one single drug that would meet
all these symptoms?*

"That would be a very different thing. But it would be in-
convenient to search for such a one; we put in one prescrip-

tion something to meet every indication, and thus we fulfil the requirements of the school."

But do you thereby satisfy the requirements of the art, of the precious human life?

" No man can serve two masters."

But do you seriously believe that your *hotch-potch* will do what you assign to each of its ingredients, just as if they were things that did not mutually react upon each other, that did not influence each other, or that would refrain from doing so at your command? Does it not occur to you that two dynamic agents given together can *never* effect that which both, given separately at different times, would do—that an *intermediate action* must ensue which could not have been foreseen beforehand—and that this must be still more the case when several are given together! Who could tell beforehand that opium given along with coffee would in most cases exert merely a strong diuretic action? who could have predicted it of these two remedies? Will opium still stupify if ipecacuan be combined with it? You perceive that they do not act according to your will, nor according to your atonic principles! The combination of these two dynamic powers causes anxiety and perspiration.

" But tartar-emetic will be more apt to excite vomiting, if on account of the weakness of the stomach I combine with it cinchona bark?"

Very little or not all, my short-sighted friend!

" Why had the white hellebore so little effect on that patient?"

Because you gave at the same time a clyster of chamomile!

" What terrific effects ought not a good extract of stramonium to have! according to medical authors. They are a pack of liars! A short time ago I gave it to a very sensitive patient in a strong dose in a draught. It had no effect, not the slightest."

Probably you mixed it with oxymel?

" Yes, I did! But what harm can that do? It was only the excipient; only four ounces."

Several ounces of that vegetable acid? Well, you need not wonder that no effect was produced.—Did I not see you the other day prescribe salt of tartar mixed with gamboge? What was your object in doing so, and what effect had the powder?

" The first was in order to loosen the mucus, and the second to expel the worms forcibly; but to my astonishment it did not cause a single evacuation of the bowels."

That does not surprise me! Know that two, not to speak of three or more substances, when *mingled together* do not produce the same result that might be expected from them if given *singly* and at different times, but a different dynamical intermediate action, whether you wish it or no. In that case the systematic arrangement of your ingredients is of no avail, nor the part you allot to the *base* and *bases*, to the *adjuvant* and *adjuvants*, to your *corrective, director* and *excipient*. Nature acts according to eternal laws, without asking your leave; she loves simplicity, and effects *much* with one remedy, whilst you effect *little* with many. Seek to imitate nature!

To write very composite recipes, and several of them in the course of the day, is the climax of parempiricism; to administer quite simple remedies, and not to give a second before the action of the first has expired—this and this alone is the direct way into the inner holy place of art. Make your choice!

FRAGMENTARY OBSERVATIONS ON BROWN'S ELEMENTS OF MEDICINE.[1]

In section XVIII he politely apologises for being obliged to make use of the phrases, *deficient, exhausted, consumed, accumulated, superfluous excitability,* owing to the novelty of the doctrine and the poverty of common language. But this is no excuse for the man who boasts (CCCXII) of having now reduced the art of medicine to an exact science which will at no distant day receive the appellation of *Doctrine of Nature* (note to DCLXXVII), and of being *the first who has made it a demonstrated science* (see end of the Preface). He who would teach a new science for which he must employ new ideas, ought to employ for them new, appropriate, unequivocal terms, or make use of the old

[1] From *Hufeland's Journal der pract. Arzneykunde,* Vol. v. Pt. 2, p. 52, 1801. [Hufeland himself puts the following note to this masterly criticism:—"These observations are from the pen of one of the most distinguished of German physicians, who, however, as he himself expresses it, 'as long as literary chouanerie makes the highways unsafe,' will not permit his name to appear, which, in my opinion, is a good plan, in cases where reason and not the authority of names are to decide. I must, however, observe that the author has read nothing either for or against the Brunonian system, and therefore we may be all the more certain that we have here the unprejudiced opinion on this subject of a practical physician of matured experience and reflection."

words, attaching new meanings to them, for the new expressions. But as Brown employs the old expressions unexplained and without attaching to them new meanings, he must permit the reader to understand them in their old signification, and when we read, *that excitability, a certain quantity or certain energy of which has been assigned to every being upon the commencement of its living state* (XVIII.), *may be worn out by stimuli* (CCCIX) *and yet afterwards be drawn forth by new stimuli,* he must not be offended if we believe that we have read nonsense.

XXI. ζ, η, " Emetics and purgatives, fear, grief, &c., diminish the sum-total of excitement, and are debilitating;—but from no other reason, not because they are other than stimulating agents, —they are stimulants but are debilitating, that is, weakly stimulant, owing their debility (he should have said, *debilitating power*) to a degree of stimulus greatly inferior to the proper one."

If all excitement, all the conditions of life and health, are owing to stimulus, and to no other cause (XXII.) no stimulus is of itself capable of diminishing the excitement. Either the external condition for life and health does not solely depend upon what is termed "stimulus," or if it do, then a stimulus, be it even a weak, an insufficient one, cannot debilitate. It is only (but Brown does not make this proviso) when it is the sole stimulus acting upon the body for a long time, all other greater stimuli being in the meantime excluded, that a debilitating effect can be produced, not, however, in consequence of the smallness of the acting stimulus, but in consequence of the absence of the greater (accustomed) stimuli. If it were otherwise, a man in good health, who would feel still more enlivened by drinking four ounces of wine, would be tremendously debilitated if at that time in place of four ounces he should take but four drops in his mouth, and would be debilitated four times as much if he took only one drop.

An addition to the condition of life, be it ever so small (a weak simple stimulus), can never become a *minus*, can never debilitate. If, however, it do debilitate (as purgatives, fear, grief, and so forth do), whilst the sum-total of the usual means requisite for sustaining life (heat, food, &c.) remains undiminished, in that case its debilitating power must be owing to quite a different cause than the smallness of the stimulating power.

Who can fail to perceive the justness of these conclusions?

A healthy, excitable girl, in the full possession of all stimuli requisite for health, dies instantaneously on suddenly hearing the tragical intelligence that her lover has been stabbed. If this was merely a simple but only a small stimulus, it must have been just a small addition to the not defective sum of all the other stimuli. How could this small addition do harm, how could it destroy life, and that instantaneously, if it merely acted as a simple stimulus and in no other manner.

Who can fail to perceive the correctness of these inferences?

He carries out his delusion so far as to assert (XXI, »), that "fear and grief are only lower degrees of confidence and joy." Were I to dare to make such allegations, I could make anything out of everything, for it is very easy to be a scholastic sophist. No, my dear friend! there are two scales; at the top of the one stands indifference, and below that come vexation, grief, despair. The other scale has indifference at its lowest part, whence it mounts up to confidence, to joy, to rapture.

If it is allowed to Brown to infer from identity of effects, identity of causes, we may be permitted to infer from opposite effects, opposite causes, and to consider cold and grief, warmth and joy, as opposite powers (because they exhibit opposite (effects), yet in such a way as that the strengthening property of the latter, like the debilitating property of the former cannot depend on their common attributes as stimuli, but must depend upon attributes that in the former are of a directly opposite nature to those in the latter.

In XX and XXI Brown reckons poisons and typhus contagions among the above powers (whose debilitating power depends on the smallness of the stimulation that they produce on the body.

Well now, if a man in the full possession of all the health-sustaining external stimuli (the sum-total of which is from 3000 to 3010 daily) should choose, after drinking his last glass of wine, to get into a pit filled with carbonic acid, and if in ten minutes thereafter he is brought out dead, irrecoverably dead, what is it in this case that prevents the continuance of life? Is it the addition of the too small and therefore debilitating stimulus of the fixed air? Let us compute the sum of its stimulating energy at 1, or if you will at $^1|_{1,000,000}$th, in that case the sum of all the stimuli that have acted upon him during the last twenty-four hours, inclusive of the carbonic acid inspired, will amount to 3001 or 3000 $^1|_{1,000,000}$th. He has been acted on every preceding day by as many (more or fewer) stimuli, there has occurred in this last day neither diminution nor increase of the stimuli up to the moment of his death. What then prevented him living?

It is evident that it was an agent that proved so excessively injurious to him, not in consequence of the smallness of its stimulating energy, but on account of its enormous power of quite a different nature.

He tries to get over the difficulty (XXI, ζ) by saying that the debilitating stimuli produce their debilitating effects *partly by means of a disagreeable relation to the excitability, or by their causing a disagreeable sensation.* But he is very inconsistent to boast in one page that he has reduced physiology and pathology to one or two principles, and in the next page *quasi aliud agendo,* to put a couple of *qualitates occultæ* in the corner, which, in case of necessity, when the defects of the vaunted chief supports of his system are exposed, he may bring forward as already established principles, and attach to them, according to his fancy, any meaning they may be required to bear. But through all these parts assigned to auxiliaries, accessory springs of action, and accessory agents, the boasted simplicity of his so-called system vanishes into nothing. Now all the specific effects of poisons, contagions, &c., when it suits the purpose of Brown and his followers, and the omnipotent words, " stimulants, weakly stimulant," will not do, can be referred to " a discordant combination of powers," and the specific remedial powers of this or that medicine, sometimes to the " agreeable relation that the exciting power bears to the excitability," sometimes to an " agreeable sensation;" and thus his retreat is covered ! How artful! but at the same time how disingenuous !

To his overstrained objections to cold in asthenic diseases—(CCXCII) " In diseases of great and direct debility, cold must be most carefully avoided, as it is *always* of a directly debilitating operation, and *never of service* but in sthenic diseases, and those that are in a progress to indirect debility"—which is repeatedly alluded to, I must oppose my experience, which is the same as that of many others, that during many years when I was still ignorant of any specific remedies for old chronic diseases, I have frequently combatted them successfully solely with cold washing, cold foot-baths, and also with immersion for one minute at a time in water of from 50° to 60° Fahr. One case however among many others is so remarkable that I cannot refrain from detailing it. A man somewhat advanced in years, but still possessing considerable strength, had had for five years from unknown cause a paralytic affection of his left arm. The movements he could perform with it were very weak and small, and

23

the sensibility of it also was much diminished. Once upon a time when he was on a visit to a relation, and there was no one to fetch the fish for the supper out of a frozen tank, he gets up quietly, breaks the ice, leans over it and passes nearly one hour with both arms in the ice-cold water before he can get out the required number of fish. He comes and brings them to the great delight of his host, but immediately complains of pains in the affected arm, which in the course of a few hours inflames. The following day the pain and inflammation were gone, and his arm had acquired its healthy sensibility and all the powers of health. The paralysis was cured and remained so. Should he have remained uncured to support Brown's erroneous maxims?

Brown, like all short-sighted, unpractical physicians, always looked only to the primary and incipient action of the remedy, but not to the after effect, which is, however, the chief thing.

CCXCVIII. "In spasms and convulsions, in the internal, in the external parts, in bleeding discharges, in the direful delirium of fevers and other very violent diseases, in asthenic inflammation; when those stimuli, which have a more permanent influence, fail, or act to no good purpose; the virtue of the diffusible stimulants, *the principal of which is opium,* is eminent." What a general way of speaking, and how empirical! What an immense deal the man can do with opium! I only wish I could do the like. To *cure internal and external spasms* with opium better than with any other remedy, any one else would find somewhat difficult.

CCXCIX. "When the action of all the other powers by which life is supported, is of no effect, they (that is, wine, brandy, opium) turn aside the instant stroke of death." No one took them more copiously and more variously than the Master who wrote this; how is it that they did not turn aside the stroke of death from himself (at his moderate age), and so avert the stigma from his doctrine?

CCCI. "A higher place in the scale is claimed by musk, volatile alkali, camphor;—however, in every respect the preparations of opium are sufficient for most purposes of high stimulating." According to this, opium ought to be quite adequate for the cure of most chronic diseases, and of others that he ascribes to a high degree of debility, as poisonings of all sorts, &c. In that case it would be a real panacea, and we should scarcely require any other remedy. He could certainly have seen and treated but few chronic diseases, and assuredly no cases of poisoning with white hellebore, arsenic, &c., otherwise he would not have asserted such falsehoods.

According to this paragraph, camphor should possess the same powers as opium, only in a somewhat less degree; and yet *actual experience* shows that their effects are exactly opposed; the one removes the effects of the other. How little Brown knew about the things whereof he speaks so confidently!

CCCII. "In diseases depending upon great debility [consequently according to him, in acute typhus, putrid and bilious fevers, the Levantine plague, &c.] animal soups should be given." But animal soups are utterly abhorred by them; will he in spite of the disgust they occasion force them upon the patients? They would agree with them admirably!

CCCIII. In the case of a convalescent in whom stimulants should be continued, he recommends that "in his movements he should first use *gestation.*" The old school, profoundly ignorant of nature, with whose fables Brown, the reformer of medicine, is still so chokefull, also considered riding without succussion as coming under the category of strengthening remedies, and ranged this passive motion alongside the active ones (such as walking, digging, and other manual exercises), and yet the former acts antagonistically to the latter, and is antiphlogistic, antisthenic, debilitating (at all events in its primary effect), greatly diminishing the pulse, causing vomiting and nausea, &c. The reader will easily perceive how opposed this is to truth and nature.

CCCVII, φ, "The remedies of asthenic diathesis, to whatever part they are applied, stimulate that part more than any other." This is also one of his maxims that carries us away by its god-like simplicity. Pity that it is fundamentally false—that it is completely opposed to all true experience. Tincture of opium applied to the pit of the stomach causes no sensation on the spot to which it is applied, but speedily relieves hysterical vomiting. When applied there, or to the neck, or to any other sensitive part of the body, it checks (in a palliative manner) some diarrhœas, removes the apoplectic death-like coldness, stiffness and unconsciousness caused by large doses of camphor, the abdominal pains produced by belladonna, and the sopor of typhus, though at the seat of its application no perceptible change is observable. And I could adduce a hundred other examples opposed to the generality of the maxim "that medicines act more strongly at the part where they are applied than elsewhere." This is a pure invention of his own.

CCCVIII. "Inanition of the vessels (penury of blood) takes place in asthenic diseases in an *exact* proportion to their degree." In pestilential typhus fevers, where sometimes only a few hours elapse in the transition from health to death, or in the sudden fatal cases caused by cherry-laurel water, by carburetted hydrogen, by exposure to the exhalations from cesspools, by the vapour of charcoal, by carbonic acid, by fright, where the interval betwixt health and death often scarcely amounts to a couple of minutes, how could such an enormous deficiency of blood "in an *exact* proportion to the degree of these asthenic diseases" have occurred in such a short time? Whither has the blood gone? It would be ridiculous to expose still further the absurdity of this assertion on which he prides himself so much.

According to this paragraph he considers the most efficacious remedy for asthenic diseases to be (artificial) filling of the vessels with blood! Just as if healthy blood could be prepared in a diseased body, just as if blood could be manufactured all at once by means of opium, wine, and forced-down animal soups, in such diseases, in the same way as butter is made in a churn, or beer in a brewing vat! What sort of blood? How different is chlorotic blood from that of phthisical subjects! *Ast parva non curat philosophus.*

CCCIX. "When the excitability is worn out by any one stimulus, any new stimulus finds excitability and draws it forth, and thereby produces a further variation of the effect." The fact is no doubt true, that a second medicine again acts when the one just given no longer does any thing. But the cause of this phenomenon, what is it? It is impossible that it can be as Brown says.

If stimulants do not differ among each other *in kind, but only in degree and strength* (an unconditional main dogma of Brown's, CCCXII, CCCXIII), then it is *impossible* that the second stimulant could act anew, after the first stimulant has ceased to be able to act. An increased dose of the first must necessarily effect all that could be expected from the second stimulant, if they differed from each other only in degree and strength; but the first, even when given in a stronger dose, now does nothing more, whereas the second acts anew, consequently they cannot differ merely in degree, they must differ *in kind* (*modo*). If however, this be the case, the whole Brunonian system falls to the ground.

Moreover, how can the second stimulus still find excitability and draw it forth, as he here asserts, when it has been already worn out by the first? Whence came the new excitability? from his fancy, or from the resources of the animal economy, whose existence he will not acknowledge? *Tertium non datur.* If it come from the latter source, then indeed it may sometimes flow more slowly and with greater difficulty, sometimes too quickly and impetuously. But then the second and only remaining mainstay of his system breaks down. Behold there a more natural origin of diseases, which these words of his betray against his will. Had he wished or been able to be consistent, he would not have ventured to touch this ticklish point, which gives him a slap in the face.

That all this nonsense is his actual meaning, is evident from the following assertions in

CCCXII, CCCXIII. "The effects of all external powers upon us do not differ among themselves; they produce life, activity, health and disease, by the same operation, by the same stimulus. Hence it follows that things which restore health cannot act otherwise than by one and the same stimulus."

"Several things that produce the same effect are then identical with each other, are one and the same thing."

This is far from being the case when the action is *complex ;* for even according to Brown, the medicines do not establish health in the system so very immediately, so unconditionally, so independently of the corporeal powers, so entirely without previous reaction, as the apple-tree lets the apple fall on the grass.

But if the effect be brought about by composite actions, the prime agent on which the action depends may certainly be very different.

Windmills, horse-power, steam-engines and capstans worked by men, may all empty a reservoir of water; the dry atmospheric air also that extends over the reservoir empties it; but does it therefore follow that wind, horses, fire, men and the dry atmosphere are one and the same thing? There are also many powers that exercise a double action, a primary and a secondary, and several among them that *resemble* each other in their primary action, and not a few that do so in their secondary action. If then the careless observer looks only to the resemblance of the primary action of some powers (as Brown often did), or only to their secondary actions, or to similarity of actions, be they primary or secondary, he may often be misled to infer an identity of cause from some similarity of these one-sided actions, as usually happened to Brown. In making deductions from similar false premises, I might with equal justice say, that a watery vegetable diet, and strong animal soups were one and the same thing, for they both (in their primary action on the body) cause satiety. The same effects have the same cause, therefore watery vegetable nutriment and beef-tea are one and the same thing. And thus the false scholastic deduction is made.

CCCXIV. " In asthenic diseases the administration first of diffusible stimulants, for the purpose of bringing back the appetite [even in every diseased body?] for the greatest remedy, food, as well as keeping the food on the stomach and assisting in the digestion of it [will they do so in every diseased body?], then the application of heat, then the use of less diffusible and more durable stimulants: as animal food, without and with seasoning, wine, gestation, gentle exercise, moderate sleep, pure air, exertion of mind, [can the mind of one affected with melancholia be exerted?] exertion in passion and emotion, [even in idiots and raving maniacs?] an agreeable exercise of the senses; all those reproduce health, by no other operation but that of only increasing excitement."

This then sums up all Brown's therapeutics for diseases of, and accompanied by, weakness! That kind nature and youth will, assisted by such an appropriate regimen, (for it is nothing more) and even by itself, cure diseases having far other producing causes than deficiency and excess of excitability, is a phenomenon daily witnessed by the unprejudiced observer, which, however, must be explained away or denied by Brown in order to support his scholastic system.

But without reckoning this divine power, and granting that all these diseases depended on a morbid degree of excitability, and could *only* be removed by the remedies indicated by him (but which were used long before his time), what becomes of the myriads of diseases that cannot be cured by these remedies? It avails us little that he ascribes them all also to deficiency or excess of excitability. All that we want is that he should cure them. We shall see if by this regimen, the large number of mental diseases, the epilepsies, the venereal lues, the mercurial wasting, the pellagra, the plica polonica, (I reject the name of local diseases, the refuge of the Brunonians, for these affections) will be cured. *Hic Rhodus! hic salta!*

Or will this regimen, whose curative effect cannot be looked for under a considerable time, cure asthenia which often kills healthy individuals in a few hours or even minutes (the bad kinds of typhus fevers, the Levantine plague, apoplexy, the accidents caused by laurocerasus, azotic and carbonic acid gas, carburetted hydrogen, veratrum album, arsenical vapour, &c.)?

DCLXXVII. "As it now happens, that either direct or indirect debility proves hurtful, hence we have a third case given, where we have to combat both sorts of debility."

Who could have believed that a scholastic pedant who plumes himself so much on his logical forms, who reckons for us in figures on a scale of his own exactly the degree of the exciting power and excitability, would have so far forgotten himself, as Master Brown does here at the end of his immortal work? How! both kinds of debility conspiring to make one disease in one body?

In the first place, I should like to know, as he (notes to XLVII and LXXXII) fixes the standard of health at 40 degrees of excitability—the predisposition to direct debility in the degrees below 40 down to 25,—complete and extreme direct debility from 25 to 0,—the predisposition to sthenia in the degrees from 40 to 55,—sthenia itself in the degrees from 55 to 70,—and indirect debility in the degrees from 70 to 80;—I should like to know in what part of this scale (which he is so proud of) he could place the mixed form of debility he speaks of, by what figures he would expound this supposed excitability? Here he says nothing about the figures of his table, which he is so fond of putting forward elsewhere.

Here he prudently ignores them and attempts in a note, by means of mere words, I know not whether I should say to conceal or to increase the hiatus. He brings forward many examples where in one disease direct debility occurs along with indirect, indirect with direct debility. Granted that the man whom he there supposes to be affected with typhus had got thereby a direct debility of 10 (30 degrees below 40) that is 40—30, but in the meantime, by means of great corporeal motion, had contracted an indirect debility of 70 (30 degrees above 40) that is 40+30, can the man thereby have aggravated his state and be now labouring under indirect and at the same time direct debility? If Brown's excitement theory be not entirely false and his scales not the mere offspring of his fancy, must not instantaneous health or the degree of 40 ensue, since 40 minus 30 and plus 30, gives 40, the sum of excitability?

If this be not the result of the meeting of the two opposed debilities, I should like to know what it is then? What part of his excitability-scale is not already occupied?

Either there is not a spark of truth in his excitement theory or his scale of excitability, or the man must, although already affected by typhus, be instantly restored completely to health or nearly so by the added corporeal exertion, according to Brown's whole theory and his vaunted scale. But if, as must naturally happen, the man visibly aggravates his malady by this fatigue, as Brown himself confesses, this circumstance overthrows his whole system.

If the extraordinary accumulation of excitability in a case of typhus, imagined by Brown, can and must be aggravated by corporeal exertion, as experience teaches and as he here admits, then either the corporeal motion cannot remove the excitability, otherwise in this case health would ensue or almost ensue, or there can be in typhus no accumulation of excitability. Plus and minus cannot co-exist without mutually annihilating one another.

It is impossible that a state of accumulation of excitability can be aggravated by a power that diminishes excitability (according to his whole theory), therefore the aggravation that ensues is a refutation of his whole beautiful excitement theory and his tabularly expressed accumulation and exhaustion of excitability, to which, according to him, all the conditions of life may be referred.

Brown gives us no information as to the state (and degree) in which we must suppose the excitability to exist when the two debilities meet together. That he himself did not know how to conceive this state is obvious from his extraordinary and ambiguous assertions relative to this point.

Thus, as the direct debility of the man affected with typhus must amount to at least 70 degrees of accumulation of excitability, to what height did the degrees rise since his state was aggravated by corporeal exertion? The degrees of the accumulation could certainly not be the least diminished, otherwise the disease had not been aggravated, at all events it had been transformed into a sthenic disease (at 60); the state must then have sunk suddenly and far below 40 into indirect debility, in order to be able to express the great aggravation that has ensued at least by the degree 10. In the former case, seeing that for the commencement of the treatment of the simple direct debility Brown prescribes ten drops of laudanum, he must prescribe for its cure eight drops or less; in the latter case, however, as he orders for the commencement of the treatment of the simple indirect debility 150 drops, he must for a worse degree have administered 200 drops and upwards. But no! his vaunted consistency forsakes him here.

"When the affection," he says (DCLXXXVI), "is more a mixture of both sorts of debility, these proportions of the doses must be blended together."

Though this is purposely worded so as to be incomprehensible, it can only have this one meaning, that we should from the two select an intermediate number betwixt the dose increasing from a few drops and that decreasing from many drops. Therefore a medium proportion betwixt an increasing and decreasing progression. Very strange! In this case, from the beginning to the end (if both debilities were pretty equal in point of strength) 80 drops should be given uninterruptedly, which is contrary to his other modes of treatment and opposed to the nature of the thing. And how if the direct debility was greater than the indirect, or the latter greater than the former, what state is present, what is to be done for it? He himself does not actually know what he should direct to be done for cases which he can make clear neither to himself nor to others, and what would he advise to be done in this dilemma? He prudently forbears giving any detailed information on the subject, and merely in the note to DCLXXVII cunningly says, (possibly in order to escape observation in the confusion?) "A judicious physician will find plenty of scope for the exercise of his judgment in these mixed states." In a word, he leaves us, with a bow to the reader, in the lurch, not only here but in the *treatment of all asthenias*, "*because*," as he assures us in this paragraph, "*there is scarcely any asthenic disease where such a mixed state is not present*," So almost *all* asthenic diseases consist of an unknown mixture of both debilities, whereof he knows not how to impart any information in reference to the change therefrom resulting in the body, and to the accompanying state of excitement and excitability, nor to give us any advice on the subject! Heaven help us! throughout the whole transparent work he has dazzled as with a flaring straw fire, here it sinks down into ashes, and he leaves us, with a smile, surrounded by a howling wilderness in the darkness of night.

VIEW OF PROFESSIONAL LIBERALITY AT THE COMMENCEMENT OF THE NINETEENTH CENTURY.[1]

I do not here refer to that low, envious trading spirit, for which the pressure of want is often the cause that can best be pleaded in excuse; I wish to say a few words about the professional jealousy of medical men among themselves, which is the prevalent custom in Germany (in the southern more than the northern parts), a *bellum omnium contra omnes*, which has had a most injurious influence on the prosperity of one of the noblest arts, and the one which stands most in need of improvement—medicine. For no sooner has a colleague made a suggestion that must be for the general good, put forward a perhaps useful proposition, discovered something profitable, than instantly the professional jealousy of his colleagues (with very few exceptions) falls foul of him in order to bury in oblivion, or if possible, to destroy the novelty by spoken or written depreciations, insinuations, sophistries, or even injurious aspersions, and all because—*it did not originate with themselves*.[2] Instead of seeing, as we do in England and Scotland, fraternal meetings, and societies of physicians and surgeons, animated by the desire to promote the welfare of humanity, and investigating medical subjects for the purpose of mutual improvement and perfection, without party-spirit, without seeking self-aggrandisement, without ministering to individual vanity—we see the German medical men (with few exceptions) completely divided among themselves, each acting by himself, *pro modulo ingenii*, occasionally appropriating the useful discoveries of others, but quite silently, without betraying by the slightest sign that any one else has any thing to recommend him, or that they were in-

---

[1] From the *Allgemeiner Anzeiger d. D.* No. 32. 1801. [This article is interesting in reference to the history of the discovery of Belladonna as a prophylactic for scarlatina. It will be seen that in the first instance Hahnemann did not reveal the name of the remedy he employed for that purpose, which may possibly account in some degree for the unwillingness of his colleagues to test the efficacy of the remedy he furnished with them, but they had not this excuse after 1801, for in that year he announced the prophylactic to be belladonna, as will be seen in the next essay, and yet many years elapsed before they put his prophylactic to the test, whereby its utility was, as is well known, signally verified by some of the best physicians of the day.]

[2] [May these remarks of the illustrious master ever be remembered by American physicians, and whenever envy or other unworthy feelings prompt them to calumniate their brethren, may this lash of Hahnemann fall upon their unworthy backs.] —*Am. P.*

debted for anything whatsoever to this one or the other. Not only do they make use of the propositions and inventions of others without betraying the least thankfulness, but they often throw out spiteful insinuations against the originator, at all events always (few are the exceptions!) *without taking any public part in promoting and perfecting the proposition or discovery*, particularly if it proceed from a German physician; far more likely are they to do so if it belong to a foreign physician. How much this egotistical professional jealousy prevents the shooting forth and vigorous growth of our divine healing art, which is still in the condition of an undeveloped bud, must be evident to every non-professional person. Were it not for this paltry self-seeking spirit, of a truth Germany alone, with its great intellectual talents, could affect a regeneration of the great art.

How spitefully Wichmann was assailed when he exposed the prevalent fallacies respecting difficult teething! How infamously the same clique calumniated that unenvious favourite of the Asclepiadean muse—Hufeland, whose soul is animated by truth alone! How was Tode, how was Sömmering treated! Were the men that could act in this manner exclusively devoted to the beneficent art whose aim is the weal of humanity?

Ever sadder, ever more gloomy are the prospects of the development of our art in the new century; without friendliness and good-fellowship among its professors, it will remain but a bungling art for another century.

Let it not be retorted that there now exists, at least among the followers of the Brunonian system, an *esprit de corps*. The rallying motto of a sectarian name is incapable of exciting to sober, calm scientific investigation; it only rouses the explosive spirit of accusations of heresy to a fierce volcanic flame. Truth and the weal of humanity should be the only motto of the genuine elucidators of the art and the watch-word of their brotherly, peaceful bond of union, without slavish adherence to any sectarian leader, if we would not see the little good that we know completely sacrificed to party-spirit and discord. In these times, when accusations of heresy are so rife, the most important question that is ever put is, "Art thou of Paul, art thou of Cephas or Apollos?" Would it not be far better to say, "Brother! what is the peculiar mode of action of cinchona bark on the healthy individual? so that we may at length learn how to employ it with confidence in diseases, seeing that we have hitherto blindly wasted many thousand hundred-weights of it, at one time doing good, at another harm, without knowing what it was we did." Would it not be better to say, "Dear colleague! let us together investigate and observe the many and various kinds of intermittent fevers, and let us unite in laying before the world the discoveries we thus make, as to which kind among them may be, cæteris paribus, *always cured* by cinchona, which by sal-ammoniac, which by chamomile, which by ignatia, which by capsicum, &c."—"God forbid! who would consent to such an exposure of himself as to confess to his colleagues or to the public that he did know everything? Those around me must be impressed with the belief that I am infallible, that I embrace the whole sphere of the art, as I hold a ball in my hand, that the inmost secrets of medical science lie clearly open to my all-seeing eye, like the seed-recepticle of an apple cut through the middle. I dare not say one word that could betray that something was still to be discovered or that there was any room for improvement. But the notion that another and more especially a German colleague could teach us something more, or could make any fresh discovery, must not be uttered, must be to the best of our ability scouted."

Such is the spirit that has prevailed in Germany during the latter half until the end of the bygone century ; the benefactors of their race, and with them the good spirit that inspired them with zeal for the common weal, were sought to be kept down and set aside. Just as theological polemics have never produced a desire for truth, a perception of the high object of our existence or genuine virtue and devotional feeling—just as the personal squabbles of literary men have never succeeded in developing the love of art, the true æsthetic feeling, enlightened taste, and artistic skill—in like manner it needs no great sagacity to understand that the mutual detractions of medical men can have no other result but the depreciation and obscuration of their art, which is, without that, the most obscure of all arts.

Honourable, non-medical friends, endowed with a desire to promote the well-being of mankind and who have had the advantage of a scientific education!—the energies of my life, which have been devoted to promote the welfare of the community, have also been cramped and kept under by this unpatriotic spirit of many of the medical men of Germany.

As soon as I stepped forth among my colleagues, not without nearly twenty years of preparation, not without many long years of Pythagorean silence, to contribute here and there something to the improvement of our art, I found that I had lost my accustomed peace and quietness, and had fallen among a crowd of professional brethren, who (with few exceptions) regard nothing impartially; I was maligned. And how easy it is to persecute, to malign an art, which has hitherto been founded on ever-changing maxims, in which by the force of authorities, learned, empty terminology, sophistry, scholastic, stereotyped dogmas, and imaginary experience, black was made to appear white, just as any one pleased, especially where the judgment was perverted by depravity of heart, egotism and illiberality.

It is undoubtedly true that truth penetrates even through the thickest clouds of prejudice, but the often too tedious conflict of the opposing elements conveys a disagreeable, a discouraging impression to the mind. Thus at the commencement of my career, on account of my discovery of the best anti-venereal medicine, the soluble mercury, I was abused in the most vulgar manner in a journal notorious for its outrageous vituperations, and also elsewhere, but the common experience of Europe in a few years removed the slander from this remedy and worthily appreciated a discovery that I had unselfishly revealed for the good of humanity, in order to make amends for the death of thousands who had been literally dissolved by the abuse of the feebly anti-venereal preparations of corrosive mercury. The same thing happened when I was afterwards again (to pass over the bad reception some other useful truths met with) abused in the same vituperative journal on account of my " *new principle,*" where I taught a mode of learning to look at diseases from a point of view that directs us *almost unmistakeably* to the appropriate remedy for every case—shewing how to discover from the positive nature of medicinal agents the diseases for which they are suitable. But because this kind of system differed so much from the ordinary one, because it was so simple, so unartificial and (purposely) so free from the sacred arabesques of the learned language of the schools, it made very little impression, it was not cultivated by German medical men, but was sought to be quietly shelved by them.

Now, once more, at the end of the century that has just expired, my zeal for the welfare of mankind misled me to announce a prophylactic remedy for one of the most destructive of children's diseases, *scarlet-fever.* Scarcely a fourth part of the number I might have expected subscribed for it. This lukewarm interest shown for such an important affair discouraged me, and I arranged that the subscribers should receive a portion of the medicine itself, in order to satisfy them, in case my book on the subject should not be published. The subscribers consisted chiefly of physicians' who had epidemics of scarlet-fever in their neighbourhood. At least thirty of these, whom I begged by letter to testify to the truth, and to publish the result (be it what it might) in the *Reichs-Anzeiger*, made *no reply*.

Two others, unsolicited by me, Dr. Jani in Gera and Dr. Müller in Plauen, wrote something on the subject, but, good heavens! in what a spirit! Is this the way one colleague treats another in Germany? Is an affair of such importance for mankind to be so readily dismissed?

After the latter had said in No. 215 of the *R.A.*, 1800, "that in the epidemic he witnessed no child took scarlet-fever who had used this medicine for two or three weeks," he repents of his honesty and feels himself compelled in No. 239 "to deny the truth of his former declaration (the facts brought forward by himself!) because *one* child took the scarlet-fever. This case proves more against the efficacy of the remedy than 500, where the individuals seem to have been protected by it, prove for it."

What monstrous logic! Mercury is, as is well known, the best and sole remedy in the venereal disease; thousands have been cured by its means. "No," quoth Bavius, "I could shew you at least twenty cases where it did no good. Mercury is of no use; these twenty cases certainly prove more against the efficacy of the remedy than your thousands of successful cases prove for it. Therefore we should rather let ourselves be eaten up by the venereal disease than have it cured by mercury, because out of many thousand cases there are twenty where it does no good."—"A single case in which cinchona bark failed in intermittent fever proves more for the worthlessness of this bark than 500 cases in which it was efficacious for it." What a delirium of logic! The good Dr. Müller has once upon a time heard of the deduction *a minori ad majus*, and seeks to apply that here. In like manner the wag made the deduction *a minori ad majus* in the Müllerean fashion: "Since it feels hard to lie upon a single feather on the bare floor, this proves more against the softness of feathers than a bed filled with millions of

---

¹ A good many private individuals got the medicine sent them; but the basest mendacious insinuations of their ordinary medical attendants prevented them from *saving* their children by its means.

eider-feathers for their softness; I will therefore never more sleep upon feather-beds after having lain so hard upon one feather."

But perhaps Dr. Müller invented this pleasant piece of sophistry only in order to eradicate from the minds of the uniniated, by one (philanthropic) blow, this *German* invention, *not proceeding from himself.* Be it so, my friend! But have you anything better to substitute for the remedy? Is there to be found in medical writings a single mode of treating scarlet-fever on which we may rely? We shall not say a word about a preventive remedy. According to the directions usually given, there is not a single symptom that can be removed without several worse ones being excited. It may be said of the old mode of treatment of every acute disease: " *With* our medicines and *without* our medicines the primary fever goes off in twenty-one days, or the patient dies in the meantime, he might not have died had he not taken our medicines."

Dr. Jani, on the other hand, says in No. 255, that his scarlet-fever was complicated with malignant typhus-fever and acute herpetic-fever, and very rarely ran a regular course.

He then seeks to prove "that my preservative does not protect unconditionally." He might have spared himself the pains. *God himself cannot create a remedy that shall be unconditionally efficacious, that when used wrongly, at an inappropriate time, in an improper place, or under adverse circumstances, shall yet of necessity do good.*

" After it became *universally prevalent,* and was raging among them like an evil demon, he allowed ten families, consisting of thirty-six children, to use my remedy. *Three* children in one family were attacked by scarlet fever whilst using it (?). Of the thirty children of the remaining nine families who used it for a month, none was attacked by scarlet-fever. *But as far as was known none of them were exposed to infection.*"

Therefore it was no merit of Hahnemann's prophylactic that just those nine families with their thirty children remained free amidst all the others. This miracle is owing solely to the fact that they were not exposed to infection (*scilicet*) at a period when, as he asserts, scarlet-fever was *universally prevalent.* When an epidemic of scarlet-fever (which generally does not spare two out of a hundred children in the place) is *universally* prevalent, does the mere circumstance " of not having been exposed to the infection as far as was known" suffice to preserve from infection? Were that the case, it were impossible that any epidemic of scarlet-fever could ever arise, because no child of sensible or at least of timorous parents would ever be knowingly exposed to infection!

"But because it was not I, but another, and what is worse, a German physician who discovered the remedy, it must be allowed us, in order that the honour may not be given to the preservative, to ascribe the wonderful, unheard-of exemption of the nine families, to a notoriously inefficient cause, in order that we may be enabled to shelve Hahnemann's prophylactic remedy before the very eyes of the all-seeing public."

Here are striking features of the professional liberality among the physicians of our time! Here is a fine specimen of zealous endeavour to clear up the truth, of warm interest in promoting an affair of infinite importance to humanity.

The furtherance of every means, be it ever so small, that can save human life, that can bring health and security (a God of love invented this blessed and most wondrous of arts!) should be a sacred object to the true physician; chance, or the labour of a physician, has discovered this one. Away, then, with all grovelling passions at the altar of this sublime God-head, whose priests we are!

We all strive after a common, holy object; but it is not easy to be attained. It is only by joining hand in hand, only by a brotherly union of our powers, only by a mutual intercommunication and a common dispassionate development of all our knowledge, views, inventions and observations, that this high aim can be attained :—*the perfecting of the medical art.*

*   *   *   *

But why the most trustworthy remedy sometimes does not answer in our private practice—this every observant physician who has grown gray in his profession, and who possesses at the same time a knowledge of mankind, can easily account for from his own experience. Hospital patients, whom the unprejudiced clear-sighted physician never loses sight of, are certainly much more favourable for determining the truth, though even with them, deceptions, mistakes, insufficiency, and a thousand other opposing accessory circumstances, are *unavoidable.*

But how we may fail to attain our object in private practice, particularly as regards my preservative, and how failure is to be avoided, I shall explain in my forthcoming little work.

*   *   *   *

Physicians of Germany, be brothers, be fair, be just!

CURE AND PREVENTION OF SCARLET FEVER.[1]

PREFACE

Had I compiled a large book upon scarlet fever, I should have obtained, through the usual channels of publication, at least as much in the way of honorarium as by the subscription for this little book. But as, according to Callimachus, a great book is a great evil, and is soon laid aside, one of my chief aims, to wit, *to excite a great interest in a subject of so much importance to humanity as this is, in order clearly to ascertain the truth, by bringing the observations of many to bear upon it*—could not have been fulfilled so well by the large book as by the mode I have adopted.

Up to this period it is impossible that the corroboration of my assertion could be complete. The extract of belladonna, which I caused to be delivered to my subscribers, might have lost its power by the great distances it was sent, and by the long period it had been kept. Occasionally it fell into the hands of some who had neither the ability nor the good will to administer its solution in an appropriate manner. The precautions laid down in this book could not all be enumerated in a small paper of directions, where on account of the danger of misusing the medicine, it was necessary to direct that only the very smallest dose should be administered. Moreover it is probable, that the *thorough* admixture of the few drops with a sufficient quantity of the fluid in which it should be taken, was generally neglected; a circumstance the neglect of which makes this and every other medicine many hundred times less powerful than they would be were they properly combined with the diluting fluid. The hurry and inaccuracy of young doctors of the present day are well known, and we know also how little dependence we can place on our private patients.

In addition, *very inclement weather*, and in general what is understood *a chill* (which I have forgotten to allude to in the text), present obstacles by no means slight to the power of belladonna as a preventative of scarlet-fever. Children should be carefully preserved from it, without however completely excluding them from the open air, and if this precaution be neglected, the dose of the remedy should at all events be increased.

There may also be many other circumstances unknown to me

---

[1] This was published as a pamphlet at Gotha, in 1801.

to diminish the power of belladonna. The philanthropic physician ought to endeavour to discover and to avoid them.

It is only in accordance with my well known maxim (the new principle) that small-pox, to give one example from among many, has an important prophylactic in the cow-pox, which is an exanthematous disease, whose pustules break out after the sixth day of innoculation, with pain and swelling of the axillary glands, pain in the back and loins, and fever, and surrounded by an erythematous inflammation—that is to say, constituting altogether a disease very similar to variola. And, in like manner, a medicine which causes symptoms so similar to those of the invasion of scarlet-fever, as belladonna does, must be one of the best preventive remedies for this children's pestilence. It should however be put to the test with candour, carefulness and impartiality—not cursorily or hurriedly, not with the design of depreciating the originator of it at the expense of truth.

But if its efficacious prophylactic power has incurred and may still incur opposition from prejudiced, ill-disposed, weak-minded and cursory observers, I may be allowed to appeal against their conduct to the more matured investigation of the clear-sighted, dispassionate portion of the public, and to trust to time for a just verdict. I should esteem myself happy if I should see, some years hence, this scourge of mankind in any measure diminished by my labours.

CURE AND PREVENTION OF SCARLET FEVER.

At the commencement of the year 1799 small-pox came from the neighbourhood of Helmstädt to Königslutter[1] which spread slowly around, and though not mild in character, the eruption was small, warty looking, and accompanied with serious symptoms, especially of an atonic kind. In the village it came from, the scarlet fever was prevalent at the same time, and, mixed up with the latter, the small-pox made its appearance in Königslutter. About the middle of the year the small-pox ceased almost entirely, and the scarlet-fever then commenced to appear alone and more frequently.

HISTORY OF THE SCARLATINA EPIDEMIC.

In this as in all other epidemics the scarlet-fever shewed itself to be the most spreading and contagious of all the maladies that befal children. If a single child was affected with it, not

---

[1] [Where Hahnemann at that time resided.]

one of its brothers and sisters remained exempt, nor did it fail to effect other children who came too close to the patients, or to things that had come in contact with their exhalations.[1] Parents above thirty years of age who are in the midst of many children affected with scarlet fever, usually in dirty damp rooms, get now and then in place of the general eruption a very painful pustular erysipelas of the face, or the peculiar scarlatina sore-throat—always along with some degree of fever.

In its main symptoms this epidemic of scarlet-fever resembled the scarlatina of Plenciz.[2] In some families the disease was of a mild form, but generally it was of a bad kind.

When it occurred in the mild form it generally remained mild in the whole family living together. There occurred a slight feeling of weariness, a kind of faint-heartedness, some difficulty of swallowing, some fever, red face and hot hands. There then appeared, usually the very first day, alone with slight itching, the spots of various shape, and sometimes paler, sometimes redder, on the neck, the chest, the arms, &c., which disappeared again in from three to four days, and the desquamation that followed was scarcely observable on the fingers, and almost nowhere else. Towards evening only the patients laid down in bed for a short time, but the rest of the day they went about. The sleep was pretty tranquil, the bowels usually somewhat less open than when in health, the appetite usually not much diminished.

Very different was the course of the *bad form* of scarlet-fever that prevailed in most families. *Generally*[3] *the seventh day after the infection had been communicated it broke out* suddenly and unexpectedly, without any previous feeling of illness seldom was it that *horrible dreams* on the previous night served as a prelude to it. All at once there occurred an unusual *timidity* and *fearfulness, rigour with general coldness, especially in the face, the hands and the feet,* violent *pressive* headache, *especially in the forehead, above the orbits. Pressure in the hypochondria, chiefly in the region*

---

[1] Among children under fifteen years of age that may be exposed to contagion in epidemics of scarlatina, hardly one in a thousand escapes the disease, though they may only be affected by the specific sore throat, or a combination of some of the other symptoms; from fifteen to twenty years of age scarcely one in five hundred is spared; from twenty to thirty years the infection becomes always rarer. It is very seldom that persons above thirty are affected by the perfect scarlet-fever exanthema, and then only in the most malignant and fatal epidemics.

[2] *Opera medico-physica.* Tract iii, Sect. iii. Vindob. 1762.

[3] Those symptoms not described by Plenciz I have had printed in *italics*, but those that correspond with his are in the usual Roman type.

of the stomach ; in most cases there occurs *a very unexpected attack of violent vomiting, first of mucus, then of bile, then of water* recurring at intervals of from twelve to twenty-four hours, accompanied by an ever increasing weakness and anxiety, *with trembling. The parotid and sub-maxilliary glands swell and become hard and painful,* swallowing becomes very difficult, *with shooting pains. After rigours that last from twelve to twenty-four hours,* the body becomes excessively hot, *accompanied with itching burning, the head, neck, hands* (forearms) *and feet* (legs) *are hottest, and swollen so as to present a shining appearance, which lasts to the end of the disease.*[1] (*Almost every paroxysm of heat terminates in profuse sweat, which, however, only affects the rest of the body, but not the head, hands and feet.*) On these swollen parts, but first in the pit of the throat, then on the arms and legs, there appear about the second day variously shaped *cinnabar coloured* spots of various sizes *that readily grow pale on any slight chill;* these spots are scarcely raised above the level of the skin, *and are always accompanied by smarting, itching, burning;* as the disease advances they spread out into a connected, but less vivid redness. *On the outburst of the eruption, the fever does not diminish ; on the contrary, the greater the redness the more violent is the fever.* In the meantime the sore-throat increases, swallowing becomes very painful, in the worst cases almost impossible. The interior of the mouth, the tongue and the palate are inflamed, very painful, raw, *and as if ulcerated all over.* In very bad cases the swelling of the cervical glands almost closes the jaws, and *from between the teeth, which can be but slightly separated, there flows almost incessantly a very viscid and very fetid saliva,* which can scarcely be expelled from the mouth in consequence of the tongue being so painful. In like manner, in the worst cases the lining membrane of the nose is ulcerated. At this period the voice becomes weak, suppressed and unintelligible, and respiration difficult. The taste in the mouth is putrid; the stools, *which are usually rarely passed,* have the odour of assafœtida. A *drawing pain in the back and cutting bellyache* are characteristic symptoms, which, together with pressive headache, in bad cases persist in alternation day and night, but in less dangerous cases

---

[1] The sudden disappearance of the redness with the fatal termination without obvious cause observed in some of the epidemics of 1800, I had not an opportunity of seeing. Probably this depended on a peculiar complication, and I am not aware if my preservative, which is only for pure scarlatina, would have the power of averting this.

only recur in the evening after sunset, along with increase of anxiety and timidity. In the very worst cases there are alternate paroxyms of *agonising tossing about,* raving, *groaning, grinding of the teeth, floccitations, general or partial convulsions* and comatose stupefaction or sopor, with half-shut eyes *and head bent backwards.* The urine, which is light-coloured, and the fæces, are passed involuntarily, and the patient sinks down to the bottom of the bed. The *grumbling,* complaining disposition increases from day to day. *The smallest quantity of food,* even in the slighter cases, *perceptibly and immediately increases the anxiety, more than in any other disease.*

From the fourth to the seventh day, if death do not ensue, the skin rises up, or rather the pores of the skin on the reddest places become elevated, especially about the neck and the arms, in small, close, pointed miliary vesicles (somewhat resembling goose's skin), which at first, as the redness of the rest of the skin declines, appear extremely red, but afterwards, or when cold is applied, grow pale and at length quite white; they are however empty, and contain no fluid.

Neither the greater intensity nor the more general extension of the redness of the skin, nor yet the occurrence of these empty miliary vesicles, diminish the fever after the manner of a critical eruption; the former indeed is rather a sign of an increased intensity of fever which can only subside as this redness decreases.

The bad form of scarlatina lasts from nine to fourteen days, and the disgust at food lasts about the same time. As the appetite returns, the patient first wishes for fruit, then meat, he generally prefers pork.

As the convalescence progresses, there is, in addition to the uncommon emaciation, a *stiffness,* causing the patient to go half bent, that lasts several days, sometimes weeks; *it is a kind of contraction* of the joints, *especially the knees, with a feeling of stiffness in the abdomen.*

During the fever, blood-red spots now and then appeared on the sclerotic; in some the cornea of one or both eyes was completely obscured; others (probably badly treated patients) were rendered imbecile.

At length the epidermis gradually peels off on the places where the redness appeared, and even where there was only burning itching without subsequent redness; on the hands and feet it comes off in large pieces, like pieces of a torn glove, but on the other parts only in larger or smaller scales. In one case

the nails of the fingers and toes also fell off. The falling off of
the hair only commenced some weeks or months after the fever;
in one case it went the length of total baldness.

Among the after-sufferings the following were prominent :
long-continued debility, a very disagreeable feeling in the back,
as if it were asleep (narcosis), pressive headache, a painful sensation of constriction in the abdomen only felt on bending backwards, abscesses in the interior of the ear, ulceration of the lining
membrane of the nose, ulcerated angles of the mouth, other
spreading ulcers in the face and other parts of the body, and
generally a great tendency of the whole skin to ulceration
(*unhealthy skin* as it is termed). In addition to the above, a great
hurriedness in speaking and acting, fits of sleepiness by day,
crying out in sleep, shuddering in the evening, puffiness and
earthy colour of the countenance,[1] swelling of the hands, feet
and loins, &c.

TREATMENT OF SCARLET-FEVER.

Any one who chooses may read for himself in the works of
the various authors the infinity of medicines and modes of treatment invented for this disease (from blood-letting and leeches
to bark, from gargles and clysters to blisters, from antispasmodic, derivative, antiseptic to refrigerant, resolvent, purgative,
involvent, humectant, alexiteric, incitant, asthenic, and God
knows what other ingenious modes of treatment) intended to
meet the thousand imaginary indications. Here we often see
the *ne plus ultra* of the grossest empiricism: *for each single
symptom a particular remedy* in the motley, mixed, and repeated
prescriptions ; a sight that cannot fail to inspire the unprejudiced
observer with feelings at once of pity and indignation !

For my own part, when summoned to cases of the fully developed disease (where there was no question of prevention or
suppressing its commencement), I found I had to combat two
different *states of body* that sometimes rapidly alternated with
one another, each of which was composed of a convolute of
symptoms.

The first: the burning heat, the drowsy stupefaction, the
agonising tossing about with vomiting, diarrhœa, and even convulsions, was subdued in a very short time (at most an hour)
by a very small quantity of opium, either *externally* by means

---

[1] Neither Plenciz nor I observed the jaundice symptoms that were noticed in some
of the epidemics of 1800.

of a piece of paper (according to the size of the child, from a half to a whole inch in length and breath) moistened with strong tincture of opium, laid upon the pit of the stomach and left there until it dries;[1] or if there is no vomiting, *internally*, by giving a small quantity of a solution of opium.

For external use I employed a tincture formed by adding one part of finely pulverised crude opium to twenty parts of weak alcohol, letting it stand in a cool place for a week, and shaking it occasionally to promote the solution. For internal use, I take a drop of this tincture and mix it intimately with 500 drops of diluted alcohol, and one drop of this mixture likewise with other 500 drops of diluted alcohol, shaking the whole well. Of this diluted tincture of opium (which contains in every drop one five-millionth part of a grain of opium) one drop given internally was amply sufficient in the case of a child of four years of age,[2] and two drops in that of a child of ten years, to remove the above state. It is unnecessary to repeat these doses oftener than every four or eight hours, in some cases not more than every twenty-four hours, and that sometimes only a couple of times throughout the whole fever, for which the more frequent or more rare occurrence of these symptoms must be our guide.

Where also, during the further progress of the disease, the same symptoms appeared accompanied by constipation of the bowels, opium so applied externally, or given internally in such doses,[3] never failed to produce the desired effect. The result, by no means of a transient character, appeared at most in an hour, sometimes within a quarter of an hour, and just as rapidly from the external application as from the internal administration.

Larger doses than the above, occasion raving, hiccough, unappeasable peevishness, weeping, &c.—an array of factitious symptoms which, when they are not severe, disappear spontaneously

---

[1] For infants and other children who will not lie still long enough, we should hold the paper on with the point of the finger until it is dry, (which requires about a minute) and then we should throw away the paper, in case they swallow it.

[2] For younger children I mixed one drop of this with ten teaspoonfuls of water and gave them, according to their age, one, two, or more spoonfuls.

[3] The smallness of the dose in which the medicine that acts upon the whole system of the living organism, when it is suitable to the case, produces its desired effect, is incredible, at least it is incredible to my colleagues, who think it requisite to give to infants at the breast opium in half-grain doses, and who are ready enough to attribute the sudden death by poisoning that often ensues to a multitude of other causes. The drops for internal use must be intimately mixed with from one to four tablespoonfuls of fluid (water or beer) just before they are administered.

in a few hours, or may be more speedily removed by smelling at a solution of camphor.

The second morbid condition that occurs in the course of this disease: the increase of fever towards evening, the sleeplessness, the total loss of appetite, the nausea, the intolerable lacrymose peevishness, the groaning, that is, the state where opium does and must do harm,—this state was removed in a few quarters of an hour by ipecacuanha.

For this end, immediately on the occurrence of this state, or during its persistence, I gave, according to the age of the child, ipecacuanha, either in substance in the dose of a tenth to half a grain in fine powder; or I employed the tincture prepared by digesting in the cold for some days one part of the powder with twenty parts of alcohol, of this one drop was mixed with a hundred drops of weak alcohol, and to the youngest children a drop of this last was given, but to the oldest ones ten drops were given for a dose.

I found these two remedies as indispensable as they were generally *completely sufficient*[1] not only to ward off the fatal termination, but also to shorten, diminish and alleviate the scarlet-fever. I cannot imagine a more suitable mode of treatment, so rapid and certain in its results I found it.

As regards moral and physical accessory dietetic means in the treatment of a fully developed case of scarlet-fever, I would advise that we should try to *dispel all fear* by means of kind and cheering words, by nice little presents, by holding out hopes of a speedy recovery—and on the other hand, we should allow the patient *a free choice of all kinds of drinks*, and warmer or cooler *coverings* to suit his feelings. The patient's own feelings are a much surer guide than all the maxims of the schools. We must only take care kindly to keep the patient from taking solid nutriment too soon, or in too great quantity during his convalesence.

PROTECTION AGAINST SCARLET-FEVER.

I. *Prophylaxis.*

But even under the most appropriate and certain medical treatment of developed scarlatina of a bad type there is always

---

[1] Even in the very worst cases I never employed either gargles, or fomentations, or vesicatories, or sinapisms, or clysters, or venesections, or leeches. When the urgent febrile symptoms in their whole connexion were fully met, the result which is (*vainly*) sought to be obtained by each of these appliances occurred spontaneously The illusory and meddling, pedantic *opus operatum* should, in this enlightened century, never constitute the *chief business* of the earnest practitioner.

risk of death, of the most miserable death, and the amount of
the countless sufferings of the patients is not unfrequently so
great that a philanthropist must wish that a means could be discovered by which those in health might be protected from this
murderous children's pestilence, and be rendered secure from it,
more especially as the virus is so extremely communicable that
it inevitably penetrates to the most carefully guarded children
of the great ones of the earth. Who can deny that the perfect
prevention of infection from this devastating scourge, and the discovery of a means whereby this divine aim may be surely attained, would offer infinite advantages over any mode of treatment, be it of the most incomparable kind soever?

The remedy capable of maintaining the healthy uninfectable by the
miasm of scarlatina, I was so fortunate as to discover. *I found*
also that the same remedy given at the period when the symptoms in-
dicative of the invasion of the disease occurs, stifles the fever in its
very birth; and, moreover, is more efficacious than other known
medicaments in removing the greater part of the *after-sufferings*
following scarlatina that has run its natural course, which are
often worse than the disease itself.

I shall now relate the mode in which I made the discovery of
this specific preservative remedy.

The mother of a large family, at the commencement of July,
1799, when the scarlet-fever was most prevalent and fatal, had
got a new counterpane made up by a semptress, who (without
the knowledge of the former) had in her small chamber a boy
just recovering of scarlet-fever. The first mentioned woman on
receiving it, examined it and smelt it in order to ascertain
whether it might not have a bad smell that would render it
necessary to hang it in the open air, but as she could detect
nothing of the sort, she laid it beside her on the pillow of the
sofa, on which some hours later she lay down for her afternoon's
nap.—She had unconsciously, in this way only (for the family
had no other near or remote connexion with scarlatina patients),
imbibed this miasm.—A week subsequently she suddenly fell
ill of a bad quinsy, with the characteristic shooting pains in
the throat, which could only be subdued after four days of
threatening symptoms.

Several days thereafter, her daughter, ten years of age, infected most probably by the morbific exhalations of the mother
or by the emanations from the counterpane, was attacked in the
evening by severe pressive pain in the abdomen, with biting itch-

ing on the body and head, and rigour over the head and arms, and with paralytic stiffness of the joints. She slept very restlessly during the night, with frightful dreams and perspiration all over the body, excepting the head. I found her in the morning with pressive headache, dimness of vision, slimy tongue, some ptyalism, the submaxillary glands hard, swollen, painful to the touch, shooting pains in the throat on swallowing and at other times. She had not the slightest thirst, her pulse was quick and small, breathing hurried and anxious; though she was very pale, she felt hot to the touch, yet complained of horripilation over the face and hairy scalp; she sat leaning somewhat forwards in order to avoid the shooting in the abdomen which she felt most acutely when stretching or bending back the body; she complained of a paralytic stiffness of the limbs with an air of the most dejected pusillanimity, and shunned all conversation; "she felt," she said, "as if she could only speak in a whisper." Her look was dull and yet staring, the eyelids inordinately wide open, the face pale, features sunk.

Now I knew only too well that the ordinary favourite remedies, as in many other cases, so also in scarlatina, in the most favourable cases leave everything unchanged, and therefore I resolved in this case of scarlet-fever just in the act of breaking out, not to act as usual in reference to individual symptoms, but if possible (in accordance with my new synthetical principle) to obtain a remedy whose peculiar mode of action was calculated to produce in the healthy body most of the morbid symptoms which I observed *combined* in this disease. My memory and my written collection of the peculiar effects of some medicines, furnished me with no remedy so capable of producing a counterpart of the symptoms here present, as *belladonna*.

It alone could fulfil most of the indications of this disease, seeing that in its primary action it has, according to my observations, a tendency to excite even in healthy persons great dejected pusillanimity, dull staring (stupid) look, with inordinately opened eyelids, obscuration of vision, coldness and paleness of the face, want of thirst, excessively small, rapid pulse, paralytic immobility of the limbs, obstructed swallowing, with shooting pains in the parotid gland, pressive headache, constrictive pains in the abdomen, which become intolerable in any other posture of the body besides bending forwards, rigour and heat of certain parts to the exclusion of others, *e. g.*, of the head alone, of the arms alone, &c. If, thought I, this was a case of approaching scarlet-fever, as I considered was most probable, the subsequent effects peculiar to this plant—its power to produce synochus, with erysipelatous spots on the skin, sopor, swollen, hot face, &c.—could not fail to be extremely appropriate to the symptoms of fully developed scarlatina.

I therefore gave this girl of ten years of age, who was already affected by the first symptoms of scarlet-fever, a dose of this medicine, ($^1\backslash_{432,000}$th part of a grain of the extract, which, according to my subsequent experience, is rather too large a dose.)[1] She remained quietly seated all day, without lying down; the heat of her body became but little observable; she drank but little; none of her other symptoms increased that day and no new ones occurred. She slept pretty quietly during the night, and the following morning, twenty hours after taking the medicine, most of the symptoms had disappeared without any crisis, the sore throat alone persisted, but with diminished severity, until evening, when it too went off. The following day she was lively, ate and played again, and complained of nothing. I now gave her another dose, and she remained well, perfectly well—whilst two other children of the family fell ill of bad scarlet-fever without my knowledge, whom I could only treat according to my general plan detailed above; I gave my convalescent a smaller dose of belladonna every three or four days, and she remained in perfect health.

I now earnestly desired to be able if possible to preserve the other five children of the family perfectly free from infection. Their removal was impossible and would have been too late.

I reasoned thus: a remedy that is capable of quickly checking a disease in its onset, must be its best preventive; and the following occurrence strengthened me in the correctness of this conclusion. Some weeks previously, three children of another family lay ill of a very bad scarlet-fever; the eldest daughter alone, who, up to that period, had been taking belladonna internally for an external affection on the joints of her fingers, to my great astonishment did not catch the fever, although during the prevalence of other epidemics she had always been the first to take them.

---

[1] At least, if given for a preventive object, too large a dose for a child of this age, but probably exactly appropriate for the so far advanced symptoms of scarlet-fever, but this I do not know for certain. I cannot therefore advise an exact imitation of this case, but yet neither can I advise that it should not be copied, for the scarlet-fever is a much more serious evil than a few troublesome symptoms produced by a somewhat too large dose of belladonna.

This circumstance completely confirmed my idea.   I now hesitated not to administer to the other five children of this numerous family this divine remedy, as a preservative, in very small doses, and, as the peculiar action of this plant does not last above three days, I repeated the dose every 72 hours, and they all remained perfectly well without the slightest symptoms throughout the whole course of the epidemic, and amid the most virulent scarlatina emanations from their sisters who lay ill with the disease.

In the mean time I was called in to attend in another family, where the eldest son was ill of scarlet-fever. I found him in the height of the fever, and with the eruption on the chest and arms.   He was seriously ill, and the time was consequently past to give him the specific prophylactic remedy.   But I wished to keep the other three children free from this malignant disease: one of them was nine months, another two years, and the third four years of age. The parents did what I ordered, gave each of the children the requisite quantity of belladonna every three days, and had the happiness to preserve these three children free from the pestilential disease, free from all its symptoms, although they had unrestricted intercourse with their sick brother.

And a number of other opportunities presented themselves to me where this specific preventive remedy never failed.

In order to prepare this remedy for preventing the infection of scarlet-fever, we take a handful of the fresh leaves of the *wild*[1] *belladonna* (*atropa belladonna*, Linn.) at the season when the flowers are not yet blown ; these we bruise in a mortar to a pap, and press the juice through linen, and immediately (without any previous purification) spread it out scarcely as thick as the back of a knife, on flat porcelain plates, and expose it to a draught of dry air, where it will be evaporated in the course of a few hours. We stir it about and spread it again with the spatula, so that it may harden in a uniform manner until it becomes so dry that it may be pulverized.   The powder is to be kept in a well stopped and warmed bottle.

If we now wish to prepare from this the prophylactic remedy, we dissolve a grain of this powder (prepared from well preserved belladonna extract evaporated at an ordinary temperature) in

---

[1] For my experiments I have only employed the wild belladonna gathered in its natural habitat, but I doubt not that the cultivated sort will display the same powers, f it be grown in a situation very analogous as to soil and position to the natural one : vide *Hahnemann's Apotheker Lexicon.*   Art. *Belladonna-schlaf-beere.*

one hundred drops of common distilled water, by rubbing it up in a small mortar; we pour the thick solution into a one-ounce bottle, and rinse the mortar and the pestle with three hundred drops of diluted alcohol (five parts of water to one of spirit), and we then add this to the solution, and render the union perfect, by diligently shaking the liquid. We label the bottle *strong solution of belladonna.* One drop of this is intimately mixed with three hundred drops of diluted alcohol by shaking it for a minute, and this is marked *medium solution of belladonna.* Of this second mixture one drop is mixed with two hundred drops of the diluted alcohol, by shaking for a minute, and marked *weak solution of belladonna;* and this is our prophylactic remedy for scarlet-fever, each drop of which contains the twenty-four millionth part of a grain of the dry belladonna juice.

Of this weak solution of belladonna we give to those not affected with scarlet-fever, with the intention *to make them uninfectable by the disease,*—to a child one year old, two drops (to a younger child one drop), to one two years old, three—to one three years old, four—to a child four years old (according to the strength of his constitution), from five to six,—to a five years old child, from six to seven,—to a six years old child, from seven to eight,—to a seven years old child, from nine to ten,—to an eight years old child, from eleven to thirteen,—to a nine years old child, from fourteen to sixteen drops; and with each successive year up to the twentieth, two drops more (from the twentieth to the thirtieth, not above forty drops)—*a dose every seventy-two hours* (well stirred for a minute with a teaspoon in any kind of drink) as long as the epidemic lasts, and four (to five) weeks thereafter.[1]

Should the epidemic be very violent, it would be safer, if the children could bear it, to let the second dose be taken twenty-four hours after the first, the third dose thirty-six hours after the second, the fourth forty-eight hours after the third, and thereafter to let the subsequent doses be taken every seventy-two hours until the end, in order that the system may not at first be taken by surprise by the miasm.

This course of medicine does not disturb the health of the children. They may and indeed ought to follow the mode of life of healthy individuals, and keep to their usual drinks, food,

---

[1] It seems to me somewhat probable that a similar employment of belladonna would also preserve from *measles.*

and ordinary recreation and exercise in the open air, but they must take care to avoid excess in any of these things.

The only thing I must prohibit is the use of too much vegetable acid, of sour fruits, of vinegar, &c. The action of belladonna is thereby enormously increased, as my experience (contrary to the assertions of ancient writers) has taught me.

In case of the occurrence of such a case of the injurious and too violent action of belladonna (from this or any other cause), we should make use of its peculiar (according to my observations specific) antidote, opium, externally or internally, in doses similar to those I have above indicated, for the external or internal treatment of natural scarlatina.

There are, however, cases in which we are forced to give the above doses of belladonna oftener than every seventy-two hours. A delicate girl, three years of age, who was successfully using the belladonna as a preservative, in the above dose, beside her sister who had scarlet-fever, bruised her hand severely one day with the door of the room, and thereby fell into a mental and bodily condition so favourable to the reception of the infection, that, notwithstanding that she had taken the prophylactic the day before, she presented in a few hours all the signs of approaching scarlet-fever; but two drops of the weak solution of belladonna given immediately removed these symptoms just as quickly, without any further effects. From that time forward she took the medicine only every three days (as previously), and she remained quite free from the scarlet-fever and well.

We would therefore do well in the event of such sudden accession of *violent mental depressions*, occasionally, when requisite, to give one or two extra doses. We will also sometimes meet with children who possess naturally such timorous, tranquil dispositions, that in them the dose above indicated for children of their age will not suffice to protect them from scarlet-fever; the physician may therefore be allowed to increase it somewhat, and to stir the drops up with somewhat more fluid, and for a minute longer. I may observe, that it is scarcely credible how much this and every other medicine loses in power (so as even to be unserviceable for protecting from scarlet-fever), if we allow it to be licked simply and unmixed with anything from a spoon, or give it only on sugar, or, though dropping it into a fluid, administer it without stirring it well up with it. It is only by stirring, by *brisk*, long-continued stirring, that a liquid medicine obtains the largest number of points of contact for the living fibre, thereby alone does it become right powerful. But the well stirred dose should not be allowed to stand for several hours before it is administered. Water, beer, milk, and all such excipient fluids, when allowed to stand, undergo some decomposition, and thereby weaken the vegetable medicinal agent mixed with them, or even destroy it completely.

I would, moreover, advise that the medicine bottle should be locked up after every time of using it. I once saw a little girl of four years old fill up a medicine bottle with brandy, whence, as she confessed to me, she had previously drunk out all the medicine, which was also made with spirit and colourless. She had mounted on the table, had taken the bottle down from a high cupboard in the wall, and was about to fill it up with what she supposed to be a similar fluid, in order that her parents might not discover what she had done, when I entered the room.

II. *Suppression of the Scarlet-fever in its first germs.*

Although a practitioner will seldom be so fortunate as to accomplish this extinction of the fever in question in its birth by means of belladonna, because it is not usual to send for him at the very beginning when the miasm attempts its first partial onslaught, and when uneasy dreams, paralytic stiffness of the limbs, pressive headache, rigour over one or other limb and over the head, constitute almost the only symptoms of the still feeble reaction of the system, yet it is a real fact, and, according to my by no means small experience, beyond all doubt, that it is capable of extinguishing the approaching fever with all its concomitant symptoms in the course of from twenty-four to forty-eight hours, and of restoring the previous state of health without the slightest bad consequences. To accomplish this object I found it best in this case to administer the half of the dose recommended above as a preventative every three hours, until all the symptoms had disappeared, and then to continue giving a full dose only every seventy-two hours in order to protect the patient from all further infection.

I have, indeed, even in cases where there was already shooting pain and swelling of the cervical glands and increased heat of skin,[1] that is, when a more considerable degree of natural reaction against the miasm was present, always succeeded in attaining my object by similar doses given at similar intervals

---

[1] But without increased redness.

of time, but I cannot recommend this practice to any practioner who is not a most accurate observer, because should he chance to overlook symptoms of a more advanced stage that may be present, it must always remain a doubtful matter, whether, in such a case, by the addition of a new and powerful agent, the advanced disease would be suppressed and extinguished, or a tumultuous commotion be excited in the diseased system without any good result.

But least of all is it probable that our object would be attained by giving belladonna, and it *is certainly not advisable to attempt it*, if there are present greater heat, redness of face, great thirst, inability to leave the bed, vomiting and cinnabar-coloured eruption, in other words, fully developed scarlatina. It does not seem suited for administration in the height of the fever, just as Peruvian bark cannot be given in the middle of the hot stage of a paroxysm of intermittent fever with advantage or without producing a bad effect on the system.

AFTER-SUFFERINGS.

On the other hand, belladonna displays a valuable and specific power in removing the after-sufferings remaining from scarlet-fever—an object that our forefathers, as we know, vainly strove to attain. *Most medical men have hitherto regarded the consequences of scarlatina as at least as dangerous as the fever itself, and there have been many epidemics, where more died of the after-affections than of the fever.*

The puffiness of the face, the swelling of the hands and feet, &c., the cachexy, the slow evening fever with shuddering, the stiffness of the limbs, the sense of constriction of the abdomen on holding the body erect, the formication and sleeping (*narcosis*) in the spine, the inflammation of the glands, the suppuration inside the ears, the ulcers on the face, on the lining membrane of the nose, at the angles of the mouth, &c., the extraordinary debility of the whole body, the sleepy, dull disposition, alternating with excessive hurry in talking and acting, the calling out in sleep, the pressive headaches, &c., will be specifically and rapidly removed by the same doses of this remedy as suffice (*v. supra*) for prophylactic purposes, or accordingly as the practitioner judges expedient by smaller or larger doses of it. Sometimes all that is required is to give the doses somewhat more frequently.

It is only in some particular cases, where the original disease was very violent, and advice has been sought for the after-sufferings too late, that I have witnessed what is termed the unhealthy skin, that is, the tendency to a solution of continuity in the solid parts, to ulceration, sometimes to such a degree, that belladonna is no longer of service. In such and other similar cases the most excellent remedy was the inspissated juice of the *matricaria chamomilla*, dried at a natural temperature in the air —of this a grain was first of all dissolved in 500 drops of water and mixed intimately with 500 drops of alcohol, and of this solution one drop was mixed with 800 drops of diluted alcohol—of this last diluted solution one drop ($\frac{1}{800000}$th of a grain of the inspissated juice) was given every day to a child of a few years old, two drops to one of ten years of age, and so forth; the medicine being well mixed with any liquid, and in a few days all tendency to ulceration of the skin was removed, the so-called unhealthy skin was cured—a disease in every case much dreaded by every medical man who does not know of this excellent but very heroic remedy.

The suffocating cough that sometimes follows the disease is also removed by chamomilla, especially if there is at the same time a tendency to flushing of the face, accompanied by horipilation over the limbs or back.

ON THE
POWER OF SMALL DOSES OF MEDICINE IN GENERAL,
AND
OF BELLADONNA IN PARTICULAR.[1]

You ask me urgently, *what effect can* $\frac{1}{100,000}$*th part of a grain of belladonna have?* The word *can* is repugnant to me, and apt to lead to misconceptions. Our compendiums have already decided what medicines and certain doses of them *can* do, and have told us exactly what we are to use; they have determined these matters so decidedly that we might consider them to be symbolic books, if medical dogmas were to be believed as articles of faith. But, thank God, they are not yet; it is well known that our materia medicas owe their origin to anything but pure experience, that they are often the inanities of our great-grandfathers, uninquiringly repeated by their great-grandsons. Let us not, then, interrogate the compendiums, let us ask nature:

---

[1] From *Hufeland's Journal.* Vol. vi. Pt. 2. 1801.

what effect has $^1\backslash_{\text{100,000}}th$ *of a grain of belladonna?* But even in this shape the question is too wide, and it can only become more definite and answerable by stating the *ubi, quomodo, quando, quibus auxiliis.*

A very hard dry pill of extract of belladonna produces in a robust, *perfectly healthy* countryman or labourer usually *no effect.* But from this it by no means follows that a grain of this extract would be a proper, or too weak a dose for this or a similar stout man *if he was ill, or if the grain were given in solution,*—certainly not! On this point let the pseudo-empiricism of the compendiums hold its tongue; let us hear what experience says. The most healthy robust thresher will be affected with the most violent and dangerous symptoms from one grain of extract of belladonna, if this grain be dissolved thoroughly in much (*e. g.* two pounds of) water by rubbing, the mixture (a little alcohol being added, for all vegetable solutions are rapidly decomposed[1]) made *very intimate* by shaking the fluid in a bottle for five minutes, and if he be made to take it by spoonfuls within six or eight hours. These two pounds will contain about 10,000 drops. Now if one of these drops be mixed with other 2000 drops (six oz.) of water (mixed with a little alcohol), by being vigorously shaken, one tea-spoonful (about twenty drops) of this mixture given every two hours, will produce not much less violent symptoms in a strong man, *if he is ill.* Such a dose contains about the millionth part of a grain. A few tea-spoonsful of this mixture, will, I assert, bring him to the brink of the grave, if he was previously regularly ill, and if his disease was of such a description as belladonna is suitable for.

The hard grain-pill finds few points of contact in the healthy body; it slides almost completely undissolved over the surface of the intestinal canal invested with a layer of mucus, until it (in this manner itself covered with mucus), completely buried in excrement, is speedily expelled in the natural manner.

Very different is it with a solution, and particularly with a thorough solution. Let this be as weak as it may, in its passage

---

[1] Plain water even is liable to constant fermentation, especially when vegetable substances are mingled with it, and these lose their medicinal power in a few hours. Without the addition of a little spirit we cannot preserve them half a day in their integrity. Exposed vegetable juices go on to fermentation a minute after their exposure. We might drink a large quantity of hemlock juice without injury if it has stood for twenty-four hours in a moderate temperature; it then is changed into a kind of vinegar. To some vegetable juices I have had to add one-third, to others as much as equal parts of spirits of wine, in order to prevent their fermentation.

through the stomach it comes in contact with many more points of the living fibre, and as the medicine does not act atomically but only dynamically, it excites much more severe symptoms than the compact pill, containing a million times more medicine (that rests inactive), is capable of doing.

But how is it, I am asked, that excepting yourself no other physician has ever observed that remarkable action from belladonna (and other medicines) in so small a dose? The answer is not difficult. In the first place, because many may only have experimented with watery solutions, whose medicinal power, as above stated, is gone in a few hours, destroyed by the internal fermentation of the water; secondly, because many physicians, ignorant of the purely dynamical action of medicines, are prevented from instituting any experiments of this nature by their invincible prejudiced incredulity; thirdly, because no physician designs to observe and to study the positive and absolute effects of medicines, most of them being content to learn by rote the traditions in the works on materia medica, in other words, the general, often imaginary, use of the medicines—"*belladonna is of use* (and is of no use) *in hydrophobia* "—" *is of use* (and is of no use) *in cancer of the face*," &c. " We don't need to know any thing more." What organs it deranges functionally, what it modifies in other ways, what nerves it principally benumbs or excites, what alterations it effects in the circulation and digestive operations, how it affects the mind, how the disposition, what influence it exerts over some secretions, what modification the muscular fibre receives from it, how long its action lasts, and by what means it is rendered powerless; all this the ordinary physician wishes not to know, and therefore—he does not know it. Such being his ignorance, he often regards the peculiar effects of small doses of belladonna as natural morbid changes, and thus he will never know what small doses, not to speak of the very smallest doses, of belladonna do, since he does not know what effects belladonna produces, nor does he desire to know them.

To the ordinary practitioner it is incredible that a given person, when sick, needs only to take a millionth part of the same drug that he swallowed when well without it having any particular effect, in order to be violently acted on; and yet this is undeniably the case. It is a fact, that in disease the preservative power, together with all the subordinate, nameless forces (some of them almost resemble the instinct of animals), is much more excitable than in health, when the reason and the power of the animal machine being in their complete integrity stand in no need of such anxious guardians. How well the patient distinguishes betwixt drinks that will do him good, and such as would be prejudicial to him! An individual affected with an acute fever, smells from afar the approach of an animal soup, to which his now wakeful, still unknown life-preserving faculty evinces the greatest repugnance. He would vomit violently were we to bring it too near him.

If lemon-juice is good for him—see! at the very mention of it, his countenance expresses pleasure and desire, and yet when he was well how indifferent were they both to him!

In a word, all the powers, whose very names we are ignorant of, which have reference to the preservation of life and the avoidance of destruction, are infinitely more excited in disease. What an enormous quantity of freshly made soup it would take to excite a healthy stomach to violent vomiting! But look, the patient ill of an acute fever does not require a drop for this purpose; the mere smell of it, perhaps the millionth part of a drop, coming in contact with the mucous membrane of the nose, suffices to produce this result.

Will medical men ever learn, how small, how infinitely small, the doses of medicines may be in order to affect the system powerfully when it is in a morbid state? Yes, they affect it powerfully when they are chosen *improperly ;* new violent symptoms are added, and it is usual to say (whether correctly or not, this is not the place to decide), the disease has undergone an aggravation. They affect it equally powerfully when they are *suitably* selected; the most serious disease often yields in a few hours. The nearer the disease approaches the acute character, the smaller are the doses of medicines) I mean of the best selected one) it requires in order to disappear. Chronic diseases also combined with debility and general derangement of the health, do not require larger ones. It is only in cases where along with a local affection, the general health seems to be good that we must proceed from the at first small doses to larger ones, to the very largest however in those cases where the medicine only can act in a palliative manner.

Those who are satisfied with these general hints, will believe me when I assert, that I have removed various paralytic affections by employing for some weeks a quantity of diluted solution of belladonna, where for the whole treatment not quite a hundred-thousandth part of a grain of the extract of belladonna was required, and that I have cured some periodical nervous diseases, tendency to boils, &c., by not quite a millionth of a grain, for the whole treatment.

If the appropriate medicine in solution is efficacicus in such a small dose, as it assuredly is—how highly important on the other hand is it, that in the event of the remedy being improperly selected, such a small dose can seldom excite such serious symptoms (ordinarily termed aggravations of the disease) as that they shall not soon disappear spontaneously, or be readily removed by some trifling antidote.

THOUGHTS SUGGESTED BY THE RECOMMENDATION OF A REMEDY FOR THE EFFECTS OF THE BITE OF MAD DOGS.[']

SINCE the most remote times a number of remedies have been recommended as preventives of this horrible disease, accompanied by numerous certificates to attest their efficacy for several generations. The arcanum generously purchased some years ago by the Prussian government, which received the sanction of a medical commission and was at last authoritively disclosed—I mean the worthless electuary of the *meloë majalis* may serve as a specimen of all the rest.

All were at length found to be valueless, one was worth just as much as another, that is to say, worth nothing! What a fearful condition to find one's self at a moment of such imminent danger to life, left in the lurch by a remedy publicly and universally vaunted as infallible! The drowning man clutches at the rope thrown to him—the only one at hand—it breaks, and see, he sinks to rise no more!

But how is it that men have been so universally, so completely deceived in all these nostrums for rabies?

Had the real cause of the deception in all these cases been known, the πρῶτον ψευδος—assuredly not the slightest attention would have been paid even at their first announcement to any of these nostrums, which have now been proved to be powerless —we should, on the other hand, have long since discovered a true remedy for the disease.

The source of the delusion that contributed to the celebrity of all the nostrums hitherto advised, was the circumstance that is was deemed sufficient to bring forward proofs *that the remedy in question preserved from hydrophobia so many persons who had been bitten by supposed mad dogs.*

But of ten dogs that have bitten persons and animals, and which, from dread of injury, people are more disposed to consider mad than not, frequently not two are really rabid. But it is very rare that any one takes the trouble to obtain a regular verification of the fact of their being really rabid, they are pursued, slaughtered, and all the ten are held to be mad. Whether the dog really had the disease, remains in most instances undecided and improbable.

Now out of a hundred persons bitten, who can prove that a single one among them was wounded by a really rabid dog?

And on the other hand, it is well known *that of persons bitten, nay, lacerated by dogs really mad, it is very far from the case that all will be affected by hydrophobia.* Instances are known of twenty persons having been bitten by a rabid dog, of whom only one or two were seized with the disease, whilst the eighteen or nineteen used no medical or surgical preventive and yet retained their health. (Had the nostrum been given to these latter eighteen or nineteen, many would have sworn that the remedy had destroyed the virus and preserved them from the disease.)

Both these circumstances—the frequency with which dogs are considered and killed as mad (*i. e.*, the rarity of really mad dogs,) and the rarity of the inoculation of the really rabid saliva, have furnished the material for the thousand empty testimonials as to the prophylactic power of those vaunted nostrums. We should now, however, once for all cease to pin our faith on such remedies, for which a mere (delusive) *prophylactic power* is alleged; we should once for all cease to grasp at shadows in an affair of such importance, and fraught with so much danger to mankind!

If the vapour of nitric acid, in a state of ebullition, were not at the same time one of the most trustworthy *remedies* for the jail-fever, Smith would have exerted himself in vain to assert its *prophylactic power for the contagion* of this typhoid fever.

In like manner there cannot be any *prophylactic* of hydrophobia, that does not prove itself to be at the same time a really efficacious *remedy for the fully developed hydrophobia.*

Let us begin at this as our starting point. Let a remedy be

discovered that has already cured at least ten persons, really affected with hydrophobia, without exception and permanently; this will, this must be, likewise the best prophylactic; but any substance that cannot stand this test, can never, in the eyes of reason and experience, be considered as a trustworthy prophylactic. Let the best extinguisher of burning wooden buildings be discovered (be it vitriol or potash) and this will also be the best preservative of wood from fire.

If the remedy of the schoolmaster of Schöneiche, announced by the philanthropic Wiesand of Pretzch, had only made a commencement such as I have indicated, and had only cured *two* persons really affected with hydrophobia, his secret would be worth a considerable reward, and had it cured a number without ever failing, his reward should be very large and his memory should always be held in honour. Then we should at length possess a genuine remedy for one of the most fearful of diseases, hydrophobia.

ON THE EFFECTS OF COFFEE.
FROM ORIGINAL OBSERVATIONS.[1]

In order to enjoy a healthy and long life, man requires foods which contain nutritious, but no irritating, medicinal, parts, and drinks which are either merely diluent, or diluent and nutritious at the same time, but which contain no medicinal and irritating component parts, such as pure spring water and milk.

In the way of accessaries to stimulate the taste, the only substances that have been found to be harmless and suitable for the human body are kitchen salt, sugar and vinegar, all three in small, or at all events, moderate quantities.

All other accessaries, which we term spices, and all spirituous and fermented liquors, bear a greater or less resemblance to medicines in their nature. The nearer they resemble medicines, the more frequently and the more copiously they are taken into our bodies, the more objectionable are they, the more prejudicial to health and long life.

Most objectionable of all is the frequent use of purely medicinal substances of great power as articles of diet.

Among the ancients, wine was the only purely medicinal drink, but the wise Greeks and Romans at least never drank it without diluting it plentifully with water.

[1] Leipzic, 1803.

In modern times many more purely medicinal drinks and condiments have been added to our diet : snuffing and smoking tobacco, chewing tobacco and hemp-leaves, eating opium and agaric, drinking brandy, several kinds of stimulating and medicinal beers, tea[1] and coffee.

Medicinal things are substances that do not nourish, but alter the healthy condition of the body; any alteration, however, in the healthy state of the body constitutes a kind of abnormal, morbid condition.[2]

Coffee is a purely medicinal substance.

All medicines have, in strong doses, a noxious action on the sensations of the healthy individual. No one ever smoked tobacco for the first time in his life without disgust; no healthy person ever drank unsugared black coffee for the first time in his life with gusto — a hint given by nature to shun the first occasion for transgressing the laws of health, and not to trample so frivolously under our feet the warning instinct implanted in us for the preservation of our life.

By continuing the use of these medicinal articles of diet (whereto fashion and example seduce us), habit gradually extinguishes the noxious impressions that they at first made upon us; they even become agreeable to us, that is to say, the disagreeable impressions their ingestion at first produced do not strike us so much as we go on using them, and their apparently agreeable effects upon our organs of sensation gradually become necessary to us. The ordinary run of mankind esteems even factitious wants as happiness, and gradually associates with their satisfaction the idea of relish.

Perhaps also, inasmuch as by their use we become to a certain degree sickly, our instinct tries from time to time at least to alleviate this indisposition occasioned by the continued use of these medicinal articles of diet, by means of the palliative relief which they are capable of affording to the malady produced from time to time by themselves.

---

[1] Chocolate belongs to the nutritious articles, when it is not too highly spiced : otherwise it is objectionable, or even hurtful.

[2] In proportion as the substances we call medicines can make the healthy body sick, so are they calculated to remove the abnormal states dangerous to life, which go by the name of diseases. The sole end of medicines consequently is, to change the abnormal, the morbid state, that is, to transform it into health. Used by themselves, and when no disease is present, they are absolutely hurtful things for health and normal life. Their frequent use as articles of diet deranges the harmonious concordance of our organs, undermines health and shortens life. A wholesome medicine for a healthy individual is a contradiction of terms.

In order to understand this proposition, we must take into consideration the fact that all medicines produce in the body conditions the opposite of one another. Their *commencing action* (*primary action*) is the direct opposite of their *secondary action*, that is, of the state they leave behind in the body when their primary action has ceased some hours.[1]

Most medicines produce, both in their primary and secondary action, disturbances in the healthy body and disagreeable sensations and pains, a certain set of these in their primary action and another opposite set in their secondary action, and even their prolonged employment excites no agreeable effects in the healthy individual.

Only the few medicinal substances that the refinement of a sensual world has chosen to introduce among articles of diet,[2] form in some degree, an exception to this, at least in their primary action. They possess the peculiar property, when continued to be used in moderation, to create in their primary action a sort of artificial exaltation of the ordinary state of health, an artificial exaltation of the life and almost only agreeable sensations, whilst the disagreeable effects their secondary action tends to develop remain for some time of little importance, *as long as the individual is pretty well in health, and leads in other respects a healthy and natural mode of life.*

To this small class of medicines introduced into our dietary belongs coffee, with its partly agreeable, partly disagreeable effects, both of which, strange though it may appear, are but little known.

Its irregular, unrestricted use in ordinary life, at almost all times of the day, its employment in such various strength and quantity, its preparation under the most dissimilar conditions, its general use by persons of the most various ages and constitutions, of the most different health and habits of life, deprives the observer of all means of seeing its action aright, and makes it excessively difficult to ascertain its true action, and thence to draw pure inferences. So a disk may be covered with the clearest characters and words, but all will be unrecognizable if the disk be whirled round with great rapidity ; in that case everything runs together, even to the eyes of the most sharp-sighted.

---

[1] For instance, to-day jalap powder purges, and to-morrow and the next day there follows constipation.

[2] These are, as before said, wine, spirits, opium, tobacco, tea, coffee, &c.

It is only by accurate, prolonged, unprejudiced observation, as free as possible from all source of deception, and by carefully tracing back the phenomena to their cause, that we can obtain accurate knowledge respecting the most important of all beverages, coffee.

Its primary action is in general a more or less agreeable exaltation of the vital activity; the animal, the natural, and the vital functions (as they are called) are artificially exalted by it during the first hours, and the secondary action that ensues gradually after the lapse of several hours is the opposite—disagreeable feeling of existence, a lower degree of vitality, a kind of paralysis of the animal, natural and vital functions.[1]

When a person unaccustomed to the use of coffee drinks a moderate quantity, or one accustomed to its use drinks an immoderate[2] quantity, for the first hours the self-consciousness, the feeling of his existence, of his life, becomes more lively. He gets a circumscribed redness of the cheeks, a redness which does not become gradually lost in the surrounding parts, but which presents the appearance of a well-defined red spot. The forehead and palms of the hands become warm and moist. He feels warmer than before; he feels agreeably, yet uneasily warm. There occurs a kind of voluptuous palpitation of the heart, somewhat resembling that occurring during great joy. The veins of the hands swell. Externally also he is warmer to the feel than natural, but this warmth never comes to the length of heat, even after a large quantity of coffee (it sooner turns into general perspiration); none ever become burning hot.

Presence of mind, attention, sympathy become more active than in the healthy natural state. All external objects appear to excite a feeling of pleasure, they take on, if I may be allowed the expression, a joyous varnish, and if the quantity of coffee

---

[1] " When I awake in the morning," writes a genteel, consummate coffee-drinking lady, " I have the power of thinking, and the activity of an oyster."

[2] The expressions *moderate* and *immoderate* must only be understood in a relative and individual sense; they cannot be defined by fixed magnitude and figures of universal acceptation. Thus a certain prince, H. C. v. C., reared in luxury, who is now dead, required for an allowance, every time he drank coffee, an infusion of fourteen ounces of the roasted bean, whereas we meet with persons who are very strongly affected by a quarter of an ounce. Each person must fix his own standard according to his peculiar corporeal system. One can bear more than another. Moreover the whole series of agreeable symptoms of the primary action of coffee I have here described does not appear in every one, at all events not all at once, but only one at a time, some in one, others in another. in this one more, in that fewer

taken was very great, they assume an almost over-pleasing lustre.[1] During the first hours the coffee drinker smiles contented with himself and with all external objects, and this property it was that mainly tended to make coffee a social beverage. All the agreeable sensations communicated are speedily increased to enthusiasm (though only for a short time). All sorts of disagreeable recollections, or disagreeable natural feelings cease during this kind of blessed fever.

In the healthy natural states of the human being, left to themselves, disagreeable sensations must alternate with agreeable ones; this is the wise arrangement of our nature. During the primary action of this medicinal beverage, however, all is delight, and even those corporeal functions which in the natural state of health are accompanied by an unpleasant sensation almost bordering on pain, are now performed with extreme ease, almost with a kind of pleasure.

In the first moments or quarters of an hour after awaking, particularly when this takes place earlier than usual, every one who is not living completely in a state of rude nature, has a disagreeable feeling of not thoroughly awakened consciousness, of confusion, of laziness, and want of pliancy in the limbs; it is difficult to move quickly, reflection is a labour.

But, see, coffee removes this natural disagreeable sensation, this discomfort of the mind and body, almost instantaneously; we suddenly become completely alive.

After completing our day's labour we must, in the course of nature, become lazy; a disagreeable feeling of weight and weariness in our bodily and mental powers make us ill-humoured and cross, and compels us to give ourselves up to the requisite rest and sleep.

This crossness and laziness, this disagreeable weariness of mind and body on the approach of natural sleep, rapidly disappears on taking this medicinal beverage, and a dispersion of sleepiness, a factitious liveliness, a wakefulness in defiance of nature occurs.

If the quantity of coffee taken be immoderately great and the body very excitable and quite unused to coffee, there occurs a semilateral headache, from the upper part of the parietal bone to the base of the brain. The cerebral membranes of this side also seem to be painfully sensitive. The hands and feet become cold; on the brow and palms cold sweat appears. The disposition becomes irritable, and intolerant; no one can do anything to please him. He is anxious and trembling restless, weeps almost without cause, or smiles almost involuntarily. After a few hours, sleep comes on, out of which he occasionally starts up in affright. I have seen this rare state two or three times.

In order to live we require food, and see! nature compels us to seek it and replace what has been lost, by hunger, or gnawing uncomfortable sensation in the stomach, a tormenting longing for food, a quarrelsome crossness, chilliness, exhaustion, &c.

Not less uncomfortable is the feeling of thirst, nor is it less a wholesome provision of nature. Besides the longing desire for liquids which our body needs for its restoration, we are tormented by a dryness of the throat and mouth, a dry heat of the whole body, that to a certain extent impedes the respiration, a restlessness, &c.

We drink coffee—and see! we feel but little or nothing more of the painful sensations of hunger, nor of the anxious, longing sensation of thirst. Genuine coffee-drinkers, especially those ladies addicted to its use, who are deprived of the opportunity of recovering from the bad effects of this drink by occasional exercise in the open air, experience little or nothing more of the real sensations of hunger and thirst. In this case the body is cheated of its nutriment and drink, and the cutaneous vessels are at the same time unnaturally forced to absorb from the atmosphere as much moisture as is requisite to carry on the functions of life. Confirmed coffee-drinkers pass much more urine than the quantity of fluids they drink. The most natural demands of nature are stifled. (Thus they gradually approach—thanks be to the divine beverage! —to the condition of the blessed spirits above; a true commencement of beatification here below.)

The all-bountiful Preserver of all living beings, made the healthy man feel uncomfortable on taking exercise immediately after having satisfied his appetite with food; this uncomfortable feeling was intended to compel us to leave off our business and to rest both the body and the mind, in order that the important function of digestion might be commenced undisturbed. A lassitude of body and mind, a constriction in the region of the stomach, a kind of disagreeable pressure, a fulness and tension in the abdomen, &c., on taking exercise, remind us when we attempt to exert our energies immediately after a meal, of the rest that is now required—and if we attempt to exercise our thinking faculty, there occurs a lassitude of the mental powers, a dulness of the head, a coldness of the limbs, accompanied by warmth of the face; and the pressive sensation in the stomach, combined with a disagreeable sensation of tension in the abdomen, becomes still more intolerable, proving that exerting the mental powers at the commencement of the process of digestion, is more unnatural and more hurtful than even exertion of the body.

Coffee puts a sudden stop to this lassitude of mind and body, and removes the disagreeable sensation in the abdomen after a meal. The more refined gourmands drink it immediately after dinner—and they obtain this unnatural effect in a high degree. They become gay, and feel as light as though they had taken little or nothing into their stomach.

The wise Regulator of our nature has also sought to compel us by disagreeable sensations to evacuate the accumulated excrement. There occurs an intolerable anxiety conjoined with a no less disagreeable feeling of straining, whereby all the agreeable sensations of life are put a stop to, and, as it were, swallowed up in it, until the evacuation is commenced. It is a necessary part of our nature that there should be some effort in the expulsion of the excrements.

But this has been provided against by the refining spirit of our age, which has sought to elude this law of nature likewise. In order artificially to promote and hasten the time required for digestion, which in the order of things is several hours, and to escape the anxious, frequently slowly increasing call to stool, the degenerate mortals of our times, who strain after enjoyment and have a childish dread of all uncomfortable sensations, find their means of escape in coffee.

Our intestines excited by coffee (in its primary action) to more rapid peristaltic movements, force their contents but half digested more quickly towards the anus, and the gourmand imagines he has discovered a splendid digestive agent. But the liquid chyme which serves to nourish the body, can in this short time neither be properly altered (digested) in the stomach, nor sufficiently taken up by the absorbents in the intestinal canal; hence the mass passes through the unnaturally active bowels, without parting with more than the half of its nutritious particles for the supply of the body, and arrives at the excretory orifice still in a half-liquid state. Of a truth a most excellent digestive agent, far surpassing nature!

Moreover, during the evacuation itself the anus is excited by the primary action of the coffee to more rapid dilatation and contraction, and the fæces pass out soft, almost without effort, and more frequently than in the case of healthy individuals who do not partake of coffee.

These and other natural pains and disagreeable sensations, which are a part of the wise ordering of our nature, are diminished and rendered almost unnoticeable by the primary action of coffee—and the disastrous effects of this are not perceived, or even dreamt of.

Even the sexual desire, which in our age has been exalted into the chief of all pleasures, is excited by the primary action of coffee more than by any other artificial means. As quick as lightning there arise voluptuous images in the mind from very moderate exciting cause, and the excitation of the genitals to complete ecstacy become the work of a few seconds; the ejaculation of the semen is almost irrestrainable. The sexual desire is excited by coffee from ten to fifteen years too soon, in the tenderest, immaturest age in both sexes; a refinement[1] that has the most perceptible influence on our morality and mortality—not to speak of the earlier impotence that follows as a natural consequence therefrom.[2]

In an individual of very irritable temperament, or who has already been enervated by the copious use of coffee and a sedentary life, the effects I have mentioned appear in a still more prominent light. Every unprejudiced person must perceive in the corporeal derangements and sensations effected by coffee, something unnatural, an over-stimulation. An excessive sensitiveness, or a gaiety greatly disproportioned to the object of it, a tenderness almost partaking of a convulsive character, an inordinate sorrowfulness, a wit that is not altogether under the restraints of reason, an excessive distortion of the features approaching to caricature, under circumstances where a mere smile, a little joke a slight perplexity, a moderate expression of grief or sympathy, would have sufficed.

Even the muscles of the rest of the body exhibit an unnatural excessive activity—all is life, all is motion (though there may be but little cause for it) during the first hour after partaking of strong, or (to use the often inaccurate language of the world) *good* coffee. The ideas and the pictures of the fancy flow in rapid succession and in a continuous stream before the seat of the imagination and sensation in the brain—an artificially accelerated, artificially exalted life !

---

[1] Enjoyment! enjoyment! is the cry of our age,—quicker, uninterrupted enjoyment of life at whatever cost! and this object is to a certain degree attained by means of this beverage, that accelerates and squanders the vital powers.

[2] [Who, among all the medical writers of this period (1803) has thought so justly, and written so wisely, as Hahnemann? Who among his cotemporaries has promulgated so many facts which have been confirmed by modern investigations as the founder of homœopathy ?]—*Am. P.*

In the natural state we require some effort to remember clearly things long past; immediately after taking coffee the stores of memory spring, so to speak, into our mouth—and the consequence often is loquacity, hurried chattering, and letting things escape from our lips that we ought not to have spoken about.

Moderation and purpose are entirely wanting. The cold considerate earnestness of our forefathers, the firm steadfastness of will, of resolve, and of judgment, the endurance of the not rapid but powerful movements of the body, adapted to the object in view, that used to constitute the original national character of the Germans—the whole sublime original stamp of our descent disappears before this medicinal beverage, and changes into over-hasty disclosures, hurried resolves, immatured judgments, frivolity, changeableness, talkativeness, irresolution, flighty mobility of the muscles, without the production of any durable impression, and theatrical behaviour.[1]

I well know that in order to revel in the dreams of fancy, in order to compose frivolous novels, and light, playful witticisms, the German must drink coffee—the German lady requires strong coffee in order to sparkle with wit and sentiment in fashionable circles. The ballet dancer, the improvisator, the conjurer, the juggler, the sharper, and the keeper of a faro-bank, all require coffee, as likewise the fashionable musician for his giddy rapidity of execution, and the omnipresent fashionable physician, to enable him to rush through his ninety visits in a forenoon. Let us leave to these people their unnatural stimulant, together with its evil effects to their own health and the welfare of mankind!

But this much is at least certain,—the most refined sensualist, the most devoted debauchee, could have discovered on the whole surface of the globe no other dietetic medicinal substance besides coffee,[2] capable of changing our usual feelings for some hours into agreeable ones only, of producing in us for some hours, rather a jovial, even a petulant gaiety, a livelier wit, an exalted

---

[1] Who can tell what enervating dietetic practices it was by which those admirable heroic virtues of patriotism, love of children, inviolable constancy, unshakable integrity, and strict fulfilment of duties (the well-known attributes of by-gone times) have in our days almost dwindled down into paltry egotism! Likewise the single heroic virtues of the middle ages and of remote antiquity, the antagonists of those virtues, are now-a-days (by what enervating dietetic practices?) split up into petty intrigues, concealed trickeries and artifices, and distributed over myriads of individuals —compelling the uncontaminated person to exercise much caution every step he takes! Which is the more injurious, a single bomb-shell, or a million of invisible hooks, distributed every where to catch the feet of the unwary?

[2] And to a certain extent *tea* also.

imagination above what is natural to our temperament, of quick-
ening the movement of our muscles to a kind of trembling activity, of spurring on the ordinary quiet pace of our digestive and
excretory organs to double velocity, of keeping the sexual practice in an almost involuntary state of excitation, of silencing the
useful pangs of hunger and thirst, of banishing blessed sleep
from our weary limbs, and of artificially producing in them even
a kind of liveliness when the whole creation of our hemisphere
fulfils its destiny by enjoying refreshing repose in the silent lap
of night.

Thus we despotically overthrow the wise arrangement of nature, *but not without injury to ourselves!*

When the first transient effect of coffee has departed after a
few hours, there follows gradually the opposite state, *the secondary
action*. The more striking the former was, so much the more
observable and disagreeable is the latter.

All persons do not suffer equally from the abuse of a medicinal beverage such as coffee is.

Our systems are so admirably arranged *that if we live agreeably
to nature in other respects* a few errors in diet, if they be not too
great, are tolerably harmless.

Thus, for instance, the day-labourer or peasant in Germany
drinks brandy, which is so pernicious in itself, almost every
morning; but if he only take a small portion at a time, he will
often attain a pretty considerable age. His health suffers little.
The excellence of his constitution and his otherwise healthy mode
of life counteract the injurious effects of his dram almost without
letting a trace appear.

Now, if instead of brandy the day-labourer or peasant drink
a couple of cups of weak coffee, the same thing occurs. His
robust body, the vigorous exercise of his limbs, and the quantity
of fresh air he inhales every day, repel the hurtful effects of his
beverage, and his health suffers little or nothing in consequence.

But the bad effects of coffee become much more perceptible
when these favourable circumstances are not present.

Man can, no doubt, enjoy a kind of health, though his occupation confines him to the house—or even to one room—even
though he has to live a very sedentary life in the room, and his
body is delicately constituted, provided he live in other respects
conformably with his state. Under the moderate use of only
easily digestible, mild, simple, purely nutritious, almost unspiced
food and drink, along with a prudent moderation of the passions

and frequent renewal of the air in the rooms, even women, without any great exercise,[1] enjoy a kind of health which doubtless can be readily compromised by external causes, but which, if these are avoided, may still be termed a moderate degree of health. In such persons the action of all morbific substances, that is, of all medicines, is much more striking and severe than in robust individuals accustomed to labour in the open air, who are able to bear some very hurtful things without particular injury.

These weakly dwellers in rooms live in the low level of their health but half a life, if I may use the expression; all their sensations, their energy, their vital functions, are somewhat below par, and they eagerly resort to a beverage that so powerfully exalts for some hours their vital energy and their feeling of existence, unconcerned about the results and the secondary action of this palliative.

This secondary action resembles their state before partaking of the coffee, only it is somewhat stronger.

When the few hours of the above described primary action of this medicinal beverage, that representation of artificially exalted vital energy, is gone, there then gradually creeps on a yawning drowsiness and greater inactivity than in the ordinary state, the movements of the body become more difficult than formerly, all the excessive gaiety of the previous hours changes into obtuseness of the senses. If, during the first hours after drinking the coffee, the digestion and the expulsion of the excrements were hastened, now the flatus becomes painfully incarcerated in the intestines, and the expulsion of the fæces becomes more difficult and slower than in the former state. If, in the first hours, an agreeable warmth pervaded the frame, this factitious vital-spark now gradually becomes extinguished, a shivering sensation is felt, the hands and feet become cold. All external agents appear less agreeable than before. More ill-humoured than ordinarily, they are more given to peevishness. The sexual passion which was excited by the coffee in the first hours becomes all the colder and more obtuse. A kind of speedily satiated ravenous hunger takes the place of the healthy desire for nutriment, and yet eating and drinking oppress the stomach more than previously. They have greater difficulty in getting to sleep than formerly, and the sleep is heavier than it used to be before they took

---

[1] Under such circumstances prisoners also

26

coffee, and on awaking they are more sleepy, more discouraged, more melancholy than usual.

But look! all these evils are rapidly driven away by a renewed application to this hurtful palliative—a new, artificial life commences—only it has a somewhat shorter duration than the first time, and thus its repetition becomes ever more frequently necessary, or the beverage must always be made stronger in order to enable it again to excite life for a few hours.

By such means the body of the person whose occupation confines him to his room degen rates all the more. The injurious effects of the secondary action of this medicinal drink spread farther around, and strike their roots too deeply to allow of their being again effaced, if only for a few hours, by a mere repetition of the same palliative more frequently or in stronger doses.

The skin now becomes generally more sensitive to the cold, and even to the open air though not cold; the digestion becomes obstructed, the bowels become constipated for several days at a time, flatulence occasions anxiety and causes a number of painful sensations. The constipation only alternates with diarrhœa, not with a healthy state of the bowels. Sleep is obtained with difficulty, and bears more resemblance to a slumber that causes no refreshment. On awaking there are remarkable confusion of the head, half-waking dreams, slowness of recollecting himself, helplessness of the limbs, and a kind of joylessness that throws a dark shade over all God's lovely nature. The beneficent emotions of the heart, warm philanthropy, gratitude, compassion, heroism, strength and nobility of the mind, and joyousness, change into pusillanimity, indifference, insensible hardness of heart, variable humour, melancholy.

The use of coffee as a beverage is continued, and sensitiveness alternates ever more with insensibility, over-hasty resolves with irresolution, noisy quarrelsomeness with cowardly compliance, affectation of friendship with malicious envy, transient rapture with joylessness, grinning smiling with inclination to shed tears —symptoms of constant hovering betwixt excitement and depression of the mind and the body.

It would be no easy task for me to indicate all the maladies, that under the names of debility, nervous affections and chronic diseases, prevail among the coffee-drinking set, enervating humanity and causing degeneration of mind and body.

But it must not be imagined that all the evil results I have named occur to every coffee-bibber in the same degree! No, one suffers more from this, another from that symptom of the secondary action of coffee. My description includes the whole coffee-drinking race; all their maladies which arise from this source I have arranged together, as they have from time to time come under my notice.

The palliative agreeable sensation which the coffee distributes for some hours through the finest fibres, leaves behind it, as a secondary action, an extraordinary susceptibility to painful sensations, which always becomes greater and greater, the longer, the oftener, the stronger and the greater the quantity in which the coffee is drunk. Very slight things (that would make scarcely any impression on a healthy person not accustomed to the use of coffee) cause in the coffee drinking lady megrim, a frequent often intolerable toothache, which comes on, chiefly at night, with redness of the face and at length swelling of the cheek—a painful drawing and tearing in different parts of the body, on one side of the face, or at one time in one limb, at another in another.[1] The body has a special tendency to erysipelas, either in the legs (hence the frequency of old ulcers there) or (when suckling) in the mammæ, or on one half of the face. Apprehensiveness and flying heat are her daily complaints, and nervous semilateral headache her property.[2]

---

[1] This drawing tearing in the limbs caused by coffee in its secondary action and when its use is persisted in for a long time, is not in the joints, but from one joint to the other. It appears to be more in the flesh or cellular tissue than in the bones, is unattended by swelling or other abnormal appearance, and there is scarcely any tenderness on touching the part. Our nosologists know nothing about it.

[2] The megrim above alluded to, which only appears after some exciting cause, as vexation, overloading of the stomach, a chill, &c., generally very rapidly and at all times of the day, differs entirely from the so-called nervous hemicrania. The latter occurs in the morning, soon or immediately after waking, and increases gradually. The pain is almost intolerable, often of a burning character, the external coverings of the skull are also intolerably sensitive and painful on the least touch. Body and mind seem both to be insufferably sensitive. Apparently destitute of all strength, they seek a solitary and if possible dark spot, where, in order to avoid the daylight they pass the time with closed eyes in a kind of waking slumber, usually on a couch raised in the back, or in an arm chair, quite motionless. Every movement, every noise increases their pains. They avoid speaking themselves and listening to the conversation of others. Their body is colder than usual, though without rigour; the hands and feet in particular are very cold. Everything is distasteful to them, but chiefly eating and drinking, for an incessant nausea hinders them from taking anything. In bad cases the nausea amounts to vomiting of mucus, but the headache is seldom alleviated thereby. The bowels are constipated. This headache almost never goes off until evening; in very bad cases I have seen it last thirty-six hours, so that it only disappeared the following evening. In slighter cases its original producer, coffee, shortens its duration in a palliative manner, but it communicates to the system the

From moderate errors of diet and disagreeable mental emotions there occur painful affections of the chest, stomach and abdomen (known by the inaccurate name of *spasms*)—the catamenia come on with pains, are not regular, or the discharge is less copious and at length quite scanty; it is watery or slimy; leucorrhœa (generally of an acrid character) prevails almost the whole time, from one period to another, or completely supersedes the menstrual flux—coition is often painful. The earthy, yellowish or quite pale complexion, the dull eye surrounded by blue rings, the blue lips, the flaccid muscular tissue, the shrivelled breasts, are the external signs of this miserable hidden state. Sometimes the almost suppressed menses alternate with serious uterine hemorrhages. In males there occur painful hemorrhoids and nocturnal emissions of semen. In both sexes the sexual power becomes gradually extinguished. The normal exuberant energy of the embrace of a healthy couple becomes a worthless bagatelle. Impotence of both sexes and sterility, inability to suckle a child, ensue.—The monster of nature, that hollow-eyed ghost, onanism, is generally concealed behind the coffee-table (though indulgence in the perusal of meretricious novels, over-exertion of the mind, bad company and a sedentary life in close apartments, contribute their share).

As an inordinate indulgence in coffee has for its secondary effect to dispose the body greatly to all kinds of disagreeable sensations and most acute pains, it will be readily comprehended how it, more than any other hurtful substance we are acquainted with, excites a great tendency to caries of the bones. No error of diet causes the teeth to decay more easily and certainly than indulgence in coffee. Coffee alone (with the exception of grief and the abuse of mercury) destroys the teeth in the shortest space of time.[1] The confined air of a room and overloading the stomach (especially at night) contribute their share to this effect. But coffee by itself is quite capable of destroying in a short space of time this irreparable ornament of the mouth, this indispensable accessory organ for distinct speech and for the intimate mixture of the food with the digestive saliva, or at least

---

tendency to produce it after a still shorter interval. It recurs at undetermined times, every fortnight, three, four weeks, &c. It comes on without any exciting cause, quite unexpectedly; even the night previously the patient seldom feels any premonitory signs of the nervous headache that is to come on the next morning.
I have never met with it excepting among regular coffee drinkers.

[1] Observations on which I can depend have convinced me of this.

of rendering them black and yellow. The loss of the front (incisor) teeth is chiefly due to the abuse of coffee.

If I except the true spina ventosa, there occurs scarcely a single case of caries of the bones in children (if they have not been over-dosed with mercury) from any other cause than from coffee?[1] Besides these, there are in children other deep-seated flesh abscesses that take a long time of bursting and then have but a small orifice, which are often solely to be ascribed to the action of the coffee.

As a rule, coffee acts most injuriously on children; the more tender their age, the worse its effects. Although it is incapable of itself of producing true rickets, but can only accelerate them, in conjunction with their special exciting cause (food composed of unfermented vegetable substances, and the air of close, damp rooms), yet it of itself excites in little children, even when their other food is wholesome and the air in which they live good, a kind of infantile hectic, which is not much less sad in its results. Their complexion becomes pale, their muscles quite flaccid. It is only after a long time that they learn to walk a little, but then their gait is uncertain, they easily fall, and wish always to be carried. They stammer in their speech. They wish for a great variety of things, but relish nothing heartily. The drollery, happiness and liveliness that characterize the age of childhood are changed into indolent dejection; nothing gives them pleasure, nothing makes them contented; they enjoy only a sort of half lief. They are very easily startled, and timid. Diarrhœa alternates with costiveness. Viscid mucus rattles in their chest as they breathe, especially when they are asleep, which no amount of coughing can remove: they have always got a wheezing at the chest. Their teeth come with much difficulty and with convulsion fits; they are very imperfect, and fall out decayed before the period for changing them arrives. Mostly every evening, just before bed-time or after lying down in bed, they get redness and heat on one or both cheeks. They sleep very imperfectly, toss about at night, often want to drink; they then perspire, not only on the forehead, but also on the hairy scalp, particularly at the back of the head, and whine and moan in their sleep.

---

[1] These ulcerations of the bones, which lie concealed beneath elevated, hard, bluish-red swellings of the soft parts, exude an albuminous looking mucus, mixed with some cheese-like matter. It has very little smell. The pains of the affected part are very shooting in their character. The rest of the body presents a pure picture of the coffee dyscrasia.

They get through every disease with difficulty, and their recovery is very slow and imperfect.

They are frequently subject to a chronic inflammation of the eyes, not unfrequently accompanied by an eruption in the face, along with a peculiar relaxation of the upper eyelid, which prevents them raising it, even when the redness and swelling of the lids are but moderate. This kind of ophthalmia, that often lasts for several years, making them frequently lie upon the face, with constant peevishness and crying, or conceal themselves in a dark place where they remain lying or sitting in a stooping posture; this ophthalmia, I say, chiefly affects the cornea, covers it with red vessels and at last with dark spots, or there occur phlyctenulæ and little ulcers on it, that often eat deeply into the cornea and threaten blindness.

This ophthalmia and that rattling at the chest and the other ailments above described, attack even infants at the breast, who take nothing but their mother's milk, if the mother indulges in coffee and inhabits a close room. How penetrating must not the hurtful power of this medicinal beverage be, that even infants at the breast suffer from it!

After children, coffee acts, as I have said, most injuriously on the female sex, and on literary people whose occupation is sedentary, and confines them to their rooms. To these may be added workmen engaged in a sedentary trade

The bad effects of coffee are, as I have above mentioned, most effectually diminished by great activity and exercise in the open air,—but not permanently removed.

Some individuals also find out as if by instinct, a sort of antidote to coffee in the use of spirituous liquors. It is impossible to deny that they do possess some antidotal powers. These are, however, mere stimulants, without any nutritive quality; that is to say, they are likewise medicinal substances, which, when daily used as articles of diet, produce other injurious effects, and yet are unable to prevent the hurtful action of the coffee from taking effect,—what they cause are artificial ameliorations, of the vital functions, followed by morbid effects, though of a different, more complex nature.

Leaving off the use of coffee[1] is the chief remedy for these insi-

---

[1] It is by no means easy to do away with an inveterate habit of using coffee.—I first endeavour to convince my patients seriously of the urgent and indispensable necessity of di-continuing its use. Truth grounded on obvious experience seldom

dious and deeply penetrating injurious effects, and corporeal
exercise in the open air tends to promote the subsequent recovery. If however body and mind be sunk too low, there are
some medicines very useful for that state, but this is not the
proper place to enumerate them, as I am not at present writing
for medical men. When I describe the daily use of coffee as
very prejudicial, and when I shew from observations and experience of many years that it relaxes and withers the energy
of our body and mind, some may retort upon me the appellation
"medicinal beverage," which I must unhesitatingly bestow upon
coffee.

"Medicines are surely wholesome things," says the uninitated.
They are so; but only under certain indispensable conditions.
It is only when the medicine is suitable for the case that it is
wholesome. Now no medicine is suitable for health, and to
employ a medicine as a beverage in the ordinary healthy state,
is a hurtful procedure, a self-evident contradiction.

I prize the medicinal powers of coffee when it is appropriately
employed as a medicine, as much as those of any other medica-

fails to produce conviction—almost never, when it is urged from the philanthropic
heart of a physician, who, convinced himself of the goodness of his cause, is thoroughly
penetrated by the truth of his maxims. Nothing will then prevent their reception,
there is no question of any private interest on the part of the doctor ; and nothing
but pure gain on the side of the party he wishes to convince.

If we have attained this object (whether this is the case or no, he who has a knowledge of human nature can tell by the way the patient receives his advice), we may
advise that the quantity of coffee taken be reduced by a cup every three or four days,
and allow the last breakfast-cup to be continued for a week longer, until this can
either be left off at once, or it may be continued on every alternate day for another
week, according to circumstances.

If we have to do with persons on whom we can rely, the affair is managed in the
course of four weeks. But should some faint-heartedness or indecision on the part of
slaves to coffee make its accomplishment difficult, or should the weak state of the
health make its discontinuance be too severely felt, we would do well for every cup
of coffee we take away, to allow a cup of tea to be drunk, until in the course of a
week nothing but tea (a similar but lesser evil) is drunk, and this, as it has not had
time to become a habitual beverage, may be more easily diminished, until at last
nothing more of the sort is taken, but only a couple of cups of warm milk for
breakfast, in place of coffee or tea.

Whilst thus breaking off the habit, it is indispensable that the body be refreshed
and strengthened by daily walks in the open air, by amusements of an innocent
charater, and by appropriate food, if we wish that the injurious effects of the coffee
should disappear, and the individual be confirmed in his resolution to give it up.

And if all goes on well, it will not be a bad plan for the doctor, or a friend in
his stead, to assure himself from time to time of the true conversion of his patient, and if necessary, uphold his resolution when the force of example in company
seems to cause it to waver.

ment. There is nought superfluous in God's creation; every thing is created for the weal of mankind, particularly the most powerful things, to which class coffee belongs in an especial degree. But let the following facts be borne in mind.

Every single medicine develops in the healthy human body some special alterations, that are peculiar to itself exclusively. When these are known, and when the medicine is employed in cases of disease that have an almost exact similarity with the alteration that the medicine is capable of itself producing (in the healthy body), a radical cure takes place. This employment of the medicine is the *curative* one, the only one to be relied on in chronic diseases.

In speaking of this power of a medicine to alter the human body in a manner peculiar to itself, I allude to its primary or initiatory action. I have said above that the primary action of a medicine (for some hours after it has been taken) is the direct opposite of its secondary action, or the state in which it leaves the body whenever its first action is past.

Now if the primary action of a medicine be the exact opposite of the morbid condition of the body we seek to cure, its employment is *palliative*. Almost instantaneous amendment ensues,— but a few hours afterwards the malady returns and attains a greater height than it had before the employment of the remedy, the secondary action of the medicine, which resembled the original disease, aggravates the latter. A miserable method of treatment when we have to do with a chronic malady.

I shall give an example. The primary action of opium in the healthy system is to cause a stupifying snoring sleep, and its secondary action—the opposite—sleeplessness. Now if the physician will be so foolish as treat a morbid, habitual sleeplessness with opium, he acts in a palliative manner. The stupid, snoring, unrefreshing sleep speedily follows the ingestion of the opium, but its secondary action, as I have stated, is sleeplessness, an addition to his already habitual sleeplessness, which is now accordingly aggravated. Twenty-four hours afterwards the patient sleeps still less than before he took the opium; a stronger dose of the latter must now be given, the secondary action of which is a still greater sleeplessness, that is, an aggravation of the malady, which the foolish man imagined he was curing.

In like manner, coffee proves a bad palliative remedy when it is used as a medicinal agent, for example, in cases of habitual constipation proceeding from inactivity of the bowels[1]—as is often done by medical men. Its primary action is, as I have before stated, the reverse of this state,—it therefore acts here as a palliative, and if it be used for the first time, or only on rare occasions, it speedily produces a motion of the bowels, but the following days, under the secondary action, the constipation becomes all the greater. If we again seek to remove this in the same palliative manner by means of coffee, more of it must be drunk, or it must be made stronger, and still the habitual constipation is not thereby eradicated, for it always returns more obstinately on the recurrence of the secondary action of the coffee, whenever this palliative administration of the coffee is discontinued, or stronger and more frequent potations of it are not taken, which always aggravate the disease and entail other maladies.

It will be found that the medical excuses offered by coffee-drinkers in justification of this habit almost all rest on some such palliative relief it affords them, and yet nothing is more certain than the experience that a long-continued palliative employment of a drug is injurious, but the palliative employment of drugs as articles of diet is the most injurious of all.

Therefore when I, whilst deprecating its abuse as an everyday beverage, commend the great medicinal virtues of coffee, I do the latter merely in reference to its *curative* employment for chronic ailments that bear a great resemblance to its primary action,[2] and in reference to its *palliative* employment in acute diseases threatening rapid danger, which bear a great resemblance to the secondary effects of coffee.[3] This is the only rational and wise mode of employing this medicinal beverage which is abused by hundreds of millions of individuals to their

---

[1] As is usually the case with those who lead a sedentary life in their room.

[2] For example when, in a person unaccustomed to the use of coffee, there is present (it may be a habitual) indisposition, composed of a frequent, painless evacuation of soft fæces and frequent inclination to go to stool, an unnatural sleeplessness, excessive irritability and agility, and a want of appetite and thirst, but without any diminution of the perception of the flavour of food and drink, in such a case coffee *will*, *must* effect a radical cure in the course of a short time. In like manner it is, in the frequently dangerous symptoms brought on by a sudden, great, joyful mental emotion, the most suitable, trustworthy, curative medicine, and also in a certain kind of labour-pains, which bear much resemblance to the primary effects of coffee.

[3] The following are examples of the excellent palliative employment of coffee in diseases that come on rapidly and require speedy relief: sea-sickness, poisoning by opium in those unaccustomed to the use of coffee, poisoning by veratrum album, the apparent death of drowned, suffocated, but especially of frozen persons, as I have frequently had the satisfaction of witnessing.

hurt, is understood by few, but which is extremely wholesome when used in its proper place.

ÆSCULAPIUS IN THE BALANCE.[1]

Ars autem tam conjecturalis cum sit (praesertim quo nunc habetur modo) locum ampliorum dedit non solum errori verum etiam imposturae.—BACO DE VERULAM *Augm. Scient.*

After I had discovered the weakness and errors of my teachers and books, I sank into a state of sorrowful indignation, which had nearly altogether disgusted me with the study of medicine. I was on the point of concluding that the whole art was vain and incapable of improvement. I gave myself up to solitary reflection, and resolved not to terminate my train of thought until I had arrived at a definite conclusion on the subject.

Inhabitants of earth, I thought, how short is the span of your life here below! with how many difficulties have you to contend at every step, in order to maintain a bare existence, if you would avoid the by-paths that lead astray from morality. And yet what avail all your dear-bought, dear-wrung joys, if you do not possess health?

And yet how often is this disturbed—how numerous are the lesser and greater degrees of ill-health—how innumerably great the multitude of diseases, weaknesses and pains, which bow man down as he climbs with pain and toil towards his aim, and which terrify and endanger his existence, even when he is supported by the rewards incident to fame, or reposes in the lap of luxury. And yet, oh man! how lofty is thy descent! how great and God-like thy destiny! how noble the object of thy life! Art thou not destined to approach by the ladder of hallowed impressions, ennobling deeds, all-penetrating knowledge, even towards the great Spirit whom all the inhabitants of the universe worship? Can that Divine Spirit who gave thee thy soul, and winged thee for such high enterprizes, have designed that you should be *helplessly* and *irremediably* oppressed by those trivial bodily ailments which we call diseases?

Ah, no! The Author of all good, when he allowed diseases

---

[1] Published at Leipzic in 1805.

to injure his offspring, must have laid down a means by which those torments might be lessened or removed. Let us trace the impressions of this, the noblest of all arts which has been devoted to the use of perishing mortals. This art must be possible —this art which can make so many happy ; it must not only be possible, but already exist. Every now and then a man is rescued, as by miracle, from some fatal disease ! Do we not find recorded in the writings of physicians of all ages, cures in which the disturbance of the health was so great that no other termination than a miserable death seemed possible ? Yet such cases have been rapidly and effectually cured, and perfect health restored.

But how seldom have these brilliant cures been effected when they were not rather ascribable, either to the force of youth over-mastering the disease, or to the unreckoned influence of various fortunate circumstances, than to the medicines employed. But even were the number of such perfect cures greater than I observe them to be, does it follow from that that we can imitate them with similarly happy results? They stand isolated in the history of the human race, and they can but very seldom, if at all, be reproduced as they were at first occasioned. All we see is, that great cures are possible; but *how* they are to be effected, what the power, and the particular circumstances by which they were accomplished, and how these are to be controlled so that we may transfer them to other cases, is quite beyond our ken. *Perhaps the art of healing does not consist in such transferences.* This much is certain : an art of medicine exists, but not in our heads, nor in our symptoms.

"But," it is urged in reply, "are not people cured every day in the hands of thoughtful physicians, even of very ordinary doctors, nay, even of most egregious blockheads?"

Certainly they are; but mark what happens. The majority of cases, for the treatment of which a physician is called in, are of acute diseases, that is, aberrations from health which have only a short course to run before they terminate either in recovery or death. If the patient die, the physician follows his remains modestly to the grave; if he recover, then must his natural strength have been sufficient to overcome both the force of the disease and the usually obstructing action of the drugs he took ; and the powers of nature often suffice to overcome both.

In epidemic dysentery, just as many of those who follow the

indications afforded by nature, without taking any medicine at all, recover, as of those who are treated according to the method of Brown, of Stoll, of C. L. Hoffman, of Richter, of Vogler, or by any other system. Many die, too, both of those treated by all these methods, and of those who took no medicine; on an average just as many of the one as of the other. And yet all the physicians and quacks who attended those who recovered, boasted of having effected a cure by their skill. What is the inference? Certainly not that they were all right in their mode of treatment; but perhaps, that they were all equally wrong. What presumption for each to claim, as he did, the credit of curing a disease, which in the milder cases uniformly recovered of itself, if gross errors in diet were not committed!

It were easy to run through a catalogue of similar acute diseases, and show that the restoration of persons who in the same disease were treated on wholly opposite principles could not be called cure, but a spontaneous recovery.

Until you can say, during the prevalence of an epidemic dysentery for example, "Fix upon those patients whom you and other experienced persons consider to be most dangerously ill, and these I will cure, and cure rapidly and without bad consequences." Until you can say this, and can do it, you ought not to vaunt that you can cure the dysentery. Your cures are nothing but spontaneous recovery.

Often—the thought is saddening!—patients recover as by a miracle when the multitude of anxiously changed and often repeated nauseous drugs prescribed by the physician is suddenly left off or clandestinely discontinued. For fear of giving offence, the patients frequently conceal what they have done, and appear before the public as if they had been cured by the physician. In numerous instances, many a prostrate patient has effected a miraculous cure upon himself not only by refusing the physician's medicine, but by secretly transgressing his artificial and often mischievous system of diet, in obedience to his own caprice, which is in this instance an imperious instinct impelling him to commit all sorts of dietetic paradoxes. Pork, sour-crout, potato-salad, herring, oysters, eggs, pastry, brandy, wine, punch, coffee, and other things most strongly prohibited by the physician, have effected the most rapid cure of disease in patients, who, to all appearance, would have hastened to their grave had they submitted to the system of diet prescribed by the schools.

Of such a kind are the apparent cures of acute diseases. For those beneficial and useful regulations for the arrest of pestilential epidemics, by cutting off communication with the affected district, by separation and removal of the sick from the healthy; by fumigation of the affected abodes and furniture with nitric and muriatic acid, &c., are wise police regulations, but are not medicinal cures.

In the infected spots themselves, where a further separation of the infected from the healthy is not to be thought of, there the nullity of medicine is exhibited.   There die all, if one may be allowed the expression, who can die, without being influenced by Galen, Boerhave, or Brown, and those only who are not ripe for death recover   Nurses, physicians, apothecaries, and surgeons, are all alike borne to their grave.

At the same time it is undeniable, that even in such calamities, so humiliating to the pride of our art, occasional, but rare cures occur, effected obviously by medicine, of so striking a character, that one is astonished at so daring a rescue from the very jaws of death; these are the hints afforded by the Author of Life, "THAT THERE IS A HEALING ART."

But how did it act here?   What medicine did the real good? What were the minute particulars of the disease, in order that we may imitate the procedure when such a case recurs?   Alas! these particulars are and must remain unknown; the case was either not particularly observed or not reported with sufficient exactness.   And the medicine?   No; a single medicine was not given; it was, as all learned recipes must be, an elixir, a powder, a mixture, &c., each composed of a number of medicinal substances.   Heaven knows which of them all did good.[1]   "The patient also drank an infusion of a variety of herbs; the composition of this I do not recollect, nor does the patient remember the precise quantity he took."

How can any one imitate such an experiment in an apparently similar case, since neither the remedy nor the case are accurately

---

[1] Let it not be asserted "that all the substances only did good because of their combination, that nought must be added to nothing taken from it, to enable us to repeat the fact." But many ingredients are never of equal goodness and power in any two chemists' shops, not even in the same shop at different times.   Even the same mixture will be different in the same shop to-morrow to what it was to-day, according as one ingredient was added sooner than the other, more fully pulverized, or rubbed-up more strongly with the other ingredients, according as the atmospheric temperature was lower to-day, to-morrow higher, the ingredients more accurately measured to-day than to-morrow, or according as the preparer of the prescription was more attentive to-day, less to-morrow; and many other circumstances may occur to mar human calculations.

known? Hence all the results attempted by future imitators are deceptive; the whole fact is lost for posterity. All we see is, *that* cure is possible; but *how* is it to be effected, and how an indefinite case can tend to perfect the art of medicine, that we do not see.

"But," I hear exclaimed, "you must not be too severe upon physicians, who are but men, amid the hurry and bustle which infectious diseases in circumscribed spots bring with them."

"In chronic diseases he will come off more triumphant; in these he has time and cool blood at his service in order to exhibit openly the truth of his art; and in despite of Molière, Patin, Agrippa, Valesius, Cardanus, Rosseau and Arcesilas, he will show that he can heal not only those who would get well of themselves, but that he can cure what he will and what he is asked to cure." Would to Heaven it were so! But as a proof that physicians feel themselves very weak in chronic diseases, they avoid the treatment of them as much as possible. Let a physician be called to an elderly man, paralyzed for some years, and let him be asked to exhibit his skill. Naturally he does not openly avow how impotent this art is in his hands, but he betakes himself to some by-way of escape—shrugs his shoulders—observes that the patient's strength is not sufficient to enable him to undergo the treatment (in general, a very exhausting, debilitating procedure in the hands of ordinary practitioners); speaks with a compassionate air of the unfavourable season and inclement weather, which must first be over, and of the healing herbs of spring, which must be waited for before the cure can be attempted, or of some far-distant mineral waters where such cures have been made, and whither, if his life be spared, the patient will be able to proceed in the course of six or eight months. In the meantime, not to expose himself, he orders something, of the effects of which he is not sure this he does in order to amuse the patient and to make a little money out of him at the same time; but certain relief he cannot give. At one time he wishes to remove the asthenia by internal or external stimulants; at another fortify the tone of the muscular fibre with a multitude of bitter extracts,[1] whose effects he knows not, or strengthen the digestive apparatus with cinchona bark; or he seeks to purify and cool the blood by a decoction of equally unknown plants,

---

[1] We often read in the histories of cases, even of distinguished physicians, such observations as this: "I now gave the patient the bitter extracts"—as if the bitter vegetable substances were not all very various in their peculiar actions!

or by means of saline, metallic and vegetable substance of problematic utility, to resolve and dissipate suspected but never observed obstructions in the glands and minute vessels of the abdomen; or by means of purgatives he thinks to expel certain impurities which exist only in his imagination, and thereby hasten *by a few hours* the sluggish evacuations. Now he directs his charge against the principle of gout; now against a suppressed gonorrhœa; now against a psoric acridity, anon against some other kind of acridity. He effects a change, but not the change he wished. Gradually, under the pretext of urgent business, the physician withdraws from the patient, comforting himself and at length the patient's friends when they press him for his opinion, that in such cases his art is too weak.

And that his so vaunted art is too weak, on this comfortable, soft pillow he reposes in cases of gout, consumption, old ulcers, contractions and so-called dropsies, cachexias of innumerable varieties, spasmodic asthmas, angina pectoris, pains, spasms, cutaneous eruptions, debility, mental affections of many kinds, and I know not how many other chronic diseases.

In no other case is the insufficiency of our art so strongly and so unpardonably manifested as in those distressing diseases from which hardly any family is altogether free; hardly any in which some one of the circle does not secretly sigh over ailments, for which he has tried the so-called skill of physicians far and near. In silence the afflicted sufferer steals on his melancholy way, borne down with miserable suffering, and, despairing in human aid, seeks a solace in religion.

"Yes," I hear the medical school whisper with a seeming compassionate shrug, "Yes, these are notoriously incurable evils; our books tell us they are incurable." As if it could comfort the million of sufferers to be told of the vain impotence of our art! As if the Creator of these sufferers had not provided remedies for them also, and as if for them the source of boundless goodness did not exist, compared to which the tenderest mother's love is as thick clouds beside the glory of the noonday sun!

"Yes," I hear the school continue to apologize, "the thousand defects in our civic constitution, the artificial, complicated mode of life so far removed from nature, the chameleon-like luxury enervating and deranging our natural constitution, are answerable for the incurable character of all these evils. Our art is quite excused for being incapable of the cure of such cases."

Can you then believe that the Preserver of our race, the All-wise, did not design these complexities of our civic constitution and our artificial mode of life to increase our enjoyment here, and to remove misery and suffering? What extraordinary kind of living can that be to which man cannot accustom himself without any great disturbance of his health? The fat of the seal and the train-oil eaten with bread made of dried fish bones as little prevents the Greenlander from enjoying health in general, as does the unvaried milk-diet of the shepherds on the Swiss mountains, the purely vegetable food of the poorer Germans, or the highly animal diet of the wealthy Englishman. Does not the Vienna nobleman accustom himself to his twenty or thirty covers, and does he not enjoy just as much health as the Chinese with his thin rice soup, the Saxon miner with nothing but potatoes, the South Sea Islander with his roasted bread-fruit, and the Scottish highlander with his oatmeal cakes?

I am ready to admit that the contest of conflicting passions and of many other enjoyments, the luxurious refinement, and the absence of exercise in fresh air that prevail in the labyrinth ine palaces of great cities, may give occasion to more numerous and more rare diseases than the simple uniformity that obtains in the airy hut of the humble villager. But that does not materially alter the matter. For our medical art is as impotent against the *water colic* of the peasant of lower Saxony, the *Tsömer* of Hungary and Transylvania, the *Radesyge* of Norway, the *Sibbens* of Scotland, the *Hotme* of Lapland, the *Pelagra* of Lombardy, the *Plica Polonica* of certain Sclavonic tribes, and various other diseases prevalent among the simple peasantry of various countries, as it is against the more aristocratic disorders of high life in our large towns. Must there be one kind of medical art for the former, and another for the latter: or if it were only once discovered, would it not be equally applicable to both? I should think so!

It may not certainly exist in our books, nor yet in our heads, nor be taught in our schools, but there is such a thing for all that; it is a possibility.

Occasionally a regular brother practitioner stumbles by a lucky hit upon a cure which astonishes half the world about him, and not less himself; but among the many medicines he employed he is by no means sure which did good. Not less frequently does the neck-or-nothing practitioner, without a degree, whom the world calls a quack, make as great and wonderful a cure. But neither he nor yet his worshipful brother practitioner with a diploma knows how to eliminate the evident and fruitful truth which the cure contains. Neither can separate and record the medicine which certainly was of use out of the mass of useless and obstructing ones they employed; neither precisely indicates the case in which it did good, and in which it will certainly benefit again. Neither knows how to abstract a truth which will hold good in all future time, an appropriate, certain, unfailing remedy for every such case that may occur hereafter. His experience in this case, remarkable though it seemed, will almost never be of service to him in any other. All that we learn is, that a helpful system of medicine is possible; but from these and a hundred other cases it is quite manifest that as yet it has not attained the rank of a science, that even the way has yet to be discovered how such a science is to be learned and taught. As far as we are concerned, it cannot be said to exist.

Meanwhile, among these brilliant but rare cures there are many (vulgarly called *Pferdecuren* [horse cures], which, however great the noise they might make, are not of a character to be imitated, *salti mortali*, madly desperate attempts by means of the most powerful drugs in enormous doses, which brought the patient into the most imminent danger, in which life and death wrestled for the mastery, and in which a slight unforeseen preponderance on the side of kind nature gave the fortunate turn to the case: the patient recovered himself and escaped from the very jaws of death.

A treatment with a couple of scruples of jalap-resin to the dose is by no means inferior in severity to the helleborism of the ancient Greek and Roman physicians.

Such modes of treatment are not very unlike murders, the result alone renders them uncriminal, and almost imparts to them the lustre of a good action, the saving of a life. [1]

This cannot be the divine art, that like the mighty working of nature should effect the greatest deeds simply, mildly, and unobservably, by means of the smallest agencies.

The ordinary practice of the majority of our practitioners in their treatment of diseases resembles these horrible revolutionary cures. They partially attain their object, but in a hurtful way. Thus they have to treat, for example, an unknown disease ac-

---

[1] Thus a cruel usurper vibrates betwixt the scaffold and the throne, a small unfortunate accident brings his head to the block, and he dies amidst the curses of the nation; or a small moment of luck that did not enter into his calculations puts the crown on his head, and the same nation falls down and worships him.

27

companied by general swelling.   On account of the swelling it
is in their eyes a disease of daily occurrence; without hesitation
they call it dropsy (just as if a single symptom constituted the
essential nature of the whole disease!), and they briskly set to
work with the remark : "the water must be drawn off, and then
all will be right."   Away they go at it, attacking it with a frequent repetition of drastic (so-called hydragogue) purgatives, and,
see! what a wonderful event takes place—the abdomen falls, the
arms, the legs and the face grow quite thin!   "Look what I can
do, what is in the power of my art; this most serious disease,
the dropsy, is conquered! with only this slight disadvantage,
that a new disease, which nobody anticipated, is come in its place
(properly, has been brought on by the excessive purgation), a
confounded lientery, which we must now combat with new
weapons."

Thus the worthy man comforts himself from time to time, and
yet it is impossible that such a procedure can be called a cure,
where the disease, by means of violent unsuitable medicines,
only loses a portion of its outward form and gains a new one;
the change of one disease for another is not a cure.

The more I examine the ordinary cures, the more I am convinced, that they are not direct transformations of the disease
treated into health, but revolutionizings, disturbances of the order
of things by medicines, which, without being actually appropriate, possessed power enough to give matters another (morbid)
shape.   These are what are called cures.

"The hysterical ailments of yonder lady were successfully removed by me!"

No! they were only changed into a metrorrhagia.   After some
time I am greeted by a shout of triumph : "Excuse me! I have
also succeeded in putting a stop to the uterine hæmorrhage."

But do you not see how, on the other hand, the skin has become sallow, the white of the eye has acquired a yellow hue,
the motions have become greyish-white, and the urine orange-
coloured.

And thus the so-called cures go on like the shifting scenes of
one and the same tragedy !

The most successful cases among them are still those where
the revolution effected by the drug developes a new disease of
such a sort, that nature, so to speak, is so much occupied with
it as to forget the old original disease and let it go about its
business, and is engaged with the artificial one until some lucky

circumstance liberates it from the latter. There are several kinds of such lucky circumstances. The leaving off of the medicine—youthful vigour—the commencement of the menstrual flow or its cessation at the proper periods of life—a fortunate domestic occurrence—or (but this is certainly of rare occurrence, still it sometimes happens like a ternion in the game of lotto) among the many medicines prescribed pell mell, there lay one that was appropriate and adapted to the circumstances of the case— in all these instances a cure may occur.

In like manner, mistakes of the chemist respecting the medicines and signs in prescriptions have often been the occasion of wonderful cures. But are such circumstances recommendations for the (till now) most uncertain of all arts? I should rather think not.

By treatment the ordinary physician often understands nothing more than a powerful, violent attack upon the body with things that are to be found in the chemist's shop, with an alteration of the diet, *secundum artem*, to one of a very extraordinary, very meagre character. "The patient must first be powerfully affected before I can do him any good; I wish I could but once get him regularly laid up in bed!" But that the transition from bed to the straw and the coffin is so very easy, infinitely easier than to health, he says nothing about that.

The physician of the stimulating school is in the habit of prescribing in almost every case an exactly opposite diet (such is the custom of his sect): ham, strong meat soups, brandy, &c., often in cases where the very smell of meat makes the patient sick, and he can bear nothing but cold water; but he too is by no means sparing in his use of violent remedies in enormous doses.

The schools of both the former and the latter class authorise a revolutionary procedure of this sort: "No child's play with your doses," say they, "go boldly and energetically to work, giving them strong, as strong as possible!" And they are right if treating means the same thing as knocking down.

How does it happen that, in the thirty-five centuries since Æsculapius lived, this so indispensable art of medicine has made so little progress? What was the obstacle? for what the physicians have already done is not one hundredth part of what they might and ought to have done.

All nations, even remotely approaching a state of civilization, perceived, from the first, the necessity and inestimable value of this art; they required its practice from a caste who called themselves physicians. These affected, in almost all ages, when they came in contact with the sick, to be in perfect possession of this art; but among themselves they sought to gloze over the gaps and inconsistencies of their knowledge by heaping system upon system, each made up of the diversified materials of conjectures, opinions, definitions, postulates, and predicates, linked together by scholastic syllogisms, in order to enable each leader of a sect to boast respecting his own system, that here he had built a temple for the goddess of health—a temple worthy of her—in which the inquirer would be answered by pure and salutary oracles.

It was only the most ancient times that formed an exception to this rule.

We were never nearer the discovery of the science of medicine than in the time of Hippocrates. This attentive, unsophisticated observer sought nature in nature. He saw and described the diseases before him accurately, without addition, without colouring, without speculation.[1] In the faculty of pure observation he has been surpassed by no physician that has followed him. Only one important part of the medical art was this favoured son of nature destitute of, else had he been completely master of his art; the knowledge of medicines and their application. But he did not affect such a knowledge—he acknowledged his deficiency in that he gave almost no medicines (because he knew them too imperfectly), and trusted almost entirely to diet.

All succeeding ages degenerated and wandered more or less from the indicated path, the later sects of the empirics—worthy of all respect—and to a certain degree, Aretæus,[2] excepted.

Sophistical whimsicalities were pressed into the service. Some sought the origin of disease in a universal hostile principle, in some poison which produced all maladies, and which was to be contended with and destroyed. Hence the universal antidote which was to cure all diseases, called *theriaca*, composed of an innumerable multitude of ingredients, and more lately the *mithridatium*, and similar compounds, celebrated from the time

---

[1] The speculative writings under his name are not his, neither are the three last books of the aphorisms. The want of the Hippocratic Ionicisms, the absence of the very peculiar language of this man, must convince any one of this, who knows any thing about such matters.

[2] Graphic as are his descriptions of disease, he yet only described them amalgamated together in complete classes, from many individual cases of disease: this Hippocrates did not do, but modern pathologists do it.

of Nicander down almost to our own day.   From these ancient times came the unhappy idea, that if a sufficient number of drugs were mixed in the receipt, it could scarcely fail to contain the one capable of triumphing over the enemy of health— while all the time the action of each individual ingredient was little, or not at all known.   And to this practice Galen, Celsus, the later Greek and Arabian physicians, and, on the revival of the study of medicine in Bologna, Padua, Seville, and Paris, in the middle ages, the schools there established, and *all* succeeding ones, have adhered.

In this great period of nearly two thousand years, was the pure observation of disease neglected.   The wish was to be more scientific, and to discover the hidden causes of diseases. These once discovered, then it were an easy (?) task to find out remedies for them.   Galen devised a system for this purpose, his four qualities with their different degrees; and until the last hundred and fifty years his system was worshipped over our whole hemisphere, as the *non plus ultra* of medical truth.   But these phantoms did not advance the practical art of healing by a hair's breadth; it rather retrograded.

After it had become more easy to communicate thought, to obtain a name by writing hypotheses, and when the writings of others could be more cheaply read—in a word, after the discovery of printing—the systems rapidly increased, and they have crowded one on another up to our own day.   There was now the influence of the stars, now that of evil spirits and witchcraft; anon came the alchymist with his salt, sulphur, and mercury; then Silvius, with his acids, biles, and mucus; then the iatromathematicians and mechanical sect, who explained every thing by the shape of the smallest parts, their weight, pressure, friction, &c.; to these succeeded the humoral pathologists, with certain acridities of the fluids; then the tone of the fibres and the abnormal state of the nerves was insisted on by the solidists; then, according to Reil, much was due to the internal composition and form of the most minute parts, while the chemists found a fruitful cause of disease in the development of various gases.   How Brown explained disease with his theory of excitability, and how he wished to embrace the whole art with a couple of postulates, is still fresh in our recollection; to say nothing of the ludicrously lofty, gigantic undertaking of the natural philosophers!

Physicians no longer tried to see diseases as they were; what they saw did not satisfy them, but they wished by *a priori* reasoning to find out an undiscoverable source of disease in regions of speculation which are not to be penetrated by terrestrial mortal. Our system-builders delighted in these metaphysical heights, where it was so easy to win territory; for in the boundless region of speculation every one becomes a ruler who can most effectually elevate himself beyond the domain of the senses. The superhuman aspect they derived from the erection of these stupendous castles in the air concealed their poverty in the art of healing.

"But, since the discovery of printing, the preliminary sciences of the physician, especially natural history and natural philosophy, and, in particular, the anatomy of the human body, physiology, and botany, have greatly advanced."

True : but it is worthy of the deepest reflection how it comes that these useful sciences, which have so manifestly increased the knowledge of the physician, have contributed so little to the improvement of his art; their direct influence is most insignificant, and the time was when the abuse of these sciences obstructed the practical art of healing.

Then the anatomist took upon him to explain the functions of the living body ; and, by his knowledge of the position of the internal parts, to elucidate even the phenomena of disease. Then were the membranes, or the cellular tissue of one intestine, continuations of the membranes or cellular tissue of another or of a third intestine ; and so, according to them, was the whole mystery of the metastasis of diseases unravelled to a hair. If that did not prove sufficient, they were not long in discovering some nervous filament to serve as a bridge for the transportation of a disease from one part of the body to another, or some other unfruitful speculations of the same kind. After the absorbents were discovered, anatomy immediately took upon herself to instruct physicians in what way medicines must permeate them, in order to get to that spot of the body where their remedial power was wanted; and there were many more of such material demonstrations put forward, much to the retardation of our art. It often reigned despotically, and refused to acknowledge every physician who handled his scalpel otherwise than according to the mode taught in the schools—who could not, without hesitation, give the name of each little depression on the surface of a bone, who could not, on the instant, give the origin and insertion of every smallest muscle (which sometimes only owed its individual existence to the scalpel). The examination of a physician for a degree consisted almost solely in anatomy: this he was obliged to know off by heart, with a most pedantic precision; and if he did this, then he was prepared to practise.

Physiology, until Haller's time, looked only through the spectacles of hypothetical conceits, gross mechanical explanations, and pretensions to systems, until this great man undertook the task of founding the knowledge of the phenomena of the human body upon sensible observation and truthful experience alone. Little has been added since his time, except so far as newly-discovered products, newly-discovered physical powers and laws, have conspired to explain the constitution of our frame. But from these, little has been incontrovertibly established.

In general, natural philosophy often offered its services, somewhat presumptuously, to explain the phenomena in the healthy and diseased body. Then were the manifest laws which, in the inorganic world, regulate the extrication, confinement, and diffusion of caloric, and the phenomena of electricity and galvanism, applied, without change and without any exception, to the explanation of vital operations; and there were many premature conclusions of a similar kind.

But none of the preliminary sciences has assumed so arrogant a place as chemistry. It is, indeed, a fact that chemistry explains certain appearances of the healthy as well as the diseased body, and is a guide to the preparation of various medicines; but it is incredible how often it has usurped the right of explaining all physiological and pathological phenomena, and how much it has distinguished itself by authorising this or that medicine. Gren, Tromsdorff, and Liphardt, may serve as warning examples of this.

It is, I repeat, a matter for more serious reflection, that while these accessory sciences of medicine (in themselves most commendable) have advanced within these last ten years to a height and a maturity which seems not to be capable of much further advancement, yet, notwithstanding, they have had no marked beneficial influence on the treatment of disease.

Let us consider how this has happened.

Anatomy shews us the outside of every part which can be separated with the knife, the saw, or by maceration; but the deep internal changes it does not enable us to see; even when we examine the intestines, still it is only a view of the outside of these internal surfaces that we obtain; and even were we to open live animals, or, like Herophilus, of cruel memory, dissect men alive, so little could we penetrate the minute structure of parts lying remote from view, that even the most inquisitive and attentive observer would relinquish the task in dissatisfaction. Nor do we make much greater discoveries with the microscope, unless the refracting power favour us with optical illusions. We see only the outside of organs, we see only their grosser substance; but into the innermost depths of their being, and into the connexion of their secret operations no mortal eye can ever pierce.

By means of pure observation and unprejudiced reflection, in connexion with anatomy, natural philosophy, and chemistry, we have a considerable store of very probable conclusions regarding the operations and vital phenomena of the human body (*physiology*), because the phenomena in what is called a healthy body remain pretty constant, and hence can be observed frequently and, for the purposes of comparison, from all the different points of view afforded by the various branches of knowledge bearing upon them. But it is no less true, than striking and humbling, that this anthropological or physiological knowledge begins to prove of no use as soon as the system departs from its state of health. All explanations of *morbid* processes from what we know of healthy ones, are deceptive, approaching more or less to what is untrue; at all events, positive proofs of the reality and truth of these transferred explanations are unattainable; they are from time to time refuted by the highest of all tribunals—experience. Just because an explanation answers for the healthy state of the frame, it will not answer for the diseased. We may admit it or not as we please, but it is too true, that in the moment when we attempt to regard the state of the disease physiologically, there drops before our previously clear light of physiology a thick veil—a partition which prevents all vision. Our physiological skill is quite at fault when we have to explain the phenomena of morbid action. There is almost no part of it applicable! True, we can give a sort of far-fetched explanation, by making a forced transference and application of the physiological systems to pathological phenomena; but it is only illusory and misleads into error.

Chemistry should never attempt to offer an explanation of the abnormal performances of the functions in the diseased body, since it is so unsuccessful in explaining them in the healthy state. When it predicts what, according to its laws, must happen, then something quite different takes place; and if the vitality overmasters chemistry in the healthy body, how much more must it do so in the diseased, which is exposed to the influence of so many more unknown forces. And just as little should chemistry undertake to give a decision upon the suitableness or worthlessness of medicines, for it is altogether out of its sphere of vision to determine what is properly healing or hurtful, and it possesses no principle and no standard by which the healing efficacy of medicines, in different diseases, can be measured or judged of.

Thus has the healing artist for ever stood alone—I might say forsaken—forsaken by all his renowned auxiliary sciences—forsaken by all his transcendental explanations and speculative systems. All these assistants were mute, when, for example, he stumbled upon an intermittent fever which would not yield to purgatives and cinchona bark.

"What is to be done here? what is with *sure confidence* to be set about?" he inquires of these his oracles.—Profound silence. —(And thus they remain silent up to the present hour, in most cases, these fine oracles.)

He reflects upon the matter, and comes, after the fashion of men, to the foolish notion, that his uncertainty what to do here arises from his not knowing the *internal* nature of intermittent fever.—He searches in his books, in some twenty of the most celebrated systematic works, and finds (unless they have copied from one another) as many different explanations of intermittent fever as books he examines. Which of them is he to take for his guide? They contradict one another.

By this road he finds he will make no progress.

He will let intermittent fever just be intermittent fever, and turns his attention solely to learn what medicines the experience of bygone ages has discovered for intermittent fever, besides cinchona bark and evacuants. He proceeds to search, and to his amazement discovers that an immense number of medicines have been celebrated in intermittent fever.

Where is he to begin? Which medicine is he to give first; which next, and which last? He looks round for aid, but no directing angel appears, no *Hercules in bivio*, no heavenly inspiration whispers in his ear which of all the number he ought to select.

What is more natural, what more appropriate to the weakness of man, than that he should adopt the unhappy resolution (the resolution of almost all ordinary physicians in similar cases !), "that as he has nothing to direct his choice to the best, he had better give *a number* of the most celebrated febrifuge medicines *mixed together in one prescription.* How will he ever otherwise get to the end of the long list, unless he take several at a time? As he can find no one who can tell him if there is any difference in the actions of these different substances, he considers it better to mix together many than few;[1] and if the operation of each of these different ingredients really differs from that of the .others, it would certainly, he thinks, be better, in this case, to collect several and many such reputedly antifebrile substances in one receipt."

" Among the many substances in his elixirs, pills, electuaries, mixtures, and infusions, surely (thus he philosophizes) there must be *one* which will do good. Perhaps the most effectual happens also to be the freshest and most powerful medicine therein; and perhaps the substances less adapted or even obstructive to the cure, are happily the weakest in yonder chemist's shop. Perhaps! yes we must hope for the best, and trust to good luck!"

Periculosae plenum opus aleae! What are we to think of a science, the operations of which are founded upon *perhapses* and blind chance.

But suppose the first or second, or all the trains of mixed drugs have not done any good, then I must ask, whence did your authors derive the information, that A or B, or Y or Z, was useful in intermittent fever?

" It stands written of each of these remedies in the works on Materia Medica."

But whence is their knowledge obtained? Do the authors of

---

[1] The learned excuse for the great complexity of our ordinary prescriptions, "that most of the ingredients were added from rational reasons, that is to say, on account of the particular indications in each case—and that regular prescriptions must have an orthodox form, *a basis* (fundamental medicine), *a corrective* (something added in order to correct the faults of the basis), *an adjuvant* (an auxiliary substance to support the weakness of the basis), and *an excipient* (a substance that supplies the form and vehicle)—is partly palpable school-cunning, like the latter excuse—partly fancy, like the former. For why does the opium you add not cause sleep, why do your additions of neutral salts fail to open the bowels, and your aqua sambuci to keep the skin moist? Why does that not happen, as a rule, for which you added each particular substance, if it was properly indicated as you allege?

these books anywhere assert that they themselves have given each of these substances alone and uncombined in intermittent fever?

"Oh no! Some give authorities, or quote other works on Materia Medica; others make the statement without any reference to its source."

Turn up the original authorities!

"The most of these have been convinced not by personal experience; they again refer to some antiquated works on Materia Medica, or such authorities as these: Ray, Tabernæmontanus, Trajus, Fuchs, Tournefort, Bauhin, and Lange."

And these?

"Some of them refer to the results of domestic practice;— peasants and uneducated persons, in this or that district, have found this or that medicine useful in a particular case."

And the other authorities?

"Why, they aver that they did not give the medicine by itself, but, as it became learned physicians to do, combined with other simples, and found advantage from it. Still it was their impression that it was this drug, and not the other simples, that was of service."

A fine thing to rely on, truly, a most delightful conviction, grounded upon opinions destitute even of probability!

In one word: the primary origin of almost all authorities for the action of a simple medicine is derived, either from the confused use of it, in combination with other drugs, or from domestic practice, where this or that unprofessional person had tried it with success in this or that disease (as if an unprofessional person could distinguish one disease from another).

Truly this is a most unsatisfactory and turbid source for our proud Materia Medica. For if some of the common people had not, at their own risk, undertaken experiments, and communicated the results of these, we should not have known even the little we do at present about the action of most medicines. For, with the exception of what a few distinguished men, to wit, Conrad Gesner, Stoerk, Cullen, Alexander, Coste, Willemet, have done, by administering *simple* medicines alone and uncombined, in certain diseases, or to persons in health, the rest is nothing but opinion, illusion, deception. Martin Herz thought the water-hemlock cured phthisis, although he gave it combined with various other drugs.[1] On the other hand, to me the statement of Lange

---

[1] This is the general but most unjustifiable procedure of our medical practitioners:

(in his *Med. Domest. Brunsv.*) is of much greater weight, namely, that the common people have employed it uncombined in this disease, frequently with good effect, than what the worthy doctor *thought;* and for this simple reason, because he gave it mixed with other drugs, while the others gave it simply by itself.

The Materia Medica of remote antiquity was not worse furnished. Its sources were then the histories of cures effected by simples, recorded in the votive tablets; and Dioscorides and Pliny have manifestly derived their account of the operation of simple medicines from the rude observations of the common people. Thus, after the lapse of a couple of thousands of years, we are not a step advanced! The only source of our knowledge of the powers of medicines, how troubled is it! and the learned choir of physicians in this enlightened century, contents itself with it, in the most serious contingency of mortals, when the most precious of earthly possessions—life and health—are at stake! No wonder that the consequences are what they are.

He who, after such experience of the past, still expects that the art of medicine will ever make a single step towards perfection by this road, to such a one nature has denied all capacity of distinguishing between the probable and the impossible.

To fill to the brim the measure of deception and misapprehension attending the administration of medicine to the sick, the order of apothecaries was instituted,—a guild which depends for existence on the complicated mixtures of drugs. Never will the complicated formulæ cease to prevail, as long as the powerful order of apothecaries maintains its great influence.

Unlucky period of the mediæval age, which produced a Nicolaus the ointmentmaker (Myrepsus), from whose work the *Antidotaria,* and *Codices Medicamentarii* were compiled in Italy and Paris; and in Germany, at first in Nürnberg, about the middle of the sixteenth century, the first *Dispensatorium* was written, by the well-meant zeal of the youthful Valerius Cordus. Before these unhappy events the apothecaries were merely unprivileged venders of crude drugs, dealers in simples, druggists; (at the utmost they might have some theriac, mithridate, and a few ointments, plasters, and syrups, of the Galenic stamp, ready on demand, but this was optional on their part.) The physician

---

to prescribe *nothing by itself*—no, *always in combination with several other things* in an artistic prescription! "No prescription can properly be termed such," says Hofrath Gruner, in his *Art of Prescribing,* "which does not contain several ingredients at once"—so, in order to see clearer, you had better put out your eyes!

bought only from those who had genuine and fresh materials, and mixed these for himself, according to his own fancy; but nobody prevented him from giving them to his patients in their simple and uncombined state.

But from the time when then the authorities introduced dispensatories—that is, books full of compound medicines, which were to be kept ready made—it became necessary to form the apothecaries into a close corporation, and to give them a monopoly (on condition that they should have always a stock of ready prepared medicinal mixtures), whereby their number was fixed and limited, in order that there should not be too many of them, which might cause these costly compounds to hang upon their hands and become spoiled.

It is true, that after the authorising of the complicated mixtures in dispensatories, which was the first step to mischief, had been taken, the second—the granting a privilege of the exclusive sale of these expensive mixtures to apothecaries—was neither an unexpected nor an unjust proceeeding; but had the public approval of these senseless mixtures not preceded it, then the trade in single medicinal substances would have remained as it was at first; and there would have been no need of apothecaries' privileges, from which infinite injury has gradually accrued to the healing art.

The earliest dispensatories, and those nearly down to our own time, called each compound formula by an alluring name, after the disease which it was to remove, and after each, the mode of its administration was described, and numerous commendations of its virtues. By this the young physician was led to employ these composititions in preference to the simple medicines, especially as the former were authorised by the government.

The privileged apothecaries did what they could to increase the number of these formulas, for the profit derived from these mixtures was immensely greater than would have been derived from the sale of the simple drugs employed in their composition; and thus, gradually, the small octavo dispensatory of Cordus grew into huge folios (the Vienna, Prague, Augsburg, Brandenburg, Wirtemburg, &c., dispensatories). And now there was no known disease for which the dispensatory had not certain ready-made compounds, or, at least, the formulas for them, accompanied by the most eulogistic recommendations of them. The professor of the healing art was now prepared, when he had such a receipt-book in his hand,—full of receipts for every disease, sanctioned by the highest authorities in the land! What does he want more to make him perfect as a healer of disease? How easy has the great art been made to him!

It is only quite lately that a change has taken place in the matter. The formulæ in the dispensatory have been shorn of their auctioneering titles, and the number, especially of those which were to be kept ready compounded, has been lessened. Still plenty magisterial formulæ remain.

The spirit of the advancing age had at length expunged from the list of drugs the pearls and jewels, the costly bezoar, the unicorn, and other things which were formerly so profitable to the apothecaries; simple processes for preparing the medicines were laid down; no one now required alcohol to be ten times rectified, or calomel twelve times distilled; and the establishment of more stringent price-regulations for the chemists threatened to convert their hitherto golden shops into silver ones, when things unobservedly took a turn more favourable to the apothecary, and more disastrous to the art of medicine.

The former medicinal laws[1] had already begun to restrict the compounding of the mixtures to the apothecaries, and thus, in some measure, to impose restrictions on the physicians. The more recent statutes completed the work, by preventing physicians from converting the simple drugs into compound mixtures for themselves, as well as forbidding them to give any medicine directly to the patients, and, as the expression was, "to dispense."

Nothing could have been done better adapted to ruin the true art of medicine.

Such regulations may have been adopted from one of three reasons :—

1st. Was it owing to the notorious ignorance of the physicians of the present day, which rendered them unable to prepare a tolerable combination of drugs, or even to measure out the simple medicines, that they were prevented from executing this mechanical operation on account of incompetence, as midwives are not allowed to use forceps? If this was the case (what a dreadful supposition!) how could they write a prescription, that is, directions for combining a variety of substances in a most proper manner, if they themselves were not masters of the operation which they described?

---

[1] For example, the *Constitutiones Frederici II. Imperatoris.*

2*d*. Or were they made in order to enrich the apothecaries, whose incomes suffered by the physicians themselves dispensing their medicines? If the whole system of medicine existed for the benefit of the apothecaries alone,—if people fell sick solely for the profit of apothecaries—if learned men became physicians, not so much for the purpose of curing the sick, as for the sake of assisting the apothecaries to make their fortunes—then there would be good reasons why the dispensing of medicines was forbidden to physicians, and a monopoly of it confirmed to the apothecaries alone.

3*d*. Or were they passed for the benefit of patients? One would suppose that medicinal laws would be made chiefly for the benefit of the sick! Let us see, if it were possible that patients could be benefitted by these laws.

By not himself dispensing, the physician loses all dexterity, all practice in the manipulations necessary for the compounding together of various substances which generally act chemically on each other, and decompose one another more or less in this process or the other. He gradually becomes less experienced in this art, until at last he can no longer give any detailed and consistent directions at all,[1] until at length he gives directions for compounding that are full of contradictions, and make him the laughing-stock of the apothecary. He is now completely at the mercy of the apothecary; and the doctor and patient must be content to take the medicine as the apothecary or his assistant (or even his shop-boy) pleases to compound it.

If the physician wants to order equal parts of myrrh rubbed up with camphor in the form of powder, he very likely does not know, from his want of acquaintance with pharmaceutical manipulations, that these two substances never can form a powder; but the longer these two dry substances are rubbed together, the more they become converted into a greasy mass, a kind of fluid. Then the apothecary either sends to the patient this soft mash, instead of a powder, with a sarcastic observation, much to the annoyance of the physician; or he deceives the doctor, to keep in his good graces, and gives the patient something different from what the doctor prescribed, some brown powder, smelling

[1] It soon comes to this, indeed this is almost universally the case; the physician no longer attempts to invent a prescription for himself, he must copy all his prescriptions from some well-known prescription manual, in order to avoid the danger of committing pharmaceutical blunders and contradictions, if he attempted to compose a prescription for himself.

of camphor. Or the physician, perhaps, writes a prescription for hæmoptysis, consisting of alum and kitchen-salt rubbed together. Now, although each of these substances, separately, is dry, yet out of the triturated combination no powder results, but a fluid, which the physician, not himself accustomed to dispense, could never have anticipated. What will the apothecary do in a case like this? He must either annoy or deceive the writer of the prescription.

Now, can these and a thousand other similar collisions tend to the welfare of the patient?

Errors, mistakes of every kind, which the apothecary or his assistants commit in the preparation of the compound, through ignorance, hurry, confusion, inaccuracy, or deceit from interested motives, are, to the man of science and knowledge, who wishes to test such a combination, a problem, which, when vegetable substances constitute the ingredients, it often defies his powers to solve,—how much more so for a physician who has never had an opportunity of acquiring a practical knowledge of pharmacy, or of compounding the medicines himself, indeed is prohibited from doing so! How is he ever to discover the adulterations or the mistakes which the person who makes up his prescription may have committed? If he cannot detect them, which, owing to such limitations of his knowledge, is very probable, what mischief must and does thence accrue to the patient! If he cannot detect them, what an object of ridicule he must be, when his back is turned, to the apothecary's shopboys!

By forbidding physicians themselves to dispense, the apothecary's income is secured in the most satisfactory manner. What regulations respecting the prices of drugs can check his overcharges? And even if the prices of the drugs are fixed by law, his conscience often does not prevent him from employing a cheaper substitute (*quid pro quo*), instead of the expensive one that is prescribed. Many apothecaries have carried on this kind of deception to a great extent. This practice has been in vogue for more than fifteen hundred years. We may learn something of this sort from Galen's little book, entitled περὶ ἀντιϐαλλομένων; and the multitude of books which treat of the adulteration of drugs and deceptions practised by the apothecaries, constitute of themselves no small library.

How well adapted is the whole business of treatment for the welfare of the sick!

"But the medicinal regulations do not provide only for the apothecary, they are for the interest of the physician also! The latter gets four-pence for every prescription."

So, the same for a prescription which he copies out of a printed receipt book as for one that takes him an hour to compose! Since that law was passed, of course he prefers making use of borrowed, ready-written (*i. e.*) unsuitable) prescriptions; he can write a number of such ones in the course of a forenoon—but he must write a *great many, more than are good for the patient,* because he is paid by the number of his prescriptions, and because he requires many four-pences in order to live, to live well, to live in style!

Alas! we may bid adieu to the progress of the art, to the cure of the sick!

Not to speak of the degradation to a learned man, to an artist of the highest rank, as the physician ought to be—to be paid by the number of his prescriptions (like the copyist by the number of the sheets he copies), or by the number of his courses (like a common messenger), it seems to me that the result is not commensurate with the arrangement. The physician becomes a mechanical workman, his occupation becomes a labour that requires the least reflection of all trades; he writes prescriptions (it matters not what) for whose effect he is not answerable, and he pockets his money.

How can he be made responsible for the result, when he does not prepare the medicine himself?[1] The preparation is entrusted by the state to another (the apothecary), who also is not answerable for the result (except in the case of palpable, enormous mistakes), and over whom we have no control with respect to many inaccuracies in the preparation of compound medicines, for after the mixture is made, it is absolutely impossible in many cases to prove that which ought to be proved against him.

From the very nature of the thing—it concerns the cure of the noblest of created beings, it concerns the saving of human life, the most difficult, the most sublime, the most important of

---

[1] Properly speaking, the business of treatment is a kind of contract which the patient makes with *the physician* alone; *do ut facias.* The physician solemnly promises to give his aid and to administer efficacious medicines prepared in the best way —a promise which, with such legal arrangements, he cannot redeem, and which can only be performed by a third party, the apothecary, who is not bound by any contract to the patient. What inconsistency!

all imaginable occupations!—from the very nature of the thing, I repeat, the physician should be prohibited, under the severest penalties, from allowing any other person to prepare the medicines required for his patients; he should be required, under the severest penalties, to prepare them himself, so that he may be able to vouch for the result.

But that it should be forbidden to the physician to prepare his own instruments for the saving of life—no human being could have fallen on such an idea *a priori*.

It would have been much more sensible to prohibit authoritatively Titian, Guido Reni, Michael Angelo, Raphael, Correggio or Mengs from preparing their own instruments (their expressive, beautiful and durable colours), and have ordered them to purchase them in some shop indicated! By the purchased colours, not prepared by themselves,[1] their paintings, far from being the inimitable masterpieces they are, would have been ordinary daubs and mere market goods. And even had they all become mere common market goods, the damage would not have been so great as if the life of even the meanest slave (for he too is a man!) should be endangered by untrustworthy health-instruments (medicines) purchased from and prepared by strangers.

Under these ragulations should there happen to one single physician who should wisely wish to avoid that injudicious mode of prescribing multifarious mixtures of medicines, and for the weal of his patients and the furtherance of his art should wish to prescribe simple medicines in their gonuineness, he would be abused in every apothecary's shop until he abandoned a method that was so little profitable to the apothecary's purse; he must take his choice of either being harrassed to death or of abandoning it and again writing compound prescriptions. In this case what course would ninty-nine doctors out of a hundred chose? Do you know? I do!

Therefore adieu to all progress in our art! Adieu to the successful treatment of the sick!

---

[1] I never knew any great enamel-painter who did not require to prepare his own colours, if he wished to have permanent, brilliant colours, and to produce master-pieces; if he be forbidden to prepare his own colours he will not be able to furnish any but wretched daubs.

THE MEDICINE OF EXPERIENCE.

Man, regarded as an animal, has been created more helpless than all other animals. He has no congenital weapons for his defence like the bull, no speed to enable him to flee from his enemies like the deer, no wings, no webbed feet, no fins,—no armour impenetrable to violence like the tortoise, no place of refuge provided by nature as is possessed by thousands of insects and worms for their safety, no physical provision to keep the enemy at bay, such as render the hedgehog and torpedo formidable, no sting like the gadfly, nor poison-fang like the viper;— to all the attacks of hostile animals he is exposed defenceless. He has, moreover, nothing to oppose to the violence of the elements and meteors. He is not protected from the action of the water by the shining hair of the seal, nor by the close oily feathers of the duck, nor by the smooth shield of the water beetle; his body, but a slight degree lighter than the water, floats more helplessly in that medium than that of any quadruped, and is in danger of instant death. He is not protected like the polar-bear or eider-duck by a covering impenetrable to the northern blast. At its birth the lamb knows where to seek its mother's udder, but the helpless babe would perish if its mother's breast were not presented to it. Where he is born nature nowhere furnishes his food ready made, as she provides ants for the armadillo, caterpillars for the ichneumon fly, or the open petals of flowers for the bee. Man is subject to a far larger number of diseases than animals, who are born with a secret knowledge of the remedial means for these invisible enemies of life, instinct, which man possesses not. Man alone painfully escapes from his mother's womb, soft, tender, naked, defenceless, helpless, and destitute of all that can render his existence supportable, destitute of all wherewith nature richly endows the worm of the dust, to render its life happy.

Where is the benevolence of the Creator, that could have disinherited man, and him alone of all the animals of the earth, of the bare necessities of life?

Behold, the Eternal Source of all love only disinherited man of the animal nature in order to endow him all the more richly with that spark of divinity—a mind—which enables man to elicit from himself the satisfaction of all his requirements, and a

---

[1] Published at Berlin in 1805

full measure of all conceivable benefits, and to develop from himself the innumerable advantages that exalt the children of this earth far above every other living thing—a mind that, indestructible itself, is capable of creating for its tenement, its frail animal nature, more powerful means for its sustenance, protection, defence and comfort, than any of the most favoured creatures can boast of having derived directly from nature.

The Father of mankind has chiefly reckoned on this faculty of the human mind to discover remedial agents, for his protection from the maladies and accidents to which the delicate organism of man is exposed.

The help that the body can afford itself for the removal of diseases is but small and very limited, so that the human mind is so much the more compelled to employ, for the care of the diseases of the body, remedial powers of a more efficient kind than it has seemed good in the Creator to implant in the organic tissues alone.

What crude nature presents to us should not form the limit for the relief of our necessities; no, our mind should be able to enlarge her resources to an unlimited degree for our perfect well-being.

Thus the Creator presents to us ears of corn from the bosom of the earth, not to be chewed and swallowed in a crude and unwholesome state, but in order that we should render them useful as nutriment by freeing them from the husk, grinding and depriving them of everything of an injurious and medicinal nature, by fermentation and the heat of the oven, and partaking of them in the form of bread—a preparation of an innocuous and nutritious character, ennobled by the perfecting power of our mind. Since the creation of the world the lightning's flash has destroyed animals and human beings; but the Author of the universe intended that the mind of man should invent something, as has actually been done in these latter days, whereby the fire of heaven should be prevented from touching his dwellings—that by means of metallic rods boldly reared aloft he should conduct it harmless to the ground. The waves of the angry ocean reared mountains high threaten to overwhelm his frail bark, and he calms them by pouring oil upon them.

So he permits the other powers of nature to act unhindered to our harm, until we can discover something that can secure us from their destructive force, and harmlessly avert from us their impressions.

So he allows the innumerable array of diseases to assail and seize upon the delicate corporeal frame, threatening it with death and destruction, well knowing that the animal part of our organism is incapable, in most cases, of victoriously routing the enemy, without itself suffering much loss or even succumbing in the struggle ;—the remedial resources of the organism, abandoned to itself, are weak, limited and insufficient for the dispersion of diseases, in order that our mind may employ its ennobling faculty in this case also, where the question concerns the most inestimable of all earth's goods, health and life.

The great Instructor of mankind did not intend that we should go to work in the same manner as nature ; we should do more than organic nature, but not in the same manner, not with the same means as she. He did not permit us to create a horse; but we are allowed to construct machines, each of which possesses more power than a hundred horses, and is much more obedient to our will. He permitted us to build ships, in which, secure from the monsters of the deep and the fury of the tempest, and furnished with all the comforts of the mainland, we might circumnavigate the world, which no fish could do, and therefore he denied to our body the piscine fins, branchiæ and float, that were inadequate to perform this feat He denied to our body the rustling wings of the mighty condor, but on the other hand, he allows us to invent machines filled with light gas, that with silent power lifts us into far higher regions of the atmosphere than are accessible to the feathered tenants of the air.

So also he suffers us not to employ the process of sphacelus, as the human corporeal organism does for itself, in order to remove a shattered limb, but he placed in our hand the sharp, quickly-dividing knife, which Faust moistened with oil, that is capable of performing the operation with less pain, less fever, and much less danger to life. He permits us not to make use of the so-called crisis, like nature, for the cure of a number of fevers ; we cannot imitate her critical sweat, her critical diuresis, her critical abscesses of the parotid and inguinal glands, her critical epistaxis, but he enables the investigator to discover remedies wherewith he may cure the fever more rapidly than the corporeal organism is capable of producing crises, and to cure them more certainly, more easily, and with less suffering, with less danger to life and fewer after-sufferings, than unassisted nature can do by means of crises.

I am therefore astonished that the art of medicine has so seldom raised itself above a servile imitation of these crude processes, and that it has at almost all periods been believed that hardly anything better could be done for the cure of diseases than to copy these crises, and to produce evacuations in the form of sweat, diarrhœa, vomiting, diuresis, venesections, blisters or artificial sores. (This was and remained the most favoured method of treatment from the earliest times till now : and it was always fallen back upon, when other modes of treatment founded on ingenious speculations disappointed the hopes they had raised.) Just as if these imperfect and forced imitations were the same thing as what nature effects in the hidden recesses of vitality, by her own spontaneous efforts, in the form of crises! Or as if such crises were the best possible method for overcoming the disease, and were not rather proofs of the (designed) imperfection and therapeutical powerlessness of our unaided nature! Never, never was it possible to compel these spontaneous endeavours of the organism by artificial means) the very notion implies a contradiction), never was it the Creator's will that we should do so. His design was that we should bring to unlimited perfection our whole being, as also our corporeal frame and the cure of its diseases.

This design has hitherto been in part fulfilled by pure surgery alone. Instead of acting like unassisted nature, which can often only throw off a splinter of bone in the leg by inducing a fever attended by danger to life, and a suppuration that destroys almost all the limb, the surgeon is able by a judicious division of the irritable integuments to extract it in a few minutes by means of his fingers, without occasioning any great suffering, without any considerable bad consequences, and almost without any diminution of the strength. A debilitating slow fever, accompanied by intolerable pains and uninterrupted torturing to death, is almost the sole means the organism can oppose to a large stone in the bladder; whereas an incision made by a practised hand frees the sufferer from it often in a quarter of an hour, spares him many years of torment, and rescues him from a miserable death. Or ought we to attempt to relieve a strangulated hernia by an imitation of the mortification and suppuration, which are the only means, besides death that nature possesses against it? Would it suffice for the rescue and preservation of life, did we not know of any other mode of stopping the hemorrhage from a wound in a large artery than by causing a syncope of half-an-hour's duration, as nature does? Could the tourniquet, bandage and compress be thereby dispensed with?

It has always been a matter worthy of the greatest admiration to see how nature, without having recourse to any surgical operation, without having access to any·remedy from without, does often when left quite unassisted, develop. from itself invisible operations whereby it is able,—often it is true in a very tedious, painful and dangerous manner—but still really to remove diseases and affections of many kinds. But she does not do these for our imitation! we cannot imitate them, we ought not to imitate them, for there are infinitely easier, quicker and surer remedial means which the inventive faculty implanted in our mind is destined to discover, in order to subserve the ends of medicine, that most essential and most honourable of all earthly sciences.

Ατελὲς ἀλαγος πρᾶξις καὶ λόγος ἀπρακτος.

GREG. MAG.

Medicine is a science of experience; its object is to eradicate diseases by means of remedies.

The knowledge of diseases, the knowledge of remedies, and the knowledge of their employment, constitute medicine.

As the wise and beneficent Creator has permitted those innumerable states of the human body differing from health, which we term diseases, he must at the same time have revealed to us a *distinct* mode whereby we may obtain a knowledge of diseases, that shall suffice to enable us to employ the remedies capable of subduing them; he must have shewn to us an equally distinct mode whereby we may discover in medicines those properties that render them suitable for the cure of diseases,—if he did not mean to leave his children helpless, or to require of them what was beyond their power.

This art, so indispensable to suffering humanity, cannot therefore remain concealed in the unfathomable depths of obscure speculation, or be diffused throughout the boundless void of conjecture; it must be accessible, *readily accessible* to us, within the sphere of vision of our external and internal perceptive faculties.

Two thousand years were wasted by physicians in endeavouring to discover the invisible internal changes that take place in the organism in diseases, and in searching for their proximate causes and *a priori* nature, because they imagined that they could not cure before they had attained to this *impossible* knowledge.

If the fruitlessness of these long-continued endeavours cannot be regarded as a proof of the impossibility of this undertaking, the maxim of experience that they were *unnecessary* for the cure, might suffice to shew its impossibility. For the great Spirit of the Universe, the most consistent of all beings, has made that only possible which is necessary.

Although we never can attain to a knowledge of the internal corporeal changes on which diseases depend, yet the observation of their external exciting causes has its uses.

No alteration occurs without a cause. Diseases must have their exciting causes, concealed though they may be from us in the greater number of cases.

We observe a few diseases that always arise from *one and the same* cause, *e. g.*, the miasmatic maladies; hydrophobia, the venereal disease, the plague of the Levant, yellow fever, small-pox, cow-pox, the measles and some others, which bear upon them the distinctive mark of always remaining diseases of a *peculiar character;* and, because they arise from a contagious principle that always remains the same, they also always retain the same character and pursue the same course, excepting as regards some accidental concomitant circumstances, which however do not alter their essential character.

Probably some other diseases, which we cannot shew to depend on a peculiar miasm, as gout, marsh-ague, and several other diseases that occur here and there endemically, besides a few others, also arise either from a single unvarying cause, or from the confluence of several definite causes that are liable to be associated and that are always the same, otherwise they would not produce diseases of such a specific kind, and would not occur so frequently.

These few diseases, at all events those first mentioned (the miasmatic), we may therefore term specific, and when necessary bestow on them *distinctive appellations.*

If a remedy have been discovered for one of these, it will always be able to cure it, for such a disease always remains essentially identical, both in its manifestations (the representatives of its internal nature) and in its cause.

All the other innumerable diseases exhibit such a difference in their phenomena, that we may safely assert that they arise from a combination of several dissimilar causes (varying in number and differing in nature and intensity).

The number of words that may be constructed from an alphabet of twenty-four letters may be calculated, great though that number be; but who can calculate the number of those *dissimilar* diseases, since our bodies can be affected by innumerable and still for the most part unknown influences of external agencies, and by almost as many forces from within.

All things that are capable of exercising any action (and their number is incalculable[1]), are able to act upon and to pro-

---

[1] Some of these are, *e. g.*, the innumerable varieties of odours, the more or less noxious exhalations from organic and inorganic substances, the various gases that possess such different irritating properties, that act upon our nerves in the atmosphere, in our manufactories and in our dwellings, or rise from the water, the earth, animals, and plants;—deficiency of pure, open air, the indispensable aliment of our vitality, excess or deficiency of the sun's light, excess or deficiency of both kinds of electricity, differences in the pressure of the atmosphere, in its humidity or dryness, the still unascertained peculiarities of mountainous regions compared with low-lying plains and deep valleys; peculiarities of climate or situation on large plains and on deserts destitute of plants or water, compared with the sea, with marshy districts, hills, woods, the various winds; the influence of very changeable or too uniform weather, the influence of storms and other meteoric phenomena; too great heat or cold of the air, defect or excess of warmth in our clothing, in our rooms; the constriction of various parts of the body by different articles of dress; the degree of coldness or heat of our food and drink, hunger or thirst, excessive quantities of food or drink, their noxious or medicinal nature, and their power of causing changes in the body, which are inherent in some (as wine, spirits, beer prepared with more or less hurtful plants, drinks containing foreign ingredients, coffee, tea, exotic and indigenous spices, and highly seasoned viands, sauces, liqueurs, chocolate and cakes, the unknown, noxious or health-deranging properties of some vegetables and animals when used as food), and are imparted to others by careless preparation, decomposition, falsification or adulteration (*e. g.* ill-fermented and imperfectly baked bread; underdone animal and vegetable viands, or other articles of diet spoilt in various ways, decomposed, mouldy or adulterated for the sake of gain; liquid and solid food prepared or kept in metal vessels; made up, drugged wine; vinegar sharpened with acrid substances; the flesh of diseased animals; flour adulterated with gypsum or sand; corn mixed with injurious seeds; vegetables mixed with or changed for dangerous plants, from malicious motives, ignorance or poverty); want of cleanliness of the body, of the clothing, of the dwelling, hurtful substances which get into the food during its preparation and keeping from want of cleanliness or from negligence; dust of various unwholesome kinds arising from the substances used in manufactories and workshops; the neglect of various police arrangements for the protection of the well-being of the community; excessive weakening of our corporeal powers; too violent active or passive exercise; inordinate excretions from various organs; abnormal exertion of certain organs of the senses; various unnatural positions and attitudes attendant on different kinds of work; neglect of the employment of various parts, or general inactivity of the body; irregularity in the periods devoted to rest, meals and

duce changes in our organism which is intimately connected with and in conflict with all parts of the universe—and all may produce different effects as they differ among themselves.

How various must be the effects of the action of these agencies, when several of them at once and in varied order and intensity exercise their influence on our bodies, seeing that the latter are also so variously organized and present such diversities in the various conditions of their life, that no one human being exactly resembles another in any conceivable respect!

Hence it happens that with the exception of those few diseases that are always the same, all others are *dissimilar*[1], and *innumerable*, and so different that each of them occurs scarcely more than once in the world, and each case of disease that presents itself must be regarded (and treated) as an individual malady that never before occurred in the same manner, and under the same circumstances as in the case before us, and will never again happen precisely in the same way![2]

---

labour; excess or deficiency of sleep; over-exertion in mental employments generally, or in such as especially excite or fatigue certain faculties of the mind, or which are of an injurious and forced character; overpowering or enervating passions produced by certain kinds of reading, education, bad habits and employment; abuse of the sexual function; reproaches of the conscience, uncomfortable domestic affairs, annoying family relations, fear, fright, vexation, &c.

[1] To this head belong a number of diseases which, owing to a want of accuracy in the comparison of all their symptoms, have been regarded as identical maladies, merely from the circumstance of some one striking resemblance, *e. g.*, dropsy, scrofula, wasting, hypochondriasis, rheumatism, spasms, and so forth. The very circumstance that in one case one mode of treatment was successful that was of no avail in ten others, should have shewn that the difference was not properly observed. It might, it is true, be said that there is a middle sort betwixt those specific and these dissimilar diseases of a mixed character, *e. g.*, tetanus, prosopalgia, diabetes, pneumonia, phthisis, cancer, &c., and that although a great number of cases of each of these diseases present dissimilar characters, and therefore require a different treatment, yet some cases present so much resemblance among themselves in their symptoms and mode of cure, that they should be considered as the same malady. This distinction, however, has not much practical, consequently little real, value, for we ought to observe and investigate accurately each case, in order to find out what is the suitable remedy. If I have discovered this, it is a matter of great indifference whether I then become aware that this same disease, with all its symptoms and with the same curative indications, has presented itself to me before, as this knowledge could not lead me to any other or better mode of cure (and the cure is the aim of all kinds of diagnosis of disease) than to the efficacious and best adapted one.

[2] How were it possible to arrange such *inconjungibilia* into classes, orders, genera, species, varieties and sub varieties, like organic beings, and to give *names* to such states of the extremely composite psychico-corporeal microcosm, subject as it is to such varied irritations by such innumerable agencies, that are capable of such an infinity of modifications and shades of difference! The millions of morbid cases that occur perhaps but once in the world require no names—we only require to cure

The internal essential nature of every malady, of every individual case of disease, as far as it is necessary for us to know it, for the purpose of curing it, expresses itself by the *symptoms*, as they present themselves to the investigations of the true observer in their whole extent, connexion and succession.

When the physician has discovered all the observable symptoms of the disease that exist, he has discovered the disease itself, he has attained the complete conception of it requisite to enable him to effect a cure.

In order to be able to perform a cure, it is requisite to have a faithful picture of the disease with all its manifestations, and in addition, when this can be discovered, a knowledge of its predisposing and exciting causes,[1] in order, after effecting the cure by means of medicines, to enable us to remove these also—by means of an improved regimen—and so prevent a relapse.[2]

In order to trace the picture of the disease, the physician requires to proceed in a very simple manner. All that he needs is carefulness in observing and fidelity in copying.[3] He should entirely avoid all conjectures, leading questions and suggestions.

The patient relates the history of his ailments, those about him describe what they have observed in him, the physician sees, hears, feels, &c., all that there is of an altered or unusual character about him, and notes down each particular in its order, so that he may form an accurate picture of the disease.

The chief signs are those symptoms that are most constant,

---

them. Diseases have been associated together according to some merely external resemblance, or from some similarity of cause or of one or other symptom, in order that they might be treated by the same medicine, with a small outlay of trouble !

[1] In like manner the teacher chiefly requires to observe the actions and conduct of an undisciplined new pupil, in order to lead him in the way of virtue by means of the most appropriate tuition. To effect this reformation it is not necessary either that he should know the ever inscrutable internal organization of his body, or that he should be able to inspect the equally inscrutable internal operations of his mind. In addition to this he certainly requires to know (if he can ascertain it) the cause of his moral deterioration, but only in order to be able to ward it off from him in future—and so prevent a relapse.

[2] If no obvious predisposing and exciting causes are perceptible, whose future avoidance is within the power of man, then all our aims are attained by effecting the restoration by means of remedial agents. The physician must neither invent, conjecture, nor extort from the patient any exciting cause.

[3] If we are not desirous of producing a likeness, we may draw a dozen faces on a piece of paper or canvass in an hour, but a single striking portrait requires just as much time and a much greater power of observation and fidelity in the representation.

most striking, and most annoying to the patient. The pyhsician marks them down as the strongest, the principal features of the picture. The most singular, most uncommon signs furnish the characteristic, the distinctive, the peculiar features.

He allows the patient and his attendants to relate all they have to say without interrupting them, and he notes down everything attentively—he then again inquires what were and still are the most constant, frequent, strongest and most troublesome of the symptoms—he requests the patient to describe again his exact sensations, the exact course of the symptoms, the exact seat of his sufferings, and bids the attendants once more detail, in as accurate terms as they are able, the changes they have observed in the patient, and which they had previously mentioned.[1]

The physician thus hears a second time what he had formerly noted down. If the expressions correspond with what was already related, they may be considered as true, as the voice of internal conviction; if they do not correspond, the discrepancy must be pointed out to the patient or those about him, in order that they may explain which of the two descriptions was nearest the truth, and thus what required confirmation is confirmed, and what required alteration is altered.[2]

If the picture be not yet complete, if there be parts or functions of the body regarding whose state neither the patient nor his attendants have said any thing, the physician then asks what they can remember respecting these parts or functions, but he should frame his questions in general terms, so as to cause his informant to give the special details in his own words.[3]

---

[1] The physician should *never put leading questions* in the course of his investigations. He should not suggest either to the patient, or to the attendants, the symptoms that may be present, or the words they should use to describe them, in order not to mislead them to say any thing that may be untrue, half-true, or different from what is actually the case, or, in order to please the physician, to reply in the affirmative to what is not strictly founded on truth, for in this way a false idea of the disease and an unsuitable mode of treatment must be the result.

The greatest reliance is to be placed on the accurate, although occasionally somewhat coarse expressions of the patient and his attendants, respecting his ailments.

[2] We cannot rely on the patient or his attendants possessing such an accurate memory, that after a short interval of time they should repeat in exactly the same form and manner the expressions that may at first have been inaccurately or hastily chosen. There will certainly then occur variations, which must be pointed out to them, so that they may select more accurate or definite expressions in the description of their sensations and convictions.

[3] For example: How is it as regards the fæcal evacuation?—how does the urine flow?—how is it with the sleep by day and by night?—how is his disposition?—how the thirst?—what sort of taste in the mouth?—what kinds of food and drink does

When the patient (for, except in cases of feigned diseases, most reliance is to be placed on him as regards his sensations) has, by these spontaneous or almost unprompted details, put the physician in possession of a tolerably complete picture of the disease, it is allowable for the latter to institute more particular inquiries.[1]

The answers to these last more special questions however, which have somewhat the character of suggestions, should not be accepted by the physician at the first response as perfectly true, but after making a note of them on the margin he should make fresh inquiries respecting them, in a different manner and in another order,[2] and he should warn the patient and his attendants in their answers to make accurate replies, and to make no additions, but merely to tell the exact circumstances of the case.

But an intelligent patient will often spare the physician the trouble of making these particular inquiries, and in his account of the history of his disease, will usually have made voluntary mention of these circumstances.

When the physician has completed this examination he notes down what he has silently observed in the patient during his visit,[3] and he corrects this by what the attendants tell him how

---

he relish most, what agree with him best?—has each of them its natural perfect taste?—has he any thing to state respecting the head, the limbs, or the abdomen? &c.

[1] For example: How often has he an alvine evacuation, what is the character of it, is it accompanied or not by pains? Is the sleep profound or light?—He then asks more minutely, e. g., are the sufferings complained of persistent or remitting? how often do they occur? only in the room? only in the open air? only during rest or during motion of the body? at what time of the day or under what conditions? what precedes, what accompanies, and what follows them?—And finally, he addresses quite specific questions: Does he start in his sleep? does he groan or talk in his sleep? what does he talk about? was the whitish evacuation mucus or fæces? &c.

[2] For example: How he behaved, what he did in his sleep? what the motions consisted of? does the symptom only occur only in the morning, only when at rest when lying, or when sitting? what happens when he raises himself up in bed? &c.

[3] For example: If the patient tossed restlessly about, and how he behaved; whether he was sulky or quarrelsome hasty or anxious, unconscious, comatose; whether he spoke in a low voice, or incoherently or otherwise; what kind of complexion he has, what appearance the eyes present, what expression of countenance is shewn, what is the state of the tongue, the breath, the smell from the mouth, or the hearing; how much the pupils are dilated, how rapidly and to what extent they alter in the dark and light; the state of the pulse, of the abdomen, of the skin in general, or of particular portions of it as regards moisture and temperature; whether he lies with his head thrown back, uncovered or closely covered up, whether he lies only on his back, with his mouth open, with the arms above the head, or what other position he assumes; with what amount of exertion he raises himself up; and any thing else that may strike the physician, or is observable by him.

much of this was or was not usual with the patient in his days of health.

He then inquires what medicines, domestic remedies, or other modes of treatment have been employed in former times, and what have recently been used,—and especially the state of the symptoms before the use or after the discontinuance of all medicine. The former form he regards as the original state; the latter is in fact an artificial form of the disease, which however he must sometimes accept and treat as it is, if there is any pressing emergency in the case that will not admit of any delay. But if the disease is of a chronic character, he lets the patient continue some days without taking any medicine, to allow it to resume its original form, until which time he defers his more particular examination of the morbid symptoms, in order that he may direct his treatment towards the persistent and unsophisticated symptoms of the chronic malady, but not towards the evanescent, ungenuine, accidental symptoms, produced by the medicines last used—as it will be necessary to do in acute diseases where the danger is urgent.

Finally, the physician makes general inquiries as to any exciting causes of the disease that may be known. In ten cases we shall not find one where the patient or his friends can assign a certain cause. If, however, there have happened one respecting which there can exist no dubiety, it generally occurs that has been voluntarily mentioned by them at the commencement of their account of the disease. If it is necessary to make inquiries respecting it, it usually happens that very uncertain information is elicited on this head.[1]

I except those causes of a disgraceful[2] character, which the patient or his friends are not likely to mention, at all events not of their own accord, and which, consequently, the doctor should endeavour to find out by dexterously framing his questions, or by private inquiries. With these exceptions it is a hurtful, or at

---

[1] Such a query should never have a definite character. But even when it is framed quite in a general fashion (*e. g.* how did the disease arise, what was its cause?) such a question usually only incites the patient and his friends to imagine or invent some probable cause, which might appear probable to a physician who does not possess a great knowledge of mankind, and so deceive him.

[2] For example: meditated suicide, onanism, excesses in wine, spirits or food—in unnatural debauchery—indulgence in meretricious reading; venereal disease; mortified pride; thwarted revenge; childish superstitious fear; an evil conscience; unhappy love; jealousy; domestic quarrels and grief about some family secret, about debts—straitened circumstances, hunger, unwholesome food, &c.

all events, a useless task to endeavour to ferret out other exciting causes, by means of suggestions, especially as the medicinal art knows very few of these (I shall mention them in their proper places) on which we can base a trustworthy mode of treatment, regardless of the particular signs of the disease they have induced.

By exercising all this zealous care the physician will succeed in depicting the pure picture of the disease, he will have before him *the disease itself*, as it is revealed by signs, without which man, who knows nothing save through the medium of his senses, could never discover the hidden nature of any thing, and just as little could he discover a disease.

When we have found out the disease, our next step is to search for the remedy.

Every disease is owing to some abnormal *irritation* of a peculiar character, which deranges the functions and well-being of our organs.

But the unity of the life of our organs and their concurrence to one common end does not permit two effects produced by abnormal general irritation to exist side by side and simultaneously in the human body. Hence our

First maxim of experience.

When two abnormal general irritations act simultaneously on the body, *if the two be dissimilar*, then the action of the one (the weaker) irritation will be suppressed and suspended for some time by the other (the stronger[1]); and, on the other hand, our

Second maxim of experience.

When the two irritations greatly resemble each other, then the one (the weaker) irritation, together with its effects, will be com-

---

[1] The maxim of experience will be better elucidated by another, namely: when (as is the case with palliatives) the general (medicinal) irritation that is applied is *the exact opposite* of that already existing in the body (the morbific irritation), the latter will be suppressed and suspended with remarkable rapidity—but when the general (medicinal) irritation employed is *dissimilar* and *heterogenous* to that already present in the body (the morbific irritation) *in every other respect* (as is the case in merely revolutionary modes of treatment, by revulsions and so-called general remedies), the morbific irritation will only be suppressed and suspended, provided the new irritation is much stronger than that already present in the system,—and only rapidly when this new irritation is excessively violent.

If the opposed, heterogenous, dissimilar irritations are diseases, of pretty much the same intensity, as however is rarely the case, so that they cannot suspend one another at all, or not for any length of time, then they (when uncured) unite to form a single disease which may moreover be cured as a single, uniform disease, notwithstanding that this kind has been termed *complex diseases*.

pletely extinguished and *annihilated* by the analogous power of the other (the stronger).

(*Illustration of the first maxim.*) If a person be infected at the same time by, for instance, the miasmata of measles and small-pox (two dissimilar irritations), and if the measles have appeared first, it immediately disappears on the day of the eruption of the small-pox, and it is only after the latter is completely gone that the measles again returns and completes its natural course. The red rash that had already commenced to shew itself disappeared, as I have frequently observed, on the eruption of the small-pox, and only completed its course when the small-pox was dried up.[1] According to Larrey, the plague of the Levant immediately remains stationary whenever the small-pox begins to prevail, but again returns when the latter ceases.

These two corporeal irritations are of a heterogeneous and dissimilar character, and the one is therefore suspended by the other—but only for a short time.

(*Illustration of the second maxim.*) If the two abnormal corporeal irritations be of a *similar* nature, then the weaker will be entirely removed by the stronger, so that *only one* (the stronger) completes its action, whilst the weaker was quite annihilated and extinguished. Thus the small-pox becomes an eradicator of the cow-pox; the latter is immediately interrupted in its course whenever the miasm of the small-pox that was previously latent in the system breaks out, and after the small-pox has run its course the cow-pox does not again appear.

The cow-pox miasm, which in addition to its well-known effect of developing the cow-pock with its course of two weeks' duration, has also the property of giving rise to a secondary eruption of small red pimples with red borders, particularly in the face and forearms (and under certain unknown circumstances it produces this effect usually soon after the desiccation of the pocks), permanently cures other cutaneous eruptions wherewith the inoculated person was already, though ever so long before, affected, *if this cutaneous disease was only tolerably similar to that cow-pox exanthema.*[2]

---

[1] I saw an infection of the epidemic febrile swelling of the parotid gland (mumps) immediately yield when the protective inoculation of the small pox had taken effect, and it was only after the lapse of fourteen days, when the areolar redness of the pocks had passed away, that the mumps again appeared and completed its regular course of seven days.

[2] That it is this secondary eruption (of pimples), or even the mere tendency of vaccine to cause this accessory eruption, but not the cow-pox itself which cures those

These two abnormal irritations cannot exist simultaneously in the same body, and thus the morbific irritation that appears last removes that which previously existed, not merely for a short time, but permanently, in consequence of being analogous to the latter; it extinguishes, annihilates and cures it completely.

It is the same thing in the treatment of diseases by means of medicines.

If the itch of workers in wool be treated by strong purgatives, such as jalap, it gradually yields almost completely, as long as the purgatives are continued, as the action of these two abnormal irritations cannot co-exist in the body; but as soon as the effect of the artificially excited irritation ceases, that is to say, henever the purgatives are discontinued, the suspended itch returns to its former state, because a dissimilar irritation does not remove and destroy the other, but only suppresses and suspends it for a time.

But if we introduce into a body affected by this itch a new irritant—of a different nature, it is true, but still of a very similar mode of action—as for example the calcareous liver of sulphur,[1] from which others besides myself have observed an eruption produced very similar in character to this itch, then, as two general abnormal irritations cannot co-exist in the body, the former yields to the latter, not for a short time merely, but permanently, as the last introduced was an irritation very analogous to the first; that is to say, the itch of the wool-workers is really cured by the employment of the calcareous liver of sulphur (and for the same reason by the use of sulphur powder and sulphureous baths).

Those diseases also which the casual observer considers as merely local[2] are either suppressed for some time by a fresh irri-

pustular exanthemata is evident from this, that these exanthemata remain almost unaltered as long as the proper cow-pox is running its course, and only disappear when the disease comes to the period corresponding to the occurrence of the secondary eruption of vaccinia, that is to say, after the cow-pocks are dried up. But the vaccine disease has a tendency to cause not only that secondary eruption of discrete, elevated pimples, but also another accessory eruption in the form of confluent miliary (and also exuding) tetters (but as it seems, not on the face, forearms and legs), and it is also capable of curing a similar cutaneous affection.

[1] The baths impregnated with sulphuretted hydrogen gas excite the same itch-like eruption, in the flexures of the joints especially, which itches most at night, and they therefore cure the itch of the wool-workers rapidly and radically.

[2] The unity of the life of all organs, and their concurrence to one common end, will hardly permit of a disease of the body being or remaining merely local, just as the action of no medicine can be purely local, in such a manner that the rest of the body shall take no part in it. It certainly takes a part, although in a somewhat less degree

29

tation applied to this part, where the two irritations are of dissimilar or opposite tendency, as, for example, the pain of a burnt hand is instantly suppressed and suspended by dipping it in cold water, as long as the immersion is continued, but it immediately recurs with renewed violence on withdrawing the hand from the water—or the first is entirely and permanently destroyed, that is to say, completely cured, when the last irritation is very analogous to the first.   Thus, when the action of the remedy, e. g., the artificial irritation applied to the burnt hand, is of a different nature, it is true, from the burning irritation of the fire, but of a very similar tendency, as is the case with highly concentrated alcohol, which when applied to the lips produces almost the same sensation as that caused by a flame approached to them, then the burnt skin, if it be constantly kept moistened with the spirit, is—in bad cases in the course of a few hours, in slighter ones much sooner—completely restored and permanently cured of the pain of the burn.   So true is it that two irritations, even when they are local, cannot co-exist in the body without the one suspending the other, if they are dissimilar, or the one removing the other, if the added one have a very similar mode of action and tendency.

---

than the place on which the so-called local affection is most obvious, or to which the so-called local medicine is applied.—Persons who suffer from herpes are, according to Larrey, exempted from the infection of plague, and the Europeans in Syria who have issues and perpetual blisters remain free from the infection of the Levantine plague, as observed in our own time by Larrey and in ancient times by G. F. van Hilden and F. Plater. So far are herpetic eruptions and artificial external ulcers from being purely local affections, that when they are present the system is not susceptible of such a violent and general irritation as the Levantine plague. But it is only during the continuance of this corporeal irritation, which is dissimilar to that it wards off, and no longer, that it can prevent its occurrence. Two children affected with epilepsy kept free from this disease (the epilepsy was suspended) as long as an eruption on the head that they both had persisted ; but when this healed up the epilepsy returned (N. Tulpius, lib. i. obs. 8). In like manner, obviously general diseases of the body have been—not cured, but suppressed and suspended by nature, which is powerless to cure them, by means of torpid ulcers of the legs, by the physician by means of issues, because both issues and ulcers of the legs, if they have existed some time, are abnormal general irritations ; but the attacks of apoplexy, asthma, &c., recur immediately when the ulcers of the legs and the issues heal up. An epileptic patient remained for a long time free from his attacks, as long as the issue was kept open, but the epilepsy returned immediately and in a worse shape than before, when it was allowed to close. (Pechlinus, Obs. phys. med. lib. ii, obs. 30). From this it is obvious that irritations apparently local, when they have existed some time, usually become general irritations of the body, and if they are sufficiently intense, can either suspend or cure general maladies of the body, according as the two opposed irritations were of heterogeneous or of analogous character.

In order therefore to be able *to cure,* we shall only require *to oppose to the existing abnormal irritation of the disease an appropriate medicine,* that is to say, *another morbific power whose effect is very similar to that the disease displays.*

As food is requisite for the healthy body, so medicines have been found efficacious in diseases; *medicines, however, are never in themselves and unconditionally wholesome, but only relatively so.*

The pure *aliments* of food and drink taken until hunger and thirst abate, support our strength, by replacing the parts lost in the vital processes, without disturbing the functions of our organs or impairing the health.

Those substances however which we term *medicines* are of a completely opposite nature. They afford no nourishment. They are abnormal irritants, only fitted for altering our healthy body, disturbing the vitality and the functions of the organs, and exciting disagreeable sensations, in one word, making the healthy ill.

There is no medicinal substance whatsoever that does not possess this tendency,[1] and no substance is medicinal which does not possess it.

It is only by this property of producing in the healthy body a series of specific morbid symptoms, that medicines can cure diseases, that is to say, remove and extinguish the morbid irritation by a suitable counter-irritation.

Every simple medicinal substance, like the specific morbific miasmata (small-pox, measles, the venom of vipers, the saliva of rabid animals, &c.), causes a peculiar specific disease—a series of determinate symptoms, which is not produced precisely in the same way by any other medicine in the world.

As every species of plant differs in its external form, in its peculiar mode of existence, in its taste, smell, &c., from every other species and genus of plant—as every mineral substance, every salt differs from all others both in its external and internal physical qualities, so do they all differ among themselves in

---

[1] A medicine which given to a healthy individual alone and uncombined, in sufficient quantity, causes a determinate *action,* a certain array of symptoms, retains the *tendency* to excite the same even in the very smallest dose.

The heroic medicines exhibit their action even when given in small doses, to healthy and even strong individuals. Those that have a weaker action must be given for these experiments in very considerable doses. The weakest medicines however only shew their absolute action in such subjects as are free from disease, who are delicate, irritable and sensitive;—in diseases, in like manner, they all (the weakest as well as the strongest medicines) shew their absolute actions, but so intermingled with the symptoms of the disease, that only a very experienced experimenter and fine observer can distinguish them.

their medicinal properties, that is to say, in their morbific powers; each of the substances effects an alteration in our state of health in a peculiar, determinate manner.

Most substances belonging to the animal and vegetable kingdoms,[1] are medicinal in their raw state. Those belonging to the mineral kingdom are so both in their crude and prepared state.

Medicinal substances manifest the nature of their pathogenetic power, and their absolute true action on the healthy human body, in the purest manner, when each is given singly and uncombined.

Many of the most active medicines have already occasionally found their way into the human body, and the accidents they have given rise to have been recorded.[2]

In order to follow still farther this natural guide and to penetrate more profoundly into this source of knowledge, we administer these medicines experimentally, the weaker as well as the stronger, each singly and uncombined, to healthy individuals, with caution, and carefully removing all accessory circumstances capable of exercising an influence, we note down the symptoms they occasion precisely in the order in which they occur, and thus we obtain the pure result of the form of disease that each of these medicinal substances is capable of producing, absolutely and by itself, in the human body.[3]

---

[1] Those plants and animals which we employ as food, have the advantage of containing a greater quantity of nutritious parts than the others, and moreover, their medicinal powers in their raw state are either not very great, or if they are great are destroyed and dissipated by drying (as in the case of arum-root), by the expression of the noxious juice (as in the case of the cassava), by fermentation, by smoking and by the power of the heat in roasting, baking and boiling, or are rendered innocuous by the addition of salt, sugar, and especially of vinegar (in sauces and salads). If we allow the recent expressed juice of the most deadly plants to remain only for a single day in some warm place, it undergoes the complete vinous fermentation and loses much of its medicinal power; if it stands several days, it passes through the acetous fermentation, whereby it loses all medicinal power, the sediment that is deposited from it is then perfectly harmless, and is similar to wheat starch.

[2] If we compare the occasional happy cures effected by these medicines, the most prejudiced person must be struck with the extraordinary resemblance that exists between the symptoms caused by the medicines on the healthy body, and those whereby the disease it cures is characterized.

[3] In order to ascertain the effects of less powerful medicines in this manner, we must give only one pretty strong dose to the temperate healthy person who is the subject of the experiment, and it is best to give it in solution. If we wish to ascertain the remaining symptoms, which were not revealed by the first trial, we may give to another person, or to the same individual, but only then after the lapse of several days, when the action of the first dose is fully over, a similar or even stronger portion, and note the symptoms of irritation thence resulting in the same careful and

In this way we must obtain a knowledge of a sufficient supply of artificial morbific agents (medicines) for curative implements, so that we may be able to make a selection from among them.[1]

Now, after we have accurately examined the disease to be cured, that is to say, noted down all its appreciable phenomena historically, and in the order in which they occur, marking particularly the more severe and troublesome chief symptoms, we have only to oppose to this disease another disease as like it as possible, or, in other words, a medicinal irritation analogous to the existing irritation of the disease, by the employment of a medicine which possesses the power of exciting as nearly as possible all these symptoms, or at all events, the greater number and severest, or most peculiar of them, and in the same order, —in order to cure the disease we wish to remove, certainly, quickly and permanently.

The result of a treatment so conformable to nature may be confidently depended on, it is so perfectly, without exception, certain, so rapid beyond all expectation, that no method of treating diseases can shew anything at all like it.

But here it is necessary to take into consideration the immense difference, that can never be sufficiently estimated, betwixt the positive and negative, or as they are sometimes termed, the radical (*curative*) and the *palliative* modes of treatment.

In the action of simple medicines on the healthy human body there occur in the first place phenomena and symptoms, which may be termed the *positive* disease, to be expected from the specific action of the medicinal substance, or its positive primary (first and principal) effect.

When this is past, there ensues, in hardly appreciable transi-

---

sceptical manner. For medicines that are still weaker we require, in addition to a considerable dose, individuals that are, it is true, healthy, but of very irritable delicate constitutions. The more obvious and striking symptoms must be recorded in the list, those that are of a dubious character should be marked with the sign of dubiety, until they have frequently been confirmed.

In the investigation of these medicinal symptoms, all suggestions must be as carefully avoided, as has been recommended for the investigation of the symptoms of disease. It must be chiefly the mere voluntary relation of the person who is the subject of the experiment, nothing like guess-work, nothing obtained by dint of cross questioning, that should be noted down as truth, and still less, expressions of sensations that have previously been put in the experimenter's mouth.

But how, even in diseases, amid the symptoms of the original disease, the medicinal symptoms may be discovered, is the subject for the exercise of a higher order of inductive minds, and must be left to masters only in the art of observation.

[1] My *Fragmenta de viribus medicamentorum* are something of this kind.

tions,[1] the exact opposite of the first process (especially in the case of vegetable medicines), there occur the exact opposite (negative) symptoms constituting the secondary action.

Now, if in the treatment of a disease we administer those medicines whose primary symptoms, or those of its positive action, present the greatest similarity to the phenomena of the disease, this is a *positive* or *curative* mode of treatment, that is to say, there occurs what must take place according to my second maxim of experience, rapid, permanent amelioration, for the completion of which the remedy must be given in smaller and smaller doses, repeated at longer intervals, to prevent the occurrence of a relapse; if the first, or first few doses have not already sufficed to effect a cure.[2]

Thus, to the abnormal irritation present in the body, another morbid irritation as similar to it as possible (by means of the medicine that acts in this case positively with its primary symptoms) is opposed in such a degree that the latter preponderates over the former, and (as two abnormal irritations cannot exist beside each other in the human body, and these are two irritations of the same kind) the complete extinction and annihilation of the former is effected by the latter.[2]

Here a new disease is certainly introduced (by the medicine) into the system, but with this difference in the result, that the original one is extinguished by the artificially excited one; but the course of the artificially excited one (the course of the medicinal symptoms), that has thus overcome the other, expires in a shorter time than any natural disease, be it ever so short.

It is astonishing that, when the positive (curative) medicine employed corresponds very exactly in its primary symptoms with those of the disease to be cured, not a trace of the secondary symptoms of the medicine is observable, but its whole action ceases just at the time when we might expect the commencement of the negative medicinal symptoms. The disease

---

[1] So that in this transition stage symptoms of the first order still alternate with symptoms of the second, until the second order attains the ascendancy and appears pure and unmixed.

[2] Thus, when a person accustomed to drinking brandy has heated and exhausted himself to the utmost by some rapid, violent exertion, (*e. g.* putting out a fire or reaping corn), and complains of burning heat, the most violent thirst and heaviness of the limbs, a single mouthful (half an ounce) of brandy will probably in less than half an hour, remove the thirst, heat, and heaviness of limbs, and make him quite well, because brandy given to healthy persons unaccustomed to its use, usually causes in its first action thirst, heat and heaviness of the limbs.

disappears if it belong to acute diseases in the first few hours, which are the duration allotted by nature to the primary medicinal symptoms, and the only visible result is—recovery—a real dynamic mutual extinction.

In the best cases the strength returns immediately, and the lingering period of convalescence usual under other modes of treatment is not met with.

Equally astonishing is the truth that there is no medicinal substance which, when employed in a curative manner, is weaker than the disease for which it is adapted—no morbid irritation for which the medicinal irritation of a positive and extremely analogous nature is not more than a match.

If we have not only selected the right (positive) remedy, but have also hit upon the proper dose (and for a curative purpose incredibly small doses suffice), the remedy produces within the first few hours after the dose has been taken a kind of slight aggravation (this seldom lasts so long as three hours), which the patient imagines to be an increase of his disease, but which is nothing more than the primary symptoms of the medicine, which are somewhat superior in intensity to the disease, and which ought to resemble the original malady so closely as to deceive the patient himself in the first hour, until the recovery that ensues after a few hours teaches him his mistake.

In this case the cure of an acute disease is generally accomplished by the first dose.

If, however, the first dose of the perfectly adapted curative medicine was not somewhat superior to the disease, and if that peculiar aggravation did not occur in the first hour, the disease is, notwithstanding, in a great measure extinguished, and it only requires a few and always smaller doses to annihilate it completely.[1]

If, under these circumstances, in place of smaller doses, as large or larger ones are administered, there arise (after the disappearance of the original disease) pure medicinal symptoms, a kind of unnecessary artificial disease.[2]

---

[1] In the more special part I shall discuss how far it is necessary in the treatment of chronic diseases, even after the complete restoration of health, to continue giving for some months longer a small quantity of the same medicine that cured the disease, but at ever longer and longer intervals, in order to eradicate every trace of the chronic disease in the organism that has been for years accustomed to its presence.

[2] Should we observe that the person recovering under the action of the curative medicine requires to continue taking an equally large or even larger dose in order to prevent a relapse, this is a positive sign that the cause that has produced the disease

But the case is quite different with *palliative* treatment, where *a medicine is employed whose positive, primary action is the opposite of the disease.*

Almost immediately after the administration of such a medicine there occurs a kind of alleviation, an almost instantaneous suppression of the morbid irritation for a short time,[1] as in the case cited above of the cold water applied to the burnt skin. These are called *palliative remedies.*

They prevent the impression of the morbid irritation on the organism only as long as their primary symptoms last, because they present to the body an irritation that is the reverse of the irritation of the disease; thereafter their secondary action commences, and as it is the opposite of their primary action, it coincides with the original morbid irritation and aggravates it.[2]

During the secondary action of the palliative, and when it has been left off, the disease becomes aggravated. The pain of the burn becomes worse when the hand is withdrawn from the cold water than before it was immersed.

As in the (positive) curative mode of treatment in the first

---

still exists, and this must be removed to render the recovery permanent—an error of diet (abuse of tea, coffee, wine, spirits, &c.), or some other pernicious habit [*e. g.* prolonged suckling of delicate females, the abuse of the sexual function, sedentary habits, continued quarrelling, &c.]

[1] See the first maxim of experience and the observation attached to it.

[2] Ignorance of this maxim of experience was the cause why physicians have hitherto selected, almost exclusively, palliative remedies for the treatment of diseases ; the flattering, almost instantaneously ameliorating action that first ensued deceived them. In like manner the parents of a morally diseased (naughty) child deceive themselves when they imagine that a sweet cake is the remedy for its peevishness and rudeness. It certainly grows quiet immediately after receiving the first cake, but on the occasion of another fit of wilfulness, bawling and noise from unruliness, the palliative cake again given does not prove so efficacious ; we must give it more cake, and must at last overload it with cakes, and yet at last this produces no good result. The child has, on the contrary, only become more stubborn, naughty and unruly in consequence of the palliative. The poor parents have now recourse to other palliatives ; toys, new clothes, flattering words—until at length these are no longer of any avail, and gradually induce the opposite state, an increase of the original moral disease in the child it was wished to cure, namely, confirmed naughtiness, stubbornness, wildness. If, at the beginning and on the very first occasion in which it beat or scratched its brothers or sisters or attendants, the curative agents of reprimand and the rod had been employed in adequately strong dose, and repeated a few times on the occasion of subsequent (assuredly slighter) fits of passion, they would not have failed to cure the malady positively, permanently and radically. The naughty child would, it is true, on the first application of the rod, and for the first half hour, prove somewhat more unruly, bawl and cry somewhat louder, but it would subsequently become all the more quiet and docile.

hour a slight aggravation usually ensues, followed by an amelioration and recovery all the more durable, so in the palliative method there occurs in the first hour, indeed almost instantaneously, a (deceptive) amelioration, which, however, diminishes from hour to hour, until the period of the primary, and in this case palliative, action expires, and not only allows the disease to reappear as it was before the use of the remedy, but somewhat of the secondary action of the medicine is added, which, because the primary action of the remedy was the opposite of the disease, now becomes the very reverse, that is to say, a state analogous to the disease. This state is an increase, an aggravation of the disease.

If it is wished to repeat the palliative aid, the former dose will now no longer suffice; it must be increased,[1] and always still further increased, until the medicine no longer produces relief, or until the accessory effects, whatever these may be, of the medicine continued in ever increased doses, are productive of bad consequences, that forbid its further employment, bad consequences which, when they have attained a considerable height, suppress the original malady that has hitherto been treated (in conformity with the first maxim of experience), and, in place thereof, another new and at least as troublesome disease appears.[2]

Thus, for instance, a chronic sleeplessness may be frequently suppressed for a considerable time by means of daily doses of opium given at night, because its (in this case palliative) primary action is soporific, but (in consequence of its secondary action being sleeplessness, accordingly an addition to the original

---

[1] In addition to innumerable other confirmative examples see J. H, Schulze's *Diss. qua corporis humani momentanearum alterationum specimina quaedam expenduntur.* Halae, 1741, § 18. Besides the increase of the dose, we see also that recourse is had to a frequent change of palliatives, at least in those chronic diseases for which there are many, as, for example, in hysterical fits. Thus we see the changes rung so long and so frequently on asafœtida, castor, galbanum, sagapenum, hartshorn, tincture of amber, and finally opium in ever increased doses (for each of these is in its primary action only the probable opposite of the disease and not its analogue, consequently only the first two or three doses of them give relief, but on subsequent occasions they produce less and at length no amelioration)—in order to give some alleviation as long as that can be done—until the store of palliatives is exhausted, or until the patient is tired of these undurable cures, or is afflicted with a new disease from the secondary action of these medicines, which now requires another mode of treatment.

[2] If we are so fortunate as to succeed in removing this disease caused by the palliative, the first original one generally reappears, shewing that (according to the first maxim of experience) it has only been pushed aside and suspended by the newly developed, dissimilarly irritating disease, but that it has not been destroyed or cured

disease) that only by means of ever increasing doses, until an intolerable constipation, an anasarca, an asthma, or other malady from the secondary action of opium, prohibits its further employment.

If however, but a few doses of the palliative medicine be employed for a habitual malady, and then discontinued before it can excite an important accessory affection, it is then speedily and clearly apparent, that it is not only impotent against the original malady, but that it moreover aggravated the latter by its secondary effects. This is truly but *negative* relief. If for instance, in the case of chronic agrypnia sought to be cured, the patient only obtained too little sleep, in that case the evening dose of opium will certainly immediately cause a kind of sleep, but when this remedy, which here acts only in a palliative manner, is discontinued after a few days, the patient will then not be able to sleep at all.[1]

The palliative employment of medicines is only useful and necessary in but few cases—chiefly in such as have arisen suddenly and threaten almost immediate danger!

Thus, for example, in apparent death from freezing (after friction to the skin and the gradual elevation of the temperature) nothing removes more quickly the want of irritability in the muscular fibre, and the insensibility of the nerves, than a strong infusion of coffee, which in its primary action increases the mobility of the fibre and the sensibility of all the sensitive parts of the system; and is consequently palliative as regards the case before us. But in this case there is danger in delay, and yet there is no persistent morbid state to be overcome, but whenever sensation and irritability are again excited and brought into action even by a palliative, the uninjured organism resumes its functions, and the free play of the vital processes maintains itself again, without the aid of any further medication.

In like manner, cases of chronic diseases may occur, for ex-

---

[1] If we have to combat a case of excessive sleepiness, opium, being a medicinal irritant, very analogous in its primary action to the disease before us, will remove it in the very smallest dose, and if some of the other primary effects of this medicine (*e. g.* snoring in a state of comatose sleep, with open mouth, half shut eyes, with the pupils directed upwards, talking in sleep, want of recollection on awaking, inability to recognise those around, &c.,) resemble those symptoms present in the disease, (as is not unfrequently the case in typhoid diseases) the original malady is overcome rapidly and permanently, and without any after-symptoms, the opinion being in this case a curative and positive remedy.

ample, hysterical convulsions or asphyxias, where the temporary assistance of palliatives (as *eau de luce*, burnt feathers, &c.,) may be urgently demanded, in order to restore the patient to his usual undangerous morbid state, for the cure of which, the totally different durable aid of curative medicines is required.

But where all that is capable of being affected by a palliative is not accomplished in a few hours, the bad consequences spoken of above commence to make their appearance.

In acute diseases, even such as run their course in the shortest time, we would better consult the dignity of medicine and the welfare of our patients, by treating them with curative (positive) medicines. They will thereby be overcome more certainly, and on the whole more rapidly, *and without after-complaints*.

However, the bad consequences of the palliative[1] in *slight* cases of acute diseases are *not very striking, not very considerable*. The chief symptoms disappear in a great measure after each dose of the palliative, until the natural course of the disease comes to an end, and then the organism, which has not been very seriously deranged during the short time by the secondary effects of the palliative, again resumes its sway, and gradually overcomes the consequences of the disease itself, together with the after-sufferings caused by the medicine.

If, however, the patient recover under the use of the palliative, he would also have recovered equally well and in the same space of time, without any medicine (for palliatives never shorten the natural courses of acute diseases), and would thereafter more readily regain his strength for the reasons just given. The only circumstance that can in some measure recommend the physician who practises in this way, namely, that the troublesome symptoms are occasionally subdued by his palliatives, offers to the eyes of the patient and his friends some apparent, but no real advantage over the spontaneous recovery without the use of medicine.

Hence the curative and positive treatment possesses even in diseases of a rapid course, a decided advantage over all palliative alleviations, because it abridges even the natural periods of acute diseases, really heals them before the time for completing their course has expired, and leaves behind no after-sufferings,

---

[1] This circumstance also makes palliatives unserviceable, that each of them is usually employed to subdue a single symptom only—the remaining symptoms either rest untouched, or are combatted by other palliatives, which all possess accessory actions that stand in the way of recovery.

provided the perfectly suitable curative agent has been selected.

It might be objected to this mode of treatment, "that physicians from the earliest periods of the existence of the medical art, have (to their knowledge) never employed it, and yet have cured patients."

This objection is only apparent; for ever since the existence of the art of medicine, there have been patients who have really been cured quickly, permanently, and manifestly by medicines, not by the spontaneous termination of the course of acute diseases, not in the course of time, not by the gradual preponderance of the energy of the system, but have been restored in the same manner as I have here described, by the curative action of a medicinal agent, although this was unknown to the physician.[1]

Occasionally,[2] however, physicians suspected that it was that

---

[1] In order to determine this, we must select the cases detailed by some perfectly truthful and accurate observer, where some disease not of an acute character, limited by nature to a certain short course, but some long-lasting disease, was cured permanently and without any sequelæ, not by a mixture of all sorts of different drugs, but by a single medicinal substance. This we should certainly find to have been a (curative) medicine very analogous in its primary effects to the disease. Had it been a palliative, given in ever increasing doses, the apparent cure would not have been permanent, or at least, not without some after-disease. Unless by the instrumentality of a positive (curative) medicine, no rapid, gentle, permanent cure ever took place, nor in the nature of things, could it ever occur.

In the strikingly rapid and permanent cures by means of composite prescriptions (if indeed the mixture of several drugs of unknown properties, in order to accomplish some equally unknown end, deserves a scientific notice), we shall likewise find the remedy that strongly predominates in it to be of a positive character—or the mixture constituted a medicine, of combined interminable action, in which each ingredient did not perform its own proper function, but was altered in its action by the others, and where in consequence of the mutual dynamic neutralizations that occurred, an unknown medicine remained, which effected in this case what no mortal can divine wherefore it did it, and what, for a variety of reasons (dependent on the frequently different strength of the individual drugs in different laboratories, on the mode of mixing the compound, which can hardly be performed in exactly the same way again, and on the constant variety that exists among cases of nominally the same disease) can never be imitated again; in one of the above mentioned peculiar or ' miasmatic diseases that always remain identical.

[2] Thus Hippocrates, or the author of the book entitled Περὶ τόπων τῶν κατ' ἄνθρωπων (Basil. 1538, frob. pag. 72, lin. 35.) has these remarkable words : διὰ τὰ ὅμοια νοῦσος γίνεται, καὶ διὰ τὰ ὅμοια προςφερόμενα ἐκ νοσεύντων ὑγιάνονται· ὅιον στραγγουρίην τὸ αὐτὸ ποιίει οὐκ ἐοῦσαν, καὶ ἐοῦσαν τὸ αὐτὸ παύει· καὶ βὴξ κατὰ τὸ αὐτὸ, ὥσπερ ἡ στραγγουρίη ὑπὸ τῶν αὐτῶν γίνεται καὶ παίεται—διὰ τὸ ἐμέειν ἔμετος παύεται.—In like manner, some later physicians have occasionally noticed that the power of rhubarb in producing belly-ache was the cause of its colic-subduing virtues, and that in the emetic property of ipecacuanha lay the reason why it checked vomiting in small doses. Thus Detharding (*Eph. nat. cur.*, cent. 10, obs. 76) saw that an infusion of senna-leaves, which

property of medicines (now confirmed by innumerable observations)—of exciting (positive) symptoms analogous to the disease, by virtue of a tendency inherent in them—which enabled them to effect real cures. But this ray of truth, I confess, seldom penetrated the spirit of our schools, enshrouded as they were in a cloud of systems.

When the remedy has been discovered by this mode of procedure, so conformable to nature, there still remains an important point, namely, the determination of the dose.

A medicine of a positive and curative character, may, without any fault on its part, do just the opposite to what it ought, if given in too large a dose; in that case it produces a greater disease than that already present.

If we keep a healthy hand in cold water for some minutes, we experience in it a diminution of temperature, cold; the veins become invisible, the fleshy parts become shrunken, their size is diminished, the skin is paler, duller, motion is more difficult. These are some of the primary effects of cold water on the healthy body. If we now withdraw the hand from the cold water and dry it, no long time will elapse before the opposite state ensues. The hand becomes warmer than the other (that had not been immersed), we notice considerable turgescence of the soft parts, the veins swell, the skin becomes redder, the movements more free and powerful than in the other—a kind of exalted vitality. This is the secondary or consecutive action of the cold water on the healthy body.

This is, moreover, almost the greatest dose in which cold water can be employed with a permanent good result, as a positive (curative) medicinal agent in a state of (pure) debility analagous to its above described primary effects on the healthy body. I repeat, the " greatest dose "; for if the whole body should be exposed to the action of this agent, and if the cold of the water be very considerable,[1] the duration of its application must at least be very much shortened, to a few seconds only, in order to reduce the dose sufficiently.

But if the dose of this remedy be in all respects much increased above the normal amount, the morbid symptoms peculiar

causes colic in healthy persons, cured colics in adults and he is of opinion that this must be caused by analogy of action. I need not dwell on the propositions of others (J. D. Major, A. Brendelius, A. F. Dankwerts, &c.) to cure one disease by means of another artificially excited disease.

[1] In a greater amount of debility 70° may be proportionately as considerable a degree of cold in the water, as 60° for a less amount.

to the primary action of the cold water increase to a state of actual disease, which the weak part it was intended to cure by its means cannot or can scarcely remove again. If the dose be increased still more, if the water be very cold,[1] if the surface exposed to the water be larger[2] and the duration of its application much longer than it ought to be for an ordinary curative dose of this agent,[3] there then ensue numbness of the whole limb, cramp of the muscles, often even paralysis;[4] and if the whole body have been immersed in this cold water for an hour or longer, death ensues, or at least the apparent death from freezing in healthy individuals, but much more speedily when it is applied to feeble individuals.

The same is the case with all medicines, even with internal ones.

The reaper (unaccustomed to the use of spirits) exhausted by heat, exertion and thirst, who, as I have said above, is restored in the course of an hour by a small dose, a single mouthful of brandy (whose primary action shews a state very similar to that sought to be combatted in the present instance), would fall into a state of (probably fatal) synochus, if under these circumstances he were to drink, in place of a single mouthful, a couple of pints at once;—the same positive remedial agent, only in an excessive, injurious dose.

Let it not be supposed that this injurious effect of excessively large doses appertains only to medicinal agents applied in a positive (curative) manner. Equally bad results ensue from excessive doses of *palliatives*,—for medicines are substances in themselves hurtful, that only become remedial agents by the adaptation of their natural pathogenetic power to the disease

---

[1] For example, 40° Fahr.

[2] For example, the entire leg.

[3] For example, two hours.

[4] There are, no doubt, exceptions to this, where advantage has followed from excessively large doses of the positive (curative) medicinal agent, in certain cases that occasionally come under the observation of the master in the art. Thus I saw the remedial power of the primary paralysing action of a very large dose of this agent, strikingly illustrated in the case of a man (in Thuringia) whose right arm had been for many years almost completely paralysed, and always as if numb and cold. In the Christmas season he wished to get some fish out of a frozen tank, in order to give a treat to some of his friends. He could not catch them with his left arm alone; he required to employ the lame arm also, which was not capable of so much movement. He might have been engaged with it in the ice-cold water for upwards of half-an-hour. The consequence of this was, that soon afterwards the paralysed arm inflamed and swelled, but in a few days it got quite well and as strong as the other; the paralysis was permanently cured.

(positively or negatively) analogous to them, *in the appropriate dose.*

Thus, to give an example of negative (palliative) medicines, a hand very much benumbed by cold, will soon be restored in the atmosphere of a warm room.[1] This moderate degree of warmth is efficacious in this case as an agent of antagonistic tendency to the numbness from the cold, that is to say, as a palliative; but its employment is not attended with any particular bad effects, because the dose is not too strong and the remedy need only be used for a short time, in order to remove the moderate and rapidly produced morbid state it is wished to cure.

But let the hand which has become completely benumbed and quite insensible from the cold (frost-bitten), be quickly immersed for an hour in water of 120° Fahr., which is not too great for a healthy hand, and the part will inevitably die; the hand mortifies and falls off.

A robust man, much over-heated, will soon recover in a moderately cool atmosphere (about 65° Fahr.) without experiencing any appreciable disadvantage from this palliative; but if immediately after being so over-heated he has to stand for an hour in a cold river (wherein he might probably have remained without any bad result when not in a state of heat), he will either fall down dead, or be effected by the most dangerous typhus.

A burnt part will be alleviated in a palliative manner by cool water, but will become sphacelated if ice be applied to it.

And the same is the case with internal remedies also. If a girl, excessively over-heated by dancing, swallow a quantity of ice, every one knows what usually ensues,—and yet a small tablespoonful of cold water or a minute quantity of ice would not do her any harm, although it is the same palliative, only in a smaller dose. But she would be certainly and permanently cured, even though excessively over-heated, if she were to chose a small, appropriate dose of a remedy whose primary effect is analogous (curative) to the state she is in; for instance, if she should drink a little very warm tea mixed with a small portion of heating spirituous liquor,[2] (rum, arrack or the like), in a

---

[1] For example, of 80° Fahr. at a distance from the stove.

[2] This latter example shews at the same time the correctness of the maxim, that when the morbid state is in an extreme degree, and we have only a few hours to effect the cure, the employment of the positive (curative) medicinal agent in a very small dose is infinitely preferable to that of the palliative, even though the latter be at first administered in a very small quantity. Even should the latter do no harm, it is at

moderately heated room, walking quickly about;—but a large glass of alcoholic liquor would, on the other hand, throw her into a high fever.

None but the careful observer can have any idea of the height to which the sensitiveness of the body to medicinal irritations is increased in a state of disease. It exceeds all belief, when the disease has attained a great intensity. An insensible, prostrated, comatose typhus patient, unroused by any shaking, deaf to all calling, will be rapidly restored to consciousness by the smallest dose of opium, were it a million times smaller than any mortal ever yet prescribed.

The sensitiveness of the highly diseased body to medicinal irritations increases in many cases to such a degree, that powers commence to act on and excite him, whose very existence has been denied, because they manifest no action on healthy robust bodies, nor in many diseases for which they are not suited. As an example of this, I may mentiom the heroic power of *animalism* (animal magnetism), or that immaterial influence of one living body upon another produced by certain kinds of touching or approximation, which displays such an energetic action on very sensitive, delicately formed persons of both sexes, who are disposed either to violent mental emotions or to great irritability of the muscular fibres. This animal power does not manifest itself at all between two robust healthy persons,—not because it does not exist, but because, according to the wise purposes of God, it is much too weak to shew itself betwixt healthy persons, whereas the same influence (quite imperceptible when applied by one healthy person to another) often acts with more than excessive violence in those states of morbid sensibility and irritability,—just as very small doses of other curative medicines also do in very diseased bodies.

It is analogous to the medicinal powers of the application of the magnet in disease and the contact of a morbid part with the other metals, to which the healthy body is quite insensible.

On the other hand, it is as true as it is wonderful, that even the most robust individuals, when affected by the chronic disease, notwithstanding their corporeal strength, and notwithstanding that they can bear with impunity even noxious irritants in great

---

all events certain that it does no good, whereas the smallest dose of the suitable curative agent can save life, though there may be only a few hours for the performance of the cure.

quantity (excesses in food and alcoholic liquors, purgatives, &c.)—yet as soon as the medicinal substance positively appropriate to their chronic disease is administered to them, they experience from the smallest possible dose as great an impression as if they were infants at the breast.

There are some few substances employed in medicine which act almost solely in a chemical manner—some which condense the dead fibres as well as the living (as the tannin of plants), or loosen them and diminish their cohesion or their tension (as the fatty substances)—some which form a chemical combination with hurtful substances in the body, at least in the primæ viæ (as chalk or the alkalies which combine with some deleterious metallic oxydes or some acrid acid in the stomach—sulphuretted hydrogen water with the most dangerous metals and their oxydes); others which decompose them (as alkalies or liver of sulphur do the noxious metallic salts) ; others which chemically destroy parts of the body (as the actual cautery). *With the exception* of these few things and the almost purely mechanical operations of surgery on the body, amputation which merely shortens the limb, and blood-letting which merely diminishes the amount of that fluid, together with some mechanically injurious and insoluble substances that may be introduced into the body—*all other medicinal substances act in a purely dynamic manner,*[1] and cure without causing evacuations, without producing any violent or even perceptible revolutions.

---

[1] In the change of diseases into health, as rapid and direct as it is powerful and mild, by means of the positive (curative) and dynamic mode of treatment, all those abnormal assaults on the organism called constitutional remedies, revulsions and evacuations, all emetics, purgatives, diaphoretics, and so forth, are as useless as they are injurious. The medicines employed for their production accomplish these revolutionary, disturbing, violent effects chiefly by the excessive doses in which they are given The various specific medicinal properties of tartar emetic, ipecacuanha, usarum, &c., are not perceived during their abuse as emetics, but by these properties they may become much more efficient remedial agents when used in small doses. In like manner, the many medicinal virtues of those substances abused as purgatives (for which object the true physician almost never or very rarely requires them) are designed for far more useful ends than they have hitherto been used for. It is only when they are given in excess that they cause that tumultuous, hurtful effect—and almost all other medicines may become emetics and purgatives if administered in over-doses. The so-called deranged stomach, the so-called signs of fermenting, impurities in the primæ viæ, and of disorder or disturbance of the bile, such as bitter taste, headache, anorexia, disgust, nausea, stomach-ache, and constipation, usually indicate a treatment totally different from violent emetics and purgatives ; the disease in *its whole extent* is often completely removed in a few hours by a couple of

30

This *dynamic* action of medicines, like the vitality itself, by means of which it is reflected upon the organism, is almost purely *spiritual* in its nature; that of medicines used in a positive (curative) manner is so most strikingly with this singular peculiarity, that while too strong doses do harm and produce considerable disturbance in the system, a small dose, and even the *smallest possible* dose, cannot be inefficacious, if the remedy be only otherwise indicated.

Almost the sole condition necessary for the full and helpful action is that the appropriate remedy should come in contact with the susceptible living fibre; but it is of little, almost of no importance how small the dose is which, for this purpose, is brought to act on the sensitive parts of the living body.

If a certain small dose of a diluted tincture of opium is capable of removing a certain degree of unnatural sleepiness, the hundredth or even the thousandth part of the same dose of such a solution of opium suffices almost equally well for the same end, and in this way the diminution of the dose may be carried *much farther* without the excessively minute dose ceasing to produce the same curative result as the first; of which more will be said in the special part.

I have said that the contact of the medicinal substance with the living, sensitive fibre is almost the only condition for its action. This dynamic property is so pervading, that it is quite immaterial what sensitive part of the body is touched by the medicine in order to develope its whole action, provided the part be but destitute of the coarser epidermis—immaterial whether the dissolved medicine enter the stomach or merely remain in the mouth, or be applied to a wound or other part deprived of skin.

If there be no fear of its causing any evacuation (a peculiar vital process of the living organism, which possesses a peculiar power of nullifying and destroying the dynamic efficacy of the medicines), its introduction into the rectum or application to the lining membrane of the nose, fulfils every purpose, *e. g.*, in the case of a medicine which has the power of curing a certain pain in the stomach, a particular kind of headache, or a kind of stitch

---

drops of the appropriate curative medicine, and all those threatening symptoms at once disappear, without evacuations and in such an imperceptible manner that one knows not whither they have gone.

It is only when substances of a completely indigestible, or foreign and very poisonous nature, oppress the stomach and bowels, that it is permitted in some few cases to effect their expulsion by such evacuant medicines.

in the side, or a cramp in the calves, or any other affection occurring in some part that stands in no anatomical connexion with the place to which the medicine is applied.

It is only the thicker epidermis covering the external surface of the body that presents some, but not an insurmountable obstacle to the action of medicines on the sensitive fibres underneath it. They still act through it, though somewhat less powerfully. Dry preparations of the medicine in powder act less powerfully through it; its solution acts more powerfully, and still more so if it be applied to a large surface.

The epidermis is however thinner on some parts, and consequently the action is easier in those situations. Among these the abdominal region, especially the pit of the stomach, the inguinal regions and the inner surface of the axilla, the bend of the arm, the inner surface of the wrist, the popliteal space, &c., are the parts most sensitive to the medicine.

Rubbing-in the medicines facilitates their action chiefly on this account, that the friction of itself renders the skin more sensitive, and the fibres, rendered thereby more active and susceptible, more apt to receive the impression of the specific medicinal power, which radiates thence over the whole organism.

If the groins be rubbed with a dry cloth until their sensibility is exalted, and the ointment of the black oxyde of mercury then laid upon them, the effect is the same as though we had rubbed the same place with the mercurial ointment itself, or as though the ointment had been rubbed in, as it is usually incorrectly expressed.

The peculiar medicinal power of the remedy, however, remains the same, whether it be employed outwardly or inwardly, so as to be brought into contact with the sensitive fibres.

The black oxyde of mercury taken by the mouth cures venereal buboes at least as rapidly and certainly as the rubbing-in of Naples ointment upon the groins. A foot-bath of a weak solution of muriate of mercury cures ulcers in the mouth as rapidly and certainly as its internal administration, especially if the part that is to be bathed be previously rubbed. Finely levigated cinchona powder applied to the abdomen cures the intermittent fever which it can cure by internal use.

But as the diseased organism is altogether much more sensitive for the dynamic power of all medicines, so also is the skin of diseased persons. A moderate quantity of tincture of ipecacuanha applied to the bend of the arm effectually removes the tendency to vomit in very sick individuals (by means of its primary power to excite vomiting).

The medicinal power of heat and cold alone seems not to be so exclusively dynamic as that of other medicinal substances. Where these two agents are employed in a positive manner, the smallest possible dose of them does not suffice to produce the desired effect. When it is requisite to obtain relief rapidly they both have to be employed in greater intensity, in a larger dose (up to a certain amount). But this appearance is deceptive; their power is just as dynamically medicinal as that of other medicines, and the difference in given cases depends on the already existing habituation of our body to certain doses of these stimuli, to certain degrees of heat and cold. The heat and cold to be employed in a medicinal manner must surpass this accustomed degree *by a little*, in order that it may be employed in a positive manner with success (*by a great deal*, if it is to be used in a negative or palliative manner).

The temperature of blood-heat is for most people in our climate higher than the usual degree for the skin, and consequently a footbath of 98° to 99° Fahr. is sufficiently temperate and warm enough to remove positively heat in the head (if no other morbid symptoms are present); but in order to alleviate in a palliative manner the inflammation of a burnt hand, we require to use water considerably colder than we are accustomed to bear comfortably in healthy parts of the body, and the water should be, within certain limits, so much the colder the more severe the inflammation is.[1]

What I have here stated respecting the somewhat greater dose of heat and cold for curative purposes applies also to all other medicinal agents to which the patient has already been accustomed. Thus for medicinal purposes we require to administer to persons hitherto accustomed to their use doses of wine, spirits, opium, coffee, &c., large in proportion to the amount they were previously accustomed to.

Heat and cold, together with electricity, belong to the most diffusible of all dynamic medicinal stimuli, their power is not

---

[1] At first we require for this palliative amelioration, even should the inflammation be great, only a cool water of about 70° Fahr., but from hour to hour we must use somewhat colder water; at length as much as well-cold (52° Fahr.) and even beyond that, in order to obtain the same amount of relief as at first (and provided we know no better remedy). We must from time to time increase the degree of cold, as is required in the internal employment of other palliative means.

diminished nor arrested by the epidermis, probably because its physical property serves as a conductor and vehicle for their medicinal power, and thus helps to distribute them. The same may be the case with regard to animalism (animal magnetism) the medicinal action of the magnet, and in general with regard to the power of the external contact of metals. The galvanic power is somewhat less capable of penetrating through the epidermis.

If we observe attentively we shall perceive that wise nature produces the greatest effects with simple, often with small means. To imitate her in this should be the highest aim of the reflecting mind. But the greater the number of means and appliances we heap together in order to attain a single object, the farther do we stray from the precepts of our great instructress, and the more miserable will be our work.

With a few simple means, used singly one after the other, more frequently however with one alone, we may restore to normal harmony the greatest derangements of the diseased body, we may change the most chronic, apparently incurable diseases (not unfrequently in the shortest space of time) into health—whereas we may, by the employment of a heap of ill-selected and composite remedies, see the most insignificant maladies degenerate into the greatest, most formidable, and most incurable diseases.

Which of these two methods will the professor of the healing art who strives after perfection, choose?

A single simple remedy is *always* calculated to produce the most beneficial effects, without any additional means; provided it be the best selected, the most appropriate, and in the proper dose. It is *never* requisite to mix two of them together.

We administer a medicine in order if possible to remove the whole disease by this single substance, or if this be not completely practicable, to observe from the effect of the medicine what still remains to be cured. One, two, or at most three simple medicines are sufficient for the removal of the greatest disease, and if this result does not follow, the fault lies with us; it is not nature, nor the disease, that is to blame.

If we wish to perceive clearly what the remedy effects in a disease, and what still remains to be done, we must only give one single simple substance at a time. Every addition of a second or a third only deranges the object we have in view, and when we wish to separate the effects of the remedy from the symptoms of the morbid process (seeing that at the most we may indeed be able to know the symptoms of the action of a simple medicine, but not the powers of a mixture of drugs, that either form combinations among, or are decomposed by, one another, and these it will never be possible for us to know), we now no longer see what portion of the changes that have taken place is to be ascribed to the disease,—we are unable to distinguish which of the changes and symptoms that have occurred are derived from one, which from another ingredient of the compound remedy, and consequently we are unable to determine which of the ingredients should be retained and which discarded during the subsequent treatment,—nor what other one we should substitute for one or other or for all of them. In such a treatment none of the phenomena can be referred to its true cause. Wherever we turn, nought but uncertainty and obscurity surrounds us.

Most simple medicinal substances produce in the healthy human body not few, but on the contrary, a considerable array of absolute symptoms. The appropriate remedy can consequently frequently contain among its primary effects an antitype of most of the visible symptoms in the disease to be cured (besides many others which render it suitable for the cure of other diseases).

Now the only desirable property that we can expect a medicine to possess, is this, that it should agree with the disease—in other words, that it should be capable of exciting *per se* the most of the symptoms observable in the disease, consequently, when employed antagonistically as a medicine, should also be able to destroy and extinguish the same symptoms in the diseased body.

We see that a single simple medicinal substance possesses in itself this property in its full extent, if it have been carefully selected for this purpose.

It is therefore never necessary to administer more than one single simple medicinal substance at once, if it have been chosen appropriately to the case of disease.

It is also very probable, indeed certain, that of the several medicines in a mixture, each no longer acts upon the disease in its own peculiar way, nor can it, undisturbed by the other ingredients, exert its specific effect,—but one acts in opposition to the other in the body, alters and in part destroys the action of the other, so that from this combination of several powers that dynamically decompose each other during their action in the body, an intermediate action is the result, which we cannot desire, as we cannot foresee, nor even form a conjecture respecting it.

In the action of mixtures of medicines in the body, there occurs what, indeed, must occur according to the maxim of experience given above (viz.:—that a general irritation in the body removes another, or else suppresses it, according as the one irritation is analagous or antagonistic to the other, or provided the one be much more intense than the other)—the actions of several of the medicines in the compound partially destroy one another,[1] and only the remainder of the action, which is not covered by any antagonistic irritation in the mixture, remains to oppose the disease; whether this be suitable or no, we cannot tell, as we are unable to calculate what actually will remain.

Now, as in every case, only a single simple medicinal substance is necessary; no true physician would ever think of degrading himself and his art, and defeating his own object, by giving a mixture of medicines. It will rather be a sign that he is certain of his subject if we find him prescribing only a single medicinal substance, which, if suitably chosen, cannot fail to remove the disease rapidly, gently and permanently.

If the symptoms be but slight and few in number, it is an unimportant ailment that scarcely requires any medicine, and may be removed by a mere alteration of diet or regimen.

But if—as rarely happens—only one or a couple of severe symptoms be observable, then the cure is more difficult than if many symptoms were present. In that case the medicine first prescribed may not be exactly suitable, either because the patient is incapable of describing the extent of his ailments, or because the symptoms themselves are somewhat obscure and not very observable.

In this more uncommon case we may prescribe one, or at most, two doses of the medicine that appears to be the most appropriate.

It will sometimes happen that this is the right remedy. In

---

[1] This is the reason why the frequently enormous doses of heroic medicines of various kinds in a complex prescription are often taken without any great effect. A single one of these powerful ingredients would often occasion death in the large dose.

the event of its not being exactly suitable, which is most commonly the case, symptoms not hitherto experienced will reveal themselves, or symptoms will develop themselves more fully, that the patient has not previously noticed, or only in an indistinct manner.

From these symptoms which, though slight, now shew themselves more frequently and are more distinctly perceptible, we may now obtain a more accurate picture of the disease, whereby we may be enabled to discover with greater and even the greatest certainty the most appropriate remedy for the original disease.

The repetition of the doses of a medicine is regulated by the duration of the action of each medicine. If the remedy acts in a positive (curative) manner, the amendment is still perceptible after the duration of its action has expired, and then another dose of the suitable remedy destroys the remainder of the disease. The good work will not be interrupted if the second dose be not given before the lapse of some hours after the cessation of the action of the remedy. The portion of the disease already annihilated cannot in the mean time be renewed; and even should we leave the patient several days without medicine, the amelioration resulting from the first dose of the curative medicine will always remain manifest.

So far from the good effect being delayed by not repeating the dose until after the medicine has exhausted its action, the cure may on the contrary be frustrated by its too rapid repetition, for this reason, because a dose prescribed before the cessation of the term of action of the positive medicine is to be regarded as an augmentation of the first dose, which from ignorance of this circumstance may thereby be increased to an enormous degree, and then prove hurtful by reason of its excess.

I have already stated that the smallest possible dose of a positively acting medicine will suffice to produce its full effect. If, in the case of a medicine whose action lasts a long time, as for instance digitalis where it continues to the seventh day, the dose be repeated frequently, that is to say, three or four times in the course of a day, the actual quantity of medicine will, before the seven days have expired, have increased twenty or thirty-fold, and thereby become extremely violent[1] and injuri-

---

[1] The following circumstance must also be taken into consideration. We cannot well tell how it happens, but it is not the less true, that even one and the same dose

ous; whereas the first dose (a twentieth or thirtieth part) would have amply sufficed to effect a cure without any bad consequences.

After the expiry of the term of action of the first dose of the medicine employed in a curative manner, we judge whether it will be useful to give a second dose of the same remedy. If the disease have diminished in almost its whole extent, not merely in the first half-hour after taking the medicine, but later, and during the whole duration of the action of the first dose; and if this diminution have increased all the more, the nearer the period of the action of the remedy approached its termination—or even if, as happens in very chronic diseases, or in maladies the return of whose paroxysm could not have been expected during this time, no perceptible amelioration of the disease have indeed occurred, but yet no new symptom of importance, no hitherto unfelt suffering deserving of attention have appeared, then it is in the former case almost invariably certain, and in the latter highly probable, that the medicine was the curatively helpful, the positively appropriate one, and, if requisite, ought to be followed up by a second—and finally even, after the favourable termination of the action of the second, by a third dose if it be necessary and the disease be not in the mean time completely cured,—as it often is, in the case of acute diseases, by the very first dose.

If the medicine we have chosen for the positive (curative) treatment excites almost no sufferings previously unfelt by the patient, produces no new symptom, it is the appropriate medicament and will certainly cure the original malady, even though the patient and his friends should not admit that any amendment has resulted from the commencing doses,—and so also conversely, if the amelioration of the original disease take place in its whole extent from the action of the curative medicine, the medicine cannot have excited any serious new symptoms.

Every aggravation, as it is called, of a disease that occurs

of medicine, which would suffice for the cure, provided it were not repeated before the action of the remedy had ceased—acts ten times as powerfully, if the dose be divided, and these portions taken at short intervals during the continuance of the action of the medicine; for example, if the dose of ten drops, which would have sufficed for the cure, be divided among the five days during which the action of the medicine lasts, in such a manner as that one drop of it shall be taken twice a-day, at the end of the five days the same effect is not produced as would have occurred from ten drops given at once every five days, but a far more powerful, excessive, violent effect, provided that the medicine was a curative and positive antidote to the disease.

during the use of a medicine (in doses repeated before or immediately after the expiry of its term of action), in the form of
new symptoms not hitherto proper to the disease, is owing
solely to the medicine employed (if it do not occur just a few
hours before inevitable death, if there have taken place no important error of regimen, no outbreak of violent passions, no
irresistible evolution of the course of nature by the occurrence
or cessation of the menstrual function, by puberty, conception,
or parturition) ; these symptoms are always the effect of the
medicine, which, as an unsuitably chosen positive remedy, or as
a negative (palliative) remedy, either ill-selected or given for
too long a time, and in too large doses, develops them by its
peculiar mode of action to the torment and destruction of the
patient.

An aggravation of the disease by new, violent symptoms during the first few doses of a curative medicine is *never* indicative
of feebleness of the dose (never requires the dose to be increased),
but it proves the total unfitness and worthlessness of the medicine in this case of disease.

The aggravation just alluded to by violent, new symptoms
not proper to the disease, bears no resemblance to the increase
of the apparently original symptoms of the disease during the
first few hours after the administration of a medicine selected in
a positive (curative) manner, which I formerly spoke of. This
phenomenon of the increase of what seem to be the pure symptoms of the disease, but which are actually predominant medicinal symptoms resembling those of the disease, indicates merely
that the dose of the appropriately selected curative medicine has
been too large—it disappears, if the dose has not been enormously large, after the lapse of two, three, or at most, four hours
after its administration, and makes way for a removal of the disease that will be all the more durable, generally after the expiry
of the term of the action of the first dose ; so that, in the case
of acute affections, a second dose is usually unnecessary.

However, there is no positive remedy, be it ever so well
selected, which shall not produce one, at least one slight, unusual
suffering, a slight new symptom, during its employment, in very
irritable, sensitive patients,—for it is almost impossible that
medicine and disease should correspond as accurately in their
symptoms as two triangles of equal angles and sides resemble
each other. But this unimportant difference is (in favourable
cases) more than sufficiently compensated by the inherent energy

of the vitality, and is not even perceived except by patients of excessive delicacy.

Should a patient of ordinary sensibility observe during the duration of the action of the first dose, an unusual sensation, and should the original disease appear at the same time to decline, we are unable to determine with precision (at least not in a chronic disease) from this first dose, whether or no the medicine selected was the most appropriate curative one. The effects of a second dose of equal strength, given after the first has exhausted its action, can alone decide this point. From the action of this, if the medicine was not perfectly or exceedingly appropriate, there will again appear a new symptom (but not often the same that was observed from the first dose, usually another one) of greater intensity (or even several symptoms of a like character), without any perceptible progress occurring in the cure of the disease in its whole extent;—if, however, it was the appropriate positive medicine, this second dose removes almost every trace of a new symptom, and health is restored with still greater rapidity, and without the supervention of any new ailment.

Should there occur from the second dose also some new symptom of considerable severity, and should it not be possible to find a more appropriate medicine (the fault of which may however lie either in a want of diligence on the part of the physician, or in the smallness of the supply of medicines, whose absolute effects are known) in the case of chronic diseases, or acute diseases that do not run a very rapid course, a diminution of the dose will cause this to disappear, and the cure will still go on, though somewhat more slowly. (In this case also the energy of the vitality aids the cure).

The choice of the medicine is not inappropriate if the chief and most severe symptoms of the disease are covered in a positive manner by the symptoms of the primary action of the medicine, while some of the more moderate and slighter morbid symptoms are so only in a negative (palliative) manner. The true curative power of the predominant positive action of the remedy takes place notwithstanding, and the organism regains full possession of health without accessory sufferings during the treatment, and without secondary ailments thereafter. It is not yet decided whether it is advantageous in such a case to increase the doses of the medicine during the continuance of its employment.

If, during the continued employment of a curative medicine

without increasing the doses (in a chronic disease,) fresh symptoms not proper to the disease should, in the course of time, present themselves, whereas the first two or three doses acted almost without any disturbance, we must not seek for the cause of this impediment in the inappropriateness of the medicine, but in the regimen, or in some other powerful agency from without.

If, on the other hand, as is not unfrequently the case when there is a sufficient supply of well known medicines, a positive medicine perfectly appropriate to the accurately investigated case of disease, be selected and administered in a suitably small dose, and repeated after the expiry of its special duration of action, should none of the above alluded to great obstacles come in the way, such as unavoidable evolutions of nature, violent passions, or enormous violations of regiminal rules, and should there be no serious disorganization of important viscera, the cure of acute and chronic diseases, be they ever so threatening, ever so serious, and of ever so long continuance, takes place so rapidly, so perfectly, and so imperceptibly, that the patient seems to be transformed almost immediately into the state of true health, as if by a new creation.

The influence of regimen and diet on the cure is not to be overlooked; but the physician needs to exercise a supervision over them only in chronic diseases, according to principles which I shall develop in the special part of my work. In acute diseases, however (except in the state of complete delirium), the delicate and infallible tact of the awakened internal sense that presides over the maintenance of life, speaks so clearly, so precisely, so much in conformity with nature, that the physician needs only to impress on the friends and attendants of the patient, not to oppose in any way this voice of nature, by refusing or exceeding its demands, or by an injurious officiousness and importunity.

OBJECTIONS TO A PROPOSED SUBSTITUTE FOR CINCHONA BARK,

AND TO SUCCEDANEA IN GENERAL.[1]

In the commercial world the spirit of substitution has been lately boldly stalking abroad. A large number of substitutes

---

[1] From the *Reichs-Anzeiger*, No. 77, 1806.

for coffee have been proposed and offered at low prices—and no small number of substitutes for hops in beer have been sought for.

It would have required no great experience to perceive *a priori* that infusions of burnt barley would taste like burnt barley, of burnt chicory-root and carrot would taste like burnt chicory-root and carrot, and of burnt cyperus would taste like burnt cyperus, and that each would act in its own peculiar way on the health of man, but that none of them would either taste like coffee, or yet be capable of developing on the human organism the effects to be anticipated from genuine coffee.[1]

If the substitutes for coffee had injurious effects on the health, yet they were actually, and in comparison with the injurious nature of coffee, quite inconsiderable, for before being used as drinks these substances were roasted, and thereby deprived of the greater portion of their power of deranging the health of the body.

Much more important and more objectionable as regards the health were the substitutes for *hops* in beer, which have been proposed and recommended. Notwithstanding that the hop is undoubtedly a medicinal substance, and that the daily use of its decoction in beer must affect the health, yet it has long been observed that this bitter substance in beer (though it would be better that the more *wholesome* unhopped beer made from air-dried malt, were generally used, especially that made from wheat) agreed better than any other with our constitutions, and if only a moderate quantity of it enter into the composition of the beer, it appears at length to become almost quite innocuous to us.

But what excuse can be offered for forcing us to use in our daily drink completely new medicinal substances, such as worm-wood, feverfew, and other drugs of still more unknown action, as psoralia, &c., in the form of unchanged vegetable decoctions, in place of hops in beer? What pests in the form of newly developed chronic diseases are we not threatened with, which must infallibly result from the use of decoctions of medicinal herbs in such quantities, the effects of which on the human body are quite unknown![2]

---

[1] This mistake had however an accidental, important good effect on all the inhabitants of Europe: since then some millions of dollars fewer have been drawn from our part of the world, and the very bad effects of over-indulgence in genuine coffee on the health and the morals, have been diminished.

[2] Medical men imagine, it is true, that they know the effects of, *e. g.*, wormwood

We may read the bad effects on the human nealth from the frequent use, *e. g.*, of wormwood, in Lange (*Domestica brunsv.*, p. 112), and in Vicat (*Matière med.*, p. 40). The bad effects of the other substitutes for hops are not so easily proved.

But what do the projectors of the substitutes for hops they recommend care about the injury they do, provided they only taste bitter !

It is fortunate that all these bitters, which the true physician has reason to suspect, are, when used in the preparation of beer, suspected also by the drinkers, and are usually rejected by them from a sort of instinct.

        *   *   *   *

Of a not less injurious tendency are all the so-called succedanea for powerful, established medicinal substances, particularly for cinchona-bark.

I have nothing more to say respecting *Breitfeld's substitute for cinchona* than the following :

1. That there is no such thing as a succedaneum or substitute for bark, nor is it possible that there can be ;

   a. Because every plant has its own peculiar medicinal mode of action that is not to be found in any other plant in the world—and no other plant is cinchona; therefore *it stands to reason* that cinchona can be replaced by nothing but by cinchona itself.

   As little as a willow, an ash, or a horse-chesnut-tree, corresponds in external and botanical respects with a cinchona tree, so little do the medicinal powers of the barks of said trees resemble the cinchona bark. In like manner a mixture of calmus, gentian and gall-nuts may indeed be much more aromatic, more bitter and more astringent than cinchona bark; but it can never be cinchona bark.

   b. Because all the substitutes for cinchona that have hitherto been proposed, inclusive of Breitfeld's, were only useful where cinchona would have been of no use, and consequently would do no good where cinchona is indicated, and could do no good—therefore they cannot replace the latter.

and feverfew. They consider them as absolutely wholesome. This is however a delusion. They have employed both these substances only in diseases in which the slow recovery was dependent often on quite other circumstances than the medicines given; they have used them only in combination with other drugs. But few know what harm these herbs can do to the human body when given singly in large quantities.

2. That Breitfeld's is undeserving of consideration because it is composed of several vegetable substances—a circumstance that, owing to the ever-varying quality of the different ingredients, the different modes in which they are dried and preserved, the coarser or finer pulverization of the several substances, and even the impossibility of mingling them always in the same manner, must always give a different product, as is the case with all compound medicines.

3. That no one has yet determined the accessory medicinal effects of the several ingredients of his mixture, whereby they must evidently excite an accessory action different from that of cinchona, and of an injurious nature, which the prescribing physician can not take into calculation, as he does not know what it is.

*　　　　*　　　　*　　　　*

Provided the cinchona bark be not employed in excessive doses, nor given repeatedly where it can be dispensed with, nor where it can do no good, nor yet where it must do much and often irremediable injury—not one tenth part of the valuable bark that has been hitherto wasted will be required. Then it would not be too dear; then the two millions and a half of dollars which Europe yearly pays to South America for bark might be diminished to 250,000, and if we were wiser physicians, to 50,000 dollars, *to the great advantage of our patients.*

Would it be very difficult to cultivate this invaluable tree in Europe, seeing that it grows on the Andes [1] at a height of 7692 feet above the level of the sea?

In conclusion I must express my regret that Mr. Breitfeld has not devoted his well-meant labours to a less thankless subject.

OBSERVATIONS ON THE SCARLET-FEVER.[2]

The malignant scarlet-fever that has prevailed in Germany for eight years and proved fatal to many thousands of children and older persons, often so unexpectedly, so rapidly, and with symptoms never before heard of under such circumstances, this murderous disease, termed *scarlet-fever* by almost every one, is really anything but scarlet-fever; it is a new disease *never* seen in Ger-

---

[1] Properly speaking, on the *Cordilleras de los Andes,* the highest range of mountains in the known world, which includes the whole western side of South America.
[2] From the *Allg. Anzeig. der Deutschen,* No. 160. 1808.

many before the year 1800, which, on account of the red rash
that usually accompanies it, might be termed *purpura miliaris*,
and which, *then for the first time*, spread from the west, over Hesse,
Bamberg, Beyreuth, Thuringia and Voigtland, to Saxony, and
thence since that time has extended in all directions.

If it can be proved that this is a new disease and is widely
different from the old genuine scarlet-fever (which old people can
still very well remember to have noticed in their youth in themselves and others), we can very well understand how it happened,
that the medical men did not know how to act in this new disease, and that at first all who were likely to die, slipped through
their hands ; indeed that their endeavours did more harm than
good, as they were always under the delusion that they had to
do with the old genuine scarlet-fever, and thus they were misled
by this extraordinary confounding of names and things, to treat
the new disease in the same way as they had been used to treat
the true scarlet-fever (by means of keeping the patient warm,
administering elder-flower tea, &c.). Such a mistake, such a
confounding in diagnosis and treatment of two such very different
diseases, must naturally have a very unfortunate result, as experience has shewn it to have had by the many thousands who
have fallen victims to this new disease.

This disease is *new* among us, I repeat, for there is not the
slightest trace of such a purple miliary fever having ever before
prevailed in Germany.

The epidemic in Strasburg, described seventy-three years ago by
Salzmann, was a white miliary fever—white vesicles on a white
skin—and differed from our new miliary fever in this, that
children and old people were almost entirely exempted from it,
and it chiefly affected youths and adults between twenty and
forty years of age; sore throat was very rarely met with in it.

The miliary epidemic described by Welsch, of Leipzig, 150
years ago, consisted of a white, millet-seed size dexanthema, and
only affected *lying-in women ;* probably it was a disease brought
on by keeping them too warm.

The most recent miliary epidemic which Brüning observed
thirty-six years ago, in the neighbourhood of the Lower Rhine,
differs also from our new disease in this, that children of five
years and under generally remained free from it, and women
were more frequently attacked than men,—that it had its critical
days, and was likewise a white miliary rash, resting for the first
few days on red spots, which went off on the seventh day,

leaving the white miliary rash standing from three to seven days longer on the white skin.

The epidemics that bear the greatest resemblance to our present purple miliary, are those observed by David Hamilton, long ago (1710) in India, and Charles Allione (in 1758) in Turin.

Other observers only mention having occasionally observed a miliary fever in single individuals, which were usually only brought on by the use of heating) diaphoretic remedies, especially of opiates, did not prevail epidemically, and are described by them in a most vague manner.

That our miliary fever is *new* and *very different* from the true scarlet-fever, the following comparison will shew.

The new red miliary-fever (which for the last eight years has been called scarlet-fever)	*The old genuine scarlet-fever*
attacks persons of all ages ;	attacks only children until their 12th year (Sim. Schulze)—attacks only children, almost never adults (Plenciz, Sennert) ;
the eruption consists of purple-red (Jani), of dark red spots [1] (verging on brown), which on being pressed with the finger do not leave a white spot but remain unchanged, of a dark red colour,	the redness of the skin is an erysipelatous fire-coloured redness (Sennert);—a bright scarlet redness, resembling erysipelas in colour and in this, that it immediately disappears on pressure with the finger and shews a white spot, which however immediately resumes its red colour (Navier) ; the redness is like the colour of a boiled lobster (*Act. med. Berol.*) ;—a cinnabar redness (Plenciz).
of sharply defined, discrete patches of redness,	The smooth shining redness of the skin runs imperceptibly into the neighbouring white parts, in unnoticeable shades, like erysipelas, and is never well defined ;—it becomes from time to time, now a little paler, now a little redder, and almost every instant it spreads imperceptibly farther, and then retires to its original seat (Navier).
always thickly studded with dark-red miliary papulæ, which are not so much elevated above the level of the skin as stuck deep in it, yet distinctly perceptible to both the eye and the touch.	None of the above-mentioned authors allude to miliary elevations of the bright red parts of the skin;—the skin of the reddened parts is quite even and smooth (Hahnemann) ;—the red parts of the skin are quite smooth and destitute of inequalities or elevations (Plenciz, *Op. tract.*

---

[1] Hence we may unhesitatingly call it *purple miliary* (purpura miliaris). Who could confound this dark red rash with the bright fiery colour of scarlet cloth ?

This exanthema attacks in an indeterminate manner, now this, now that part of the body—there is no part of the body for which it has a peculiar affection, or to which it attaches itself in a peculiar manner (Stieglitz). Most frequently the favourite spots for its attack are the *covered* parts and flexures of the joints; most rarely the face. The rash is usually accompanied by swelling (Stieglitz).

This exanthematous fever has not a determined, regular course, like other exanthematous fevers (Stieglitz);—the eruption remains here and there for an indeterminate period, often several weeks; there is no fixed period for its departure.

The red miliary rash often disappears suddenly at indeterminate times, with increased danger to life, usually followed suddenly by death.

The eruption may be copious or almost not at all present, the mildness or malignancy of the disease not depending on that (Stieglitz). Where the eruption is almost imperceptible the danger is often greatest, the fever most malignant; —where there is a general full eruption, the disease is often mild and slight.

It is only the dark red miliary patches that perspire, and it is only when the whole body is covered with it that the patient perspires all over, as in the epidemic at Wittenberg

iii, p. 49)—*and in this the scarlet-fever differs from every kind of miliary fever* (Plenciz, *ib.*, p. 58).

The redness of the true scarlet-fever prefers attacking first the *uncovered* and but slightly covered parts, which swell as far as the redness extends. At first the redness and swelling occur on the face (De Gorter, Plenciz)—at first in the face, neck, and chest (Plenciz)—the scarlet redness first appears, with some swelling, on the face (neck and chest), the hands, and the outside of the feet and from these parts it spreads out in an erysipelatous manner (in the worst cases) all over the body (Hahnemann).

In every genuine scarlet-fever the redness appears on the parts named simultaneously with the febrile heat, and in mild cases is perceptible for from three to four days (Plenciz, Sennert), in bad cases, seven days (Plenciz)—and goes off by becoming gradually paler from day to day. The parts that first became red, become first pale (Plenciz).

None of the above authors makes mention of the sudden disappearance of the redness of true scarlet fever during the fever. After the gradual fading of the redness up to the fixed days mentioned above, there occur apyrexia and desquamation (Sennert, Plenciz, De Gorter, Sim. Schulze). Even after death the hitherto red spots remain coloured and turn violet (Navier.

The fuller and more extended the redness of true scarlet-fever is, the more malignant is the fever always (Hahnemann).

None of the reddened parts in true scarlet-fever perspire during the disease (in all this the authors I have mentioned are agreed), if the skin is moist, it is so only on the parts that are not yet reddened. No erysipelas perspires, and as little does the scarlatina redness. It is only when the fever comes to an end, and the redness has gradually gone off, that there sometimes occurs general per-

This new miliary disease, falsely said to be scarlet-fever, which first appeared about the middle of the year 1800,[1] and, like every *new pestilence*, raged as a most murderous epidemic where it first appeared (there was no *mild* epidemic of it), and then from time to time recurred, often several times in a year in the same place (not unfrequently attacking the same persons a second time), during the first years still attacked several families in succession; during the last years did not, it is true, cease for any length of time, but did not prevail quite epidemically again, but rather attacked single families, or even single individuals, in one place (though it was not less fatal)—it seems in the course of a few years to have a tendency to become extinguished completely, like the English sweating-sickness at the commencement of the 16th century.

Besides the diaphoretics, elder-flower tea, &c., and the warm beds wherewith it was sought to retain the eruption on the skin (usually without success), purgatives, especially mercurial medicines, are said to have done good in this exanethematous fever; but *aconite*, along with a moderately cool regimen saved the most. It were foolish to judge of the power of belladonna from its administration in this new miliary fever, which, as we see, is anything but scarlet-fever.

spiration, and thereafter desquamation of the skin (Sim. Schulze),[2] and the disease may also go off without any perpiration.—(*Act. med. Berol.*)

The true scarlet-fever is an old disease, which has been accurately observed for two centuries in Germany and other countries, always appeared only as an epidemic and pandemic, always attacked indiscriminately, and with scarcely any exception, every child that had not had the disease (never those who had already had it), seldom prevailed in malignant, often in mild, sometimes in perfectly mild epidemics (Sydenham, De Gorter, Nenter, Junker), scarcely proving fatal to one child in a thousand, never, or very seldom, occurred sporadically, and the reason of this was, that as it almost always attacked pandemically all children who had not previously had it, there were not under 6 or 8 years enough subjects to infect in order to show its epidemic character, hence it almost never recurred in less than 6, 8, or 12 years, and on account of this rarity of its recurrence, the oldest practitioners scarcely ever saw it oftener than three times in their lives, and it was quite unknown to our younger practitioners.

In this old, true scarlet-fever, belladonna is useful, both as a prophylactic, and as a remedy.

---

[1] In the first half of the year 1800 true scarlet-fever still prevailed, and a couple of months thereafter the new miliary fever made its appearance.

ON THE PRESENT WANT OF FOREIGN MEDICINES.

The loud complaints that are uttered respecting the want of foreign medicines, and recently the lamentation on this subject (in No. 176 of the *All. Anz.*) from our esteemed philanthropic Faust, went to my heart, particularly as I recently got from one of the most celebrated laboratories in one of the most famed cities in Germany, in place of choicest, best myrrh which I had ordered, lumps of a gum-resin having somewhat the appearance of myrrh, but which, on being pulverized, had a most nauseous odour, apparently the product of some unknown umbelliferous plant, and which was anything but myrrh.

"What will be the result of this blockade of Europe, what the end of this deficiency of the most indispensable foreign drugs?" anxiously exclaim both physicians and patients—"particularly as the most sagacious men consider the substitution of one medicine for another to be a lamentable mistake, as no substance in nature possesses the same qualities as any other, nor is it possible that it can, for they are characteristically different in externals, and as veal cannot turn into mutton or pork, neither can quitch-grass be transformed into sarsaparilla."

Of a truth, this daily increasing deficiency of foreign drugs seems likely to become a great, an inconceivably great want.

We should no doubt find the warehouses of the druggists and apothecaries as well and constantly filled as before, notwithstanding that there is a real deficiency of most of the exotica, and a manifest want of foreign medicinal products, but—only with goods which, thanks to the known abilities of the adulterators, with the exception of an external resemblance, possess little or nothing of the actual nature of the genuine drugs, carefully stored in jars, chests, and boxes, whereon the honourable name has been for a long time painted in durable oil-colours, to guarantee the genuineness of their contents! But good heavens! what a *quid pro quo* will the connoisseur find in them! Every philanthropist must shudder at the effects such fabrications must produce on the sick.

It is not far from the truth to say, that the connoisseur can no longer meet with any genuine extra-European medicines.

---

[1] From the *Allgemeiner Anzeiger der Deutschen*, No. 207. 1898.

This want is great and incalculable, but I feel almost disposed to assert that it is a just judgment of God for the incredible abuse that has heretofore been made of these drugs. It may readily happen to the spendthrift that he may suffer from want, and that justly.

When we consider how many pounds of cinchona alone any physician in large practice has hitherto used in his practice (it is notorious that a London medical man used 500 pounds annually), and how large the number of physicians is who give large quantities of medicine, we are horrified at the quantities of foreign drugs hitherto consumed.

But, gracious God! was this not an abuse of thy noble gifts? Was the large number of draughts, teas, mixtures, electuaries, drops, powders, pills, administered at short intervals by table-spoonfuls and tea-spoonfuls, often alternated with one another several times a day, and the first one scarcely tasted, put aside, and replaced (or rather supplanted) by two or three other drugs —was the enormous quantity of drugs employed for fumigations, dry and humid applications, half and whole baths, clysters, &c. —was all this not an abuse of the noble, precious products of foreign countries brought from such great distances?

If it could be proved that such a multitude of drugs was necessary and indispensable for the patients' relief, then it would be quite a different thing. In that case the blame would rest with the Ruler of the earth, who seeing we require so much, ought to have supplied these our necessities by making them grow in larger quantities on our hazel-trees, willows, in our meadows, woods and on every hedge.

But all honour be to Him, the wise Preserver of mankind! Such an expenditure, such a waste of exotic and indigenous drugs was *never* required in order to cure the sick. It was not merely a waste (for in that case it would simply have been analogous to lighting our pipe with a bank note)—no, it was an actual sin against true art and against the welfare of sick humanity.

Do not the poor, who use no medicine at all, often recover much sooner from the same kind of disease than the well-to-do patient, who has his shelves filled with large bottles of medicine? The latter often remains much longer poorly after his treatment is finished, and must often go from one watering place to another in order to get free from the after-sufferings left in him by the monstrous quantity of powerful drugs he took,

which were usually totally inappropriate and consequently
hurtful in their character.

It must some time or other be loudly and openly declared;
and so let it now be loudly and unreservedly proclaimed before
the whole world, *that the medical art stands in need of a thorough
reform from head to foot.* What ought not to be done has been
done, and what is of the utmost importance has been totally
overlooked. The evil has become so crying that the well-
meaning mildness of a John Huss no longer avails, but the fiery
zeal of a rock-firm Martin Luther is needed to sweep away the
monstrous leaven.

There is no science, no art, not even any miserable handicraft,
that has kept pace so little with the progress of the age; no art
has remained so fixed in its original imperfection as the medical
art.

Medical men followed at one time this fashion, at another a
different one, now this school, now that, and when the more
modern method appeared unserviceable they sought to revive
some ancient one (that had formerly shewn itself worthless).
*Their treatment was never founded upon convictions, but always
upon opinions,* each of which was ingenious and learned in proportion as it was valueless, so that we are now arrived at this
point, that we have the unhappy liberty of hopelessly selecting
any one of the many methods, all of which halt in an almost
equally grievous manner, but we have actually no fixed standard for treatment, no fixed principles of practice that are acknowledged to be the best. Every physician acts according as
he has been taught by his school or as his fancy dictates, and
each finds, in the inexhaustible magazine of opinions, authorities to whom he can appeal.

The method of treating most diseases by scouring out the
stomach and bowels;—the method of treatment which aims its
medicinal darts at imaginary acridities and impurities in the
blood and other humours, at cancerous, rachitic, scrofulous,
gouty, herpetic and scorbutic acridities;—the method of treatment that presupposes in most diseases a species of fundamental
morbid action, such as dentition, or derangements of the biliary
system, or hæmorrhoids, or infarctus, or obstruction in the mesenteric glands, or worms, and directs the treatment against
these;—the method which imagines it has always to do with
debility, and conceives it is bound to stimulate and re-stimulate
(which they call *strengthen*);—the method which regards the

diseased body as a mere chemically decomposed mass which must be restored to the proper chemical condition by chemical (nitrogenous, oxygenous, hydrogenous) re-agents;—another method that supposes diseases to have no other original cause but mucosities—another that sees only inspissation of the juices —another that sees nought but acids—and yet another that thinks it has only to combat putridity;—the method that imagines it must act specially and can act absolutely on the skin, the brain, the liver, the kidneys, or some other single organ;— the method that conceives it must search for and treat only spasm or paralysis in diseases, only a derangement of the antiquated *functiones naturales, vitales, animales,* or the revival of this doctrine, the derangement of the irritability, the sensibility, or the reproductive faculty;—the method that proposes to direct its attention to the supposed remote exciting causes of disease;—the method that prescribes medicines indiscriminately in diseases, in order to be able to discard those that do harm and retain those that seem to be of use (*a juvantibus et nocentibus*);—the method that, according to the mere names that the disease before them seems to have in books, goes to work with prescriptions got out of the self-same books;—the method that merely attends to particular symptoms in diseases in order to suppress these by some palliative antidote (*contraria*),—and that method that boasts of being able to subdue the disease by assisting and promoting the efforts of nature and the natural crises; —all these modes of treatment, many directly opposite to one another, have each their authorities and illustrious supporters; but nowhere do we find a universally applicable, efficacious standard of treatment accredited in all ages.

Imagine the embarrassment in which a physician must be placed when he comes to the sick-bed, as to whether he should follow this method or the other, in what perplexity he must be when neither the one nor the other mode of treatment avails him; how he, misled now by this, now by that view, feels himself constrained to prescribe now one, now another medicinal formula, again to abandon them and administer something totally different, and finding that none will suit the case, he thinks to effect, by the strength of the doses of the most powerful and costly medicines, that cure which he knows not (nor any of his colleagues either) how to bring about mildly by means of small, rare doses of the simple but appropriate medicine. All this he does the more readily seeing that the prevailing system derived from England commands him to assail his poor patients with large, with enormous doses of the most active medicines. He is thus in the habit of *forcing* the disease to take itself off by administering repeated, frequently alternated and varied mixtures of large doses of very powerful, expensive medicines. The disease no doubt is removed, it yields to the force brought against it; but if death be not the result, there arise other diseases, new maladies, that entail the necessity of a long, expensive after-treatment, because all these numerous, dear, strong drugs were for the most part unsuitable, were not accurately adapted to the cure of disease in all its parts.

Thus the ruination of human health goes hand in hand with the lavish waste of so many costly foreign drugs—the way of destruction! This was assuredly not the intention of the all-bountiful, wise Creator, who in nature effects many and great and multifarious objects with few, simple means, and apparently insignificant appliances, and has certainly so ordained the medicines he created, that each should have its own immutably fixed uses, its certain, unvarying curative power, with which it should be able to effect, in excessively small doses, many and great things for the weal of (God-beloved) man, if we, instead of interminably talking and writing mere empty conjectures and hypotheses, would but endeavour to become better and more accurately acquainted with it. *Dixi et salvavi animam.* Let us become better, and all will soon go better.

ON THE VALUE OF THE SPECULATIVE SYSTEMS OF MEDICINE,

ESPECIALLY AS VIEWED IN CONNEXION WITH THE USUAL METHODS OF PRACTICE WITH WHICH THEY HAVE BEEN ASSOCIATED.[1]

Although it has ever been man's endeavour to discover and explain the connexion of the various constituents of the living body, and the manner of their reaction upon each other, and upon external forces; to tell how they give rise to those living instruments (organs) which are requisite to the maintenance of of life; and how, out of the necessary organs, a self-contained

---

[1] From the *Allgem. Anz. der Deutschen*, No. 263. 1808.

whole—a living healthful individual—is formed and upheld; it has been found impossible, though it has been often tried, to explain these, either on the principles of mechanics, or physics, or chemistry, or the laws of liquid and solid bodies in the inorganic world; or by gravitation or friction, or by impulse, or *vis inertiæ,* or by the laws of the attraction and cohesion of several similar bodies touching each other at many points, or the repulsion of dissimilar; nor has it been explained by the forms of the individual elementary substances which compose man's body, according as these might be described as flat, or pointed, or spherical, or spiral, or capillary, or as rough or smooth, angular or hooked; or by the laws of elasticity, of the contractive and expansive power of inorganic substances, or of the diffusion of light and production of heat, or of magnetic, electric, or galvanic phenomena, or by the mode of operation of substances containing oxygen, hydrogen, carbon, or azote, or of the acids, earths, or metals, or of gelatin, albumen, starch, gluten, or sugar.

But though all the component parts of the human frame are to be found in other parts of nature, they act together in their organic union, to the full development of life, and the discharge of the other functions of man, in so *peculiar* and anomalous a manner (which can only be defined by the term *vitality*), that this peculiar (*vital*) relation of the parts to one another and the external world, cannot be judged of or explained by any other rule than that which itself supplies; therefore, by none of the known laws of mechanics, statics, or chemistry. All those theories, to which age after age has given birth, when brought in contact with simple experience, and tried by an impartial test, have ever been found to be far-fetched and unfounded.

Yet, in spite of the uniform disappointment of these innumerable attempts, the physiologists and pathologists would still return to the old leaven; not because they saw any likelihood of these hypotheses leading to useful discoveries in the art of healing, but *because they placed the essence of the medical art, and their own chief pride, in explaining much even of the inexplicable.* They imagined it impossible to treat scientifically the abnormal states of the human body (diseases), without possessing a *tangible* idea of the fundamental laws of the normal and abnormal conditions of the human frame.

This was the first and great delusion they practised on themselves and on the world. This was the unhappy conceit which, from Galen's days down to our own, made the medical art a stage for the display of the most fantastic, often most self-contradictory, hypotheses, explanations, demonstrations, conjectures, dogmas, and systems, whose evil consequences are not to be overlooked. Even the student was taught to think he was master of the art of discovering and removing disease, when he had stuffed his head with these baseless hypotheses, which seemed made for the express purpose of distracting his brains, and leading him as far as possible away from a true conception of disease and its cure.

From time to time, it is true, an accumulation of facts, often of a nature to arrest the least attentive observer, forced on men the conviction that the doctrine of the structure and functions of the human body in the healthy state (physiology), and of the inward changes consequent on the generation of disease (pathology) which deduces them from atomical and chemical principles, is an erroneous one; but in avoiding this error,—still misled by the *vain fancy that the business of the medicinal profession was to explain every thing,*—they fell into the opposite, but not less dangerous evil of superstition.

At one time, men created for themselves an imaginary incorporeal something, which guided and ruled the whole system in its vicissitudes of health and disease (Van Helmont's *Archœus*, Stahl's *Animal Soul*); at another, they flattered themselves they had discovered the secret of physical constitutions and temperaments, as well as the origin of particular diseases and epidemics, in the constellations of the stars, in an influence emanating from the heavenly bodies, many millions of miles distant;—or (according to the modern wide-spread notion, based on ancient absurdities), the human body, in agreement with the old mystic number three, developed itself in triplicity, presented a miniature of the universe (microcosm, macrocosm), and thus, by means of our knowledge of the great whole, miserably defective as it is, was to be explained to a hair's-breadth. That which had baffled clear chemistry and physics, dim, self-unintelligible mysticism and frenzied fancy were to bring to light: old astrology was to explain what puzzled modern natural philosophy.

Thus did the leaders of the medical sects and their followers, whenever they sought to analyse health and disease and its cure, deviate more or less widely from the truth; and the only use of piles of folios, quartos, and octavos, which cost a lamentable expenditure of time and energy, is to frighten us from indulging in a like explanation-mania, and teach us that all such immense exertions are nothing but pernicious folly.

But if these physiological refinements and pathological would-be explanations, as regards their proper object, the cure of disease, are rather prejudicial than helpful, as no unprejudiced person will deny, of what possible use are they?

" Surely the physician," I fancy I hear one exclaim, " requires a theory at once for a clue, a thread on which to string his ideas and systematic practice, and a line to direct him at the sick-bed. Every artist, who is not a mere mechanic, must desire to have some connexion of ideas in his mind as he works, concerning the character of the object on which he is to labour, and the nature of the condition into which he is to mould it."

True, I reply; but this clue must neither be a flimsy cobweb nor a false guide : for then it were worse than none.

The materials of the mechanical workman, indeed, have physical and chemical properties, and can only be fitly and fully employed by one who is well acquainted with these properties.

But it is quite otherwise with the treatment of objects whose essential nature consists in vital operations—the treatment, namely, of the living human frame, to bring it from an unhealthy to a healthy condition (which is *therapeutics*), and the discipline of the human mind to develope and exalt it (which is *education*). In both cases, the matter on which we work is not to be regarded and treated according to physical and chemical laws like the metals of the metallurgist, the wood of the turner, or the cloth and colours of the dyer.

It is impossible, therefore, that either physician or teacher, when caring for mind or body, should require such foreknowledge of his subject-matter as shall lead him by the hand, as it were, to the completion of his work, as, perhaps, a knowledge of the physical and chemical properties of the materials helps and conducts the metallurgist, the tanner, and other such craftsmen, to the perfection of theirs. The vocation of both those others demands quite another kind of knowledge, just as their object, a living individual, is quite different.

Nor are they at all more assisted by metaphysical, mystical, and supernatural speculations, which idle and self-sufficient visionaries have devised respecting the inner absolute essential nature of the animal organism; respecting life, irritability, sensibility and reproduction, and the essential nature of the mind.

Which, indeed, of the ontological systems regarding the (undiscoverable) nature of the human soul promises to afford any aid to the teacher in the execution of his noble office? He might well lose himself in the interminable labyrinth of abstract speculations on the *ego* and the *non-ego*, on the essences of the soul, &c., which extravagant self-conceit has in all ages wrung from the racked brains of hosts of sophists; but no advantage that will reward his pains will he draw from these transcendental subtleties. It has not been given to mortal man to reason *a priori* on the nature of his own soul.

The wise teacher is aware of this; he spares himself this fruitless trouble, and, in aiming at as wide an acquaintance as possible with his subject-matter, confines himself to the *a posteriori*, to *that which the mind's own acts have revealed concerning itself, to empirical psychology.* More on this subject in this stage of being he cannot, more he need not, know.

Just so is it with the physician. That which binds in so wonderful an organization the (may be originally chemical) constituents of the human frame in life—which causes them, in spite of these their original nature, to act in quite an unmechanical and unchemical manner—which excites and impels them, when thus combined, to such automatic performances (which do not obey any of the known laws of mechanics, and differ from every chemical process, and all physical phenomena); this fundamental force does not reveal itself as a distinct entity; it can only be dimly surmised from afar, and is for ever concealed from all inquiry and observation. No man is acquainted with the substratum of vitality, or the *a priori* hidden arrangement of the living organization—no mortal can ever dive into it, nor can human speech, either in prose or verse, even faintly shadow it forth: the attempt ends in fiction and sheer nonsense.

Throughout the course of the two thousand years and upwards in which men have prided themselves on the cultivation of philosophy and medical science, no single step, not the smallest, has been made towards an *a priori* knowledge of the vitality of the bodily frame or of the intellectual energy (the soul) which actuates it. All that inflated bombast, passing for demonstration, abounding in words, but void of sense—all the antics and curvets of the sophists, about indiscoverable things, are ever vain, and to the modest spirit of the true philosopher perfectly insufferable.

We cannot even conceive a path that should lead us to such knowledge.

No not a glimpse shall frail mortality ever obtain of that which lies deep hidden in the sacred recesses of the Divine Creating Mind, far, immeasurably far, beyond the grasp of human comprehension!

All, therefore, that the physician can know regarding his subject-matter, vital organization, and all that concerns him to know, is summed up in that which the wisest among us, such as Haller, Blumenbach, Wrisberg, comprehended and taught under the term physiology, and which we might designate the *empirical knowledge of vitality*, viz.: *what the appreciable phenomena are which occur in the healthy human body, and what their connexion is;* the inscrutable *how they occur*, remaining entirely excluded.

I pass on to *pathology*, a science in which that same love of system which has crazed the brains of the metaphysical physiologists, has caused a like misapplication of intellect in the attempt to search into the essential nature of diseases, that whereby affections of the system become manifest diseases. This they term the doctrine of *proximate, internal causes*.

No mortal can form a clear conception of what is here aimed at, to say nothing of the impossibility of any created intelligence, even in imagination, finding a road to an intimate view of what constitutes the essence of disease; and yet hosts of sophists with important looks, have affected to play the seer's part in the matter.

After humoral pathology (that conceit, which took especially with the vulgar, of considering the diseased body as a vessel full of impurities of all sorts, and of acidities with Greek epithets, which were supposed to cause the obstruction and vitiation of the fluids and solids, putrefaction, fever, everything, in short, whereof the patient complained, and which they fancied they could overcome by sweetening, diluting, purifying, loosening, thickening, cooling, and evacuating measures) had, now under a gross, now under a more refined form, lasted through many ages, with occasional interludes of many lesser and greater systems—(to wit, the iatro-mechanical system, the system which derives disease from the original form of the parts, that which ascribes them to spasms and paralysis, the pathology of the solids and nerves, the iatro-chemical system, &c.) the seer Brown appeared, who, as though he had explored the pent secrets of Nature, stepped forward with amazing assurance, assumed one primary principle of life (excitability), and would have it to be quantitively increased and diminished in diseases, accumulated and exhausted, made no account of any other sourse of disease, and persisted in considering all disease from the point of view of want or excess of energy. He gained the adherence of the whole German medical world, a sure proof that their previous medical notions had never convinced and satisfied their minds, and had only floated before them in dim and flickering forms. They caught eagerly at this onesidedness, which they persuaded themselves into believing was genuine simplicity. All the other fundamental, vital forces which were supposable enough (though, at the same time, little serviceable to a true view and cure), they gladly cast aside, out of love to his subtle doctrine, and found it highly convenient to be pretty nearly exempted from all further thought on disease or its cure. All they had now to do, was arbitrarily to determine, with a little help from the imagination, the degree of excitability in diseases according to the scale of their master, in order, by sedative or exciting measures —for all remedies, according to his new classification, were at once divided thus—to screw up or let down the degree of excitability assumed in each case. And what was after all, this his onesided excitability? Could he attach any definite and intelligible idea to it? Did he not overwhelm us with a flood of words destitute of any clear meaning? Did he not draw us into a treatment of disease, which, while it answers in but few instances, and then imperfectly, could not but in the preponderating remainder give rise to an aggravation or speedy death?

The transcendental school repudiated the idea of having but one fundamental, vital force. The reign of dualism commenced. Now we were fooled by the natural philosophers. For of such seers there was no lack; each fell on a new aspect of things— each wove a different system, having nothing in common but the morbid propensity, by inward self-contemplation not only to give an exact *a priori* account of the nature and universal constitution of things, but, moreover, to look on themselves as the authors of the whole, and, according to their own fashion, to construct it for and out of themselves. Every hint they deemed themselves to have gathered on life in the abstract, and the essential nature of man was—like their whole conception—so unintelligible, so hollow and unmeaning, that no clear sense could be drawn from it. Human speech, which is only fitted to convey the impressions of sense, and the ideas immediately flowing from them—generalizations, each one of which is easily insulated into concrete examples, and thus brought home and typified to the sense—refused to embody their conceits, their extravagant fantastic visions ; and, therefore, they had to babble them forth in new-fangled, highsounding words, superlunary collocations, eccentric rhapsodies, and unheard-of phrases without any sense, and got involved in such gossamer subtleties, that one felt at a loss to know which was the most appropriate—a satire on such a misdirection of mental energy, or an elegy on its ill success. We have to thank the natural philosophers for the disorder and dislocation of many a young doctor's understanding. Moreover, their self-conceit was yet too much inflated for them to bring forward many views on diseases or their cure, except what they now and then put forth on their dualism, their polarization, and representation, their reflex, their differentizing, and indifferentizing, their potentizing and depotentizing. This natural philosophy still lives and flourishes in a forced animation of matter, and in ecstatic hallucinations concerning the modelling and ordering of the world and its epitome—man. Incorporeal and ethereal, it still soars aloft beyond our solar system, beyond the bounds of the actual ; and does not seem likely yet awhile to descend from its super-sublime elevation to the lowly sphere of practice (the cure of man's diseases), nor indeed—so far has it overstrained its power—to be able to do so.

But lately there has shot out a branch from this tree, that seemed to have more reference to the medical art. This new doctrine, to give us an insight into the nature of disease, bethought itself of serving up afresh the old *functiones, animales, naturales, vitales,* though under new names. But what imaginable expedient have they for ascertaining *the exact degree* in which the sensibility, irritability, or reproduction, they themselves (arbitrarily) dealt out to each of the organs, are, in individual cases, increased, diminished, or changed in quality—to *which* of these, preferably to the rest—and (for there is scarcely an organ in the human frame to which any one of these three properties can be denied) what is the part played by each organ with reference to these three great divisions in any given case of disease, and what intimate and absolute condition of the whole system thence arises, whence it may be clearly seen what is the appropriate, and in every respect suitable, remedy ? What an unsolvable problem! And yet its solution is indispensable to the practitioner, if he is to make any use of the system.[1]   And—lest we should,

[1] If, indeed, this laying down of three prime organic functions, means nothing more than an approximative view, on which nothing is intended to be built, and least

after all, be only quibbling about words—what do these three words, sensibility, irritability, and reproduction, precisely stand for, in concrete ideas?

How impossible is it by all these barren *a prioris* to obtain such a just view of the different maladies as shall point out the remedy suited to each—the sole genuine aim of the healing art! How can one justify to a sound judgment the seeking to make these speculative subtleties, which can never be made concrete and applicable, the chief study of the practical physician?

It is one of the regulations that most clearly mark the wisdom of the all-consistent, all-merciful Creator, that what would be useless to man has been rendered impossible to him.

The teacher is well aware, that as he is shut out from an ontological acquaintance with the absolute nature of the soul (since it would profit him nothing), besides empirical psychology, he needs to know nothing but the practical aberrations of the human mind and heart, and the methods whereby to lead each misguided wanderer back to the paths of virtue—to carry his noble work to its highest perfection.

Socrates, the instructor of men, with his practical knowledge of mankind, his delicate moral sense, and fine perception of what makes the true happiness of man, needed but a historical knowledge of the faults of those with whom he had to do, in order, by the application of the fittest arguments, and his own better example, to allure them back to virtue. He was informed of Aristodemus that he slighted the Deity ; he gathered from some of his expressions the symptoms of this perversion of mind, and the particular prejudices that held him back from religious feeling ; and this sufficed him to teach him better, and to elicit from his own confessions, the arguments that were to shut him up to reverence for the Deity. Assuredly he needed not to institute any researches on the essence of the human mind, or the metaphysical nature of this or that delinquency of heart to attain the godlike aim.

And, in like manner, besides a historical acquaintance with the constitution of the human frame in a healthy state, the physician needs but in the same way to know the symptoms of the particular malady (further, indeed, he cannot explore, as it would serve him nothing), *in order to remove it, supposing he then knows the right remedy.*

---

of all, medical practice, in this case, I can find no fault with this antiquated scheme, which simply, *as a view*, is rational and harmless enough, though of no practical utility

Or, after all, is this all a mistake, and does the design and dignity of the medical art lie rather in vapoury theorizing, than in skill in curing diseases? Then, indeed, those word-mongers, who neither do nor cure, must bear away the palm!

Yet, if these metaphysical speculations and systems concerning the essential nature of disease (supposing they possessed some, though it were the veriest shadow of probability) were of some, the least possible value to the physician, (and some value, methinks, that, after all, must surely possess, which has been the cause of so much ado), then we cannot but conclude that this race of system-framers and system-followers must, at any rate, form the better and more successful practitioners, since they are possessed of that which—to believe them—is the true and only solid basis of the art of medicine!

But alas! it is these very men who refute, at the sick-bed, their own bragging boast of being the confidants of Nature; it is these very men who are the most helpless, when they are not the most disastrous, practitioners.

Not a single founder or follower of any of the many medical systems could or (if he could, as now and then, perhaps, he might) would dare to carry out his system faithfully and vigorously into practice, without doing the greatest injury to his patients; so that they would have been far better off wanting medical aid altogether.[1] They were obliged, if they did not wish to see all die before them, either to betake themselves to the do-nothing (expectant system; or, contrary to the professed tenets of their school, to return secretly to the least harmless expedients of earlier times, the revulsive, purgative, and palliative measures of humoralism and suburralism.

But we need not very particularly examine their method to perceive, that, at any rate, it did not take its rise in true philosophy, nor lift its aspirations to the lofty heights of reason and consistency.

One might have expected, that, in the cure of disorders which, in their own opinion, they had right learnedly defined à priori, and reduced to most simple principles, they would only have each time employed a single simple medicine (and watched its effect,) a substance whose action was quite known to them in extenso, the best known, most appropriate, only applicable—according to the

---

[1] I may refer, in place of any other of the thousand well-known instances, to that notorious instance of the Brunonian treatment, in the case of one of the sons of the renowned Peter Frank, of Vienna.

32

general rule binding on all: what may be effected by a simple remedy one should not seek to attain by means of compound ones: *quod potest fieri per pauca, &c.*

But nothing was farther from their thoughts. In the main thing, the *application* of the beautiful simple theory—in *practice* —they kept faithfully to the old beaten track (though with the constant addition of the newest, most fashionable remedies), a plain proof that their system was framed for show—for a make-believe, and not for use.

In direct opposition to plain common sense, they attack disease by *complex mixtures* of medicines, none of which they are more than superficially acquainted with, and of these medicinal *pots pourris* they often give several together, and many in one day: "haud leve obstaculum penitiori virium in medicamentis cognitioni objicit, quod *rarissime simplicia, sed ut plurimum composita, nec haec sola, sed aliorum usu interpolata usurpentur.*" [1]

Such a mode of proceeding, of itself, knocks all the pretensions to philosophical simplicity and consistency of these *a-priorists* [*a priori* men] on the head. No single physician on the face of the globe, neither the framer of the system nor his followers, uses a simple unmixed medicamant, and then waits, till its action is exhausted before giving another!

Even supposing the virtues of each single medicine were exactly known, this employment of the many-mixed, this pell-mell adminstration of several substances at once, each of which must have a different action, would in itself be highly absurd, and produce a blind and confused practice. For how complicated must the interaction be of so many ingredients; how impossible to trace back the combined effect on the patient to them each individually, in order, in the subsequent treatment, to omit or diminish the one and increase the other! But this will not do with these hotch-potch doses; they produce, thus united, such a resultant, that no one can tell what is owing to this or the other ingredient in the combined effect. No one can tell which ingredient vitiated the action in such and such a manner, or which altogether antagonized the other, and neutralized its effect.

But the case is worse still, and the proceeding more reprehensible, when we consider that the action of each, or, at any rate, of the most of these substances thus huddled together, *is individually great and yet unascertained.*

---

[1] Fr. Hoffmann, *Med. Rat.*, vol. iii, s. ii, c. 37, § 10.

Now, to mix in a prescription a number of such strong disordering substances, whose separate action is often unknown, and only guessed and arbitrarily assumed, and then forthwith, at a venture, to administer this mixture, and many more besides, thick upon one another, without letting a single one do its work out upon the patient, whose complaint and abnormal state of body has only been viewed through illusive theories, and through the spectacles of manufactured systems—if this is medical art, if this is not hurtful irrationality, I do not know what we are to understand by an art, nor what is hurtful or irrational.

It is usual at this point, for want of anything else to say, to excuse one's self by saying, " the several ingredients in a prescription are to be chosen with reference to the various aspects of the (hypothetically assumed) inward condition of the body, or, indeed, of the symptoms."

Just as if one single simple substance, if it were but rightly known, might not conform to several, many, all of the (un-ideal) aspects of the complaint,—as if all the numerous symptoms could be covered by a medley, whose ingredients, so unknown in their action, in combination counteract and, in an unforeseen manner, vitiate and neutralize each other !

This motley mixing system is nothing but a convenient shift for one who, having but a slender acquaintance with the properties of a single substance, flatters himself, though he cannot find any one simple suitable remedy to remove the complaint, that by heaping a great many together there may be one amongst them that by a happy chance shall hit the mark.

Whether this mode of treatment be successful, or the reverse, in neither case is any thing to be learnt from it, nor can it cause the medical art to make a hair's-breadth of progress.

Has there been a change for the better—to which of the ingredients of the medley, or the many successive medleys, treading on each other's heels, is it owing? This must ever remain a problem.

" All you have to do, in a similar case, is to repeat the same mixture, or succession of mixtures, in the same order."

Fond fool! The case exactly coinciding with that will never occur—*can never occur again.*

Moreover, it is always difficult to prepare mixtures a second time precisely the same as the first, and how much more so when a long interval intervenes. The same recipe often brings out a very dissimilar compound, when it is given to several apothecacaries at the same time to make up. This results from many causes.

It is not likely, either, often to happen that the patient will take these mixtures, not unfrequently disgusting both to taste and smell, in the exact quantity and time prescribed. Are you quite sure that he has even tasted this or that nauseous dose, and that he has not substituted for it a less disagreeable domestic remedy, to which his improvement is due?

And now, on the contrary supposition, that he is no better for the medley dose, or even somewhat worse, which ingredient, among so many, is to be blamed for this result, that it may be omitted in the recipe on a future occasion?

"That is what no one can tell, so it is better never to repeat the whole mixture."

I should regret much thus to throw away the gold with the dross. Have I not happily cured the disease by the employment of a single ingredient, which I picked out from the prescription of my predecessor, which had long been used with bad effects, because I knew that it must be the only efficacious one for the case before me?

How unwise is it, therefore, to prescribe such mixtures—uninviting often to the eye, the smell, and the taste—of drugs, not one of which is rightly known in itself, or in connexion with the rest!

Am I told "The properties of the medicines are not unknown"? I ask: Are the half-dozen words which the Materia Medica contains regarding each to be called information, exact information?[1] Often it is nothing more than a list of names of diseases, in all of which the substance in question is said to have been useful (frequently a long list, so that the falsehood is manifest.[2]) Names of diseases, did I say? Heaven knows to what states of body these names were given, and what wisdom presided over the assigning of them!

---

[1] How honestly our Friedrich Hoffman speaks on this subject:—

"Quomagis in artis exercitio utile est, veras et non fictas medicamentorum, pro tam diversa corporum et morborum ratione, virus intimius nosse, eo magis utique dolendum, immo mirandum est, quod, si dicere licet, quod res est, *perpauca sint remedia*, quorum virtutes et operationes certe ac recte perspectae, sed pleraeque spem atque expectationem, curantis frustrentur, *quia verae pharmacorum facultates in Democriti quasi puteo adhuc latitent !*—pauca certe supersunt, quae fidae et expertae virtutis, *plurima* vero infida, suspecta, fallacia, *ficta*." (*Med rat.*, t. iii., s. ii, c. 3, § 1.)

[2] And how dangerous are such falsehoods! "In nullo mendacio majus est periculum, quam in medico." (Plin., *Hist. Nat.* lib. 29, c. 1.)

And whence do these medical authorities draw their data? Surely not from an immediate revelation? In truth, one would almost be induced to believe they must have flowed to them from a direct inspiration, for they cannot be derived from the practice of the physicians, who, it is well known, hold it beneath their dignity to prescribe one single, simple medicament, and nothing more, in a disease, and would let the patient die, and the medical art ever remain as a no-art, sooner than part with their learned prerogative of prescribing *artistically compounded receipts.*

As, therefore, the authorities in materia medica, if I may speak out a little, cannot have obtained the greater part of their data as to the supposed virtues of the pure, simple medicinal substance from the experience [1] of learned physicians, since scarcely

---

[1] Although it is certain that the Materia Medica can and must be the daughter of experience, yet even it has given way to arbitrary opinions, ideal and dreamy hypotheses, and has allowed itself to be moulded to-day into one form, and on the morrow into a new form, exactly as the dominant medical system for the time being commanded. The remedies employed by the ancients, as *alexipharmaca, cephalica splenica, uterina,* had afterwards to undertake the office of antispasmodic and antinervous remedies. When the prevailing system assumed tension and laxity of the fibres as the foundation of disease, the very same medicines which had hitherto performed a different part were forced to be twisted into one of these two directions. But did the reigning system require blood cleansing or morbid-acridity-destroying means, then the quondam *tonica,* or *sedantia,* or *diaphoretica,* or *eccoprotica,* or *diuretica,* were quickly transformed into *mundificantia, antiscorbutica, antiscrophulosa, antiphorica, &c.* Then, when Brown needed for his system only *stimulating and debilitating remedies,* those very remedies which formerly had been marshalled under many other titles, are immediately enlisted in the two new regiments, and at will drafted into one or the other; and as he more particularly required *diffusible* and *permanent* stimuli, unfettered fancy was not long at a loss—medicines were speedily raised to one or the other rank, just as if one had but to utter the fiat, and the substances could not choose but obey the commands of the exalted man, at his pleasure to enter on one or the other function. Just as if the primary action of *cinchona* would spread more slowly through the system, or its secondary action last much longer than that of the equally little understood opium! As matters till then had stood, the system maker had only to dictate which new part this or the other medicine had to assume, whether it was to be an *invertens,* a *revertens,* or a *torpens* (Darwin); and, see, it must suffer itself to be so employed, until for the behoof of a new system, it is christened anew, and is as peremptorily required to discharge another office.

"But if you refer the action of the medicines to their chemical bases, as the very newest system does," I hear some one reply, "then, assuredly, you will act conformably to nature." In this way some medicines are (as arbitrarily as before) reckoned carbonaceous and others hydrogeneous, and to each of these summarily-divided classes peculiar (fictitious) modes of action despotically assigned. But cabbage, roast-beef, and wheaten cakes, contain also plenty of nitrogen, carbon or hydrogen—where then do we discover in them those properties which were so liberally allotted to these elementary substances?

What is to become of an art (to which the charge of human life has been committed) *if fancy and caprice are to have the upper hand in it?*

anything of the kind is to be obtained from them, whence do they get it ?

Most of the imputed virtues of the simple drugs have, in the first place, obtained a footing in domestic practice, and been brought into vogue by the vulgar and non-professional, who often cannot judge of the genuineness of the medicine; often do not give it the right name ; least of all, can correctly determine the state of the body in which it is said to have been useful. I say "said," for even with them, if needs be, now this now that, family recipe has been outwardly or inwardly applied ; so that at last it is impossible to say what has really been beneficial, granting the complaint itself has been perfectly recognised, which, however, by such observers, it never is.

Barren information of this sort was collected by the old herbalists, Matthioli, Tabernæmontanus, Gesner, Fuchs, Lonicer, Ray, Tournefort, Bock, Lobel, Thurneisser, Clusius, Bauhin, &c., very briefly, superficially, and confusedly, and interwoven with baseless and superstitious conjectures, intermingled with that which the unciting Dioscorides had in a similar manner collected; and from this unsifted catalogue was our learned-looking *Materia Medica* supplied. One authority copied another, down to our own times. Such is its not very authentic origin.[1]

---

[1] How uninquiringly our writers on materia medica have adopted the statements proceeding from these impure sources is evident, among other things, from this, that they enumerate among the virtues of crude medicines such as were originally derived from the mere suppositions of our superstitious forefathers, who had childishly enough asserted certain medicinal substances to be the remedies of certain diseases, merely on account of some external resemblance of those medicines with something appreciable by the senses in those diseases (*signature*), or whose efficacy rested only on the authority of old women's tales, or was deduced from certain of their properties that had no essential connexion with their fabulous medicinal powers. Thus the roots of the *orchis* and of the *saloop*, merely because, on account of their resemblance in shape to a pair of testicles, the ancients perceived in this an augury of their utility in aiding the sexual function, are still said to be analeptics and aphrodisiacs. The *hypericum* is still esteemed as a vulnerary, because the ancients stamped it with this character on account of the trifling circumstance that its yellow flowers, when rubbed betwixt the fingers, give out a blood-red juice, which procured for it the name of *John's blood.* Whence do the *chelidonium*, the *berberis-bark* and the *turmeric* derive the reputation they enjoy in our Materia Medica as remedies for the jaundice, but from this, that formerly it was imagined that the yellow milk of the first and the yellow colour contained in the two last was a sure sign (signature) that they must be useful in a yellow disease ? And whence does *chelidonium* in particular get its name and its fabled efficacy in dimness of vision, if not from the old story that the swallows restore the sight of their young ones by means of this plant ! The tasteless *dragon's-blood* is still, merely on account of its name and blood-red colour, said to be good for bleeding gums and hæmorrhages ! *Ranunculus ficaria* and *scrophularia*

The few books that form an exception to this (Bergius and Cullen), are all the more meagre in data respecting the properties of the medicine; consequently, as they for the most part, the latter especially, reject the vague and doubtful, we can gain *little positive* knowledge from them.

One only among thousands, Murray, gives the cases in which the medicines were used. But on this point the authorities generally clash with one another, one affirming one thing and another another, and so the decision still remains frequently quite doubtful. In many of the cases he lamented – oh that he had done so in most of the cases!—that the medicine was not employed alone, but in combination with several others, so that we are once more plunged into darkness.

The authorities cited even here leave the reader often in doubt as to the nature and exact constitution of the disease in which they employed the remedy.

---

nodosa are said to be useful for piles, merely because the roots of both these vegetables present a knotty appearance similar to the hemorrhoidal tumours. *Madder* obtained its reputation as an emenagogue on account of its containing a dark red colour; and because animals, when fed upon it, have the red colouring matter deposited in their bones, therefore it is celebrated in the Materia Medica as especially useful in diseases of the bones! *Saponaria* is still always celebrated in our books as a valuable solvent and detergent medicine, because the decoction of its root, when beaten up, forms a froth like a solution of soap, although otherwise it is totally different in its nature from soap, and it loses its frothing property not like the latter by the addition of acid, but on the contrary but adding alkali to it. And does soap itself derive its reputation for dissolving obstructions and indurations in the body, from any other source except from the conceit, that as in household operations and chemical manipulations it exercises a solvent property, it must do the same in the living organism also? Because the cabinet-makers make use of three coloured woods in their trade under the common name of *Sandal woods*, they must therefore enjoy in medicine a common power (in the so-called blood purifying drinks), although the yellow (and white) kind (*santalum album*) is obtained from a totally different tree from the red kind (*pterocarpus santalinus*), and causes very violent and serious effects, of which, however the materia medica knows nothing. Because the bark of *cinchona* tastes bitter and astringent, therefore the bitter and astringent barks of the *ash, horsechesnut, willow,* &c., were considered to possess the same action as cinchona bark,—just as though the taste could determine the action! Because some plants have a bitter taste, especially *gentiana centaureum,* called *fel terrae,* for that reason only practitioners were convinced that they could act as substitutes for the bile! From the circumstance of the root of the *carex arenaria* possessing an external resemblance to *sarsaparilla root,* it was inferred that the former must possess the same properties as the latter. Therapeutists have attributed to the *stellated anise* the same expectorant qualities as are possessed by anise seeds, merely because the latter have a resemblance in taste and smell to the seed capsules of the former, and yet some parts of the tree (*iliceum anisatum*) that bears these capsules is used in the Philippine islands as a poison for suicidal purposes.—This is what I call a philosophical and experimental origin of the materia medica!

How little the greater number of these observers are to be relied on, is evident, were it only from this, that they commonly assert, that "the remedy in their hands had never been detrimental, never done the least harm, even when it had done no good;" for every powerful medicine must invariably do injury where it fails to do good; a proposition which does not admit of a *single* exception. Behold again, then, manifest untruth!

But what is the anxious reader to learn even from this sole critically sifting and best of all *materia medicas?* Certainly little of a positive character!—little of a positive character concerning the only implements of healing! Righteous heaven!

Consider how uncertain must be the use of drugs so extremely imperfectly known, against diseases which are as diverse as the clouds in the sky, whose recognition, even by the best of methods, is tedious, and whose number is legion!

Nay more. Consider how extremely precarious, I might say, blind, that practice must be, where states of disease, misviewed through the coloured medium of ideal systems, are attacked by means of many such almost unknown medicines, mingled together in such a prescription, or in many such! On this I let the curtain drop. —

*   *   *   *

Thus we find, spite of the well nigh uninterrupted revolutions of the physiological, pathological, and therapeutic theories, during two thousand years and more, according to mechanical, atomical, chemical, ideal, pneumatical, and mystical theories, and owing to this infantile state of knowledge as to the real properties of simple medicines,—we still find—even in this century which in every other respect is hastening towards perfection—we *still find*, I repeat, that only a *very small* proportion of human ailments can in such a manner be removed as shall leave the physician the merit of having been the undoubted author of the cure. Either the remaining maladies remained as uncured as before the days of Galen. or, thanks to medical practice, in the room of the original ones there have arisen new distempers of a different aspect: or the energy of the still vigorous life, backed usually by the secret *disease of drugs*, itself got the better, in the course of time, of the disease that oppressed it; or single symptoms, hitherto stubborn, yielded to some lucky accident, wherein no one could trace the connexion of cause and effect; or else the unfailing termination of all earthly woes stepped in to settle the matter.

Such is the fearful but too true condition of the medical art hitherto, which under the treacherous promise of recovery and health, has been gnawing at the life of so many of the inhabitants of earth.

Oh! that it were mine to direct the better portion of the medical world, who can feel for the sufferings of our brethren of mankind, and long to know how they may relieve them, to those purer principles which lead directly to the desired goal!

Infamy be the award of history to him who by deceit and fiction, maims this art of ours, which is intended to succour the wretched!

All-compensating, divine self-approval, and an unfading civic crown to him who helps to make our art *more beneficial* to mankind!

ON SUBSTITUTES FOR FOREIGN DRUGS,

AND ON THE RECENT ANNOUNCEMENT OF THE MEDICAL FACUL-
TY IN VIENNA RELATIVE TO THE SUPERFLUOUSNESS OF THE
LATTER.[1]

When the imperial government of Austria exerts itself to supply the want of foreign drugs that is to be feared by indigenous substitutes, the intention is certainly patriotic; but when the medical Faculty thereupon utters an oracular deliverance as to which of the foreign drugs are quite superfluous, which may be in some measure dispensed with, and which are quite indispensable, it is in many points decidedly wrong.

The utility or superfluousness of a medicine is not a thing to be *decreed* by any medical faculty, just as it was absurd of the Parisian parliament to take upon itself to forbid the use of antimony as a medicine in 1566, and by a contrary edict to allow of its employment in 1669. Neither parliament nor faculty can do such a thing. The art of healing the sick remains a free art, which can make use of all substances in the whole of the great kingdom of nature, without any exception, for the relief of the sick.

Let us only teach physicians *principles of universal applicability*, according to which the powers of drugs may be ascertained and tested with certainty, as to what each is incontrovertibly useful and suitable for, to what cases of disease each is unex-

---

[1] From the *Allgemeiner Anzeiger der Deutschen*, No. 327. 1808.

ceptionably adapted, and what is the proper dose; and then each physician would naturally only make use of those, which are most certainly the most suitable for each case of disease and the most serviceable, whether they come from the east or from the west,[1] or are found at home,—and then he would, from his own perfect conviction, and from irrefragable reasons, of his own accord leave many foreign drugs totally unemployed in his practice, or only use them in a few well defined cases.

But we are by a long way not so far advanced as this. No principles are yet universally recognized, according to which the curative powers of medicines (even of such as have never yet been employed at the sick-bed), can with certainty be ascertained, *a priori*, without first subjecting them to the infinitely tedious process of *testing them in hap-hazard fashion at the sick-bed*, which is almost never convincing, and is usually attended with injurious effects. This obscure mode *ab effectu in morbis*, whereby little or nothing is determined, has, moreover, the cruel and unpardonable disadvantage, that the individual, naturally so irritable in disease, is readily aggravated by so many blindly instituted experiments, and may even fall a victim to them, especially since the recent fashion of prescribing large doses of powerful medicines has been adopted.

But as long as the former better way is not established in the state, and the latter mode only is so, which has been from the beginning acknowledged to be unserviceable and insufficient— so long will contradictory opinions of physicians relative to the curative powers of the different medicines continue; none will be able to convince the other of the fallacy of his opinion, none will be able to bring forward irrefragable proofs of the correctness of his own views. Almost every one entertains a different idea respecting the power of this medicine and of that, and no one can shew any proofs for his particular opinion.

---

[1] But if from the obstruction of our maritime commerce he is deprived of this medicine or the other, he is naturally deprived of what he can no longer obtain, and so he does what he can in diseases with those medicines that are still at his command, *which he must also know accurately as respects their internal properties and powers.* But if he can obtain them, then no Faculty in the world has any right to prohibit him using them, or decree their rejection. But if a Faculty can *shew on satisfactory grounds, e. g.,* that pearls are exactly the same substance as muscle and oyster shells, in that case no sensible physician *who is convinced of the fact* will employ the costly pearls, but will voluntarily use in place of them, oyster and muscle shells. The identity of salts, earths, and metals may, however, be ascertained by well-known chemical principles, but the curative powers of vegetable medicines do not depend upon their chemically cognizable constituents, but upon principles of quite a different sort, which have not yet been ascertained.

So also the present declaration of the faculty is nothing more than the private opinion of certain individuals as to what they consider to be the probable properties of the medicines in question, founded upon what they have heard or read somewhere about them, or upon what each may have experienced in his individual practice, wherefrom they pretend to *guess* that such and such is the case.

In order that a judgment should be valid much more is required, generally recognised principles are requisite, to which the judicial court may be able to appeal. If it can shew none, then its judgment must be merely a collective individual opinion, principally of those colleges that act as spokesmen, which can no more be considered absolute truth, than the private opinion of any well educated physician in the country. The majority of votes cannot in this instance determine the standard, as many may form erroneous conclusions as well as one, as long as no recognised principle proves the basis of their verdict. (So, a few years ago, many thousand physicians thought and maintained that Brown's doctrine was the only true one, and yet they all were mistaken.)

If a medicine appears to one or several practitioners never to be useful in the disease for which it has been recommended by others, no inference can be drawn from this circumstance. For it remains to be seen,—1, whether it was in each case exactly the same disease that had been treated by its eulogist (nature presents an infinite variety of diseases, that are often confounded with one another; it is excessively rare that exactly the same disease is met with twice); 2, whether it was exactly the same drug (the practitioner often is ignorant of the signs that mark the genuineness of the drug); 3, whether the medicine was always given in these experiments singly and alone, or in combination with things that were capable of altering its efficacy; (as long as physicians do not treat a determinate disease with a single unmixed medicinal substance, but, as is done by them all, mingle it with other powerful drugs, so long it is impossible to draw any, not even a probable conclusion from all their assertions relative to the curative powers of this or that medicament; they all prove *nothing at all*); 4, whether the medicine was given in the most appropriate dose; (have not the doses of most medicines been hitherto left to mere caprice! Must there not, from the very nature of such powerful substances, be a point over and under which this or that medicine cannot be prescribed, without—on account of its very quantity—producing this or that effect, or failing to produce such effect?) 5, whether it was given at a proper or improper period of the disease; 6, whether the (often nasty tasting, nasty smelling), medicine was taken at all, or taken only in part, or not at all; 7, whether some important external influences, or some circumstances peculiar to the constitution of the patient promoted the recovery, and various other considerations.

In like manner, one or several physicians may imagine that they have repeatedly cured the same disease with a certain medicine, and yet notwithstanding their honesty, this may be untrue. If we carefully investigate the above points, we shall invariably find that there is some element of inaccuracy, either that the cases of disease were different, or that the medicine was given either not alone, but in combination with other powerful drugs, or very soon after some other medicines. One or other of these imperfections, usually both, occur almost always in the treatment, whether the result was successful or the reverse.

Where then shall we be able to find a series of pure observations in the practice, that shall be able to establish the curative powers of a single medicine on sure principles? And yet the Vienna Medical Faculty in the first division of its resolutions, decrees that not only the *semen cinæ*, but *colocynth, copaiva-balsam, quassia, sabadilla, sassafras, senega,* and even *cascarilla* are *quite superfluous.* And yet but lately, the far-famed Hofrath Hecker, of Berlin, asserted in a voluminous essay published in *Allg. Anzeiger der D. (No.* 221), "that cascarilla is not only equal in curative virtues to cinchona bark, but is much superior to it." I say *asserted,* for in a thousand words he did nothing more than what the Faculty did in two words; he only *asserted,* but *proved* nothing. He does not adduce a single case (*and could not adduce one*) in which cascarilla had been used *alone* in ague, still less does he shew, in which of the infinitely numerous varieties of ague, cascarilla proved serviceable, when given purely and alone, in order that we may see whether it ʼwas certainly and really alone useful in *the same* cases in which cinchona is, or whether in other cases also, where the latter is of no use, or perhaps might be useful *only* in certain other (what?) cases of ague, but just not such ones as cinchona is alone suitable for. He has, consequently, just as all the rest of the herd of our medical authors are in the habit of doing, deduced with much prolixity: that he has *asserted,* and not that he has *proved* and made the matter clear;—*transeat cum cæteris.*

Now as both parties, the Vienna Faculty and Hofrath Hecker, so flatly contradict each other, which is in the right?

Unhappy art, in which such direct contradictions are possible! What incalculable evil may not daily and hourly be poured forth on suffering humanity from thy cornucopia, which is as vast as the whole range of opinions!

The Faculty rejects this first class as quite superfluous, " because either they are powerless (that they cannot say of the substances named) or any physician can substitute for them indigenous drugs, their well known succedanea." What are these indigenous succedanea; why does not the Faculty name them? It says they are well known. But how can such succedanea be known when they are simply *impossible?*

Among vegetable drugs there are no true succedanea, there can be none. The powers of each of these medicinal substances accurately speaking (and what friend to humanity would not try to be accurate when dealing with substances on which depend the sickness and health, the pains, the death and the life of suffering mankind?) are so multifarious, so peculiar, so different from those of any other drug, that a vegetable medicinal substance can only be replaced by itself, that is by a plant of exactly the same genus and species. There are, no doubt, substances which have one property or another in common with that which it is required to replace. But what becomes of the many other properties that each possesses *peculiarly* by itself?

He who is ignorant of the whole range of properties of the one drug, and likewise of the individual powers of the other which is to be used as its substitute, will certainly find it an easy matter to substitute the one for the other! Hence we see that apothecaries, because they have no more than a superficial acquaintance with the one and the other drug, in respect to their power of altering the organism, find it so easy when their own interests are concerned, to substitute the one for the other in making up their prescriptions.—Poor patients!—" We believe," so the apothecaries have always said in their hearts, " that turpentine is the same as copaiba—we believe that gentian is as good as quassia ; therefore let us substitute the one for the other." *If, as we know but too well, in the whole range of medicine, conjecture can usurp the place of conviction, if this be a mere matter of belief and guess-work,* in that case the conscience of such persons is no doubt satisfied,—before the medical authorities, before the world, —but is it so likewise before the omnicient Deity to whom human life is so precious, who endowed medicines with their inconceivable variety of wonderful properties and virtues, in order that man should investigate them and apply them for the relief of his brethren?

Hear it, our wiser, more conscientious posterity! now-a-days the substitution of one medicine for another, and the whole doctrine of succedanea, which has hitherto constituted the *partie honteuse* of the apothecary system, has even received the sanction of Faculties; different medicinal substances are decreed by high medical authorities to be all the same, to possess the same action, not the hundredth part of whose true, peculiar powers have hitherto been known!

Hear it, our wiser, more conscientious posterity! to our country practitioners, who have never been held to be too richly endowed with knowledge, the talent for careful discrimination, and a clear spirit of observation, now there is preached an indifferentism, right welcome to their habitual indolence, in the choice of remedies (those important instruments of life and death), an indifferentism the grave of all philosophy, of all conscientious discrimination, of all accurate, genuine, estimation of things!

Avaunt thou medical art, still in the babbling infancy that confounds all things with one another! Whilst thou still slumberest in thy cradle, all around thee the impulse to well-directed activity has long since been awakened, and has escaped from the trammels of ignorant credulity. Each of the devoted disciples of the new school investigates the differences and the specific properties of the things that belong to his own department; calmly and on irrefragable principles decides upon the rank that belongs to each, and assigns to it the accurately defined boundaries of its proper sphere; in order that out of all this individualization a philosophically arranged whole may proceed, in order that, consistent, incontrovertible, appropriate, living truth may thence arise.

And yet thou still continuest to sleep? Hitherto crammed to satiety with the sweet baby-food of hypotheses and pleasant figments, and stunted in thy growth by the eternal swaddling clothes of authorities that discountenance all investigations and stifle all liberty of thought, thou hast not yet, dear medicine of the past, entered the ranks of the progressive arts, nor assumed the decisive language of the other manly studies!

The deep earnest spirit of our age demands that the differences of things and of their properties should be ascertained in a

more accurate and minute manner before we can venture to in.
stitute comparisons between them, not to speak of decreeing the
substitution of one for another.   When we shall have investigated the general array of the properties and most of the powers
of every single medicinal substance, which produce such various
effects on the human organism, and when we shall have them
displayed plainly and in their rich completeness before our
view,—then, and not till then, may we be permitted to make
a relative estimate of the nature and properties of the various substances, and to institute comparisons between the curative powers of the different medicines;—to do this sooner
were presumption, that could not even be excused by the plea
of ignorance.

Succedanea of the medicines that are not chemical, but that
act specifically, which shall be *perfect* substitutes for others, there
are not and cannot be, for one medicine is not the same as another,—and succedanea that shall be *partial* and half-and-half
substitutes for others (if such were necessary), cannot be found
until the medicinal properties of the several drugs *accurately
and completely* displayed before the eyes of the world, are available for the purpose of instituting a perfect comparison among
them.   Then, and not till then, will it be possible to pronounce
incontrovertible, irrefragable judgments and verdicts.

EXTRACT FROM A LETTER TO A PHYSICIAN OF HIGH STANDING

ON THE GREAT NECESSITY OF A REGENERATION OF MEDICINE.[1]

Dearest Friend,

It is not in order to * * * you, no! it is on account of your intrinsic excellence and the irrisistible attraction
your excellent heart has for me, that I must give myself the
pleasure of exposing to you my whole course of thought and
conviction, which I have long felt a desire to do publicly.

For eighteen years I have departed from the beaten track in
medicine.   It was painful to me to grope in the dark, guided
only by our books in the treatment of the sick,—to prescribe,
according to this or that (*fanciful*) view of the nature of diseases, substances that only owed to mere opinion their place in

---

[1] From the *Allgem. Anzeiger d. D.* No. 343. 1808.   [The physician to whom this
letter was addressed is the celebrated Hufeland, with whom Hahnemann was long
on terms of intimate friendship.]

the materia medica; I had conscientious scruples about treating unknown morbid states in my suffering fellow-creatures with these unknown[1] medicines, which, being powerful substances, may, if they were not *exactly* suitable (and how could the physician know whether they were suitable or not, seeing that their peculiar, special actions were not yet elucidated) easily change life into death, or produce new affections and chronic ailments, which are often much more difficult to remove than the original disease. To become in this way a murderer, or aggravator of the sufferings of my brethren of mankind, was to me a fearful thought,—so fearful and distressing was it, that shortly after my marriage I completely abandoned practice and scarcely treated any one for fear of doing him harm, and—as you know—occupied myself solely with chemistry and literary labours.

But children were born to me, several children, and in course of time serious diseases occurred, which, because they afflicted and endangered the lives of my children—my flesh and blood— caused my conscience to reproach me still more loudly, that I had no means on which I could rely for affording them relief.

But whence could I obtain aid, *certain, positive* aid, with our doctrine of the powers of medicinal substances founded merely on vague observations, often only on fanciful conjecture, and with the infinite number of arbitrary views respecting disease in which our pathological works abound?—a labyrinth in which he only can preserve his tranquillity who accepts as gospel those assertions relative to the curative powers of medicines because they are repeated in a hundred books, and who receives, without investigation, as oracles, the arbitrary definitions of diseases given in pathological works, and their pretended treatment according to hypothetical notions, as described in our therapeutical works,—who ascribes all the cases of death that occur under his treatment, not to his own practice of shooting blindfold at the mark,—who does not attribute the aggravation and prolongation of the acute diseases he treats and their degeneration into chronic maladies, and the general fruitfulness of his efforts when he has to treat diseases of long standing, to the uncertainty and

---

[2] Respecting many medicines we have numbers of contradictory opinions, which have been repeatedly refuted by experience, and a great array of physical, chemical and natural historical information; but our books afford us no instruction as to what are the exact cases of disease for which they are adapted and in which they may be confidently relied on as curative agents. They are almost entirely unknown in a special medicinal point of view.

impotence of his art—no! he ascribes death and ill-treated disease and all, solely to the incurableness of the disease, to the disobedience of the patient, and to other insignificant circumstances, and so accommodating and obtuse is his conscience, that he satisfies himself with these excuses, though they are in many ways delusive, and can never avail before an omniscient God; and thus he goes on treating diseases (which he sees through his systematic spectacles) with medicinal substances that are far from being without influence on life and death, but of whose powers nothing is known.

Where shall I look for aid, *sure* aid? sighed the disconsolate father on hearing the moaning of his dear, inexpressibly dear, sick children. The darkness of night and the dreariness of a desert all around me; no prospect of relief for my oppressed paternal heart!

In an eight years' practice, pursued with conscientious attention, I had learned the delusive nature of the ordinary methods of treatment, and from sad experience I knew right well how far the methods of Sydenham and Frederick Hoffmann, of Boerhaave and Gaubius, of Stoll, Quarin, Cullen, and De Haen, were capable of curing.

"But perhaps it is in the very nature of this art as great men have asserted, that it is incapable of attaining any greater certainty."

"Shameful, blasphemous thought," I exclaimed.—What, shall it be said that the infinite wisdom of the eternal Spirit that animates the universe could not produce remedies to allay the sufferings of the diseases it allows to arise? The all-loving paternal goodness of Him whom no name worthily designates, who richly supplies all wants, even the scarcely conceivable ones of the insect in the dust, imperceptible by reason of its minuteness to the keenest mortal eye, and who dispenses throughout all creation life and happiness in rich abundance—shall it be said that He was capable of the tyranny of not permitting that man, made in His own image, should, even by the efforts of his penetrating mind, that has been breathed into him from above, find out the way to discover remedies in the stupendous kingdom of created things, which should be able to deliver his brethren of mankind from their sufferings often worse than death itself? Shall He, the Father of all, behold with indifference the martyrdom of his best-loved creatures by disease, and yet have rendered it impossible to the genius of man, to which all else is possible, to

33

find any method, any *easy, sure, trustworthy* method, whereby they may see diseases in their proper point of view and whereby they may interrogate medicines as to their special uses, as to what they are *really, surely,* and *positively* serviceable for?

Sooner than admit this blasphemous thought, I would have abjured all the medical systems in the world!

No! there is a God, a good God, who is all goodness and wisdom! and as surely as this is the case must there be a way of his creation whereby diseases may be seen in the right point of view, and be cured with certainty, a way not hidden in endless abstractions and fantastic speculations!

But why was it never discovered in the two or two and a half thousand years during which there have been men who called themselves physicians?

Doubtless because it was too easy—because like the καλκαγαθια in the choice of the youthful Hercules, it was quite simple, and neither capable nor standing in need of being decked in any of the tawdry tinsel of subtle sophistries and brilliant hypotheses.

Well, thought I, as there *must* a sure and trustworthy method of treatment, as certainly as God is the wisest and most beneficent of beings, I shall seek it no longer in the thorny thicket of ontological explanations, in arbitrary opinions, though these might be capable of being arranged into a splendid system, nor in the authoritative declarations of celebrated men—no, let me seek it where it lies nearest at hand, and where it has hitherto been passed over by all, because it did not seem sufficiently recondite nor sufficiently learned, and was not hung with laurels for those who displayed most talent for constructing systems, for scholastic speculations and transcendental abstractions. It only sufficed for me, whose conscience was not of that ordinary practical character that it would allow me to deliver up to death my children who were in danger, in order to please any system, any leader of a party whatsoever. Accordingly I have made no ostentatious parade of my simple little book (*Medicine of Experience*[1]) that teaches this method, quite contented with having found it myself, contented with having, in the simple style that belongs to truth, revealed it to my brethren, *as far as it was possible to do so by writing, that is, without demonstration at the sick-bed in an* hospital.

"How, then, canst thou"—(this was the mode of reasoning

---

[1] [Vide antea, p. 497.]

by which I commenced to find my way)—" ascertain what morbid states medicines have been created for? (can this be done by *experimenta per mortes in diseases themselves?* Alas! the two thousand five hundred years during which this way alone has been followed, shew that it is beset with innumerable, insurmountable illusions, and *never* leads to certainty).

"Thou must," thought I, " observe how medicines act on the human body, when it is in the tranquil state of health. The alterations that medicines produce in the healthy body, do not occur in vain, they must signify something; else why should they occur? What if these changes have an important, an extremely important signification. What if this be the only utterance whereby these substances can impart information to the observer respecting the end of their being; what if the changes and sensations which each medicine produces in the healthy human organism, be the only comprehensible language by which—if they be not smothered by severe symptoms of some existing disease—it can distinctly discourse to the unprejudiced observer respecting its specific tendencies, respecting its peculiar, pure, positive power, by means of which it is capable of effecting alterations in the body, that is, of deranging the healthy organism, and—where it can cure—of changing into health the organism that has been deranged by disease!" This was what I thought.

I carried my reflections farther. " How else could medicines effect what they do in diseases than by means of this power of theirs to alter the healthy body?"—which is most certainly different in every different mineral substance, and consequently presents in each a different series of phenomena, accidents, and sensations.[1]) Certainly, in this way alone can they cure.

But if medicinal substances effect what they do in diseases, *only* by means of the power peculiar to each of them of altering the healthy body; it follows that the medicine, among whose symptoms those characteristic of a given case of disease occur in the most complete manner, must most certainly have the power of curing that disease; and in like manner that morbid state

---

[1] Each one of the many thousand genera of plants must possess a different medicinal action; in truth, even the several species must differ from each other in this respect, for their permanent differences of appearance announce them as things differing in kind. Here, then, we have fulness and abundance, here we have a divinely rich store of curative powers! Take comfort, sick humanity! What are still required for your relief are, free sagacious men, who have the strength to emancipate themselves from the strong slave-chains of ancient prejudice and theories.

which a certain medicinal agent is capable of curing, must correspond to the symptoms this medicinal substance is capable of producing in the healthy human body! In a word, medicines must only have the power of curing diseases similar to those they produce in the healthy body, and only manifest such morbid actions as they are capable of curing in diseases!

"If I am not deceived"—I thought further—"such is really the case; otherwise how was it that those violent tertian and quotidian fevers, which I completely cured four and six weeks ago without knowing how the cure was effected, by means of a few drops of cinchona tincture, should present almost exactly the same array of symptoms, which I observed in myself yesterday and to-day, after gradually taking, while in perfect health, four drachms of good cinchona bark, by way of experiment?"

I now commenced to make a collection of the morbid phenomena which different observers had from time to time noticed as produced by medicines introduced into the stomachs of healthy individuals, and which they had casually recorded in their works. But as the number of these was not great, I set myself diligently to work to test several medicinal substances on the healthy body, and see, the carefully observed symptoms they produced corresponded wonderfully with the symptoms of the morbid states they could cure easily and permanently.

Now, it was impossible for me to avoid regarding as incontrovertible the maxim that disease was not to be made the subject of ontological and fanciful speculation as though its cure were an eternal enigma, but that it was only necessary that every disease should present itself to the practitioner as a series or group of particular symptoms, in order to enable him to infallibly extinguish and cure it by means of a medicinal substance, capable of producing of itself the same morbid symptoms in the healthy body (provided always that the patient avoids every ascertainable external cause of this disease, in order that the cure should be permanent).

I perceived that this view of diseases—regarding them always according to the sum of all the symptoms presented by each individual case—was the *only* right one, and the only one available for the curative treatment, and that the forms of disease described in our pathological works (those artistic pictures made

---

[1] The results I had collected four years ago, will be found in my book: *Fragmenta de viribus medicamentorum positivis sive in sano corpore humano observatis.* Lipsiæ apud Barth, 1805.

up of fragments of dissimilar diseases) would in future be unable to conceal from us the true aspects of the malady as nature presents it to us at the sick-bed – that the therapeutic doctrines of the numerous systems, abounding as they do in imaginary curative indications and arbitrary modes of treatment, could not henceforth mislead the conscientious practitioner, and that no metaphysical and scholastic speculation respecting the first hidden cause of diseases (that favourite plaything of rationalism) which can never be ascertained by mortal reason, would henceforth render it necessary to invent any chimerical mode of treatment.

I perceived that the only health-bringing way, without any admixture of human inventions, without any display of learning, was discovered.

But it had not yet been trodden! I had to tread it alone, depending on *my own* powers, on *my own* resources; I did so with confidence and with success.

"Take the medicines according to the symptoms careful and repeated observation has shewn they produce in the healthy body, and administer them in every case of disease that presents a group of symptoms comprised in the array of symptoms the medicine to be employed is capable of producing on the healthy body; thus will you cure the disease surely and easily. Or, in other words, find out which medicine contains most perfectly among the symptoms usually produced by it in the healthy body the sum of the symptoms of the disease before you; and this medicine will effect a certain, permanent, and easy cure.

This law, dictated to me by nature herself, I have now followed for many years, without ever having had occasion to have recourse to any one of the ordinary methods of medical practice. For twelve years I have used no purgatives for bile or mucus, no cooling drinks, no so-called solvents· or deobstruents, no general antispasmodics, sedatives, or narcotics, no general stimulants or tonics, no general diuretics or diaphoretics, no rubefacients or vesicatories, no leeches or cupping-glasses, no issues, in fact, none of the appliances prescribed by the general therapeutics of any system whatever, to fulfil indications of cure they have themselves invented. I practised *solely* in accordance with the above law of nature, and in no single instance did I deviate from it.

And with what result? As might have been expected, *the satisfaction I have derived from this mode of treatment I would not exchange for any of the most coveted of earthly goods.*

In the course of these investigations and observations, which
occupied many years, I made the new and important discovery,
that medicines in acting on the healthy body, exhibit two modes
of action and two series of symptoms entirely opposite one to
another, the *first* immediately or soon after their ingestion (or
shortly after contact with the sentient living fibre of any part of
the body)—and the *second,* the very opposite, soon after the disappearance of the first;—that moreover, when the medicines
correspond to the case of disease before us in regard to these
first, primary (medicinal) symptoms, or, in other words, when
most of the symptoms of the disease we have to combat are to
be met with among those which the medicine selected tends to
develop in the first hours of its action on the healthy subject (in
such a manner as that the symptoms of the disease and the primary symptoms of the medicine shall present the greatest possible similarity to one another), then, and then only, will a *permanent* cure result; the morbific irritation present being, as it were,
overcome, displaced and extinguished by another very similar
irritation—produced by the medicine—in an extremely, incredibly short time.   This I termed the *curative* (*radical*) method
of treatment (which produces *permanent* health, most certainly,
and without any after-sufferings.)

On the other hand I perceived,—what was now easy to be
foreseen,—that by adopting an opposite method, that is to say, if
(according to the ordinary mode of procedure, *contraria contrariis curantur*) the primary action of the medicine we employ be
just the *opposite* of the symptoms of the disease (for instance, if
we give opium for habitual sleeplessness or chronic diarrhœa,
wine for debility, or purgatives for chronic constipation), only a
palliative relief, only an amelioration for a few hours will be the
result, for, after these few hours have passed, the period for the
second stage of the medicinal action comes on, which is the contrary of the first action and the analogue of the morbid state it
is sought to cure—consequently, it causes an addition to the disease and an aggravation of it.

In the ordinary practice, whenever symptoms are attacked
with medicines,[1] this is always done, according to the principles
of art now laid down, only in this palliative manner.   The

---

[1] For in addition to the system of alleviating symptoms, there are in the ordinary
practice many others, if possible still more arbitrary, and still more unsuitable modes
of treatment.

medical art as hitherto practised, knows not the curative treatment pointed out above.

But this discovery of mine is so important, that if it were known and acted upon, experience would teach every one that it is only by the curative employment of medicines (*similia similibus*) that a permanent cure—this is especially observable in the case of chronic diseases—can be obtained by the smallest doses in a short time; whereas the ordinary palliative method, according to which every physician without exception on the face of the globe, is accustomed to combat symptoms (if any *contraria* whatsoever can be found), can only alleviate them for a few hours, and must permit the malady, after the expiry of these few hours, to shoot forth more rankly than before, unless the physician—as is not unfrequently the case—prolong the joke for a few days by giving frequently repeated and *always stronger* doses. But then, on the other hand, by such large doses of the —not curative and homœopathically adapted—medicine, and by the secondary action of these large doses, he creates new morbid states, which are often more difficult to cure than the original malady, and which often enough terminate in death.

It must be plain to all, without further demonstration on my part, that it is impossible this hurtful palliative system of treatment can avail in the case of chronic diseases, or restore unalloyed health to those suffering from them; and this is what experience also teaches us, namely, that by no system of treatment hitherto pursued could chronic maladies be removed in a short time and *health* be restored; though occasionally, after a long period of time, such a happy event might be brought about, and health be restored by the spontaneous efforts of nature, by some curatively adapted remedy accidentally prescribed among others, by some mineral water also accidentally suitable to the case, or by other fortuitous circumstances.

Besides inflicting often irreparable injury on the health of man, the palliative system wastes an incredible quantity of expensive drugs, because they must be given in large, often monstrous quantities, to the patients, in order to effect some, though but apparent good results. Thus we see Jones of London requiring three hundred pounds of cinchona bark per annum, and other physicians using several pounds of opium a-piece in the course of the year.

Precisely the contrary is the case with the physician who treats according to the curative method. As he only needs the smallest, but *analogous* medicinal irritation, in order to extinguish speedily an analogous morbid irritation, his requirements in the way of good drugs (even such as are most constantly used) are so small that I hesitate to make even a probable estimate of them, in order not to excite incredulity; so small that the blockade of Europe may be kept up for a long time to come so far as he is concerned.

By pursuing this method of treatment, which differs from all others, which is indeed almost their exact opposite in every respect, the curative physician radically cures with amazing certainty, and in an incredibly short space of time, even chronic diseases of the most ancient date, provided among the remedies he is intimately[1] acquainted with there exists a suitable one.

If the principal, the sole mission of the physician be, as I believe it is, *the cure of diseases*, the deliverance of our brethren of mankind from those innumerable tortures that disturb the tranquil enjoyment of life, that often make existence unbearable, or expose it to danger, and that even obstruct the functions of the mind; how can he, if a sensitive heart still beats within him, or if in his bosom there glows a spark of that holy fire that warms and incites the true man to aspirations for the good of humanity—how can he hesitate for a moment to choose this better, this much more efficacious method of treatment, and to trample under foot the delusions of all former medical schools, even should they be three thousand years old? They have never yet taught us how to cure our fellow-men[2] in a manner that shall satisfy our conscience, but only how we may present to the people an appearance of learned wisdom and deep pene-

---

[1] Of medicines whose action has been accurately ascertained I possess now almost thirty, and of such as are pretty well known, about the same number, without reckoning those with which I am not entirely unacquainted. Entirely unaided, it would be impossible for me to make up for all that has been neglected by my predecessors in my short life, though I have never allowed even the usual pleasures of existence to interfere with my work. I would, ere this, have communicated to the world the large number of medicines whose properties I have investigated since 1804, and have published the whole in German, were it not that the publisher of the *Fragmenta* has begged me to delay doing so on account of the badness of the times.

[2] The little of a positive character to be found amid the enormous mass of medical writings, consists in the accidentally discovered mode of cure of two or three diseases which always arise from identical miasmata; these are, the autumnal marsh ague, the lues venerea, and the itch of workers in wool; to these must be added that most fortunate discovery, the protection from variola by means of vaccination. And these three or four cures take place only according to my principle *similia similibus*. Nothing more of a positive character can be exhibited in the whole medical art since the time of Hippocrates; the cure of all other diseases remained unknow

tration. To the weak-minded alone, injurious delusions and prejudices are holy and inviolable from the circumstance of their having been once established in the world—because they are grown over with the moss of antiquity; the truly wise man on the contrary, joyfully crushes delusion and prejudice beneath his powerful tread, in order to clear the ground for the altar of everlasting truth, which needs not the rust of antiquity to serve as a guarantee of its genuineness, nor the charm of novelty or of fashion, nor any voluminous, verbose system to make it comprehensible to us, nor the sanction of imposing authorities, but which, eloquent with the voice of God, speaks aloud, in accents never to be forgotten, to the inmost heart of every unprejudiced man.

It was requisite that some one should at length beat the way, and this I did.

The way now lies open. Every attentive, zealous and conscientious physician may freely tread it.

What though this way, which alone leads with certainty and safety to the goal of health, and which I, setting aside all current prejudice, discovered by a calm observation of nature, is directly opposed to all the dogmas of our medical schools, just as the theses which Luther of yore courageously posted on the door of the Schlosskirche of Wittenberg were opposed to the mind-enslaving hierarchy—the fault lies neither with Luther's truths nor mine. Neither he nor I deserved the venom of the prejudiced.

"Refute," I cry to my contemporaries, "refute these truths if you can, by pointing out a still more efficacious, sure and agreeable mode of treatment than mine—and do not combat them with mere words, of which we have already *too* many.

"But should experience shew you, as it has me, that mine is the best, then make use of it for the benefit, for the deliverance of humanity, and give God the glory!"

But you, my dearest friend! endowed with the mild spirit of a Melancthon, that would fain unite all opposing parties, bear with me,—since illusion will not amalgamate with truth, bear with the pure-minded seeker after truth, who is inflexible in his convictions, incorruptible by the false doctrines and illusions of systems, even though you may not venture to take a bold glance into the reddening dawn, that must *inevitably* usher in the long wished-for day.

OBSERVATIONS ON THE THREE CURRENT METHODS OF TREATMENT.[1]

There have been till now but three current modes of treatment (the *treatment of diseases* having apparently not yet been discovered,) viz: *the treatment of the name, the treatment of the symptom*, and *the treatment of the cause*.

TREATMENT OF THE NAME.

Interchangeable remedies, compound prescriptions.

The method which from the remotest time has always found the most partisans, which is the most convenient of all, is the treatment of the name. "If the patient has the gout, give him sulphuric acid; the remedy for rheumatism is mercury; cinchona is good for ague, simaruba for dysentery, squills for dropsy." Here the mere name of the supposed disease is sufficient to determine the parempiric [2] for a remedy which crude, indiscriminating experience. has sometimes found useful in diseases that have been superficially termed gout, rheumatism, ague, dysentery, dropsy, but have neither been accurately described nor carefully distinguished from similar affections.

From the very frequent cases of the failure of this quackish sort of practice, which is so repulsive to me that I cannot dwell long upon it, some well-intentioned adherents of this method were from time to time induced to seek for several remedies for each name of a disease; the rude experience of domestic practice, the oracles of old herbalist books, or fantastic speculation (signature), were the gross sources whence these remedies flowed in abundance.

This was the plan pursued: "If A should not answer, try B, and if this will not do, a choice lies among C, D, E, F, G; I have often found H and K of service; others recommend most highly J and L, and I know some who cannot sufficiently praise M, U and Z, whilst others extol N, R and T. S and X also are said not to be bad in this disease. Some English physician recently recommended Q in preference to all others in this affection; I certainly would be inclined to give it a trial."

"How frequently have I formerly cured ague with cinchona," says another practitioner, "and yet of late years I have met with

---

[1] From *Hufeland's Journal of Practical Medicine*, vol. xi, pt. 4. 1809.

[2] *Parempiricism* may stand for the evil demon, *empiricism* for the good genius of experience.

some cases where I could do nothing with it. One of these, in which bark had long been used in vain, I might almost say with injury to the patient, an old woman in the neighbourhood cured with chamomile tea. One of my colleagues cut short two cases of ague with a few emetics, in which neither chamomile tea nor bark in the largest doses was of the slightest service. I tried this method in cases where neither of the two latter medicines did good, but the emetics did no good in them; I bethought myself of giving sal-ammoniac, and to my astonishment the patients recovered. Yet have I met with cases where, after bark, chamomile and emetics were tried in vain, sal-ammoniac also was of no use. Just about that time I read that gentian and sometimes nux vomica were useful in ague. I tried them. The former answered in two cases, the latter in three, where neither gentian nor the other medicines were useful. Belladonna is also said to have cured certainly and thoroughly some agues where all other remedies have been fruitless; and some assert they have met with the same result from the use of James' powder and calomel. The bark of mahogany and that of the horse-chesnut have also been lauded; but I don't believe they have much power, I can't tell why. We all know what good effects opium often has. Recently I was much struck with a case of quartan ague, that had tormented a robust peasant for a year and a half, in spite of the employment of every conceivable remedy; to my astonishment it yielded to a few drops of tincture of ignatia, sent to him by a foreign professor. And, between you and me, I must give credit to our hangman for having occasionally effected radical cures of agues that were ineffectually treated by myself and my colleagues with the above remedies, by means of some red drops, which I am credibly informed contained arsenic, although he caused with it in some cases chronic complaints, dropsy and even death. So obstinate and capricious are agues sometimes!"

My friend, do you never suspect that all these were different kinds of agues, or rather intermittent diseases differing completely from one another? If it were possible that an ague could be so capricious and obstinate, wherefore did it yield so readily to one remedy? Do you not suspect that there may be more than one, that there may be perhaps twenty different kinds of intermittent fever, which parempirical imbecility has included under one head, has asserted all to belong to a single species (intermittent fever), and has sought to combat all with a single remedy, whereas each requires its peculiar remedy, without thereby deserving to be called capricious or obstinate.

"Ah! but the practical physician has neither the inclination nor the time to draw such fine distinctions betwixt similar diseases and to assign to each its appropriate remedy. If the patient tells us he has intermittent fever, I and my colleagues give him" (you fool! do you not wish to become a bit wiser?) "at first an emetic or two; if that does no good, or does harm, we then give him cinchona; if that does not cure in large doses, neither the common sort nor the royal bark, we then give—"

Just so; you blindly give one after the other until you hit upon the right one. But you can only go on with your experiments as long as the patience, the purse, or the life of your patient lasts! Your obedient servant, doctor!

And thus there arose long lists of simple drugs (*interchangeable remedies, succedaneums*) which were all, without distinction, said to be serviceable for one disease.

Out of these lists of the names of drugs, the more elegant physicians, to give themselves an air of rationality whilst they were guilty of the grossest parempiricism, constructed their compound prescriptions,—three, four or six ague remedies, five, six or eight dropsy remedies, all jumbled together, drawn at haphazard from the list, which were recorded in their manuals under the name "Intermittent fever," "Dropsy," and used in practice by coupling them with some kind of spirit, syrup, &c. In this case, too, the mere name of the disease was combatted, but, by your leave, reader, much more methodically! with several weapons at a time. "If one ingredient in the mixture does not do any good, then the second and the third, or if all these strings break, the fourth, the sixth, the eighth, tenth, fifteenth, must effect the desired object." Thenceforth no one would look so unlearned as to prescribe only a single medicine.[1]—Thenceforth no prescription was given that did not contain a hotch-potch of simple drugs; and that not for investigated, definite diseases,

---

[1] If Brown could have the merit, though himself a practical physician, of having lifted for us the curtain which conceals the secret workings of the organism from our art, yet this merit is reduced to a nullity by that general, injurious and most erroneous maxim of his (*Elements of Medicine*, § xcii): "The cure of any disease of considerable violence, and scarce of any at all, is never to be entrusted to any one remedy; the use of several remedies is preferable to that of one"—a precept that would alone prove his incapacity as a teacher of medicine. Nothing is less known or less investigated in nature than the powers of medicinal substances, *our weapons!* How can we learn them otherwise than by using them singly? Or is a single drug, if it be the proper one, less powerful to remove a single disease than a mixture of several that counteract each other's action?

but for mere names of diseases! Parempiricism could not ascend higher, common sense could not descend lower.

TREATMENT OF THE SYMPTOM.

General indications ; general remedies. Routine remedies.

The impossibility of discovering sure remedies for vague names of diseases, induced now and then more conscientious physicians to distinguish diseases more accurately. Those that were evidently dissimilar were separated, the similarities of many of them were investigated, and those that were considered to be connected were united in classes, orders, and species, &c., according to the similarity of their exciting causes, the functions that were deranged, the identity of their seat in the body, the peculiar tone of the fibres, and some common symptoms.

By means of this historical view of the apparent relations and differences, they sought to make us better acquainted with the nature of the innumerable diseases, and to persuade us that then we knew enough about them, to enable us to cure them after that. Some resorted to generalizing (the ordinary pathologists), others to subdividing (the nosologists).

But this labour (and that at the hands of men like Rudolph Augustin Vogel or Wichmann) was only successful in so far as it had reference to the description of the course of some epidemic diseases that frequently recurred in pretty well defined characters, and to the description of endemic diseases of a fixed stamp, and of diseases whose cause was evident (the symptoms produced by some poisons—lead, charcoal-vapour—or infection by some miasms that never altered their character much—syphilis, itch). Still in all these, indescribable varieties occur, which often alter the whole affair.

(For as all other diseases, whatever be their outward resemblance—for example, the dropsies and tumours, the chronic skin diseases and ulcers, the abnormal fluxes of blood and mucus, the infinite varieties of pains, the hectic fevers, the spasms, the so-called nervous affections, &c.—present such innumerable differences among themselves in their other symptoms, that every single case of disease must as a general rule be regarded as quite distinct from all the rest, *as a peculiar individuality*, it is evident that any general descriptions of them in entire classes must not only be superfluous but must lead to error.)

However, I forbear at present from attempting to estimate their services to our art, and shall only observe that the pathological and nosological investigators who possessed this kind of historical knowledge were not much happier[1] in their treatment than those who treated mere names of diseases.

These in particular were the persons who (in combination with the therapeutists by profession), as a forlorn hope, invented the make-shift of decyphering the appropriate remedy from the description of the disease, of devising for diseases arranged in ranks and orders some general plan of treatment that should be suitable for every one of them, that is to say, the method of treatment according to general indications, the method of treatment by means of so-called *general remedies.* "The indications of impurities in the alimentary canal demand evacuations upwards and downwards, heat demands cooling medicines, fluxes demand astringents, putridity antiseptics, pains sedatives, weakness tonics, spasms antispasmodics, constipation purgatives, dysuria diuretics, a dry skin diaphoretics." Under the guidance, of the frequently misunderstood results of experience the evacuants, the cooling remedies, the astringents, the antiseptics, the sedatives, the tonics, the antispasmodics, the purgatives, the diuretics, and the diaphoretics were devised, and here was at once a complete system of therapeutics, for the over-completeness of which some other classes of remedies were invented for symptoms that were often but the offspring of fancy, such as incisives, solvents, diluents, &c.

I know not which parempiricism is preferable to the other, whether the treatment of the name of the disease, or the treatment of the name of particular symptoms. Suffice it to say, that this method had much greater attractions for the superficially instructed, much greater than most of the other methods with a trace of rationality in them, hence it was that most generally pursued by those who wished to be considered really learned physicians of a better stamp than the common herd. Of all the false methods of treatment it will undoubtedly have the longest run, because it does not necessitate much care nor much thought. It is undoubtedly very agreeable for the phy-

---

[1] Even the model of graphic description, even the most natural picture of the very constantest of all diseases, those of an endemic character, never guides us to the remedy;—the most accurate amount of pellagra, yaws, sibbens, pian, ringworm, tsömör, water-kulk, plica polonica, &c., throws no light on the specific remedy that is capable of removing each of these maladies quickly, easily, and radically; this remains still concealed from our eyes in the bosom of nature. What hint, then, could be derived for the appropriate remedy from the general description of those diseases whose character was less constant, which presented more varieties among each other, and were more vague!

sician to feel himself so powerful, or at all events to appear to be able to promote perspiration here, urine there, to lull pain here, to excite there, to bind here, to loosen there, to incise here, to expel there, to strengthen here, to cool there, to check spasms here, and putridity there, to accomplish all that he commands his cohorts of medicines to do. How often the practitioner cannot do all this, how often he finds himself deceived in his expectations relative to the medicines which have been stamped as general remedies by his teachers, he knows full well himself.

But admitting there were such general remedies that would here and there certainly promote perspiration, assuredly cause a flow of urine, strikingly soothe pain, infallibly strengthen, undeniably resolve, loosen, purge, and cause vomiting, powerfully act upon the secretion of mucus, in every case cool, allay every spasm, and check every inordinate discharge, unhesitatingly transfer congestions from a more to a less important seat, will all this, supposing it went on ever so beautifully, cure the disease? Oh, no! in most cases not. Something striking has been performed, *but health has not been restored,* and that was what had to be done.

At one time the physician soothes with his opium for a few hours cough and pains in the chest; after sixteen hours, however, the painful cough increases to a still more frightful extent —he produces a stupified sleep with it, but the patient is not refreshed thereby, his sleeplessness and anxiety become all the greater. The physician does not care for this; he increases the dose of his palliative, or he is contented with having shewn his power to allay cough and to cause sleep, though the patient is made worse thereby, though he should even die. *Fiat justitia et pereat mundus.*

Here is a case of dropsy; very little urine is passed. Our doctor will promote its flow. His squill stands at the head of his diuretic picquet. Beautiful! it instantly causes a great flow of urine, but on continuing its use, alas! always less and less water comes. Symptoms of atonic inflammation and mortification ensue, the anorexia, debility and restlessness increase with the swelling. Then if nothing more will avail, he allows the patient to die quietly, after having shewn that he has the power of causing a flow of urine for some days.

Squill has been used many thousands of times as a diuretic (during all the ages it has been employed it was never observed that it was only diuretic in a palliative sense) and yet how seldom has dropsy been *cured* by it! only when a kind of suppressed menstruation was the cause.

The physician who is consulted diagnoses this malady to be gastric; he purges, and re-purges. But behold the fever increases, the taste becomes more disagreeable, the breath and the excrements more fetid, the sclerotic yellower, the tongue more furred and browner, the ideas get confused, the lips tremble, stupifying slumber takes the place of sleep, &c. He is sorry to see his patient hurrying on towards his grave, but he is happy that he possessed the power of energetically purging away the impurities. What is the matter with you? "I put myself in a violent passion, my head is like to burst, I have spasms in my stomach, the bile rises incessantly into my mouth." You will, perhaps, take a bilious fever, take this emetic immediately. Look! he throws up bile, he vomits again and again, he will vomit up his very inside—the night of death obscures his sight, whilst he is bathed in cold perspiration. "I have done my duty," says the doctor to himself; "I have done all I could to clear away the bad bile."

And thus it is with the whole array of general remedies. The respectable doctor does much, only not what he ought;— he produces remarkable effects, but very seldom health.

Thousand-fold experience could teach him, if he would but let himself be taught, that in dropsy he only requires to remove the morbid disposition, in order to see the water disappear by ways which nature knows best how to choose for herself,—but that his designed removal of the water by the urinary organs, or by stool, effects a cure as seldom as tapping it off with the trocar; when a cure does ensue, it must be because the diuretic remedy was accidentally at the same time the proper remedy for the disease upon which that kind of dropsy depended.

Thousand-fold experience could teach him, if he would but let himself be taught, that no pain can be removed permanently and advantageously to the patient except by a remedy that affords relief to the fundamental disease; that, consequently, opium *very rarely* allays pains permanently *with desirable results,* and only when it is the true remedy for the disease on which they depended.

That opium is often the best remedy in diseases most free from pain, and attended with the greatest amount of sopor, that he does not and will not know. He is proud of his power of palliating, and of being able to allay pains for a few hours; but the after-effects—they do not trouble him. *Nil nisi quod ante pedes est.*

Where the short-sighted individual thought that it was absolutely necessary to remove bucketfuls of fetid mucus and excrement by means of all sorts of emetics and purgatives, in order to preserve life, in such a case a single drop of the tincture of arnica root will often remove, in the course of a couple of hours, all the fever, all the bilious taste, all the tormina, the tongue becomes clean, and the strength is restored before night. Short-sighted being!

But the poisonous bile, stirred up by rage and passion, how can it be subdued without causing it to be vomited clean away? My short-sighted friend! a single dose, an almost imperceptibly small quantity of the right medicine[1] will, *without any evacuation of bile*, have restored all to the right state before the second day dawns. The patient has not died as he would have done after your emetic; he has recovered.

How often are blood-letting and nitre abused, to combat symptoms of heat! Lay aside your life-shortening, temporizing remedies, remove the disease on which the accelerated pulse depends, by the appropriate remedy, and the heat ceases of its own accord. But I perceive you are not concerned about the cure of the disease, to subdue the heat is your object. Then rather open one of the large arteries until the last drop of blood is drained off, you will thereby attain your object more surely and more completely!

And thus it is always with your favourite general remedies. They render you the service of sometimes shewing you to be a mighty physician. Only it is a pity that the patient who peradventure recovers (slowly and painfully enough!) seldom, seldom owes his recovery *to them*.

But the general remedies just as often do not perform the effects they desire. Only look, how their antiphlogistic remedies often actually increase the inflammation, how their tonics increase the weakness, their purgatives the symptoms of impurities in the alimentary canal, their solvents the quantity of mucus and the hardness of the abdomen, their sedatives the pains, their derivatives the congestions, their diaphoretics the dryness of the skin, their diuretics the want of urine and oedema!

---

[1] Frequently the extract of chamomile.

34

And if they sometimes succeed in checking this or that symptom for a time, or in effecting this or that striking evacuation, how comes it that the disease notwithstanding sometimes assumes a worse turn? *Am I right in asserting that they were not the proper remedies for the disease?*

In like manner, the poor fellow unable to swim, struggles away with awkward partial movements of his arms and legs, to sink all the more certainly to the bottom.

In ordinary everyday practice, however, it is not required that we should trouble ourselves with anxiously attending to single symptoms. "When once we have got over the first irksome years incidental to young beginners—years they undoubtedly are of irksomeness and care, when we are still anxious to discover the adequate, the helpful, the best for our patients, and when the tender conscience of youth gives us much trouble—when once we have got over these pedantic years, and have got some way into the period of divine routine, then it is a real pleasure to be a practical physician. Then we have only to assume a dignified mode of carrying the head, speak in a tenor voice so as to inspire respect, give great importance to the movements of the three first fingers of the right hand, and present a certain authoritative something in the whole management of the voice and attitudes of the body, in order to be able to exercise perfectly in all its details, the golden art of the *savoir faire* of the routine physician. Of course the smallest details of the attire of the equipage, of the furniture, and of the array of servants, must all be in harmonious keeping.

"If our whole thinking power and memory during the four-and-twenty hours of each day are completely absorbed in such matters, this renders us all the more successful as physicians. Our whole practice, be it said betwixt ourselves, consists in two or three innocuous mixtures, well known to the chemist, in as many compound powders adapted for all cases, in an expensive *tinctura nervino-roborans*, a few juleps, and a couple of formulas for pills, either for acting on the blood or the bowels (*nostrums* and *routine remedies* if you will), and with these we get on capitally. My steaming horses rattle up to N.'s door, I descend from my carriage assisted by the respectful domestic, with helpful speed, but with an air of deep thought and dignified mien. The attendants of the patient throw open both wings of the door of the sick-room. In silence and with abased head stand esteem, confidence, and semi-devotion in a row, to allow the deliverer to approach the sick bed. 'How did you sleep last night, my good friend?—your tongue!—your pulse! The powders ordered yesterday may be discontinued. The mixture prescribed here is to be taken alternately with the pills indicated below, followed by the julep every half-hour.' Taking a pinch of snuff with an air of profound gravity, seizing my hat and stick and making a practised bow, the degree of which is regulated for every one in particular according to his supposed importance or rank, this constitutes the whole of the important comedy (shall I call it business?) for which we are paid as a consultation, and which we repeat as often per diem as the serious looks of the surrounding friends seem to render it necessary; for they are the barometer of the danger, since we have neither time nor inclination to ascertain it for ourselves in all our cases." And how many visits of this sort do you pay in one day? "Do you imagine, you simpleton, that I can keep up my establishment with less than several dozens of visits in a forenoon?"—What Herculean mental labour!—"Ha! ha! ha! to scribble down on a long strip of paper one of the eight or ten routine prescriptions that I can reckon up on my fingers, and can seize on in the dark without a moment's thought, the first, the best that occurs to me at the moment, without the least reflection; do you call that mental labour? It is a much more difficult matter for me to find a pair of handsome bays to supply the place of my used-up afternoon horses! *hoc opus, hic labor!*

"I have just now also much difficulty in thinking of the appropriate dishes for the sixth entrée of the entertainment we are to give to morrow fortnight, so that it may be distinguished for its rarity in respect of the season of the year, for its suitable elegance, and for its brilliant tastefulness. *Et hoc opus et hic labor!*"

The so-called favourite remedies are in great vogue; without being able to give the slightest reason for so doing, one physician of the ordinary stamp will mix with every prescription, prepared muscle-shells, a second always manages to introduce magnesia, a third invariably adds spiritus mindereri, a fourth can scarcely write a prescription from which purified nitre is excluded, a fifth brings into all his prescriptions the inspissated juice of the root of triticum repens, a sixth thinks he cannot give the extract of dandelion often enough, a seventh seasons every draught with opium, and an eighth endeavours to bring in cinchona everywhere, whether it is suitable or not, and so it goes on. Most every-day physicians have, they know not why, their favourite remedies. Anything more indo'ent and par-empirical cannot be imagined. How should all the countless array of infinitely various diseases, each of which demands a peculiar mode of treatment, always accommodate themselves to one and the same remedy, which the doctor may happen to have taken under his sublime protection? Sooner might a cabinet-minister be chosen from mere caprice, and it be taken for granted that the subjects of the prince will be sufficiently obedient and intelligent as to make harmony of the false gamut.

To stake constantly on the drawing of one and the same number always betrays a bad lotto-player. He *must* certainly occasionally win, but how much, or rather how little can he win? And does he not continually lose, these few miserable cases excepted, by not winning? Does he not render himself ridiculous to all the world?

TREATMENT OF THE CAUSE.

Treatment founded on the internal essence of the disease.

In a practically useful point of view we may divide diseases in general into two classes; diseases having a visible, simply material cause, and diseases having an immaterial dynamic cause.

The first class, the diseases having an obvious, simple, material cause, such as a splinter 'stuck in the finger, a stone swallowed, a concretion in the biliary ducts or the bladder, an accumulation of plum-stones in the cœcum, an acrid acid in the stomach, a fragment of the skull pressing on the brain, a too-prolonged frenum to the tongue, &c., are much less numerous than the diseases of the second class.

The indication for treatment is obvious. All are agreed that it consists in the removal of the material cause, be that mechanical, be it merely chemical, or a mixture of both. This generally suffices to effect a cure, provided no considerable destruction of the organ has occurred.

Its consideration does not concern us at present.

We shall occupy ourselves with *the mode of curing the second class of diseases,* the countless array of all other diseases properly so called, of an acute, sub-acute, and chronic character, together with the numerous ailments, indispositions, and abnormal states, having *an immaterial dynamic cause.*

It is the natural tendency of the human mind to seek for the exciting causes of the phenomena he sees about him, and hence we see, that no sooner does a disease show itself, than every one occupies himself with attributing it to some source, that which seems to him to be the most likely one. But we should be greatly mistaken if, from this irresistible propensity to seek a cause for an effect, we should infer a necessity for such knowledge in order to effect a cure.

For very few diseases of the latter class do we know the dynamic cause even by name, of none do we know the nature. Into the secrets of nature *no created mind can penetrate.* And yet as regards diseases, it is imagined that both can be known. The ordinary physician has this in common with the generality of people, that he imagines he can assign an exciting cause for every perceptible alteration in the health, and those physicians who were apparently the wisest, imagined that they could penetrate even to the internal essence of diseases, and that they were thereby enabled to cure them.

Owing to the very nature of the thing, it is impossible that the essential nature of most of the dynamic causes derived from without can ever be ascertained.

How much have not some attempted to demonstrate to us respecting the influence of the seasons and of the various states of the weather, as exciting causes of diseases! We were told of the variations in the thermometer and barometer, the various winds, and the alternations of moisture and dryness of the atmosphere for a whole year, or at least for several months, before the occurrence of an epidemic, and the murderous disease was attributed quite off-hand and without much consideration to the weather that prevailed during all that long period, just as if the disease could be derived from the state of the weather, or as if they bore the relation to one another of cause and effect. But granting that there was something in this, at least in the variations of the seasons, as the cause, or at least partly the cause of particular kinds of diseases, how little comfort can the physician derive from these *unalterable* accompaniments of the world's course, how little assistance do they render him in proving the indications from which he can bid defiance to the epidemic actually prevailing! Were the season of the year and the previous state of the weather really the cause of the prevailing distemper, it would avail him little or nothing to know this, seeing that from this cause the specific remedy for the pestilence cannot be deduced, cannot be decyphered.

Fright, fear, horror, anger, vexation, a chill, &c., are impressions that do not present themselves in a concrete form, that cannot be subjected to physical investigation.

How and to what extent these impressions derange the human system, what especial kind of disease they produce in it, is so entirely unknown to us, that we obtain not the slightest hint for the treatment of the diseases they give rise to, by being in-formed of the names of their probable source—fright, fear, vexation, anger, &c. The most abstract investigation into the metaphysical nature of fright affords the physician no instruc-tion relative to the proper treatment of its effects, never ex-presses the name of the appropriate remedy of the acute symp-toms arising from fright—the name of *opium.* This is not the place to indicate the shorter, more natural way by which this remedy has been discovered for these accidents.

It is very easy to say, that we may attribute itch to the itch miasm, the venereal disease to the venereal miasm, variola to the variolous miasm, ague to the marsh miasm. By pronouncing these names not the slightest advance is made to obtaining a more accurate knowledge of these diseases, nor yet to their ap-propriate treatment. The morbific miasms are as thoroughly unknown to us as regards their internal nature, as the diseases themselves they produce. Their essential nature is quite beyond the reach of our senses, and their true remedies will never be learned from what the schools can teach us regarding their ex-citing causes. All that has been discovered relative to their remedies has been discovered by mere accident, by unpremedi-tated experience. But the way to seek for them purposely and to find them will never be deducible from aught we can ascer-tain respecting the internal cause of the disease.

What amount of knowledge respecting the cause and essential nature of *endemic* diseases would suffice to reveal to us their true remedies? For us weak mortals there will ever remain an im-passable gulf betwixt such a fancied knowledge and the remedy. Reason will never discover a logical connexion betwixt the two! Were even a God to enlighten us in regard to the invisible al-terations produced in the interior of the minuest portions of our body by the miasm of that most tedious, periodical endemic dis-ease that prevails in a portion of Lunenburg and Brunswick—*the water-kulk* (water-colic) as it is termed, which the eye of the practised anatomist cannot discover, and were our mind, that is cognizant only of sensuous impressions capable of understanding such transcendental instruction, this intuitive knowledge would never guide us to the discovery of the only specific and infallible remedy—the *veratrum album.* But this is not the place to shew the shorter, more natural way in which the remedy for this disease may be sought and found.

Neither the name of goitre, nor its probable cause (a residence in mountain valleys) whispers to our mind the name of its remedy which was revealed by mere accident—the burnt sponge.

Why then should we falsely and proudly pretend that we can cure diseases from our knowledge of their dynamic causes?

For the accidents and diseases produced by commercial and pharmaceutic poisons the appropriate remedies have partially been discovered, but it was neither specu'ative investigation into the internal nature of these diseases nor physico-chemical analysis of their cause—the poisons—that taught us these specific antidotes, but a much shorter procedure, and one much more consonant with nature. It is not very long since these hurtful substances were attempted to be removed, often with very unhappy results, by emetics, diluent drinks or purgatives, as if they oppressed the stomach and bowels in a merely mechanical manner. Now, we know how to combat many of them like morbific causes of the second class, of dynamic nature, by their appropriate antidotes. They effect an alteration of the whole system in a peculiar, to us unknown manner, and their effects can never be cured like mere local mechanical irritations, as was formerly imagined.

Others went much more learnedly to work, and divided them, in an entirely apodictic manner, just as though they had been inspired thereto by a God, into acrids, narcotics, narcotico-acrids, &c., and agreeably to this arbitrary classification, dictated their remedies in an equally arbitrary manner;—*a true picture of the mode of procedure of the schools, classifying natural diseases, and assigning the remedies for them!* Arbitrariness, conceited arbitrariness, and self-satisfied pride!

Thus belladonna and nux vomica were, with arbitrary despotism, ranked among the narcotic poisons, and the vegetable acids, lemon juice and vinegar, were cavalierly appointed their antidotes. Unfortunately for them, their assumed omniscience could here be put to an infallible test, and their error detected in the very act. It was proved that vegetable acids were the very substances that most aggravated the symptoms. *And so it will usually be found, that the very opposite of what they assert is often the truth.*

Sed saeculorum commenta delet dies.

It never could have entered into the imagination of this church beyond whose pale there is no salvation, to assign opium as the antidote of the one, camphor as that of the other of these powerful substances, as experience has shewn to be the case.

But they were not content with dragging in as it were by the ears, or inventing external causes for diseases, or with arbitrarily attributing to them some peculiar nature, and, I cannot say searching for (for one can only search for a thing when there are well-grounded traces and indications of its existence), but rather imagining and inventing remedies directed against this supposed nature. They went still more learnedly to work, and concocted in their brains all sorts of *internal causes* of diseases.

The ambitious notion that they were capable of referring most diseases to one or a couple of internal causes, now became the origin of the many sects among physicians, each successive one of which was more fantastic than its predecessor.

One of these, and that not the worst, expressed the in some degree special life and the peculiarities and particular actions of each individual organ, by the figurative name of an *Archæus*, a kind of particular spirit of this or that part, and imagined that when this or that part suffered they required to soothe its particular *Archæus*, and give its thoughts another direction. It appears to me that they meant to make a confession of the incomprehensibility of all the phenomena of disease, and a confession of their inability to satisfy the requirements of these supernatural things.

Others thoughts to persuade us that a predominance of acid was the proximate cause of all diseases, and they prescribed nothing but alkalies. An attempt to ally itself with them was made by the old sect which referred all kinds of acute diseases, especially the epidemic maladies, to a common poison which they contended often developed itself in the interior of the body, and sought for the antidote of this poison, which they believed to be the general excitant of most diseases, in absorbent alkaline earths, but especially in the stony concretions found in the stomach of an antelope (bezoar) and in the most heating spices mixed with opium (mithridate, theriac, philonium, &c.). Their abuse of the earthy powders has extended down to modern times, and their evil demon, the empirical universal abuse of opium, has now possessed some sects of the present time, who have thought of other reasons for their misapplication of this remedy for special cases as a positively universal remedy.

C. L. Hoffmann imagined that he had an equal right to set

forth as a universal truth his own particular notion that almost all diseases arose from a kind of putridity, and were to be cured with remedies which his school denominates antiseptics.

No one will question his right any more than they will that of the other leaders of sects, who perceived in diseases nothing but acridities in the blood; demonstrated these for our edification by far fetched, scholastic arguments, and in an off-hand manner at once invented the remedies for the black bile, for the psoric, arthritic, scrofulous, rachitic, muriatic and God knows what other kinds of imaginary acridities, until the moderns, unmindful of the *medio tutissimus*, founded a religion equally exaggerated in the opposite direction, in which the fluids were entirely banished from the list of morbific causes, and the production of disease was attributed to the solids alone.

In this way the poor diseases were ascribed now by this pigheaded fellow and now by that, at one time to this, at another to that cause. All this time they remained in quiet possession, and never suffered themselves to be disturbed.

Let it not be supposed that on the whole more diseases were cured by one sect than by another. To excogitate causes of diseases, speculative modes of their production, and to found systems thereon, were what was aimed at; but not *to cure* them. The former undertaking exalts the artist much nearer the stars than the latter, and thus diseases remained just as before, uncured, except such of them as would get as well of their own accord, that is, under any arbitrary treatment whatsoever.

The doctrine of bad humours long enchained mankind, the dominion of acridities and perverted juices long prevailed. But as the specific anti-acridity remedies could not so readily be found out, the whole joke usually and principally consisted in producing evacuations. With the exception of a few empirical drinks and several kinds of mineral waters prescribed at haphazard, which the humoral physician commanded to enter the blood, to sweeten it, to correct it, and to expel by sweat and urine the impure parts of it separated from the good portion as if by magic, the principal manœuvre of the humoral school consisted in the evacuation of the bad blood (bleeding mania) and in the expulsion of the impure fluids by the mouth and anus (stercoralism, saburralism.)

How? did they pretend to let out the impure blood only? What magician's hand could separate, as through a sieve, the depraved from the good blood within the blood-vessels, so that only the bad would be drawn off and the good remain? What head is so rudely organized as to believe that they could effect this? Sufficient for them that streams of blood were spilt, of that vital fluid for which even Moses shewed so much respect, and that justly.

The more refined humoralists, in addition to the impurities in the blood, alleged besides, the existence of a pretended, almost universal plethora, as an excuse for their frightful, merciless blood-lettings; they also gave out that these acted derivatively, depressed the tone, and ascribed many other subtle scientific effects to them. They acted, as we see, like other sects, quite arbitrarily, but obviously with an endeavour (not indeed to cure, that would be vulgar, no!) to give to their arbitrary procedures the highest possible colouring of rationality.

Reasons equally excellent, aims equally sage, had the humoral-saburral physicians for their innumerable emetics and their strong and mild purgatives. "Consider the quantity of impurities that are thereby purged from the blood, only look at the contents of the chamber utensil! When all that has been removed, then the body will be purified from all bad humours. Consider, moreover, what a quantity of impurities must daily remain and collect in the body from the food and drink we take in;—it must be purged away, and that repeatedly, if we do not wish the patient to die. Observe also how most patients complain of tense or at all events painful abdomen, or at least of unnaturally shaped hypochondria, furred tongue and bad taste; who can fail to perceive from these signs that the germs of all fevers, the actual cause of all diseases, lie in the impurities of the first passages? Yes, we must certainly purge, and that frequently and strongly, in order to bring away the material cause of the disease. The excellence of our method is shewn by this, that we are in high estimation as skilful physicians. The patient feels that he gets a good equivalent for his money, he perceives how the medicine acts on his body, and he sees with his own eyes the impurities that are expelled from him! Who can deny that all this speaks to the convictions of the people, who can doubt that our church alone holds the true faith?"

"I cannot quite agree with you, brother," says another branch of the saburral school, "when you ascribe all diseases to the bile. I maintain that they all depend upon the phlegm in the first passages. The phlegm must be energetically cut into, diligently dissolved; the phlegm, I say, must be properly purged away, in order to extirpate the disease by the roots. All your bilious and putrid fevers are masked pituitous fevers, all conceivable diseases now-a-days depend upon phlegm, and if patients treated according to our method are long in recovering, we yet can boast of our system that it is radical and lucrative."

Thus would Blennophilos (in the style of his whole art) descant still more discursively upon the advantages of his system, whilst Eucholos, greatly displeased at hearing the bile denied to be the universal cause of diseases, could not refrain from making an equally vigorous speech in defence of bile, which demands a general employment of emetics and purgatives. "Bile, bile must be expelled," was the conclusion of his philippic, "diligently and universally, upwards and downwards must it be expelled, for it is the originating cause of all diseases!"

Accordingly the poor world was for more than half a century properly cleared out upwards and downwards, so that any one must have thought that it was thoroughly cleansed of all impurities. All a mistake, said Kämpf they are not nearly enough dissolved and purged, at least they have not had half enough of the only efficacious process from below. The source of all diseases has been sought for in an entirely wrong place. Whence proceed the many hundreds of hypochondriacal and hysterical nervous diseases, the hitherto mysterious chronic diseases of the better classes, whence all the pulmonary, hepatic, splenic, cutaneous and cephalic diseases, and I may say all other diseases, whence do they all proceed if not from infarctus and lodgments in the abdomen? By means of solvent clysters in hundreds must these be dissolved and purged away if we wish to avert death. Heavens! how purblind the world has been not to have discovered before now, this the only possible remedy for the only possible cause of all diseases! And verily, there could scarcely be a more lucrative method for the practitioner; by no other could he so beautifully get over the difficulties of his indications as by this, by which, without requiring to give any further reason, holding up the fearful talisman of infarctus in order to work uncontrolled in the dark, beyond the ken of the common sense of the uninitiated, and with the hocus-pocus of several hundred clysters (composed of a number of unintelligible ingredients) he could—how wonderful!—bring bodily to light the dreaded infarctus in all its hideous deformity. Making omelettes in a hat is child's play to this.

If, sighed Tyro, I only knew all the external signs by which lodgments could be diagnosed in any human being, If I only knew what infarctus really is, what part of the intestines (of so many, of almost all persons!) is constituted so torpid, as to harbour in such an imperceptible manner these Protean masses, and what causes their greyish colours, their various shapes, consistences, and odours, as they are to be found arranged in a tabular form in Kämpf's work! The difficulties of the subject make me quite ill! since there are no sure external signs of their existence, who can tell whether some such horrors do not lurk in my own entrails!

Grieve not, dear Tyro! that your five senses are inadequate to enable you to discover all this. The game of infarctus and infarctus-clysters is already played out. It was only a financial manœuvre, if it was not a pious self-deception of the inventor. By a succession of clysters we may make the bowels of even the healthiest peasant into an organ for the production of unnatural fæces, of masses of mucus of every variety of form and colour.

Other modern visionaries attributed almost all diseases they could not cure to a step-sister of the infarctus, I mean to obstruction in the minutest vessels of the abdomen. They have not mentioned any signs by which this may *with certainty* be recognised. Here, therefore, was another subject of panic terror for the poor easily frightened patients, another rich draught of fish in the dark! But be comforted! They immediately discovered in their nightcap the most effectual remedies for it. The vast number of mineral waters and baths that still continue daily to gush forth from the bosom of the earth to the great advantage of the presiding physicians of each watering-place, which, like the waters of Bethesda, are good (we know not how) for all conceivable maladies, must consequently be also capable of clearing away the obstructions of the finest vessels of the abdomen and of the mesenteric glands—*id quod erat demonstrandum.* Moreover, the saponaria, the taraxacum, the antimonial medicines, especially the antimonial soaps, invented in defiance of all chemistry, as they become spoilt in an hour, soap itself, ox-gall, the triticum repens, and above all, ye, our more than harrow and plough, noble *neutral salts,* known to us at least by name! What can resist your solvent powers!

Bravely spoken!

But have you ever witnessed, whether and how they perform this solvent action? What divine revelation has pointed them out to you as solvent remedies, since experience teaches nothing thereof to our senses, can shew no proofs of it—since all is hidden from our view? Are you convinced of the existence of your imaginary obstructions? Are you aware that Sömmering found the enlarged glands, which you consider obstructed, actually the most pervious to injections of mercury? Do you know that when you successfully employed muriate of baryta, or muriate of lime in some cases of scrofulous disease, you did not dissolve, as you fondly dreamt, but only separated the saccharine acid in them, discovered by Fischer, which was the cause of the tumefaction in the glands? Where, now, are your obstructions? Of what value are your solvent remedies, seeing that there is nothing to dissolve?

But whence proceed the great number of children's diseases, that carry off one-half of all that are born, before their fifth year? One replies, " I consider the process of dentition as almost the sole cause of the diseases and the mortality of children. We shall find, if we view the matter aright, that from the very first weeks of their existence they begin to suffer from this troublesome teething, and thus it goes on for several years. The poor creatures are always engaged in this teething process, some one tooth or other is always attempting to come through. Hence we refer all their whining, their capricious tempers, their working with the fingers in the mouth, their pallor, their bowel-complaints, their enlarged abdomens, their starting in their sleep, their restlessness, their turning and twisting, their convulsions, all their febrile symptoms, in short, everything that can happen to them, if we are unable to cure it, not to our ignorance, by no means!—but to one sole cause, that is as inevitable as the Turkish fate. The parents have nothing to blame us for. For if the dear child gets some well-known disease, hooping-cough, measles, small-pox, &c., and dies of it, we always have the capital excuse, that the process of dentition had something to do with it. We have the same excuse when secondary diseases occur after these maladies, as marasmus, cough, diarrhœa, ophthalmia, deafness, ulcers of this or the other part. For all these tedious convalescences no one is ever to blame, the troublesome dentition is alone in fault. God bless that man who invented this difficult teething! For, thank heaven! it always gives us something to do with children! Only it is shocking that the stupid peasant children get their rows of white teeth with no bad symptoms, quite unawares, as it were, without any aid from us, or, indeed, any medical assistance. For it might so happen that the families that employ us might fall upon the horrible idea, that kind nature knows how to bring through the teeth without the aid of man, and can actually place them quite silently in the mouth, like rows of pearls, if the awkward officiousness of medical men, and a town-life, that great producer of children's diseases, did not hinder her."—

This opinion is flatly contradicted by a colleague, who, with the usual exaggeration, attributes the whole array of children's diseases to no other cause but worms. He carries this delusion so far as to attribute a number of epidemic fevers prevalent among children solely to worms, "because they so often pass worms when affected by them." I am very much astonished that he does not begin to seek the exciting cause of small-pox, measles, and scarlet-fever in intestinal worms only, for in them also worms often are expelled (in consequence of matters repugnant to them being present in the bowels). If he cures children's diseases by means of iron, semen contra, jalap-powder or calomel, and worms have thereby been expelled, in that case the disease, according to his notion (*fallasia causae, non causae ut causae*) must have been produced by worms, and this even if no worms but only mucus is passed (purging with jalap and calomel always causes a discharge of mucus). That must undoubtedly have been worm-mucus, he alleges.—What peculiar kind of mucus have the lumbrici, that it can be distinguished from all other kinds of mucus? And the seeds of the Persian artemesia, jalap, iron, and calomel, can they cure no other diseases besides those that arise from worms? With regard to the first, experience has shewn me that it can, and as for the others the whole medical world is convinced that they can.

And are you sure that your worm-symptoms, a distended abdomen, bulimy alternating with anorexia, itching of the nose, blue rings surrounding the eyes, dilated pupils, &c., and even the discharge of lumbrici, are incontestible symptoms of vermicular disease? May they not rather be symptoms of a state of ill-health co-existing along with an accumulation of lumbrici, which may be the cause and not the effect of the collection of worms? Does not this ill-health persist even after the expulsion of many worms, does not this cachexy often last till death, and yet sometimes no worms may be discovered on dissection?

Should the intestines sometimes be found to be perforated

and should we assume that these creatures have themselves effected the perforation (and not rather have merely crept through it), it seems to be so foreign to their nature thus to bore through their place of abode, that we often find them quietly remaining in the intestines of robust children up to the period of manhood, frequently in considerable numbers, without causing any inconvenience, and apparently doing nothing so unnatural as perforating the bowels unless they are excessively irritated by some totally different disease of the child (which ought to have been removed in time by other remedies).

"Away with such gross exciting-causes of diseases!" exclaims the solidist in the narrow sense of the term, "such doctrines are not suited to our metaphysical age! Nervous debility is alone the cause of most of the diseases of our degenerated race now-a-days. Nervous debility and relaxed tone of the fibre, nothing else. All the diseases of our time may be referred to this!',— And the remedies for this nervous debility, that excludes all other causes? Tell us, my friend, what are they?—"What else except those incomparable remedies, cinchona bark, steel, and the bitter extracts?"—And how so?—"Why, look you, that every thing that is bitter, as Cullen has justly remarked, acts as a tonic; whatever corrugates the tongue, like the salts of iron, must strengthen the fibre, and what can resist bark, with which we can tan hides? Now we have almost nothing else to do in diseases than to remove the nervous debility and to raise the tone of the fibre, consequently these medicines fulfil all our ends."— This would be all very fine if it were all true. If only the innumerable varieties of diseases did not produce innumerable varieties in the functions and states of the *solidum vivum*, which short-sightedness alone could dream of comprehending in a single word! If you only knew the infinite varieties of the effects of the various bitter substances! If cinchona-bark only ceased to be a powerful remedy when all its tanning properties were extracted from it by means of lime-water! If you could but attribute all the various effects of iron to its astringent property!

"Even these causes of diseases," I hear some one say, "are not subtle enough for our superfine decennium, but as regards the mode of treatment, that smells strongly of crude notions. Far more subtle is the nature of diseases, far more subtle let their mode of treatment be! Nothing less forms the basis of both than substrata of the various gases. The new system of chemistry alone opens the portals of life.

"Know, that all the derangements that occur in our functions
arise from a deficiency or excess of oxygen, of caloric, of hydrogen, of azote, or of phosphorus, consequently that they can
only be cured by superoxydating or disoxydating, by superca-
lorifying or decalorifying, by superhydrogenizing or dehydro-
genizing, by superazotizing and disazotizing, by superphospho-
rizing or dephosphorizing remedies."

This sounds very finely in theory and reads well on paper; it
is also in the spirit of the prevailing ideas. But for every case
of disease I should require the supernatural existence of a seer,
to make for me all these generalities concrete, in every case to
reveal to me whether the disease depends on deficiency or excess of azote, oxygen, &c., and what the chemical antidotes of
this particular chemical state are, for these subjects may indeed
be speculatively excogitated with some semblance of probability,
but being mere products of reason are not cognizable by the
senses in individual cases. *Every assertion that has some truth at
bottom* (all medical systems contain a portion of truth) *is not of
practical utility.*

"We must go still higher," insists a celebrated teacher of
dynamology, who has been reared on the ethereal milk of
critical philosophy, "we must mount up to the original source
of diseases, *the altered composition and form of matter.*" This ontological maxim, however near to the truth it may appear *a
priori* to the thinker conversant with natural science in general,
and with the probable arrangement of our organism, is entirely
useless to the practitioner; it cannot be applied to the treatment
of individual diseases. In like manner, what Bruce says about
the remotest source of the Nile is of no practical utility at its Delta.
Still this teacher of natural science has approximated much
more closely than we might have expected to what pure experience teaches, in his special views relative to diseases, and particularly fevers, and given much less scope to mere probabilities
than his dogmatical and credulous predecessors. Though a love
of system guides all his steps, he always honestly points out
where his deductions run counter to the maxims of experience,
and has a wise respect for the latter. The medical thinker may
educate himself under him, but when he is at the sick-bed, let
him not forget that these views are mere individual ideas, mere
hints, and that from them no remedial means can be deduced.

The view of the medical art that Wilmans presents to the reflecting physician seems to be that most consistent with nature

of all others, but if we would not wander from the right way, we must confine ourselves to his preliminary observations.

The schools have already adopted his classifications. All speculations in medicine, that proceed from pure empiricism, lead to particulars and not to the philosopher's stone, if I may be allowed to borrow a metaphor from a false art.

In dialectic sophistries, in bold assertions, (in shameless self-praise), and in disregard of the infinite multiplicity of nature, manifested in the varieties presented by diseases and by their remedies, all known founders of medical sects were, however, far surpassed by that deceiving parempiric, Brown, who, though not himself engaged in the treatment of diseases, limited all possible curative considerations to exciting and diminishing excitement, and presented to the eyes of the world the greatest of all medical absurdities, " that there can only be two or three diseases, which are distinguished from each other by no other difference besides a plus and minus of excitement, and a corresponding accumulation of excitability." The therapeutics adapted to this notion were easily supplied: " seek for stimulating substances and for such as are as little stimulant[1] as possible; these are the true remedies." And for the first of these objects I should imagine, one or two drugs would amply suffice. Had he wished to avoid contradictions, he should only have named one of the volatile and one of the fixed stimuli *instar omnium*, and not several; for if one can effect every thing, what is the object of having several?

Perhaps, however, he felt the untenableness of his simplifications, perhaps he himself had experienced that the drunkard could not exchange his brandy for musk or camphor. In order to complete his edifice, he must have ignored even patent facts and daily experience.

But I need not enter into all the contradictions he must have felt within himself, nor what it cost him to deny the most palpable facts, in order to become the founder of a bran-new, unheard-of sect; suffice it to say, no medical sectarian, *apparently*, knew less about nature than he, but none understood better

---

[1] It surprises me that his adherents have of their own accord substituted an explanation of the latter substances, which was not that of their master, and could not be his, if he wished to be consistent. He nowhere makes mention of remedies that abstract stimulation. His sthenia-lessening substances were such as debilitated solely by the smallness of their stimulus (*Elements of Medicine*, § xc., cclii).

35

than he, by means of illusory syllogistic ratiocination, to elevate a few true (and from the novel point of view in which
he placed them, apparently new) maxims into the only ones, to
weave over all defects by his obscurity of stating them, and to
assert so despotically the superiority of his subtle mind in secu-
larizing all other incontrovertible truths. Probably he would
himself have confessed that he had made fools of the world, had
his excessive use of his diffusible stimuli allowed him to live
longer.

There is no absurdity that has not already been maintained
by some sophist, and in all ages the mania for simplification has
been the chief stalking horse of system manufactures of the first
rank.

Thus one in his theories asserted that the world was formed
exclusively by fire, another that it was produced by water
only;—a third contended that all living beings were formed
from one egg;—thus Descartes ascribed the universe to his imaginary vertebræ; thus the Alchemists forced the infinite multiplicity of chemical substances into the triangle, salt, sulphur
and mercury. What cared they for the numerous varieties of
metals? They prided themselves on dictatorially fixing the
number of metals at seven, and these they falsely and boldly
referred to a single original substance, their metal-seed. What
else was it but proud simplifying mania, to decree our little terrestrial globe to be the end and centre of all creation, and to
imagine the thirty thousand suns scattered throughout space to
be scarcely more than lamps for its illumination?

Still, I feel provoked at the wiseacre who sought to measure
the great science of medicine with a span, himself acquainted
with hardly any other diseases than perhaps the gout,[1] a few
rheumatisms, some catarrhs, some hæmorrhages, and the malignant croup.

From his theoretical sins, of which I must not speak in this
place, I revert to those immediately concerning the treatment of
diseases.

There never was a doctrine so calculated to mislead the practical physician, nor one so dangerous for the beginner.

According to him we must not trust any thing to the powers of

---

[1] It is remarkable how Brown treats of gout with disproportionate prolixity, I
might almost say pragmatically (§ dci, et seq.), whilst he has scarcely a couple of
empty, superficial words to say about other special diseases of the greatest importance.

nature (XCV.), we must never rest with our remedies, we must always either stimulate or debilitate. What a calumniation of nature, what a dangerous insinuation for the ordinary half-instructed practitioner, already too officious! What a ministration to his pride to be deemed the lord and master of nature!

"We should never use one single remedy alone, but always several at once in every disease"! (XCII.) This is the true sign of a spurious system of medicine. Quackery goes *always* hand in hand with complex mixtures of medicines, and he who can inculcate (not merely permit) such a system, is *toto cœlo* removed from the simple ways of nature and her rule, to effect many objects by one single means. This single axiom, invented for the purpose of confusing men's minds and making a mystification of treatment, must already have cost many their lives.

He makes no distinction betwixt palliative and curative remedies. Like a bungler, he always recommends only such as are of a palliative character,[1] which, by an action the direct opposite of the state of the malady (LXXXIII, LXIV), at first subdues the symptoms (for a few hours), to leave afterwards a state the opposite of that produced by the temporary remedy. Thus opium is his true panacea in all diseases arising from and attended by debility. What a climax of parempiricism and what a mistake —to recommend a medicine as a general strengthener which after the lapse of a few hours, during which it excites the strength, subsequently allows it to sink all the deeper, deeper than before its employment, to prevent which stronger and ever stronger doses must be given! And what experienced practitioner is ignorant of the effects resulting from a continued employment of opium in elevated doses. This drug that strengthens only in a palliative manner, but that is, more than any other remedy, in its after-effects weakening and productive of an increased sensitiveness to pain, Brown could recommend universally and without any limitation as the universal and appropriate remedy for all sorts of diseases, whose character is weakness, even such as are of a most obstinate and chronic character (CCCI, CCXCVIII). He who fails to perceive in all this the perfect picture of a parempiric has lost the use of his eyes. It is only in the special and very rare cases in which opium is at the same time the specific

---

[1] I am not ignorant of the great value of palliatives. For sudden accidents that have a tendency to run a rapid course, they are not only often quite sufficient, but even possess advantages where aid must not be delayed an hour or even a minute In such cases and *in such alone* are they useful.

remedy for the disease, that it cannot debilitate, and when it is employed in very small doses as a palliative in robust constitutions and along with strengthening regimen, it *apparently* does not weaken. This is the source of the delusion. But of really curative drugs, the true weapons of the true physician,—which remove the disease *permanently and radically*, by first exciting an affection similar to the disease present,—of these he says never a word, he does not even know their names. He that knows them I term a restorer, a discoverer of the medical art, as he calls himself. Thus he had not the most distant idea—to give a single example—that a burnt finger may be held for a long time in cold water before it (when taken out and dried) shall cause no more pain—indeed vesication occurs all the more certainly if so-called antiphlogistic, debilitating remedies be applied to this local inflammation. He has not the least idea that the opposite of all this occurs if the burnt finger be held in alcohol.[1] Where now are your palliative anti-sthenic, where your palliative anti-asthenic remedies? How far they are behind!

What true, experienced physician knows not the palliative debilitating power of cold and of cold water? Brown had no need to put forward as a novelty the debilitating property of cold and of the cold bath. But when he announces it to be a positively debilitating thing, he shews that he does not know it, just as he views many other things in a false manner. It is only for the moment during its application that it debilitates (palliatively), whilst in its subsequent effects it manifests itself as one of the most excellent of strengthening remedies (as a curative and permanently remedi. ¹ means). The greatest weakness of a limb, a frost-bite, is confessedly cured by nothing more quickly than by cold water. This may stand for one of the thousands of instances of the curatively strengthening effects of cold water.

He knows no other cause of diseases besides either a too violent excitement by means of stimuli (sthenia), the continued action of which causes indirect weakness, or too little excitement by means of too weak stimuli (direct debility). The former includes all purely inflammatory diseases, and the latter all other diseases that bear the stamp of debility. The former are cured by venesections, cold, water-drinking, &c., the latter by heat,

---

[1] Look at the reaper excessively heated by working in the heat of the sun; with what does he allay his thirst most certainly and most effectually, with what can he do this better than with a little brandy. Brown's antisthenic palliatives, cold water, &c., could scarcely refresh him for an instant.

soups, wine, brandy, and particularly opium. In this manner all the countless diseases, varying infinitely in kind, are cured by him (on paper) or directed to be cured. The crudest parempiricism, the most audacious ignorance, could not go farther than this. According to this all epilepsies,[1] all dropsies, all endemic diseases, all melancholias, are to be certainly cured by opium, brandy, heat and beef tea! Has any one ever experienced a certain, radically good result from such treatment in such diseases? Is he making game of us? Does he want to consign completely to the tomb the medical art, sunk as it already is down to the administration of a few routine drugs?

But no! he is in the highest degree rational. He permits no treatment to be undertaken before ascertaining all the inimical influences that have preceded the disease, whether they could act in a too exciting or in a debilitating manner, and from these alone he will allow the nature of the disease and its treatment can be determined (but always only for two objects, viz., whether we should debilitate or strengthen). But the very circumstance of his making this investigation the only indispensable indication, betrays that he has treated disease in his study only, that he speaks as a blind man would do about colours. In all the cases of sudden disease and such as occur among the common people, who could ascertain in every instance and in the most exact manner, before commencing the treatment of any disease, what was the kind of injurious agency (as Brown affects to discover in every case) had occurred long before; whether the malady was preceded entirely or only in some degree by an excess of stimuli, or entirely or only in some degree by too weak stimuli, or in how far it was preceded by greater stimuli mingled with deficiency of stimuli (and in what proportion?); whether a sthenia has changed into an indirect or direct debility, or the latter into the former, or whether one sort of asthenia has conjoined with another, and (what nonsense!) brought about a *mixed state*, in which the excitability of eighty degrees, that divine revelation to the inspired Brown, is exhausted or accumulated? Who can always institute a comparison between the strength of these noxious influences and the sum total of excitability assigned to the individual, modified as it is said to be by age, sex, constitution, climate, country, &c.? What experienced practitioner can assert that a tenth part of his patients or the friends of his

---

[1] He knows of no epilepsy with excess of good blood, no sthenic dropsy, no sthenic hæmorrhages, no asthenic catarrhs, though nature knows them and not unfrequently produces them.

patients could, would or should give accurate information on all these hyberbolical or hair-splitting questions, give a detail of all previous agreeable or disagreeable mental emotions, of the impressions of the various degrees of temperature to which they may have been exposed throughout a considerable lapse of time, of the exposures to too much or too little sunlight (a stimulus of no mean intensity!) or to a more or less dry, moist, impure or pure air for some considerable period, of the divers kinds of more or less nutritive, sapid, seasoned or unseasoned articles of food that may have been indulged in, the quantity of more or less strong, vinous or watery drinks that may have been taken, the frequency of indulgence in venereal excitement, the degree and quantity of exercise that has been taken, the nature of the amount, the degree and the frequency of all previous mental excitement by means of reading, conversation, amusement, music, &c.? And even supposing among many families one could be found who after *some weeks* of interrogation (for it is impossible that such a variety of questions could be asked in one day) was able and willing (supposing the greater part had not been already forgotten) to answer the most of these questions, how painfully, how fruitlessly I may say, must not the poor doctor rack his brains, in order to estimate and compare these hundreds of thousands of various influences, to calculate their exact effect on the patient whose excitability was at first so and so much, to estimate the resulting sum total, and to discover the amount in Brunonian degrees of the excess of the noxious powers of over-stimulation over those of the deficiency of excitement, of the excess of the powers of the latter over those of the former, and all this in connexion with the particular subject before him! No single circumstance of importance must remain unascertained, or be left out of the list, or be omitted in the calculation, neither must the lesser circumstances (which constitute something considerable by virtue of their number) be forgotten, unascertained, omitted or unestimated, otherwise the whole reckoning will turn out false!

I need scarcely remark, how vain, how impossible, how senseless, such a mode of procedure (which, according to Brown's maxims, § XI, XII, LXXVIII, C, &c., cannot be pushed too far, seeing that all the investigation of disease depends on it) must be in every-day practice—what an enormous amount of trouble and time must be expended in the investigation and consideration, before the treatment of a single case can be commenced; and in the time thereby lost the disease must unobservedly pass into another stage, if it do not in the interim terminate in death.

A *conscientious* Brunonian would probably never arrive at the period when he would commence the treatment, with all this investigation and effort to form a just estimate. And after all, nothing more would have been ascertained but the point respecting the sthenia on which the disease depends, or respecting the direct or indirect debility! Is this the only thing we require to know in order to effect a cure? Well then, know that debility is present in all endemic diseases. Now, quick? cure me all the countries affected with ringworm, pellagra, plica polonica, sibbens, yaws, pian, water-colic, &c. Do you want nothing but fixed and diffusible stimuli? Here you have opium, caloric, brandy, bark, beef-tea.—Cure me them quickly!

God help us! what a mass of nonsense a single unpractical book-maker can rake together and inflict on weak lamb-like mortality, in defiance of all common sense!

But let us do him justice! whilst we see that the glory which was to constitute the apotheosis of this original head vanishes, whilst the Titan who sought aimlessly to heap Pelion on Ossa, quietly descends from the rank of heroes—whilst we see that his colossal plan to turn everything topsy-turvy in the domain of Æsculapius is dashed to pieces, and that the myriads of special diseases cannot be referred by him to one or two causes, or what is the same thing, be decreed by him to consist of two or three similar diseases only varying in degree, nor their infinite variety be cured by two or three stimulants or non-stimulants;—whilst we consign all these arabesque eccentricities to the domain of fable, let us not forget to do him the justice to acknowledge that with a powerful arm he dispersed the whole gang of humoral, acridity, and saburral physicians, who with lancet, tepid drinks, miserable diet, emetics, purgatives, and all the nameless varieties of solvents, threatened to destroy our generation, or at least to deteriorate it radically, and reduce it to the lowest possible condition,—that he reduced the number of diseases requiring antiphlogistic treatment to three per cent. of their former amount (§ CCCCXCIII), that he determined more accurately the influence of the six so-called non-natural things on our health, that he refuted the imaginary advantage of vegetable over animal diet, to the advantage of mankind;—that he restored to the rank of a medicinal agent a judicious diet, and that he reintroduced the old distinction between diseases from defect of stimulus and those from excess of stimulus, and taught with some degree of truth, the difference of their treatment in a general way.

This may reconcile us with his manes!

His disciples, proudly wrapt in the mantle of their Elijah, support his doctrine *utcunque* with much noise (the sign of a not very good cause), deafen us with the Brunonian cant about degrees of excitability, which they consider to be exalted and depressed by previous noxious agencies just as they please, prate about simple and compound, direct and indirect debility, about diotheses and predispositions as (imaginary) distinguishing signs of the general from the local diseases, about (pretended) diffusible and fixed stimuli—and treat their patients right and left with compulsory soups, wine and opium; they are become sufficiently cunning to engraft from vulgar medicine what is requisite and indispensable, and when beef-tea, rum and opium do not suffice, they employ the excellent bark (which their master decried) in intermittent fever (protesting all the while that they use it only in its quality of a fixed stimulus), and turpentine oil in dropsy, but under cover of the Brunonian explanatory formula: " that turpentine possesses the exact degree of stimulant power necessary in this case." Thus have I seen the devout monks in a monastery dine upon partridges on a Friday, but not before the prior had made the sign of the cross over them, accompanied by the transmuting blessing—*fiat piscis !*

TO A CANDIDATE FOR THE DEGREE OF M. D.[1]

I have read your notes of the lectures on therapeutics of your celebrated professor. You are quite right to learn all these things, and to take notes of them. We ought to know what our predecessors and contemporaries have imagined. In like manner I often allow my patients to tell me what they think their disease is and what it proceeds from, what sort of witchcraft produced it and what were the sympathetic remedies and foolish means they have used for it. I like to know what sort of ideas people form of things. The same with you in your college, where you learn the fables those people who imagine themselves to be sagacious physicians have invented respecting all those things which they do not understand, and which no one in the world can know *a priori*. Of course there will be many extraordinary freaks of imagination and daring maxims that find no

[1] From the *Allgem. Anzeig. der Deutschen*, No. 227. 1806.

corroboration in nature, and much more learned stuff, which at all events sounds very profound and wise, because it is paraded in grand, florid and metaphorical language,—there the oxygen and hydrogen poles in the human body, intensified factors, the ganglionic system, the centre of vegetative life, a peculiar irritable or a totally distinct sensitive system within us, must play parts in the comedy we have ourselves invented. Beautiful shadows on the wall! But when they come to the bedside of the patient, one will see a *synochus systematis irritabilis*, where the other, who has been taught by the self-same master, firmly and obstinately asserts he finds the exact opposite, for the signs of the one and of the other as taught *ex cathedra* are as non-essential and undecisive as they are vague and indeterminate. Now should it so happen that one of them has divined the real meaning of the system-monger, what advantage does the healing art thereby gain? None at all! No subtle theorizing respecting the essential nature of fever ever points directly to what should and must be useful for it. The theoretical house of cards stands quite isolated in its imposing majesty, but is hollow and empty within, and does not even contain an indication for the appropriate remedy for the disease, the inspired revelation of whose essential nature is here solemnly announced. *O quanta species, cerebrum not habet !* The whole jingle of theoretical flourishes is far from being of the same use to the directions appended to it as to what is to be used in the disease, that the premises are to the deduction in a logical syllogism—no! they more nearly resemble the sound of the trumpet and drum in the street wherewith the mountebank seeks to announce the *quid pro quo* which he proposes to juggle before his delighted spectators in the afternoon. For see, what the professor imagines to be of service in this case or the other is just as arbitrary, has no firm foundation, and is not the result of experience, but *is inferred from the most superficial view* of the case, and *only asserted* with the satisfactory ἀντὸς ἔφα. For a single genus of fevers there will be found almost the whole materia medica: give the patient, gentlemen, draughts of bitter and aromatic plants (does this mean that we are to give colocynth, squills, ignatia, nux vomica, aloes? also yellow sandal-wood, dittany, abelmochus seeds, rose-wood?), or saccharine oils in tea (including the oil of laurocerasus and the distilled oil of bitter almonds?).

The whole concern with its many definitions of fever and its superfine pedantry in pulse-feeling—which every one finds to

vary almost every hour, and which feels different at every modification of the patient's temper—all these are no doubt glittering things, but they are at the same time utterly vain, affording
no comfort and no assistance, obscuring our vision like a mist
when we seek to cure our patients. On account of the learned
mist which obscures and does not illuminate, we neither perceive
the true state of the patient, nor that wherewith we might afford
him relief.

Only ask yourself, if you knew all that off by heart, would
you be able by means of it to form an accurate conception of
the disease, and could it aid you to cure the disease? No doubt
you would be able to treat it with all the array of proposed remedies, but *whether* one of these is the best and most suitable,
and *which* among them it is that solely and especially can and
must be of service, that you will not know; the professor himself does not know it, otherwise he would only have mentioned
this sole best and most suitable remedy, and no other. When
the therapeutic professor can put together a number of general
artistic, flowery, phrases respecting things that none can know,
and can dash a learned-looking varnish over the hypothesis of
his own invention, the whole affair appears to be all right; but
when he attempts to apply it to the relief of disease—the proper
object of the medical art—his learned, theoretical apparatus
leaves him in the lurch; he then runs over, in a purely empirical manner, just like the most unreflecting, routine practitioner,
a number of names of medicines—"there, make what you can
of that! you may put all the names together into a bag, and
according to your fancy draw out one or several, it is quite immaterial, you may use this one or that one!" Here, where the
question is to afford relief, we find the most stupid sincretism
and empiricism, and there, where theorizing is the question, we
find the most sublime, mystical, and incomprehensible phrases
in use, as elevated as if they had been solemnly delivered by a
divinely inspired oracle from the cave beneath the tripod of the
Delphian Apollo. But cease to entertain a reverential awe for
these magic mutterings; they are mere empty sounds that have
no connexion with the simple, certain and rapid delivery of your
fellow-creatures from the pangs of disease; they are but sounding brass and a tinkling cymbal. [1]

---

[1] [Let the students of our modern medical colleges, ponder well upon these
just remarks, and ascertain if they are not applicable to the schools of our own
country.] Am. P.

ON THE PREVAILING FEVER.[1]

The medical men of the present time, by regarding the fever that has prevailed for a year past in Germany, and indeed throughout the greater part of Europe, as a common ague or intermittent fever of some other ordinary kind, and by treating it as such (every one knows with how little success!) have given a fresh proof of the imperfection of the ordinary medical art, I might almost say of its absolute futility.

When one thing expresses itself differently from another, and exhibits different properties and actions, it requires very little discriminating skill to regard it as a thing of a different character! And when one disease shews itself in its course, its symptoms and all its phenomena quite different from another well known disease, surely every person endowed with ordinary reason must perceive that the former must be another, a peculiar disease, differing completely from the one already known; and, as a necessary consequence, to be treated quite differently, and entirely according to its peculiar properties.

Not so our dear ordinary system of medicine, whose maxim seems to be to leave every thing in the old way, to take everything quite easily, and to spare ourselves as much reflection as possible. Our ordinary medical system, I say, felt no hesitation in declaring this new peculiar fever to be an ague and (what should prevent it?) treating it accordingly. For mark! dear reader, the medical art has but a single intermittent fever, what is called *ague* in the books; therefore there must be in nature no other typical fever. *Quasi vero.*

And thus the misunderstood fever at present prevailing is treated by practitioners like the ordinary ague that occurs in autumn and in marshy districts,—right away with emetics and purgatives, with sal-ammoniac (opium), millefoil, buckbean, centuary, and cinchona-bark, which has been considered as almost omnipotent. By means of the first mentioned, the (imaginary) febrile matter was to be dissolved, or expelled, but by the last the type was to be extinguished. But what was the effect of this general plan of operation (which was long since introduced for the ordinary autumnal marsh intermittent fever) when

---

[1] From the *Allgem. Anz. der Deutschen*, No. 261. 1809

employed against the misunderstood fever at present prevailing? I appeal to the experience of all countries where it has raged, if it was not attended with bad effects, if it was not often the case that more disease (even death) and long-lasting indisposition were not often thereby promoted, than would have been the case without all those unsuitable medicines, and actually was the case among poor people who used none of them?

These substances, and particularly the bark given in large quantities, certainly sometimes suppressed the paroxysms (when they did not change the fever into an acute rapidly fatal one) for a longer or shorter time,—but they did not thereby generally restore the patients to health; they generally became in other respects worse, they became subject to *very* painful local diseases in place of the suppressed paroxysms, or they languished with nervous symptoms and wasting affections, which were worse than the typical fever itself.

These dangerous mistakes were in the first place owing to this, that practitioners as usual did not distinguish the disease, did not examine what particular, peculiar symptoms were proper to this prevailing fever as distinguished from all other kinds of intermittent fevers, whereby it was rendered quite a distinct, peculiar disease; and, in the second place, that they did not know how to discover the peculiar, specifically suitable remedy for this peculiar fever.

Can that be termed a medical art which has no power to perform its two sole duties—the discriminating observation of diseases, and the discovery of the appropriate, specific remedy?

In ordinary diseases which (God be praised!) tend to get well of themselves, the ordinary practice of medicine can contrive to conceal its inefficiency and hurtfulness—there it can, to use its own language, dissolve, purge, depress, stimulate, and do whatever else it will with remedies, that the most unreflecting caprice suggests to it;—some persons certainly get well under the treatment, let the doctor act as madly as he pleases. Good constitutions often even then gain the victory (not unfrequently with the aid of throwing away unsuitable, injurious medicinal mixtures) not only over the disease itself, but also over the newly added malady—over the blind treatment of the unknown disease by means of inappropriate, therefore hurtful medicines, and out of the number of those that die no one can tell how many who had originally a moderate attack of the disease succumbed solely in consequence of the interference of the art.

But in the diseases that do not soon go off spontaneously, that will not allow themselves so complaisantly to be overcome by the dear *vis medicatrix naturæ*—such as the fever at present raging—in them it will be quite obvious that the ordinary medical art is not very far from being a scientifically propped-up monster and a misleading phantom, and its practice with few exceptions a futile injurious procedure. Almost all its efforts tend but to aggravate (when the reverse does not happen, as it does sometimes, in consequence of the accidental and lucky admixture of some addition to the methodical medicinal compound) or to excite new maladies, often not less to be dreaded than the original disease. Thus, in the present instance, by the injudicious suppression of the paroxysms of the prevailing fever there are produced a continued morbid, chronic febrile state, periodical spasmodic nervous affections, asthma, stiffness of the joints, swelling of the glands, constant or periodical discharges of blood, or long continued suppression of the menses, but particularly excessively painful local diseases, and many other wasting affections, which no sensible person can term a cure.

I shall endeavour to describe the peculiarities of this fever, as they present themselves, *when it has not been altered by drugs*, and then I shall shew what medicines must be suitable for it, afford, relief, and restore health.—

A difference of sex, of constitution, of age and of the immediate exciting cause (whether it was anger, grief, a fright, excess in sensual indulgence, a debauch, &c., that first caused the fever to break out),—also, to a certain extent, the climate and the state of the weather, sometimes occasion at first some variety in the course and form of the fever. But the following is its general course.

Often for several days or weeks before it breaks out there are observed, headache in the evening, bitter taste in the mouth, and heaviness in the legs.

1. In bad cases the fever commences as a continued one, and goes on without intermission in almost equal violence day and night, constituting, as it were, a single paroxysm, which ends, if inadequately treated, the ninth, eleventh or fourteenth day with death—or it subsides (and this it is very apt to do) into a continued chronic state, wherein certain sufferings are more severe at one time of the day than at another;

2. Or it resolves itself (either spontaneously or by the com-

mencement of appropriate treatment) into tertian or quotidian fits. The remissions, however, do not in the most cases constitute a genuine intermission, not a state of absolute freedom from disease ; a few or many of the sufferings persist (though in a less degree) and the fever is therefore only to be regarded as a remittent one, which is especially the case in its worse forms, the paroxysms of which do not terminate under eight, twelve, sixteen, and even twenty-four hours.

(It is only a very small minority of these fevers that have true intermissions, but, notwithstanding this, their nature is the same, and they require the same mode of treatment.)

In both kinds, which often pass into one another, the *shivering* or *rigour* (which sometimes passes into violent shaking and chattering of the teeth) is not (as it is in ordinary agues) accompanied by real external coldness, but it is a merely internal shuddering sensation of cold (internal rigour), during which the patient is hot (in some cases only naturally warm) to the touch all over, but chiefly so on the hands and feet.

This cold stage commences with thirst, vertigo, and a drawing tearing (mixed with shooting) from the legs upwards, which, when it, according to the patient's sensation, gets up into the head, produces heat of the head, headache, nausea, &c.

In the continued kind the sensation of flying heat in the head alternates almost unremittingly with rigour ; often both are present at once (the patients complain of "internal rigour, and of their head being at the same time so warm that the heat mounts up into their head, with nausea"). At the same time the patients feel hot all over the body, without themselves being aware that they are so, on the contrary, they wish the room to be strongly heated, wrap themselves closely up, and only complain of the so-called flying heat rising up into the head.

In the chronic, degenerated kind of the continued fever, the rigours with external heat of the body and of the hands are not unfrequently conjoined with actual coldness of the feet, then the patients complain that after going to bed at night they cannot get warm, whereas when they waken in the morning they feel so hot.

As a rule, the rigours in the continued variety come on from very slight causes, on getting up, even on sitting up in bed and on the slightest movement, often even every time the patient drinks, even warm beverages.

In the paroxysms of the remitting sort also, the so-called heat is, according to the patient's description, generally only a feeling of strong warmth rising to the head, often accompanied by burning in the eyes and redness of the face (this is the only heat they feel, not that of the rest of the body), with which is conjoined a series of other affections of the sensibility and irritability, which together constitute the so-called hot stage.

The most frequent complaint is the *headache*, which they usually describe as a tearing pain in the skull, mingled with shootings, also as a bursting pain, often also as a digging in the brain and as if it would be forced out superiorly, whereby a throbbing in the occiput not unfrequently supervenes, which deprives them of consciousness, or jerks in the head from before backwards. They have this headache even while lying, but on rising up, or even moving the head, either the shoots or the blows (jerks) in the head increase to an intolerable degree.

Patients of a different constitution complain, instead of this headache, that their head feels so heavy, so stupid, so dizzy, that they are so forgetful and intoxicated, that every thing appears to them wrong, that there is hissing and roaring in the brain. This state in the hot stage often turns into real unconsciousness and loss of reason, that often lasts many hours and even degenerates into violent mania and raving madness.

But an equally frequent symptom in the hot stage is the *anxiety* (generally combined with palpitation of the heart and sweat on the brow), which often rises to the most fearful height, during which the patients complain that they cannot control themselves, and not unfrequently in these dreadful moments they commit suicide, either by strangling or hanging themselves.

In the continued variety of this fever, this anxiety usually becomes aggravated after midnight, especially after three o'clock, when the patient cannot endure to remain in bed, but must walk about, until they sink down exhausted. In this kind of fever the kind of pain which the patient experiences during the day is at the same time aggravated so as to be intolerable, whether it be in the head, the chest, one of the limbs, the uterus, the urinary organs or elsewhere. In the slighter degrees of this continued fever there occur after midnight, half remembered, anxious phantasies, deliria, tossing about of the body and limbs.

The disposition of our fever-patients is also very much affected by precordial anxiety even when no fit is present. They are timorous and easily vexed by trifles, and, according to their temperament, either very dismal and full of fears of impending death, or intolerant, impatient and weary of life, occasionally so much so as to induce them to commit suicide.

A third symptom occurring along with the hot stage of the paroxysms is *nausea*, a *faint feeling*, such as is apt to accompany horrible pain, which often tends to increase into retching for several hours, and vomiting of sour, bitter or watery fluid.

In the continued kind the nausea often often comes on in conjunction with the anxiety, vertigo, faintness and trembling. Even when no actual retching is present the patient has a constant feeling in his stomach as if he could vomit incessantly.

The *vertigo* is one of the most frequent symptoms of this fever. It often comes on at the commencement of the rigour, on any slight movement, and is accompanied by the nausea, the noise in the ears, the obscuration of the vision and the faintness. The patients feel as if they would fall rather sideways and forwards than backwards. In the chronic continued variety the vertigo happens chiefly in the morning.

Not less characteristic of this fever and a very frequent phenomenon is the *trembling*, especially of the limbs, which sometimes occurs alone, sometimes conjoined with the anxiety, the heat of head, the attacks of faintness and vertigo, and also with the sickness. Most frequently of all, the trembling shews itself at the commencement of the hot stage. In the chronic, continued variety it sometimes becomes the most prominent symptom, and then attacks only one limb at a time; it occasionally appears only when lying down, and not at all when moving.

The paroxysms of some children are ushered in with *clonic spasms* and *epileptic convulsions;* seldom are they mere tonic continued flexures of their limbs at the commencement of the heat.

The *perspiration* (which usually smells sour or sourish) usually occurs in the paroxysms of the remittent kind, not, as is the case in the autumnal intermittent fever, during the heat, but (very characteristically) afterwards, often only some, several or even many hours afterwards, [1] often also not until the patients get up, or move about, or when they fall asleep some hours after the heat. In the mean time the worst symptoms of the fits, the precordial anxiety, the pains of the head and other parts, the weight and stupid feeling in the head, the loss of reason, &c., go off, but usually not until the perspiration comes on, however long it

---

Generally the flow of urine remains suppressed just as long.

may delay.[1] In the chronic continued variety of this fever, the perspiration comes on when moving slightly, even when eating, but especially on the recurrence of the pains, and whenever the patients go to bed and cover themselves up. During the slightest sleep most of them become immediately covered with perspiration.

In the kind of fever consisting of repeated paroxysms, the *thirst* from the very commencement of the fit, even before it comes on, until the end, is unquenchable, but though the patients drink very often, they take but little at a time, for every liquid becomes repulsive to them the moment they partake of it; there also often occurs immediately after drinking either shuddering or nausea and retching; this kind of thirst is also not unfrequent during the remissions. If the fever assumes the chronic type, there sometimes occurs complete adypsia, though not often.

Along with the sinking feeling and retching sickness there is conjoined *disgust* at all kinds of food, chiefly at meat, butter, &c. Even when, in the fevers that pass into the chronic form, food and drink begins to taste tolerably, there still occurs after it is partaken of, sinking and nausea—or anxiety, as if from difficulty of breathing, so that there is a desire felt to open the doors and windows. In the chronic continued fever, periods of annorexia and bulimy sometimes occur alternately.

On taking any food, *the sense of taste appears as if extinguished*; food tastes, even during the remission, just like hay or straw; but immediately after partaking of it the mouth becomes completely filled with a bitterness like gall, just like after vomiting from taking an emetic; and there occur nausea, or bitter or sourish-bitter eructations. In some there occur even whilst eating, especially eating bread, bitterness in the mouth. More rarely does it happen that there is constant bitterness of the mouth, and in that case the bitterness is much increased after every meal. At the commencement of a paroxysm the bitter or bitter-sour eructations are of frequent occurrence.

The usual sensation in the mouth is dryness of the fauces with feeling of mucus upon the tongue, not unfrequently combined with a feeling of rawness in the fauces. Frequently, after awaking in the morning, the taste in the mouth is bitter, rarely like that of rotten eggs.

---

[1] There are some of these fevers where perspiration never ensues, only during the anxiety there may be a little on the head; in these cases the perspiration is sometimes replaced by clonic spasms.

The urine is generally dark and of a greenish-brown colour.

There often appear burning itching eruptions all over the body, or on different parts of it; sometimes a very frequently occurring cough.

The sleepiness by day in the continued kind of this fever is great. Even in the morning soon after awaking, whether they are seated or standing, their eyes often close, frequently in the act of talking.

Very characteristic of all the states of this fever is the *intolerance of movement or of muscular exertion*. Immediately on the occurrence of a fit their limbs appear stiff, as if *paralysed;* they must instantly lie down, and even when lying they feel as if paralysed. If the patients get up during the heat, then shuddering occurs, not unfrequently with sudden chilling of the hands and feet, they feel sinking, the vision becomes obscured, a faintness supervenes. Also when the paroxysm is not upon them, the least movement deprives them in a few moments of all strength. Trembling, vertigo, nausea, obscuration of vision, roaring in the ears and fainting, these symptoms so characteristic of our fevers, frequently come on on the least movement, and the strongest men often fall to the ground before we are aware of it. Also in the intermission and in the chronic continued state, the patients cannot bear to stand even for a short time; obscuration of vision and vertigo, shortness of breath, and even fainting, are the result. All the pains they usually suffer are especially increased by movement of the body, or of single limbs. On putting their foot to the ground they feel the shock in their head, or shootings go through it.

All the symptoms are alleviated by lying.

But still more injurious to them in every condition of this fever is movement *in the open air;* this deprives them suddenly of strength, produces in them either shuddering and rigour (followed by perspiration) or shortness of breath, or drawing in the limbs, or increased tearing shooting headaches; at the same time it diminishes the dizziness, maziness and intoxicated feeling in the head, which however soon recur on coming back into the room. A kind of pressive *pain in the chest*, or rather *in the scrobiculus cordis, with sense of suffocation,* is a not unusual symptom at the commencement of and during the heat; it often occurs simultaneously with the precordial anxiety. Pain, like rawness in the chest, is far from being rare, and the same may be said of *drawing pains in the back, as if from a strain.*

This fever seems sometimes to cease suddenly of its own accord, but more frequently by the use of some medicines unsuitable for it, especially cinchona-bark; but on the other hand,
there occur at the same time vicarious affections, periodical nervous maladies, suppression of the menses, or periodical, very
painful discharge of coagulated blood and mucus from the womb
or urinary organs, or anus, and other intolerable painful local
affections, and even aberrations of the mind. In proof of their
origin and that they are only degenerated and masked forms of
this fever, there remain several of the above-named characteristic
affections peculiar to this fever, and the vicarious maladies themselves become aggravated at certain times of the day. The aggravations usually occur from four o'clock in the afternoon until
three or four o'clock in the morning in some, but in others from
three in the morning until four in the afternoon. The other
twelve hours are much more endurable.

For these vicarious maladies (masked fever) the only efficacious
medicines are those that are capable of curing the original fever.

Nothing can do good and restore health but the medicines specially suitable (specific) for this fever, that is, such as are capable
of exciting similar symptoms in the healthy human body.

Let my readers endeavour to find out in Hahnemann's *Fragmenta de viribus medicamentorum positivis* what medicine it is
that causes the following symptoms characteristic of this fever:
Rigiditas artuum—juncturarum mobilitas diminuta—torpor omnium membrorum—instabilitas, infirmitas pedum, genuum—
lassitudo ingens—tremor—tremor pedis alterutrius et genuum—
lapsus virium subitus—syncope—gravitas capitis ebriosa, verti-
ginosa—ebriosa capitis obtenebratio—vertigo cum scotomia—
nisus in decubitum—impotentia caput erigendi, in dorso recli-
nati ob vertiginem et scotomiam—respiratio extra lectum angus-
ta, difficilis; in lecto justa—dolor pectoris respirationem suffo-
cans—anxietas ingens—palpitatio—anxietas autochiriae cupida
—mortis timor—mortem instare putat—anxietas diaphoresin
gignens, ad minimum frontis—post anxietatem nausea, vomitu-
ritio—deliquescentia cordis—horripilatio primo, tum calor ango-
rem creans—horrescentia—genae calidae cum horrore interno—
faciei caloris sensus cum horrore corporis caeteri—calor internus
capitis cum frigore corporis—ardor in oculis sine inflammatione
—calor cum lecti appetentia—dilacerans capitis dolor eundo
auctus—pulsationes vel ictus aliqui in capite—aëro libero auctus
capitis dolor et crurum lassitudo—anorexia cibi—anorexia
maxime panis—regurgitatio amari et acidi saporis—impatientia

parvorum malorum—pavor—phantasiae nocturnae semi-vigiles —phantasiae delirae terribiles—eruptio miliaris ardenti pruriens —ardens pruritus per totum corpus.

The seed[1] which is capable of producing these symptoms, is of all known vegetable medicines the only one that is also capable of curing a great part of this prevalent fever in a short time, that is, of transforming it into health,[2] but this is only to be done by giving at first about every fourth day, afterwards every sixth or eighth day, a very small dose of it. The smallest particle of it in powder, or a small portion of a drop of a solution of it, every drop of which contains a trillionth of a grain of this seed, is an amply sufficient dose and suited for the purpose; *no* other medicine, of course, being used intercurrently, either inwardly or outwardly.

It will, however, be noticed, that in the enumeration of the symptoms of our fever there are some not perfectly contained in this plant, consequently which cannot be perfectly covered by it, and this is especially the case with regard to the worst form of this fever.

On the other hand, there is a mineral[3] which, in its extraordinary action on the human body, is capable of exciting those symptoms which make up our fever, in a much more perfect manner, and consequently of curing it with much greater certainty and completeness, particularly those kinds in which every action is followed immediately by shuddering or nausea, or bitter taste; in which the taste of food and drink is extinguished, but still there is no constant bad or bitter taste in the mouth, and in which only whilst eating or soon thereafter there occurs some bitterness in the mouth for a short time; in which vertigo, nausea, trembling, and rapid sinking of the strength increase to the greatest degree; in which drink is often desired, but little is drunk at a time; in which perspiration only occurs some time after the heat, or not at all; in which paralysis of the irritable or sensitive fibre prevails, and pains of the most intolerable kind unite, are conjoined with great anxiety of heart; for all these symptoms are completely contained in the sphere of action of this mineral on the human body, therefore it can cure these when it is brought to bear upon them, it can cure the greatest and worst portion of our fevers quickly, easily, and with the greatest certainty.

---

[1] [Strychnos nux vomica.]

[2] Especially when the sinking of the forces is not so striking, the food still tastes naturally, and there is only a continual bitter taste in the mouth.

[Arsenicum album

But what do I say? Has not this mineral almost irretrievably incurred the ban of the medical art? But what cares the free investigator of truth, who only sees in the whole kingdom of nature the fatherly love of God dispensing blessings with a liberal hand? Nothing is unconditionally to be rejected; everything is a beneficent gift of God; and among God's good gifts, the greatest are just those that are injurious to the world in the hands of fools; they were only created for the use of the wise, who alone are capable of employing them for the weal of mankind, and to the glory of the beneficent Deity.

How can it be imputed to the very powerful medicinal substances as a fault, that when given in our gross medicinal weights, in drachms, scruples and grains, they are still much too large for wholesome use? so that the ordinary drachm, scruple and grain practitioners, must almost abandon their employment in consequence of their enormous powerfulness, whilst the smallest quantity which these shortsighted beings can think of employing must still be something that they can measure in their medicine scales.

But if a tenth part of a grain of this mineral was still often found to be dangerous, in other words, too powerful, what was to have prevented physicians, if they had but but reflected a little, from trying whether a thousandth, a millionth of a grain, or still less, was not a moderate dose, and if even such a small fragment of a grain was found to be too gross a dose of this most powerful of all medicinal agents (as it is in fact), what should have prevented them from diminishing this fractional quantity still more, until they found that a sextillionth of a grain in solution becomes a mild and yet sufficiently powerful (in our case specifically curative) dose, when administered every five to ten days? Here also, of course, it must be employed singly and alone, and without the administration of any intercurrent medicine whatever.

In the immoderate perspirations in the worst kind of the fever, and in the continued unconsciousness when a remedy is required, camphor affords speedy relief, but only in a palliative manner; it cannot be continued without injury, nor used as a permanent remedy. The excessive perspirations which it here suddenly diminishes, it is capable of exciting itself in the healthy body, but only in its secondary action; hence its employment in this case is only palliative.

SIGNS OF THE TIMES IN THE ORDINARY SYSTEM OF MEDICINE.[1]

Art of physic is a most appropriate name for designating the practice hitherto pursued by physicians, of whom we might say that they (in place of *healing*) only *physic*, that is, give medicines —it matters not what—in diseases.

Such a procedure can never, until it alters for the better, be termed *healing art.*

But that this drugging business has not altered up to this time, and gives no sign of wishing to alter and better itself, we learn from innumerable circumstances occurring every day, and also from the following:

Who would have believed that in the nineteenth century a physician with a real degree in a *university town* (Dr. Becker of Leipsic) could give a commission to another regular physician in a university town (Dr. Nöthlich of Jena) for the sale of his quack medicines,[2] and could puff off his rubbish as infallible in these terms: *they effect a certain cure*, &c. This has been done in No. 293 of this journal.

A quack nostrum is a medicinal agent prepared in a certain invariable manner for public sale, which is puffed off as efficacious for several named diseases, or for one disease, whose name includes several morbid states, differing from each other, each of which will require for its cure an essentially different peculiar remedy.

Such are Dr. Becker's dental medicines, offered for sale by Dr. Nöthlich.

Now, who would have believed that a physician would have publicly advertised a *spirit for the toothache as certain to cure?* Mark, one and the same spirit as certainly efficacious for the innumerable array of the very different kinds of pains in the teeth!

When the toothache does not arise from the effects of an external injury immediately preceding it (for then only is the toothache merely local and idiopathic),—its aching always represents only the chief symptom of a malady of very various character distributed throughout the whole system, arising from

---

[1] From the *Allgemeiner Anzeiger der Deutschen*, No. 326. 1809.

[2] Essence for scurvy of the teeth, tincture for caries of the teeth, tooth-powder and spirit for toothache,

such things as suckling a child too long, abuse of the sexual function, of spirituous liquors, of coffee or tea, from fright, from anger, from grief, from too violent exercises and overheating of the body, or from fatigue, from a chill, from over-exertion of the mind, from a sedentary life, from working among warm damps things, &c.

The toothache is as various in character as are the internal maladies that produce it. Hence as those different kinds of internal malady cannot be removed by one and the same medicament, neither can the varieties of toothache depending upon them.

Hence one medicine is useful only in one kind, another in another kind of toothache;—one[1] is only of service in those toothaches that occur in fits, most violently at night, with redness of the cheek, that during the fit seem to be quite unbearable, that do not effect any one tooth in particular, that in their slightest degree consists of formicating pecking pains, when more severe cause a tearing pain, and in their greatest severity occasion a shooting pain extending often into the ear, that most frequently come on soon after eating and drinking, are somewhat relieved by the application of the finger that has been dipped in water, but are much increased by drinking cold things, and that generally leave a swelling of the cheek. This kind affects persons of capricious disposition who are very much disposed to anger, and have been rendered irritable by means of coffee.

Quite another medicine[2] is of service in those cases where the pain in the gum is of a gnawing, fine shooting character, but that in the nerve of the tooth is drawing, jerking (as if the nerve were violently drawn and suddenly let loose again) with chilly feeling, combined with paleness of the face, occuring most frequently in the evening, more rarely in the morning, increased by a warm room and the heat of the bed, relieved by cool air blowing upon it, not increased by chewing, but brought on by the use of the toothpick. It effects persons of mild, quiet disposition, disposed to shed tears.

Another totally different, peculiar medicine[3] is required for the cure of that toothache that only effects a hollow carious tooth, with a drawing, boring pain as if it were being forced out of its socket, and single, rare, coarse shoots, which cause a shock

---

[1] Chamomilla.   [2] Pulsatilla.   [3] Nux vomica.

through the whole body, with painful, frequently suppurating swelling (epulis) in the gum. It generally comes on quite early in the morning in bed, does not permit of chewing, is generally renewed and aggravated most by opening the mouth in the open air, and by exertion of the mind in reading or reflecting. It usually attacks only persons of hasty choleric temper, who render themselves irritable by the use of spirituous liquors and coffee, and are not much in the open air.

Besides these three most common kinds of toothache there are many other not rare kinds, one of which only occurs in the morning on the partaking of warm fluids, another where the tooth only pains whilst chewing, still another which only affects the front teeth with obtuse pain, another where the tooth aches chiefly when touched which causes a pressive throbbing pain, again another all the carious teeth at once, where the gums are swollen and painfully sensitive to the touch, whilst single jerks dart through the periosteum of the jaw, which, in its slighter form, consists of jerking pressure, but in its more severe form of a digging tearing pain and burning stitches, and along with which the incisor teeth are often painful on respiring through the mouth, and yet another kind that occurs only from cold air, mostly in the morning, with rush of blood to the interior of the head, that makes the tooth loose with a formicating pain in it, and on chewing there occurs a sensation as if it would fall out, whilst at the same time there is a tearing pain in the gum.

When the state of the system otherwise indicates them, *hyoscyamus* is the sole, peculiar remedy of the last form of toothache, and the *north pole of the magnet* the sole remedy for the second last one : but both these remedies are unserviceable in all other kinds of toothache, which, as peculiar diseases of different kinds, require for their certain permanent cure each its own peculiar appropriate remedy, but they are aggravated or rendered more lasting by every other medicine not specifically suitable for them.

I say *remedy*, and do not thereby imply any palliative, which merely deadens the pain somewhat for one or more quarters of an hour, only to return subsequently all the more severely, and with fresh annoying symptoms in its train, but I imply a medicinal agent which is quite appropriate to the disease, and completely eradicates and removes the pain in the course of a few hours, so that for a long time, often as long as life lasts, it does not again occur Of such a character must the medicines be,

each of which is *certainly* and *permanently* curative for a particular kind of toothache, and at the same time for the internal
malady of the system on which it depends.

What a self-deception, then, it is, which can only be excused
by the plea of *total ignorance*, for a physician, without knowing
the many essentially different kinds of toothache, to imagine
that there is *but one toothache*, and that but a *single toothache-
medicine* is required (and that *his own*)—and thus by means of
opium (the chief ingredient of all nostrums for the toothache)
he only sometimes, and for a short time, deadens the general
sensibility, whilst he creates many new sufferings—and yet in
his puffing advertisement he dares to assert, that his *spirit* is a
certain remedy for the toothache!

What a palpable falsehood this is, for it is *impossible* that
essentially different diseases (in the very nature of things) can
be cured by one and the same medicine, and *every medicine*
which does not do good, that is, which is unsuitable, *does harm*.

MEDICAL HISTORICAL DISSERTATION ON THE HELLEBORISM OF THE ANCIENTS.[1]

INTRODUCTION.

1. It is my intention to speak of the helleborism of the ancients, that very celebrated operation by which the ancient
physicians were accustomed to treat with great daring the
greater number of chronic diseases of the most obstinate character by a medicament of excessive violence, the *veratrum.
album*, and not unfrequently effected, as if by a miracle, a radical cure. This ancient method is most worthy of attention, and
the more so as in our days the use of this grand remedy has
been more completely abandoned, both in general and in particular in the treatment of chronic diseases, so neglected by

----

[1] [The original of this, which is in the Latin language, and is the thesis presented
by Hahnemann to the Leipzic Faculty of Medicine in order to obtain the license to
practice, bears the following title, *Dissertatio historico-medica de helleborismo veterum.
Lipsiae*, MDCCCXII. I have thought it best to translate it, because the Latin language
is so little cultivated now among medical men, that the original would be but little
read by them, and this essay is too valuable to be cast aside unread, if we would
wish to form a just estimate of the learning and genius of Hahnemann.]

modern physicians who are in the habit of giving *any* medicine for *any* chronic disease.[1]

2. In this essay we shall proceed in the following order: first, we shall inquire into the antiquity of this drug and its primitive employment; then we shall examine if our veratrum is the same plant that the ancients used for the production of helleborism; then we shall indicate the places which were celebrated for the growth of the best kinds of this plant, and the signs by which its good quality was distinguished; and finally, we shall speak of the employment of veratrum, both in general, in ordinary cases, and for the great treatment, the helleborism itself. The period when its employment was first introduced, that in which its use was abandoned, the most favourable season for the treatment, the circumstances that contra-indicated its use, the maladies that demanded helleborism, then the preliminary treatment to which the patient was subjected, the preparation of the medicament, its form, its dose, the substances that were combined with it, the regimen prescribed to the patient after taking the veratrum, the remedies used to obviate and correct the evils and dangers that usually accompanied its use, in order to ensure a safe and perfect cure; such are the subjects that will come under our attention. In conclusion, we shall briefly mention the employment of the *helleborus niger* among the ancients.

3. In my researches into this ancient mode of treating diseases, I shall proceed only up to the middle ages, I shall leave it to others to treat of the employment of veratrum album and helleborus niger in modern times.

Earliest medicinal employment of hellebore.

4. In the remotest periods of Grecian history, the people, robust in body but of uncultivated mind, when oppressed by calamities or afflicted by diseases, trembling with a vain and childish superstitious dread of the anger of the gods and with a fear of demons, were less solicitious about warding off evils than about ascertaining the will of the gods with respect to the

---

[1] Thus Ernst Horn, Medical Vice-Director of the Charité hospital, and Professor of Physic at the Medico-Chirurgical College of Berlin, asserts (*Anfangsgründe der med. Klinik*, pt, ii. ch. 7) that he knows of only one treatment for all chronic diseases whatsoever, which is to remove the debility by any excitant, *it matters not what*, the indications for the use of which are left almost to chance (*i. e.* no account being taken of the specific quality of such medicine, and of the immense variety of chronic diseases.) This is the manner in which the *rational* physicians of our days have mingled together and confounded medicines and diseases, and whilst they pretend to find in every medicine a remedy for every disease, they actually cure none at all.

issue of the evil or their future fate, and only demanded of physicians vaticinations and prognostications respecting the periods of the crises, the convalescence or death—in those times I say, physicians were looked upon rather as augurs than as practical sustainers of health, that is to say, as men who removed diseases by means of remedies.

5. At that time the art of medicine could scarcely be said to exist, the number of medicaments was most insignificant.

6. Among this small number of medicines however, veratrum album is found, and occupies the first rank, thus being one of the most ancient as well as efficacious of remedies.

7. Thus, about the year 1500 before our era, a certain Melampus, son of Amithaon, a most celebrated augur and physician, first at Pylos, then among the Argivans, is said to have cured the daughters of Proetus, king of the Argivans, who in consequence of remaining unmarried,[1] were seized with an amorous furor[2] and affected by a wandering mania;[3] they were cured chiefly by means of veratrum album,[4] given in the milk of goats fed upon veratrum, which Melampus had observed to produce purgative effects on these animals.[5] From this circumstance the great fame of this plant is derived.

8. In later times, it was stated by a certain interpolator of Theophrastus' *History of plants*,[6] repeated in the self-same words by Rufus the Ephesian,[7] and Diascorides,[8] that this cure effected by Melampus was due to the helleborus niger, hence this plant was denominated *Melampodium*. But that this is an error[9] we shall shew in a few words.

9. I shall not waste time by citing in corroboration the testi-

---

Appolodor., *Biblioth.* Lib. ii, cap. 2.

[2] Avicenna, Lib. ii, *de medicamentis simplicibus.* Artic. *Charbak,* (in Oper. Roma, 1593, fol. p. 269) corroborates this in these words :—

فوسوس من ساحية لبنات فروطس

[3] They wandered through the woods like cattle.

[4] Galen, in the book *de atra bile,* cap. 7.

[5] C. Plinii sec. *Hist. nat.,* lib. xxv, cap. 5, sec. 24. He seems to indicate that Melampus fed the goats upon veratrum album (in order to render their milk medicinal for the treatment), this we may infer from what he adds: "nigro (elleboro) equi, boves, sues necantur, itaque cavent id ; cum candido vescantur."

[6] See below in the note to § 17.

[7] In Oribasii, *Collectorum medicinalium* (Venet. op. Ald. 8), lib. vii, cap. 27, p. 251.

[8] *Mater. Med.,* lib. iv, cap. 151.

[9] This has already been suspected by J. H. Shulze. in his *Diss. de Elleborismis veterum,* p. 3, 4. (Halae, 1717, 4).

mony of Herodotus, whom Sprengel, otherwise a most weighty authority in medical history, affirms, though erroneously,[1] to have attributed the cure of the daughters of Proetus to *veratrum album.*

10. Suffice to say, that in the earliest period of Grecian history no other evacuant medicine seems to have been known to the physicians, who were still tyros in their art, and therefore that none other could have been used by Melampus for this treatment except this plant, which is now termed veratrum album, and that it was termed by them *hellebore*, κατ'ἐξοχην, thereby denoting that it was their sole and well known *evacuant* (purgative.)[2]

11. But in process of time, and if I am not deceived, soon after the time of Hippocrates the son of Heraclides, another evacuant medicine having been discovered, the physicians of that time seem to have applied to this new purgative plant the name that had been used for the most ancient and hitherto unique purgative (*hellebore*), adding by way of distinction the word black, as though they should say *purgans* (helleborum)[3] *nigrum.* And thus in all probability the appellation *black hellebore* arose, as indicating the later discovered plant.

12. That such was actually the case, appears from this : that no writer is found prior to the 100th Olympiad, who makes mention of black hellebore, because it had not yet been discovered, or, which comes to the same thing, it had not yet come into use ;[4] there is no writer, about and before that time, who

---

[1] *Geschichte der Arzneikunde*, pt. i, p. 121. The passage of Herodotus which he cites (lib, ix, cap. 33) says nothing but that Melampus was offered a reward by the Argivans to cure the Argivan women who were affected with mania, that he demanded the half of the kingdom for his remuneration, and that he at length obtained it. Herodotus does not say a word about the remedy used by Melampus in the treatment.

[2] The word *Hellebore*, the name of the sole and universally known emetic, received by use such an extended signification that it was applied to the operation itself, and sometimes signifies *vomiting.* Thus Hippocrates (sect. iv, aph. 13) πρὸς τοὺς ἐλλεβόρους, &c.

[3] *Helleborus* and *Helleborum* are used indifferently.

[4] The *Praenotiones Coacae* attributed to Hippocrates, are so full of archaisms, and written in such a hard, rough and abrupt style, that Grimm in the index to his German version (vol. ii, p. 586) suggests that they were probably the writings which, long before the time of Hippocrates, were preserved in the temple of Æsculapius at Cos. In this very ancient monument of the art of medicine, there is frequent mention made of ἐλλέβορος, as the root that causes evacuation by vomiting (veratrum album),—but in none of these places do we find black hellebore spoken of, because, most likely, it had not at that time been discovered (as we shall shew hereafter

applies to the plant which was the only one employed by the ancients for evacuating (vomiting), anything but the *bare* term, hellebore.[1]

13. Thus, as I have stated in a note, the very ancient authors of the *Praenotiones coacae*, and also Ctesias,[2] who was almost contemporaneous with Hippocrates, when they are evidently speaking of the veratrum album, make use of the bare term *hellebore* only. Moreover, in the genuine writings of Hippocrates[3] there is not a single passage where he uses the word ἰλλέβορος without meaning the veratrum album, and none in which he adds the word λευκὸς, for this simple reason, that there was as yet no occasion for applying this distinctive epithet to the plant which was the only evacuant at that period, the black hellebore not having been discovered, or no name having yet been given to it. In his genuine writings the expression ἰλλέβορος μέλας is never used, as I shall shew hereafter.

14. Even in the times shortly posterior to the age of Hippocrates, (as we see in the pseudo-Hippocratic writings of his sons and disciples), though mention is made of ἰλλέβορος μέλας, still the most ancient veratrum is always only alluded to under the simple appellation of *hellebore*.

15. It is indeed certain, that in almost all human affairs, the *primitive* thing is denoted specially by the *simple* word, whilst the *derived* and *compound* name is applied to a thing that is similar, but that has been *discovered later*; and is, consequently, *newer* than to which the simple word is applied.

16. Hence it is obvious that in the earlier times of Greece there was but one single hellebore (and that the veratrum album); and that if the so-called black hellebore, after Hippocrates' time, became known, the word "black" was added to it, but it was

when treating of the helleborus niger), nor is the word λευκὸς ever found a ded to ἐλλεβόρος, that being the only one known.

[1] Thus Galen (in Comment ad Hippocr., Sect. v, aph. 1) says: ἐλλέβορον λευκὸν ἁπλῶς ἰώθασι ὑνομάζειν ἐλλέβορον, οὐχ, ὥσπερ τὸν μέλανα, μετὰ προσθήκης, "they (the ancients) were accustomed to call (the white) hellebore by that simple word and not with any addition, as they did the black hellebore."

[2] A fragment of Ctesias in Oribasii, *Collect.*, lib, viii, cap. 8.

[3] Sect. iv, aphor. 13, 14, 15, 16.—Sect. v, aphor. 1.—In the book, *de fracturis* (op. edit. Chart. t. xii. p. 203 and 257), and in the book, *de articulis*, (ibid. p. 434)—These two books are both genuine writings of Hippocrates or of his grandfather, and are written in the same unadorned style. As regards the latter book (which is merely a continuation of the book *de fracturis*, as Galen has demonstrated in his preface to the book *de articulis*) Ctesias the Coan, refuses to admit it as a work of his relative Hippocrates (a lucid testimony to the genuineness of the book), as Galen also relates (Comment. iv. in lib. *de Articulis*, Op. edit. chart xii, p. 452).

not till after the lapse of a considerable time, and after the black hellebore had long been in use that the original hellebore could and did receive the addition of λευκος.[1]

17. Another proof of the greater antiquity of the (white) hellebore is, that in times now remote (when the more recent origin of the *black hellebore* could not be unknown) an author worthy of all confidence, Theophrastus the Eresian, distinctly refers Melampus' cure to the veratrum album, when he says, that it could not have been effected by the use of the black hellebore, which is deleterious to most animals, in consequence of which they will not touch it, but rather by that of the veratrum album, which the sheep (and also the goats) eat, and thereby purge themselves, which led to the discovery of its medicinal power: ἀναιρεῖν δὲ τὸν μὲν μέλανα, says he,[2] καὶ ἵππους, καὶ βοῦς, καὶ ὗς, διὸ καὶ οὐδέ νέμεσθαί τοῦτον· τον λευκὸν δὲ νέμεσθαί τὰ πρόβατα,[3] καὶ ἐκ τούτου πρῶτον συνοφθῆναι τὴν δύναμιν καθαιρομένων ἐκείνων.[4]

---

[1] The primitive signification of the word *hellebore* in the age of Hippocrates and some time afterwards, remained so strongly impressed on the memory of all who then flourished, that the physicians of that age (*i. e.* the immediate successors and disciples of Hippocrates, in the Writings termed pseudo-Hippocratic) although they commenced to give the name of black hellebore to the new plant, always continued to designate the first one by the simple word ἐλλέβορος, nor did it ever occur to them to distinguish by any adjective that med *e* e which had hitherto been the sole and was the most ancient evacuant. Had the black hellebore been discovered before the time of Hippocrates, and had it long been employed (concurrently with veratrum album) the simple appellation of the primitive hellebore would have long since become obsolete, and they would have been forced immediately after Hippocrates to employ the distinctive appellation "*white*;" but at that time this appellation had not come into use, and was only commenced a century later, after the black hellebore had already been employed for upwards of half a century. Indeed Theophrastus the Eresian (about the year 330 before our era) in his *history of plants* often denominates it by the single word, but sometimes he calls it ἐλλέβορος λευκὸς. In like manner it is called λευκὸς in the apocryphal continuation or the book attributed to Hippocrates, *De victu acutorum*, commencing from the words: καῦσος δὲ γαρ—(Op., t. xi, p. 175) by an anonymous author (one of the empirical sect rendered famous by Serapion of Alexandria), who in all probability composed the appendix about two centuries after Hippocrates. At length in more recent times the veratrum is more often mentioned with the distinctive adjective, under the name of ἐλλέβορος λευκὸς and that the more frequently as the use of the helleborus niger became more common.

[2] Theophrastus, *Hist. plant.* ed Stapelii, lib. x. cap. ii. (In this edition among other marks of haste and error, the fourth and fifth books are condensed into one, the *numerical order* of the subsequent books is consequently designated by lower numbers than they ought, thus that which ought to be the tenth and last is here termed the ninth.)

[3] In ancient times this word πρόβατα was used to signify all sorts of cattle, oxen sheep and goats, as Galen teaches us (Comment. i, ad Hippocr. lib. de articulis, ed. Chart. t. xii, p. 306).

[4] The appendix to this sentence in the same chapter of Theophrastus—καλοῦσι δὲ

18. This passage agrees with the words of Pliny: "alterum genus (hellebori, Melampodem) invenisse tradunt, capras purgari pasto illo amimadvertentem, datoque lacte earum sanasse Proetidas furentes,"[1] (although a little further on he again refers the plant of Melampus to helleborus niger, led into error probably by his compiling habits.)

19. The observations of Theophrastus are corroborated by this passage of Haller: "Not only do mules freely eat of this plant, but even the cattle feed in spring on the tender leaves of the veratrum album, whereby they purge themselves, but when the leaves become more expanded they cease eating them, until the tender leaves again appear the following spring."[2]   Pallas[3]

τὸν μέλανά τινες ἐκ τοῦ τεμόντος καὶ ἀνευρόντος Μελαμπόδιον, ὡς ἐκείνου πρώτου τεμοντος καθαίρουσι δὲ καὶ ὗας αὐτῷ καὶ πρόβατα, συνεπᾴδοντές τινα ἐπῳδὴν, καὶ εἰς ἄλλα δὲ πλείω χρῶνται—is said to be a spurious passage introduced by some sciolist. For it is contradicted by what Theophrastus says before, viz., *that hellebore is abhorred by swine and that it kills them.* But if by the word καθαίρουσι is to be understood not a medicinal purgation but a sort of bath by aspersion only—this would suffice to make us reject the passage as spurious, for it is an expression unworthy of such an illustrious man (Theophrastus) and repugnant to common sense, as must be evident to every reader. The origin of this old woman's tale is hereby revealed, and it is this, that *Blackfoot* (Μελάμπους) could not possibly have employed for the cure any other than *black* (μέλας) hellebore. Certainly a most extraordinary sort of argument! This clumsily attached patch, is then to be rejected, it smells of the mysticism of the Therapeutists, who piqued themselves on treating diseases by prayers and incantations. This school flourished at Alexandria a century and a half before our era (two centuries after Theophrastus), just at the time when the rivalry of the Kings of Egypt and Pergamus about their libraries encouraged by hopes of gain the interpolators of books and the Diascevastæ of manuscripts, to manufacture whole books, or to insert or add supposititious parts to genuine works, in order that they might appear more complete (see Galen, *Comment.* ii, *in lib.* iii, *Epidem.* p. 411.—*Comment.* i, *in lib. de. nat. hom.* p. 127, and his preface to *Comment.* ii, of the same book, p. 128.)

Therefore (it may be said *en passant*) it appears more than probable, not only that the whole ninth chapter (of the tenth book of Theophrastus') History of Plants) is spurious, but that it proceeds from the pen of the same interpolator. For the falsifier not only relates, but actually *approves* and *commends* the ridiculous superstitions and magical incantations of the doctrines of his own time (which could never have entered into the imagination of Theophrastus, who was imbued with the philosophy of Aristotle, and of the author of the *Moral Character*), which proceeded from the fertile brains of the Therapeutists, who were nourished on the absurdities of the East. In fact the whole style of the passage is that of this stamp of men. Moreover, the end of the eighth chapter is connected with the beginning of the tenth *much more naturally and logically*, and passes into it, as it were, in a continuous stream, if we expunge that jejune ninth chapter, so unworthy of Theophrastus, the production of a perverted mind, stuffed full of magic, incantations, and divinations.

[1] *Histor. natur.*, lib. xxv, sect. 21.

[2] *Hist. stirp. Helv.* N. 1204 ; and in Vicat's *Matière médicale tirée de Halleri hist. stirp.* Berne, 1776. 8.

[3] *Russische Reise.* Vol. II. 190.

also asserts that in Russia the horses eat the young leaves of the veratrum album, without any other effect than the production of looseness of the bowels.

20. But the chief thing, and that on which the whole affair turns, is that *goats* feed upon the veratrum, which Lucretius' testifies to when he sings :

> "Praeterea nobis veratrum est acre venenum,
> At *capris* adipes et coturnicibus auget."

21. But the most lucid testimony to this fact is furnished by Galen, a most weighty authority on the subject of the history of medicine among the ancients, and an author worthy of all confidence. He speaks of the treatment we have related as of a thing very generally known and admitting of no doubt. "Until now," he says,[2] "physicians have attempted to cure melancholia by means of vomiting produced by veratrum album. Indeed none who is acquainted with Greek literature could have failed to read or hear of the story of the maniacal daughters of Proetus who were cured by Melampus by means of this evacuant; from which circumstance this evacuation (viz. helleborism) remained celebrated for two or three centuries and more, but during that time all physicians have employed this medicine (veratrum album)."

From the description given by the ancients of the white hellebore does it follow that it is the same plant as our veratrum album ?

22. But we must inquire further if the (white) *hellebore*, used by the ancients for helleborism, is indeed the *veratrum album*[3] or not.

23. And first let us look at the description[4] of this plant left us by Theophrastus, who was an intelligent and learned naturalist, which it is to be regretted is so short, and buried as it were in a corrupted text.

---

[1] In his *Carmen de natura rerum*, lib. iv, v. 642. This celebrated poet flourished a century before our era.

[2] Ἰατρῶν—πάθος μελαγχολικὸν—ἐπιχειρούντων—τῇ θεραπείᾳ δι' ἐλλεβόρου τοῦ λευκοῦ καθάρσεως. Οὐδεὶς γὰρ οὕτως ἀπαίδευτός ἐστι τῶν ἐν Ἕλλησι τεθραμμένων, ὡς μήτ' ἀνεγνωκέναι, μήτ' ἀκηκοέναι, τὰς Προίτου θυγατέρας μανείσας ὑπὸ Μελάμποδος ἰαθῆναι καθαρθείσας οὕτως, ὥστε οὐ πρὸ διακοσίων ἐτῶν ἢ τριακοσίων ἀλλὰ πολὺ πλειόνων ἐνδόξου τῆς καθάρσεως ταύτης οὔσης, καὶ πάντων τῶν ἐν τῷ μεταξὺ χρόνῳ κεχρημένων τῷ φαρμάκῳ. Galen, *De atra bile*, cap. 7.

[3] Cornelius Celsus already employed this name in his *Libri de Medicina*.

[4] *Hist. plant.* lib. x, cap. 11.

24. He treats of both kinds of hellebore in one and the same chapter. "The helebores," he says, "both the black and the white species, bear a common equivocal name, but authors differ respecting their form and appearance. Some say they are similar, except as to colour, which in the root of one is white, in that of the other black, but the leaves of the black kind resemble in colour those of the laurel, whilst those of the white kind resemble in colour the leaves of the pear-tree." Then there follows a most corrupted text: οἱ δ᾽ οὖν ὁμοίας λέγοντες, τοιάνδε φασὶν εἶναι τὴν μορφὴν· καυλὸν δὲ ἀνθερικώδη, βραχὺν σφόδρα· φύλλον δὲ πλατύσχιστον ὅμοιον τῷ τοῦ νάρθηκος, μῆκος ἔχον εὔμηκες, &c. The first words of this sentence have been very properly changed by Scaliger and the editor Stapel into οἱ δ᾽ ἀνομοίας λέγοντες, in order that they should present a kind of *opposition* to the words in the principal period: οἱ μὲν γὰρ ὁμοίας εἶναι. As regards the rest of the sentence, καυλὸν δὲ &c., these writers, in other respects very sagacious, suppose it to allude solely to the black helebore, and do not think that in this description Theophrastus ever refers to the white, but in this they greatly err, for some of these words refer to the black, others to the white; moreover it is impossible but that Theophrastus must allude in this place to the white, because throughout the chapter he continually speaks alternately of the white and of the black, and describes the one after the other in such a manner as to demonstrate the distinction between them, and wherein they differ in their various parts. Therefore if he wished to be consistent it was necessary that he should in this place insert some description of the white helebore before proceeding to describe the black.

25. The following is the mode in which it seems to me possible to restore the words, mutilated as they have been by the injury of time, and mixed up among each other in a most confused manner: οἱ δ᾽ ἀνομοίως λέγοντες, τοιάνδε φασὶν εἶναι τὴν μορφήν· καυλὸν μὲν (τοῦ λευκοῦ)[1] ἀνθερικώδη, ὅμοιον τῷ τοῦ νάρθηκος· (τοῦ δὲ μέλανος)[2] βραχὺν σφόδρα φύλλον πλατύσχιστον, μῆκος ἔχον εὔμηκες.

26. Indeed it is the veratrum album only whose stem, with its attached flowers, could be likened to the flowery stem of the asphodel (which Theophrastus himself, lib. viii, cap. 12, calls ἀνθέρικον[3]): certainly not the helleborus niger, which has almost

---

[1] I have only added these two words; the remainder of the text of Theophrastus I have preserved in its integrity, only somewhat changing the order of the words.

[2] These three words have very properly been supplied by Scaliger.

[3] Μέγιστον δὲ πάντων (the bulbous plants) ὁ ἀσφόδελος, ὁ γὰρ ἀνθέρικος μέγιστος. In

37

no stem. But as regards the character of this stem, "which rises singly from the root, and in which moreover the leaves grow alternately [1] from protuberances," Theophrastus speaks of it under the general term ferulaceus [like a ferule] or *ὅμοιον τῷ νάρθηκι* (see lib. vii, cap. 2, *where he applies this character expressly to the hellebore,* that is to say, to the white hellebore.) This is the character that specially distinguishes the stem of the veratrum album, and is not at all applicable to the helloborus niger, which has hardly any stem.

27. Therefore we see that Theophrastus writes in this manner: "Those who allege that they (the white and black hellebore) are different, thus describe their respective forms: *The stem of the white hellebore resembles* (in its florescence) *that of the asphodel, and* (on account of the single stem that ascends from its root, and the disposition of its leaves) *has the appearance of a ferule; but the black hellebore, on the contrary, has a very short stem, large leaves, divided into broad lobes,*" &c.

28. To this rather superficial description of Theophrastus, let us add the brief one of Dioscorides, whereby it will be better apparent, that by their white hellebore the ancients understood nothing else than veratrum album, and that all the signs they mention as proper to it prove it to be the very same plant.

29. The words [2] that bear upon our subject are: Ἑλλέβορος λευκὸς φύλλα ἔχει ὅμοια τοῖς τοῦ ἀρνογλώσσου[3]—καυλὸν δὲ παλαιστιαῖον, κοῖλον περιφλοιζόμενον, ὅτε ἄρξεται ξηραίνεσθαι· ῥίζαι δ᾽ ὕπεισι πολλαὶ, λεπτα ἀπὸ κεφαλίου μικροῦ καὶ ἐπιμήκους, ὡσπερεὶ χρομμύου συμπεφυκυῖαι. These words, with a slight change, putting, for example, κοῖλον after περιφλοιζόμενον, will read thus: "*The white hellebore has leaves resembling those of the greater plantain, a stalk a palm in height, enveloped in*

like manner Dioscorides (lib. ii, cap. 199,) gives to the stem of the asphodel, with its flowers, the name of "*ἀνθέρικος*": ἀσφόδελος—ἔχων—καυλὸν—λεῖον ἔχοντα ἐπ᾽ ἄκρου ἄνθος, καλούμενον ἀνθέρικον.

[1] Not oppositely. Τὸ ναρθηκώδες, he says, μομονόκαυλον—βλαστάνει δὲ παραλλὰξ τὰ φύλλα—οὐκ ἐκ τοῦ αὐτοῦ μέρους τῶν γονάτων, ἀλλ᾽ ἐναλλὰξ—ὁμοιότερον τούτῳ τὸν καυλὸν ἔχει —ὁ ἐλλέβορος (καὶ ὁ ἀνθέρικος.) *Hist. pl.,* lib. 7, c. 2.

[2] *Materia Med.,* lib. iv, c. 150; written as it would seem before Pliny's work on *Natural History;* the latter translates and copies whole passages from Dioscorides without ever mentioning his name, shewing *a kind of envy and rivalry by no means rare among contemporaries.*

[3] Murray (*Apparat. Medicam.,* vol. v, p. 149) doubts whether the plantain of the ancients was the same as ours, but he is wrong to do so, for that by the word *arnoglossus* Dioscorides really implies our greater *plantain,* is obvious from several things: first, because the title of the chapter that treats of *arnoglossus* (Dios. *Mat. Med.,* lib. ii, c. 153) is, in some ancient manuscripts, περὶ ἀρνογλώσσου ἑπταπλεύρου, *i. e., on the seven-nerved plantain* (and that is precisely the number of nerves the leaf of the great

coats [1] (the sheaths of the leaves), *and hollow when it commences to dry. Its roots are numerous, delicate* (the fibrils), *fixed to a small and oblong bulb like an onion.*

30. If he says that the stalk is only a palm in height, whilst in reality it often attains the height of a cubit and two cubits, this error is to be attributed to the writers from whom he has compiled. He himself being a Cilician, does not seem to have known the plant from actual inspection, because (ὁ λευκὸς ὀλιγαχοῦ φύεται, as Theophrastus in his *Hist. Plant.*, lib. x, c. 11, calls it) it grows in but few parts of Greece. For the same reason, viz., not having himself seen the plant, he does not give an accurate description of the colour of the leaves. Moreover, it grows, as he says, in mountainous districts, not ἐν τραχέσι (in rugged places), but in the alpine and subalpine meadows and moist plains. [2]

31. The description which the ancients have left us of the white hellebore, though very superficial, still proves clearly that it is the same plant as our veratrum album, although the ancient works on natural history generally describe natural objects in a loose and superficial manner.

32. To the above we may add the very weighty authority of Avicenna, who describes the Dioscoridean veratrum album under the name of خربق ابيض, by which very name, as Forskal an eye-witness testifies, the veratrum album is still called in those regions. [3]

33. But the most important argument to prove the identity of the white hellebore of the ancients with our veratrum album, still remains, viz.—

The effects of both are not only similar but absolutely identical.

34. Among those who doubt if the plant which the most ancient Greeks designated by the single word ἐλλέβορος, but after-

---

plantain possesses) : second, because the Arabic version of Avicenna (*Lib. de Simpl. Medicam. Art. Charbak-Abiadh. Opera*, Romae 1593, fol. cit.) expresses the word ἀρνογλῶσσος by لسان الحمل —a word which to this day, in Arabic, signifies our plantain, as Forskal testifies, who saw it *Plant. Aegypt. et Arab.*, p. lxii,), and who himself gives it that name.

[1] Jacquinus, in his description of veratrum album, *Flora Austriaca*, plate 135. p. 18, says, "almost all the stem is enveloped in the sheaths of the leaves."

[2] The description of Pliny *Hist. Nat.*, lib 25, sect. 21) is evidently taken from that of Theophrastus and Dioscorides (thus, for instance, he attributes to the white hellebore the leaves of wild beet—*beta incipiens*, as he calls it—thus rendering the σεῦτλον ἄγριον of Dioscorides), it is therefore not much to be relied on.

[3] *Materia Medica Kahirini*, in the appendix to *Descript. Anim. in itinere orientali*, Hafn. 1775, 4, p. 152.

wards termed *white hellebore*, was actually our veraturm album, the most distinguished is a man who formerly rendered great service to the materia medica, John Andrew Murray,[1] who complains "*that the arguments to prove that it is the same plant are sought for rather in the similarity of its effects, which may be identical in many different plants,* than in the description of the plant, which is very imperfect."

35. As to what relates to the description and delineation of the plant by the ancients, we have already seen that it is not absolutely imperfect.

36. But with respect to that doctrine (the unhappy source, alas! of *succedanea* and *substitutes*)—"that no plant possesses peculiar properties of its own, but that a host of different plants produce the same effects on the human body, which are therefore, vague and uncertain," here this man, great and distinguished as he was, errs in common with most of the physicians of this age.

37. For the great Creator of the universe has implanted in every medicament *a constant rule of action ;* to each he has given *peculiar, specific, certain* powers, which are of the most constant and unvarying character, although, unfortunately, medical men have not investigated, and have almost entirely neglected them hitherto. The properties that existed in a medicament a thousand years ago are the same as they now possess, and as they will possess for ever.

38. But I would ask, what reason have you for affirming so confidently, that many different plants have the same effects, when it is well known that the peculiar and positive effects of all medicines have been so little investigated by medical men, that they are almost unknown to them, and it seems as though they thought their ignorance on this subject to be something quite legitimate and meritorious? How do they know then, that many plants possess the same properties? In place of devoting themselves to experimental investigation they delude themselves with their vain conceits and preconceived opinions.

39. No one species of plants has the same external form and appearance as another, and in like manner, each possesses a certain peculiar power proper to itself, which is not to be found in any other *species* of the same genus, and still less in any other

---

[1] *Appar. medicam.* Vol. v, p. 149. Cl. Salmasius also (in *Exercit. de homonymis hyles iatricae, Traj. ad Rhen.* 1689 fol.) thinks that "the hellebore of the ancients is lost and does not exist among us."

genus. As the external appearance differs, so also does the internal medicinal power!

40. This peculiar and specific power of acting on the system, which the great Creator has implanted in every medicine, is proved to be of such a constant character that it cannot be doubted—that the *oxyde of copper*, for example, when taken internally, excited many thousands of years ago, when it was first discovered, the same anxious vomiting which it caused eighteen centuries ago,[1] and the same which it causes to day,—that the *oxyde of lead* and *cerussa*, when applied externally, shewed in the earliest times the same refrigerating qualities, and the same power of constricting the pores of the skin,[2] that it manifests at the present day,—that the *cantharis* taken by the mouth caused in ancient times the same dysuria, the same hematuria, the same dysenteric affection of the bowels,[3] that it does now,—that *opium* exhibited in the most remote times the same specific quality, that, taken in a large dose, it caused the same prostration, with chilliness of the external parts of the body,[4] as it does to-day ; and so with all other medicaments.

41. From the collection of the peculiar and specific powers of any medicine observed from its use in ancient times, are we not justified in inferring, that a medicine which in our own days produces the same effects on the human body must be identical with the ancient one? There is certainly nothing that should prevent us coming to this conclusion.

42. I may here be permitted to compare the properties of the white hellebore of the ancients with those of our own veratrum album.

43. *The properties of the white hellebore as observed by the ancient physicians.*	*The properties of the veratrum album as observed by more modern physicians.*
At first there occurs heat of the throat and stomach.[5]	Internal heat with dislike to drinks.[6] Burning about the precordial region.[7]

---

[1] Diosc. *Mat. Med.* lib. v., cap. 87.

[2] Δύναμιν ἔχει ψυκτικὴν, ἐμπλαστικὴν—Diosc., *Mat. Med.*, lib. v, cap. 103.

[3] Δυσουροῦσι· πολλάκις δὲ αἷμα προΐενται δι' οὔρων· φέρεται δ' αὐτοῖς κατὰ κοιλίαν ὅμοια τοῖς ἐπὶ δυσεντερικῶν.—Diosc., ἀλεξ., cap. i.

[4] Μήκωνος δὲ ὅπου ποθέντος· παρακολουθεῖ καταφορὰ μετὰ καταψύξεος.—Diosc., ἀλεξ., cap. xvii.

[5] Antyllus in Oribas., *Collect.*, lib. viii, cap. 6, p. 278.

[6] S. Grassius, *Misc. Nat. Cur.*, dec. i, an. 4, p. 93.

[7] J. de Muralto, *Misc. Nat. Cur.*, dec. ii, an. 2, p. 240.

Many are *suffocated.*[1]

After violent and ineffectual efforts to vomit, *suffocation ;*[2] the face swells, the eyes are prominent, the tongue protruded from the mouth.

If vomiting comes on late, *strangulation.*[3] The face excessively red.

The parts belonging to respiration are constricted, with great difficulty of breathing.[4]

Often deprived of their voice.[5]

Loss of the voice and the senses.[6]

Gnashing of the teeth; the mind is deranged.[7]

Delirium.[8]

Heat of the tongue and throat.[1]

Heat of the fauces.[2]

Inflammation in the interior of the mouth.[3]

Constriction of the throat.[4]

Strangulation of the fauces.[5]

Strangulation about the throat.[6]

Strangulation, spasm, constriction of the throat.[7]

Swelling of the œsophagus, with dread of suffocation.[8]

Loss of breath.[9]

As if strangled, they are in great danger of suffocation.[10]

Inspiration very laboured and difficult.[11]

Stammering.[12]

Loss of voice.[13]

Loss of vision.[14]

Almost complete loss of the senses.[15]

Delirium.[16]

---

[1] Ctesias, apud Orib., loc. cit.

[2] Herodotus, in Orib., *Collect.,* lib. viii, cap. 7, p. 284.

[3] Antyllus, loc. cit.

[4] Herodotus, loc. cit.

[5] Antyllus, loc. cit., p. 280.

[6] Antyllus, loc. cit., p. 281.

[7] Herodotus, loc. cit.

[8] Antyllus, loc. cit.

[1] C. Gesner, *Epist. Med.,* p. 69.

[2] Bergius, *Mat. Med.,* p. 872.

[3] Greding, *Vermischte Schriften,* pp. 31, 36.

[4] Winter, in *Bresl. Samml.,* 1724, p. 268.

[5] Lorry, *de Melanchol.,* ii. pp. 312, 315.

[6] J. de Muralto, loc. cit.

[7] Reimann, *Bresl. Samml.,* 1724, p. 535.

[8] C. Gesner, loc. cit.

[9] P. Forestus, l. xviii, obs. 44.

[10] L. Scholzius, ap. P. Schenk, lib. vii, obs. 178.

[11] Benivenius, ap. Schenk, loc. cit. obs. 174.

[12] S. Grassius, loc. cit.

[13] Rödder, in *Alberti Jurispr. Med.,* obs. 15.

[14] O. Borrichius, *Acta Hafn.,* t. vi, p. 145.

[15] Vicat, *Plantes venen. de la Suisse,* p. 167.

[16] S. Grassius, loc. cit.; Greding, loc. it., pp. 35, 41, 42, 43, 49, 51, 54, 66, 69, 86.

In almost every case hiccough; in many the mouth quivers and twitches.[1]	Hiccough.[1]
Continual and violent hiccough.[2]	Hiccough for half an hour.[2]
Muscular contractions (cramp), especially in the muscles of the calves, thighs, arms, extremities of the feet, and chiefly in the hands,[3]	Hiccough all day.[3]
	Spasm.[4]
	Cramp of the calves.[5]
	Spasms in the hands, in the fingers.[6]
Also in the muscles of mastication.[4]	Attempts to vomit, with trismus.[7]
As if strangled, he falls down with his *teeth clenched* like a strangled victim.[5]	
Prostration of the strength.[6]	
Loss of consciousness.[7]	Excessive weakness.[8]
	Pulse almost extinct, imperceptible.[9]
	Threatening of syncope.[10]
	Loss of consciousness [11]
	Enormous efforts to vomit, even to syncope.[12]
Excessive vomiting.[8]	Enormous, horrible, severe, most violent vomiting.[13]

44. In the face of such a remarkable resemblance of the symptoms caused by these two plants, who can deny that the very same plant which now grows in our gardens was that which the ancients made use of for the production of helleborism? Where, I ask, can another plant be found which shall shew these same peculiar effects on the human body that are produced by the (white) hellebore of the ancients, and our veratrum album? The external character of the plant resembles that described by the ancients, the name is the same as that given to it by the Romans,* it has the same properties now

[1] Antyllus, loc. cit., pp. 281, 282.
[2] Antyllus, loc. cit., p. 282.
[3] The second day after taking the white hellebore.
[4] Antyllus, loc. cit., p. 282.
[5] Herodotus, loc. cit.
[6] Antyllus, loc. cit., p. 278.
[7] Antyllus, loc. cit.
[8] Antyllus, loc. cit., p. 283.

[1] J. de Muralto, loc. cit.; Smyth, in *Medic. Communic.*, vol. i, p. 207.
[2] C. Gesner, loc. cit.
[3] Greding, loc. cit., p. 43.
[4] J. de Muralto, loc. cit.
[5] Reimann, loc. cit.; Lorry, loc. cit.
[6] Greding, loc. cit., pp. 62, 71.
[7] Greding, loc. cit., pp. 82, 83.
[8] Benevenius, Smith, Vicat, loc. cit.
[9] Vicat, Rödder, loc. cit.
[10] Lorry, loc. cit.
[11] Forestus, loc. cit.
[12] Greding, loc. cit., p. 68.
[13] Many observations of Forestus, Lorry, Vicat, loc. cit., and Lentilius, *Misc. Nat. Cur.*, dec. iii, an. 1, app. p. 130, and Ettmüller, *Oper.*, tom. ii, pt. 2, p. 435.

* Cornelius Celsus, who wrote in the time of Augustus in his books on medicine always speaks of it under the name of *veratrum album.*

as formerly, there is the same danger attending its use now as formerly, it is undoubtedly the *same plant*.

Parts of Greece where the best grew.

45. The white hellebore grew in few parts of Greece, and, as I have above stated, in the moist plains of high mountainous regions. In the most remote times Theophrastus approved most of that which grew most abundantly in the Oeta hills near Pylaea in Pyra;[1] then that of Pontus; then that from Elaea; and lastly, that which grew in the bay of Malia;[2] he disapproves of those from Parnassus and Aetolia as being hard and dangerous in their effects.

46. In later times the two towns of Anticyra were celebrated for their white hellebore, namely, the town of Anticyra on the Phocian coast,[3] where the helleborian medicine was best prepared for medicinal use, and the other town of the same name in the gulf of Malia near Mount Oeta, and not far from Thermopylæ, which attained much celebrity on account of the excellence of the hellebore that came from this part.[4]

47. It is probable that the hellebore did not grow naturally in the country about the Phocian Anticyra, because the range of Mount Oeta did not extend that length,[5] but that it was

---

[1] Pyra was a plain near Pylaea in the chain of Mount Oeta (which, running from Thermopylae to the Ambracian gulf, extended as far as Doris) where Hercules is said to have burned himself on a funeral pile (Pliny, *Hist. nat.*, lib. xxxv. cap. 11) in order to obtain the honour of being received among the gods.

[2] In Stapel's edition of Theophrastus the reading μασσαλιώτης (ἐλλέβορος) is wrong. There was no place of that name in Greece (for it could not be referred to the river Massalia in Crete); the Massaliotic country was situated on the frontiers of Gaul, of which there can be no question here. We should read μαλιώτης, from the country about the gulf of Malia, where excellent hellebore was procured, as Strabo testifies. The derivation of κόλπος μαλιώτης is from the ancient but destroyed city Μαλία just as σικελιώτης is derived from σικελία, or μασσαλιώτης from μασσαλία, as Strabo tells us (*Geogr.*, lib. iv, 270), a Phocian colony in Gaul, now called *Marseilles*.

[3] Situated between the town of Crissa and Marathon (and the Pharygian promontory) (Strabo, *Geogr.*, lib ix. edit. Amst. p. 640, collated with p. 647), but in D'Anville's map it is placed wrong.

[4] Strabo (*Geogr.*, lib. ix, p. 640)—Εἶτα (after the gulf of Crissa) Ἀντίκυρα (in Phocis) ὁμώνυμος τῇ κατὰ τὸν μαλιακὸν κόλπον, καὶ τὴν Οἴτην· καὶ δή φασιν, ἐκεῖ τὸν ἐλλέβορον φύεσθαι τὸν ἀστεῖον, ἐνταῦθα δὲ σκευάζεσθαι βέλτιον, καὶ διὰ τοῦτο ἀποδημεῖν δεῦρο πολλοὺς καθάρσεως καὶ θεραπείας χάριν· γίνεσθαι γάρ τι σησαμοειδὲς φάρμακον ἐν τῇ, φωκικῇ, μεθ' οὗ σκευάζεσθαι, τὸν οἰταῖον ἐλλέβορον.. In like manner Stephanus, the Byzantine, (*Libr. de urbibus*) says: Ἀντίκυραι πόλεις δύο, ἡ μία Φωκίδος, ἡ δὲ ἐν Μαλιεύσιν· ἐνταῦθα φασι τὸν ἐλλέβορον φύεσθαι τον ἀστεῖον.

[5] The nature of the country about Phocian Anticyra, which Pausanias (*Graec. descr.*, p. 652, ed. Hanoviae, 1613) describes thus: τά δὲ ὄρη τὰ ὑπὲρ Ἀντίκυραν πετρώδη - —was such, that the black hellebore might grow there *spontaneously*, but not

either brought from there or cultivated by the inhabitants in gardens, and proved to them a source of profit. In the time of Pliny[1] the white hellebore used still to be cultivated in the island of Thasos.

48. In the time of Rufus, a Galatian white hellebore used to be sold, which, however, he condemns as being very bad.[2] Pliny pronounces the hellebore of Parnassus to be the fourth best, and says it used to be adulterated with the Aetolian.[3] Dioscorides tells us that the veratrum of Galatia and Cappadocia was white and resembled a rush, and that it possessed a greater suffocating power;[4] it does not appear to have been disliked in his time. After the time of Dioscorides, the Galatian veratrum commenced to be reckoned one of the good kinds, the Sicilian kind then also got into notice; but it was not considered so good.[5] Thus in the course of time several kinds of white hellebore, some from one country and some from another, were considered good and sought after, and less care than previously was exercised in their selection.

Signs of its good quality.

49. The ancient physicians selected for employment those fibres of the roots that were moderately rigid,[6] friable, soon causing sneezing when brought near the nose,[7] fleshy, of equal thickness throughout,[8] and they rejected those that were too pointed, like the fibrils of a rush, and from which, when broken, dust escaped, (for this was a sign that the root was old). They ought to have a narrow medulla and taste moderately hot.

50. But of all who have described the way to choose the veratrum album the most accurate is Aëtius (who seems to have

---

the veratrum album; the veratrum of Phocian Anticyra must therefore either have been brought from Doris, where it grows and where mount Oeta extends, or cultivated in the garden.

[1] *Hist. nat.*, lib. xiv, cap. 16.

[2] See a fragment in *Oribasii Collect.*, lib. vii, cap. 27, p. 249.

[3] *Hist. nat.*, lib. xxx, sect. 21.

[4] *Mat. Med.*, lib. iv, cap. 150.

[5] See a fragment in *Oribasii Collect.*, lib. viii, cap. i. p. 271.

[6] Dioscorides, in the place already cited, has : μετρίως τεταμένος, or as other manuscripts have it : τετανώδης, which Sarrazin renders moderately *extended;* but this is certainly an obscure if not a false reading. Rasarius after Archigenes (ap. *Oribas.*, l. c. lib. viii, c. 2) more clearly renders this quality of the good fibres by the term *rigid.* Aëtius likewise makes use of the term : κάρφη τέτανα.

[7] Herodotus, apud *Oribas. Collect.*, lib. viii, cap. 4, p. 276.

[8] Herodotus, loc cit.

drawn his description from Posidonius); these are his words—
"The best hellebore is that which, from one root, sends forth
many fibres, which are short, rigid, not rough, nor thin at their
ends, nor ending in a point like the tail of a mouse, very white
internally, but externally of a yellowish colour, heavy, having
a friable medulla not so soft as to be able to be bent, but apt to
break across, and when broken, diffusing around a sort of smoky
and pure cloud (if, however, they emit dust, this is a sign of the
oldness of the hellebore). Good hellebore has at first a sweetish[1]
taste, which then becomes acrid for a short time, and afterwards
excites a great heat in the mouth, causes a great flow of saliva
and deranges the stomach."[2]

51. Others condemn that kind which produces a copious flow
of saliva, because it causes too easily the strangulating sensation
in the throat; but they are wrong, for this is only a sign of the
greater medicinal virtue of the hellebore, and indicates that a
smaller dose of it should be given.

52. The earliest physicians preferred that which was gathered
during the wheat harvest, but Aëtius rightly gives the preference
to that which has been collected in the spring, for at that season
of the year the plant still contains all its juices.[3]

Medicinal uses of Veratrum album.

53. The ancient physicians used veratrum album in two different ways—first, the *ordinary use* for obtaining speedy and
obvious effect; the second, the *grand cure* for inveterate chronic
diseases, the latter they termed *helleborism*.

54. In general the ancient physicians employed the veratrum
album for the purpose of exciting vomiting, and the helleborus
niger for purging.[4]   Throughout the writings of the most ancient

---

[1] Archigenes (loc. cit., lib. viii, cap. 2, p. 272,) also says: "all kinds of hellebore
have a sweetish taste.

[2] Aëtius (lib. iii, cap. 126, ed. Ald.): Κράτιστος ἐλλέβορος ὁ ἀπὸ μιᾶς ῥίζης πάνυ πολλὰ
ἔχων κάρφη καὶ ταῦτα σμικρὰ καὶ τέτανα καὶ ἀρυσα (read ἄρρυσσα) καὶ οὐκ ἀπολήγοντα εἰς
ὀξὺ, οὐδὲ μειουρίζοντα· λευκὰ δὲ σφόδρα ἔντοθεν, ἐκτὸς δὲ ὠχρότερα ὑπάρχῃ, βαρέα, ἐντερίωνην
ἔχοντα εὔθρυπτα (read εὔθρυπτον·) οὐ καμπτόμενα διὰ μαλακότητα, ἀλλὰ καταγνύμενα καυληδὸν,
καπνῶδες τι ἐν τῇ θραύσει περιέχοντα καὶ ἀνιέντα, καὶ τοῦτο καθαρόν· τὸ γὰρ κονιορτῶδες παλαιὸν
δηλοῖ τὸν ἐλλέβορον· ὁ δὲ ἀγαθὸς διαμασσηθεὶς, πρῶτον μὲν γλυκύτητος ἔμφασιν παρέχει, αὖθις
δὲ δριμύτητος βραχείας· μετὰ δὲ τοῦτο πύρωσιν ἰσχυρὰν ἐμποιεῖ περὶ τὸ στόμα καὶ σίελον ἄγει
πολὺν, καὶ τὸν στόμαχον ἀνατρέπει.

[3] Loc. cit. Δεῖ δὲ ἔαρος ἀναλέσθαι τον ἐλλέβορον, ἔτι τῆς ῥίζης ἐγκυμονούσης.

[4] See Aretaeus, *Curat. chronic. morb.*, lib. ii. cap, 13, p. 136, edit. Boerhavii.—Pliny,
(lib. 25, sect. 22) says: "Nigrum purgat per inferna, candidum autem per vomitum.
In like manner Rufus (loc. cit., lib. vii, cap. 26, p. 250) and many others testify to the
same effect; but the thing speaks for itself in all the writings of the ancient physi-

physicians, when they speak of purging upwards,[1] they always allude to the veratrum album, even though the word "hellebore" is not added; but when they speak of purging downwards either the black hellebore is understood, or they mention the name of the purgative to be administered. But in the latter times[2] the remedy used to produce the one or the other operation is not understood, but usually mentioned expressly.

Of the lesser treatment with veratrum album, without preparatory treatment of the patient.

55. The earliest physicians seem to have employed this medicine, without *previous preparation* of the patient, in ordinary and acute diseases when they wished to procure evacuation upwards, as they termed it, that is, vomiting.

56. Hippocrates used to give the veratrum album at once, and without preliminary treatment of the patient in urgent cases,[3] and whenever he wished to evacuate quickly by vomiting.

57. The symptoms which he considered to indicate veratrum were—want of appetite, corroding sensation in the stomach, vertigo with obscuration of sight and bitter taste in the mouth, without fever;[4] in general he ordered it to be given in cases where the pains and morbid symptoms were in the upper part of the body, and when the other symptoms seemed to demand evacuation.[5]

---

cians. One only, the author of the pseudo-Hippocratic book *De affectibus internis* (Opera Hippocr., edit. Foesii, sect. v, p. 118), orders (if the text be genuine) the black hellebore to be used for promoting evacuation upwards, but he has found no imitators among all the physicians of antiquity.

[1] Thus before, during and immediately after the time of Hippocrates the words ἐλλέβορος and vomiting were synonymous terms. Therefore the Latin versions of the Greek medical writings are wrong, when the question is concerning the evacuation by veratrum album (which was always by vomiting) to render the work καθαίρειν by "*purgare*," because the Roman physicians never employed this word alone (*i. e.* without the addition of "*per superiora*") to express "to excite vomiting," or to evacuate by vomiting," although the Greeks could employ καθαίρειν alone to express vomiting.

[2] From and a little before our era.

[3] See the book *De Fracturis* (ed. Chart. t. xii, p. 203). He there says: ἄμεινον ἐλλέβορον πιπίσκειν αὐθήμερον, ἢ τῇ ὑστερίῃ; in this place he speaks of the employment of vomiting by hellebore in order to guard as rapidly as possible against swelling, trismus, acute fever and sphacelus from a bruise in the sensitive parts in the vicinity of the calcaneum. This recommendation he confirms in another place (sect. iv, aph. 10) where he says: φαρμακεύειν ἐν τῇσι λίην ὀξέασι, ἢν ὀργᾷ αὐθήμερον· χρονίζειν γὰρ ἐν τοῖσι τοιούτοισι, κακον.

[4] Sect. iv, aphor. 17.

[5] Sect. iv, aphor. 18.

58. In this manner his successors up to the time of Galen ordinarily employed the veratrum in order to cause vomiting, as we find in the pseudo-Hippocratic and other writings.

59. That the veratrum was then given in a smaller and even in a very small dose is a mere conjecture, for Hippocrates nowhere makes mention of the dose. It was only at a later period that physicians mentioned the dose of veratrum album which they employed for common use, as well as for the production of helleborism.

60. As the earliest physicians up to the time of Hippocrates neither knew nor employed any other emetic besides veratrum album; when they wished to evacuate upwards, they could only make use of this medicine for obtaining prompt and immediate relief by diminishing the dose;[1] they would have to diminish the dose whether of the crude root, or of the infusion, or of the decoction.

61. Those physicians who immediately followed Hippocrates, in order to mitigate the effects of veratrum in its ordinary employment, imagined various ways of administering it without giving it by the mouth, a mode of administration very repugnant to the dogmatic school of that age, which was more intent on theorizing upon the nature of things than on practising rationally.[2]

62. Accordingly, Plistonicus and Dieuches, followers of this sect,[3] as also Diocles (who flourished thirty years before them) strove to excite mild vomiting by means of this medicine introduced as a suppository by the anus, or as a pessary by the vulva, or employed as an epithem.[4]

63. But the principal mode of mitigating the effects of helle-

---

[1] This milder treatment by diminished doses seems to be alluded to by Hippocrates himself in the following place (*De fracturis.* Operum edit. Chart. tom. xii, p. 257): ἐλλέβορον μαλθακὸν πικίσαι χρῆ αὐθήμερον; the expression γαλθακὸν—slight—applied to hellebore would seem to indicate a smaller dose of it. Also in another place (*De Artic.*, tom. xii, p. 362) ἢν δὲ καὶ εὐήμετος ἔη, ἐμέειν ἀπὸ συρμισμοῦ—if the person vomit easily, he should get a slight emetic ("which does not exhaust him too much," according to Galen's explanation).

[2] Mnesitheus (one of this sect who lived about 320 years B. C.) shews some fear of this kind. The following are his words (in *Oribas. Collect.*, lib. viii. cap. 9): "There is great danger attending the drinking of hellebore; for either the patient is restored immediately to health, or he is subject to much and long-continued suffering: remedies of this sort should not therefore be given unless all the safer modes of treatment have been exhausted."

[3] Contemporaries of Mnesitheus.

[4] As Rufus mentions (apud *Oribas.*, l. c. lib. vii, cap. 27, p. 266).

bore wast that invented by Philotimus,[2] a physican of the same school, and contemporary of the above, which was adopted by all the practitioners of the succeeding ages. When it was drsired to produce a milder and more expeditious vomiting, he introduced a root of veratrum album into a radish,[3] and (as we are informed by the physicians who immediately followed him) háving extracted the veratrum the following day, he gave the radish thus impregnated with the medicinal power of the veratrum to be eaten either alone or with oxymel.[4] "By this means," says Rufus, "vomiting was most rapidly excited, which would not have occurred so successfully by the employment of hellebore alone."

64. Rufus likewise mentions that in his timo evacuations upwards were produced by employing footballs of hellebore.[5]

65. For the same object Herodotus, a pneumatic physician contemporary of Rufus, gave two spoonfuls of the decoction of hellebore to those who did not require violent evacuation.[6]

66. On the other hand Galen, who gave hellebore with considerable timidity, ingenuously confesses, "that it seemed to him dangerous[7] to give the veratrum album to sick persons in his time without preparing them for it, as their juices, which had been rendered viscid by idleness and luxury, required first to be purified."

67. Antyllus gave to old men, children, &c., a small quantity of the infusion of hellebore.[8]

68. But I shall now proceed to give the more important treatment of chronic diseases by means of veratrum album, to which the ancients gave the name of

---

[1] See Rufus, l. c.

[2] Aëtius (as we learn from Antyllus and Posidonius) gives the following prescription:—"Six drachms of the fibres of the root of veratrum are to be inserted into a radish which has been pierced with a reed, the following day they are to be taken out, care being taken not to leave any of the bark of the veratrum inside; the radish is to be cut in pieces and then eaten along with oxymel."—(lib, iii. c. 120).

[3] Loc. cit. The same method is recommended by Pliny (*Hist. nat.* lib. xxv., sec. 24) and Galen (lib. i, *de method. med.*, ad Glauc. cap. 12). It is, however easy to perceive that from such a process it is impossible that the medicine can always be the same, or in the same quantity, as Murrray observes (*Apparat. med.*, tom. v. p. 158)

[4] Rufus, loc. cit.

[5] In *Oribas.*, loc. cit., lib. viii. cap. 3, p. 276.

[6] Τὸ τοίνυν διδόναι ἐλλέβορον ἄνευ τοῦ προδιαιτῆσαι, σφαλερὸν, &c. See Galen, *Comment.* ii, in Hippocrat. lib. *de fracturis*, (edit. Chart. t. xii, p. 203).

[7] In *Oribas.*, l. c. lib. viii, cap. 5, p. 277.

Helleborism.[1]

69. Serious and inveterate diseases in general the earliest physicians endeavoured to cure by means of large doses of veratrum, but they shewed a great deal of caution and care in their employment of it, partly because they sought to overcome a disease, as they imagined, by a medicine of a more violent character[2] than the disease itself; partly because they sought to produce the least possible amount of inconvenience from its use.

70. In the earliest times, physicians knew of no other medicine for combatting chronic diseases, with the exception of a few, except the veratrum album, to which, when all common resources had failed, they resorted as to an anchor of safety.

71. "The white hellebore," says Aretaeus,[3] "is the most efficacious, not only of the emetics, but also of all evacuant medicines, not indeed by the quantity and variety of the excretions it occasions (for cholera does the same), nor yet by the intensity and violence of the vomitings (in this it is surpassed by sea-sickness), but by the quality and remarkable power with which it restores the sick to health by means of a slight and far from violent evacuation. It is moreover the sole remedy of all chronic diseases which have already taken deep root in the constitution, if other remedies fail. It resembles the power of fire; and what is effected by the combustion of fire, that hellebore does still more

---

[1] We find the word ἐλλεβορίζειν used by the anonymous continuer of the Hippocratic book, *De diaeta acut.* (edit. Chart. t. xi. p. 165), and the author of the sixth book, *De Epid.* (l. c. t. ix. p. 360); in these places it refers to the use of hellebore in diseases as an emetic; but the substantive ἐλλεβορισμὸς, referring to the grand cure was first employed by Aretaeus (*de curatione diuturnorum morborum*, lib. ii, cap. 13) and later, Caelius Aurelianus (*Chronic.* lib. i, cap. 4), in his barbarous language improperly applies the term *helleborismus* to the *decoction of veratrum.*

[2] Galen explains the operation of the larger doses of hellebore in a much too mechanical and gross manner when (in his *Comment.* i, on the *Epidem.* vi. of Hippocr. he says—"If the disease is of very long standing and cannot be eradicated as *with a lever,* we employ the veratrum album," (ἐλλεβορίζειν μὲν ἐὰν πάνυ χρόνιον ᾖ τὸ πάθος, καὶ ὡς ἂν ἔποι τις μοχλεῖ ις δεόμενον, εἰς ταῦτα γὰρ ἐλλεβόρῳ χρώμεθα).

[3] Ἔστι ὁ λευκὸς (ἐλλέβος) οὐκ ἐμετηρίων (conjecture of Wigan for ἐμετήριον of the text)πόνον, ἀλλὰ καὶ ξυμπάντων ὁμοῦ καθαρτηρίων ὁ δυνατώτατος, οὐ τῷ πλήθει καὶ τῇ ποικιλίῃ τῆς ἐκκρίσιος· τόδε γὰρ καὶ χολέρη πρήσσει· οὐδ᾽ ἐντάσει καὶ βίῃ τῇσι ἐπὶ τοῖσι ἐμέτοισι· ἐς τόδε γὰρ ναυτίη καὶ θάλασσα κρέσσον· ἀλλὰ δυνάμι καὶ ποιότητι οὔτι φαύλῃ· Τῇπερ ὑγιέας τοὺς κάμνοντας ποιέει, καὶ ἐπ᾽ ὀλίγῃ καθάρσι, καὶ ἐπὶ σμικρῇ ἐντάσι. Ἀτὰρ καὶ πάντων τῶν χρονίων νούσων ἐς; ῥίζαν ἱδρυμένων, ἢν ἀπαυδήσῃ τὰ λοιπὰ ἄκεα, τόδε μούνον ἰητήριον· πυρὶ ἴκελον γὰρ, ἐς δύναμιν λευκὸς ἐλλέβορος, καὶ ὅ, τι περ πῦρ ἐργάζεται ἐκκαίον τοῦδε πλέον ἐλλέβορος εἴσω παρεκθέων πρήσσει, εὔπνοιαν μὲν ἐκ δυσπνοίας, ἐξ ἀχροίης δὲ εὐχροίην καὶ ἀπὸ σκελετίης, εὐσαρκίην. (*De curat. chronic.*, lib. ii, cap. 10, ed. Boerh., p. 136.)

completely in the interior of the body, giving to the asthmatical an easy respiration, to the pale faced a florid complexion, and to the emaciated a robust body."

When helleborism began to be practised, and how long its use was continued.

72. Before the age of Hippocrates many physicians were afraid to employ this "grand cure," because they were ignorant of the doses and of the caution necessary to be employed in the use of Hellebore; those who used it, however, not unfrequently did harm by their rude mode of exhibiting it.

73. This we learn from Ctesias, a physician of the Cnidian school, a relation and almost a contemporary of Hippocrates, but a little his junior: "In the times of my father and grandfather,"[1] says he, "no physician administered hellebore, for they knew not the proper mode of administering it, nor the proper dose in which it should be given. If, however, they sometimes gave a patient a draught of hellebore, they warned him that he ran a great risk. Of those who took it many were suffocated, few benefitted. But now we see it given with perfect safety.

74. After the authors of the *Praenotiones Coacae*, Hippocrates himself, who flourished about the year 436 B. C., employed helleborism boldly, and taught the precautions it was requisite to take in its use, but as was his wont, in very few words, which I shall quote when I come to treat of the mode of employing it.

75. In later times helleborism underwent various changes of fortune. For the medical sects that arose after the time of Hippocrates, applied their minds more to obtain a paltry renown for vain speculations and theoretic subtleties, than to the careful treatment of diseases; therefore in consequence of their ignorance or neglect of the precautions requisite in employing hellebore, the use of this root came to be regarded as dangerous and fell into disrepute.[2]

76. Still it was employed by many physicians of those times, as may be learned from the writings that were given out under the name of Hippocrates (called pseudo-Hippocratic).[3]

---

[1] In a fragment preserved by Oribasius, *Collect.*, lib. viii, cap. viii, p. 285.

[2] See above, in the note to § 61, the observation of Mnesitheus, the dogmatic physician.

[3] See the apocryphal continuation of Hippocrates' book, *De victu acut.* (edit. Chart. t. xi, pp. 165, 175, 180),—as also the pseudo-Hippocratic books, *De Morb. popula.*

77. But it was principally the Anticyran physicians of this period who practised helleborism, *ex professo*, if I may be allowed to use the expression, and they pursued it vigorously for several centuries. A great number of sick persons from other countries who had been given up by other physicians, travelled to both Anticyras (towns, as I before stated, in great repute for this treatment), in order to be cured of the most protracted and serious diseases by means of the potent employment of hellebore.

78. Afterwards Themison,[1] founder of the methodic sect, began to recommend this mode of treatment by means of large doses of veratrum,[2] but his books on chronic diseases[3] have been lost.

79. Cornelius Celsus,[4] who followed him, says very little in his writings respecting the use of veratrum album, but he mentions it incidentally; it is doubtful if he employed it himself.

80. Thereafter Aretaeus of Cappadocia, a man gifted with the genius of Hippocrates, who flourished in the reign of Domitian, wrote a good deal of useful matter relative to helleborism.

81. Then Rufus (apparently the Ephesian[5]) and the pneumatic physicians, Herodotus and Archigenes, who flourished at the close of the first century of the Christian era, made great efforts to propagate and teach the use of hellebore, as the fragments of their writings preserved by Oribasius clearly testify.

82. But not long after them appeared Claudius Galen[6] of Pergamus, founder of a sect, the torch and trumpet of general therapeutics, a man more desirous of inventing a subtle system than of consulting experience. Disdaining to learn the powers of medicines by instituting experiments, he gave the bad example of generalizing and framing hypotheses.[7] He neglected the em-

---

especially the fifth (which was most probably written by a Coan physician, perhaps by the son of Draco), the sixth (probably written by Thessalus), and the seventh (written by several hands)—and finally, the books *De affectionibus* and *De internis affectibus*, in many places.

[1] About the year 63 B. C.

[2] Pliny, *Hist. natur.*, lib. xxv, sect. 53.

[3] Quoted by Caelius Aurelianus (*Tard. Passionum.* lib. i, cap. 1).

[4] In the commencement of our era.

[5] That the fragments quoted by Oribasius are from the works of Rufus of Ephesus seems to be borne out by this, that a part of them is to be found in a manuscript containing the anatomical works of Rufus of Ephesus, translated into Latin by J. P. Grassus, in the *Principes artis Medicae* of Henr. Stephanus, 1567, fol. p. 128.

[6] This, the greatest celebrity in the medical schools, and almost the only authority for thirteen centuries, flourished at Rome after the middle of the second century of our era.

He indicated all the powers and qualities of all simple medicaments, not by exployment of veratrum album, or rather he dreaded it. In very few places of his most copious writings (which certainly prove the fecundity and subtlety of his mind) is mention made of this celebrated medicine. To be sure, in his book, *Quos purgare oporteat*, he repeats, principally from Hippocrates and Rufus, the preliminary precautions and rules for the employment of helleborism, but he adds nothing of his own which would lead us to infer that he approved of it himself; on the contrary, he says: "We have sometimes given in oxymel, radishes in which the fibres of white hellebore had been left for twenty-four hours, in order to excite gentle vomiting by this means"; which is as much as to say, that he did not employ the grand cure, but only sometimes used the gentle method of Philotimus. He elsewhere [1] recommends the same gentle use of veratrum. Moreover, in his commentaries on the Hippocratic writings he now and then says something about hellebore in a superficial and imperfect manner. thereby shewing that he had a great objection to the serious employment of this root. Thus when Hippocrates [2] orders, for a contusion of the heel got by leaping from a height, apparently for the purpose of preventing tetanus and gangrene, hellebore to be given, that same day or the next, before the fever comes on, or when it is slight or not continued, Galen confesses that "he would not dare to give hellebore, even if there was no fever," [3] so far was he from making use of the helleborism of the early physicians.

83. I know not whether it was the mere example of Galen, or the dogmatic style of his writings which were repeated literally in all medical writings as though they had been the oracles of an infallible God, or if it was from other causes, that the physicians who immediately followed [4] him almost entirely neglected helleborism ; thus much however is certain, that for almost two centuries it was very little used, until a man distinguished

---

periments upon the human body, but by mere conjecture : thus he arbitrarily placed both the hellebores *in the third order of hot and dry substances* (in the 11th book *De simpl. med. facultate*, t, xiii, p. 173), whereas it is impossible that these two medicines, which have a totally opposite medical action on the human body, can be of the same quality.

[1] In the first book of the *Method. medend.* ad Glauconem, cap. 12.

[2] Or his grandfather, who by some is thought to be the author of the books *De fracturis* and *De articulis*.

[3] Ἡμεῖς δὲ οὐδ' ἀπυρέτῳ τολμῶμεν διδόναι (ἑλλέβορον). *Comment.* ii, in librum *De Fracturis* (edit. cit., tom. xii, p. 204).

[4] Caelius Aurelianus, who seems to have been a contemporary of Galen, and not to have lived after him, recommends the employment of helleborism in epilepsy (l. c. lib. i cap. 4). His dialect is African, not pure Roman, but rude and rough.

equally in medicine and in surgery, Antillus,[1] paid so much attention to this mode of treatment that he is justly regarded as the greatest authority in laying down the precautions it was requisite to use in the employment of this means.

84. Shortly after him Posidonius, a physician of no mean reputation, as may be seen from the fragments of his writings preserved by Aëtius, rivalled Antyllus in the attention he devoted to helleborism.[2]

85. Thereafter the grand cure by hellebore again declined sensibly and fell into disuse. In fact Oribasius, about the year 362, in his *Collecta*, dedicated to the emperor Julian (called the apostate), has brought together many observations of the ancients on the subject of helleborism, but where he ought to have given instructions concerning it himself (in the *Synopsis* to his son Eustathius), he does not say a word about it.

86. But in the following century Asclepiodotus, abandoning in a great measure the doctrines of his fanatical preceptor Jacobus Psychrestus (about the year 460), revived the practice of helleborism, which had long been neglected and discontinued, and gained great reputation by his wonderful cures of very obstinate and serious diseases by means of this medicine.[3] But of all the physicians of antiquity he was the last who practised this way, for after him the employment of helleborism fell into oblivion, nor was it afterwards restored by any of the Arabian physicians.[4]

---

[1] This author flourished about the year 330 of our era; fragments of his writings have been preserved by Oribasius} and Aëtius ; Sprengel has published a separate edition of them.

[2] That he wrote in the time of Oribasius, and some time before him (about the year 360), is apparent from this, that Oribasius in his chapter on epilepsy (*Synopsis*, lib. viii, cap. 6), transcribes word for word, without mentioning his authority, Posidonius' method of treating this disease, which Aëtius (*Tetrab.* ii, Serm. ii, cap. 13) ascribes to Posidonius. But our Posidonius (whom some, for what reason I know not, call Possidonius, though the etymology of the word, as well as the Aldine edition of the Greek text, and Photius also—p. 565—all make the word Ποσειδώνιος) must not be confounded with the more ancient philosopher of the same name, whom Strabo calls the *friend of Ptolemy* (Geogr., lib. xi, p. 491).

[3] Ἀσκληπιόδοτος—τοῦ λευκοῦ ἐλλεβόρου πάλαι τὴν χρῆσιν ἀπολωλυῖαν—αὐτὸς ἀνεκαίνησε, καὶ δι᾽ αὐτοῦ ἀγιάτους νόσους ἰάσατο (Photii Μυριόβιβλον, p. 1054, edit. Schotti, Rothomagi, 1653, fol.)

[4] Mesue, who flourished during the reign of the caliph Al Rashid, about the year 800, a man of such celebrity that he was termed the evangelist of physicians, contributed much to the almost complete abandonment of the use of veratrum album. In his book *De Simpl.*, cap. 30, he says, "There are two kinds of hellebore, the white

87. So also Aëtius the Amidenian, who about the year 545 [1] arranged in sixteen books, with much order and clear method, all the writings of the ancients on the treatment of diseases that remained, carefully extracts from Antyllus and Posidonius what relates to helleborism, but adds nothing from his own experience.

88. In like manner Alexander of Tralles, who composed twelve books in the Greek language on the art of medicine, about the year 555, in the time of Justinian, was so prejudiced, like the rest of his contemporaneous colleagues,[2] against the use of this root, that he greatly prefers the Armenian stone (fossil oxyde of copper) to veratrum album, "as an evacuant medicine without the harm and danger that attend the employment of veratrum album." [3]

89. Afterwards indeed Paulus of Aegina, who wrote his seven books on medicine about the year 640, in Greek, describes cursorily the mode of practising helleborism among the ancients, but as far as can be understood he does not seem to have employed it himself.[4]

90. Finally Johannes, the son of Zacharias, surnamed Actuarius,[5] only makes mention of veratrum album incidentally,[6] and only after the description of others.

Of the seasons of the year, the diseases, and the subjects in which the ancients considered helleborism suitable or unsuitable.

91. The earliest physicians considered the spring the most suitable season for the evacuations by hellebore, next to that the autumn, and if a choice were capable of being made betwixt winter and summer, they preferred the latter for the evacuations, upwards, the former for those downwards.[7]

---

and the black; the latter is more wholesome than the white, which produces most terrible symptoms."

[1] The learned Dr. Carl Weigel (*Aëtianarum exercitationem specimen*, Lips, 1791, 4, p. 8) proves that Aëtius flourished about the years 540 and 550, but that Alexander of Tralles is to be referred to the sixth decenium of that century.

J. Friend (*Hist. de la med.*, t. i, p. 160) says : "Ce médicament, si renommé parmi les anciens, etait (du temps d'Alexandre de Tralles) déjà devenu tout-à-fait hors d'usage."

[3] Book i, at the end of the chapter *De melancholicis.*

[4] Lib. vii, cap. 10.

[5] From a passage in Myrepsus, who wrote about the end of the thirteenth century, quoted from Actuarius, it seems that the latter could not have flourished after the year 1280 (see Freind, loc. cit., p. 463, 464).

[6] *Method. med.*, libr. v, cap. 8.

[7] Hippocr., sect. iv. aph. 4 and 6.

92. They prohibited the employment of helleborism in asthmas, coughs, and internal ulcers (such as pulmonary consumption [1] and suppuration of the liver); also in cases of hemoptysis, even when the patient seemed to be in good health, they feared lest its use should occasion the rupture of a blood-vessel in the lungs, especially of those who were thin, had a narrow chest, and a long neck, *i. e.* were of a phthisical habit (for persons of that description have generally tubercles in the lungs, breathe with difficulty, and are harrassed by cough[2]); also in diseases of the throat and neck, in the pain at the opening into the stomach of those who had a difficulty of vomiting,[3] also of lientery,[4] in commencing amaurosis, in affections of the head that were accompanied by violent pains at intervals, with redness of the face and congestion of the vessels; and lastly, in the hysterical suffocation.[5]

93. It was not allowed to use it in any febrile disease, except some cases of quartan ague.[6]

94. Moreover, the vomitings provoked by hellebore were not thought to be suitable for obese persons,[7] nor for the plethoric,[8] nor for those subject to syncope.

95. It was with difficulty borne by persons of a timid or pusillanimous disposition; this treatment requires a greater amount of fortitude than almost any other thing; wherefore it was not considered suitable for women, or old men or children.

96. It was chiefly employed in diseases of long-standing without fever, in insanity,[10] melancholia, [11]in inveterate pains of the

---

[1] Hippocr., sect. iv, aph. 8.—Rufus quoted by Oribasius, *Collect.*, lib, vii, cap. 26, p 244.

[2] Rufus, l. c., p. 245.

[3] Rufus, l. c., pp. 244, 245.

[4] Hippocr. l. c., aph. 12.

[5] Aëtius, quoting from Antyllus and Posidonius, lib, iii, cap. 121.

[6] Galen, lib. i., *De method. med.* ad Glauconem, cap. 12.—Rufus, l. c., cap. 121.

[7] Rufus, l. c., p. 245.—Hippocrates seems to me to allude to this when he says (sect. iv., aph. 16): Ἑλλέβορος ἐπικίνδυνος τοῖσι τὰς σαρκάς ὑγιέας (as though he had said " fleshy persons ") ἴχουσι, σπασμὸν γὰο ἐμποιίει,—wherefore for this same reason he orders (sect. iv., aph. 6) *thin persons to be evacuated upwards:* τοὺς ἰσχνοὺς—ἄνω φαρμακεύειν.

[8] Aëtius, lib. iii. cap, 124.

[9] Rufus, l. c., p. 245.

[10] C. Celsus, *De medicina*, lib. ii., cap. 13, with whom all ancient medical authors agree.

[11] Aretaeus, *Curat. diut.*, lib. i., cap. 5.—Galen. *De atra bile*, cap. 7. Pliny, *Hist. nat.*, lib. xxv., sect. 94.—" Efficacius elleborum," he says, " ad vomitiones et ad bilem nigram extrahendam."

feet and hips, pains of the joints,[1] the commencement of the gout,[2] epilepsy,[3] spasms of the facial muscles,[4] laziness of the mind,[5] loss of consciousness (apoplexy), vertigo which caused confusion of the head, (fanatics,[6]) inveterate paralysis,[7] obstinate headache,[8] lethargy, vertigo, white leprosy,[9] and elephantiasis[10] and other cutaneous diseases; also in baldness, falling out of the beard, nightmare, developed hydrophobia,[11] renal calculi,

---

[1] Rufus, l. c., p. 263. Aëtius l. c., cap. 121.

[2] Aretaeus, *Curat. diut.* lib. ii., cap. 12, καὶ γάρ τοῖσι ποδαγρικοῖσι ἐλλέβορος τὸ μέγα ἄκος ἀλλὰ ἐν τοῖσι πρώτησι προσβολῇσι τοῦ πάθεος.

[3] Celsus, l. c.—and Caelius Aurelianus, *Tard. poss*, lib. i., cap. 4, §108—111.

[4] Celsus, lib. iv., cap. 2.

[5] It was not only employed for mental imbecility, but remarkable to relate, it was also used for healthy individuals given to literary studies in order to sharpen their intellect, as Pliny informs us (*Hist. nat.*, lib. xxv., sect. 21): "Ad pervidenda acrius," he says, "quae commentabantur, saepius sumptitabatur veratrum;" as an example, I may mention the case of Carneades the Academician, who (see A. Gellius, *Noct. Att.*, lib. xvii., cap. 15) "scripturus adversus Stoici Zenonis libros superiora corporis elleboro candido purgavit." The same Carneades, we are told by Valerius Maximus (lib. viii., cap. 7), "cum Chrysippo disputaturus helleboro se ante purgabat ad exprimendum ingenium suum attentius et illius refellendum acrius." It is to this employment of veratrum album for the purpose of sharpening the intellect that Lucian of Samosata refers (βίων πρᾶσις, Op., tom. i., p. 564, edit: Reitzii): οὐ θέλις, γενέσθαι σοφὸν, ἢν μὴ τρὶς ἐφεξῆς τοῦ ἐλλεβόρου πίῃς—" thou canst not become *wise* unless thou *thrice* usest hellebore;" and in like manner Horace, by the words: "Tribus Anticyris insanabile caput," means to ridicule a dullard whose stupidity could not be removed by *three* courses of hellebore.

So frequent and so well known was the treatment of mental infirmities by hellebore at Anticyra in ancient times that the name of this town was often used to denote the process of helleborism itself, and the word Anticyra was used when helleborism and hellebore were meant. Hence that sarcasm which Horace directs against misers (lib. ii., *Sat.* iii., v. 82, 83):—

"Dando est ellebori multo pars maxima avaris;
"Nescio an Anticyram ratio illis destinet omnem"—

i. e. I should think that all the hellebore that can be found should be devoted to the treatment of misers.

Persius also says (*Sat.* iv., v. 16)—

"Anticyrae melior sorbere meracas,"

it were better that thou shouldst swallow pure hellebore.—This is an imitation of Horace (*Epist.* ii., v. 137.)—

"Expulit elleboro morbum bilemque meraco."

[6] Rufus, l. c.

[7] Aëtius, l. c., cap. 12. Cael. Aurelianus, l. c., lib. ii., cap. 1.

[8] Rufus, l. c. Aretaeus, *Cur. diut.*, lib. i., cap. 2.

[9] Rufus, l. c.

[10] Pliny, l. c., lib. xxv., sect. 24.

[11] Rufus, l. c., p. 263, "It causes," he says, "those who already have a dread of water, to dread it no longer; and this fact was anciently known to the peasants who, when their dogs became affected by the disease, purged them with hellebore, and this led physicians sometime after to give hellebore to a man affected with the same disease."

ancient crudities,[1] the coeliac disease,[2] leucophlegmasia, diseases
of the spleen,[3] struma,[4] concealed cancer, though it seems to
have been less suitable for the ulcers themselves;[5] in a word,
in an almost innumerable multitude of diseases.[6]

97. In a disease which from its nature is of a chronic character, it was considered much better to administer the veratrum in
the commencement of the malady before it had acquired greater
power, because most such diseases became from long habit in
the course of time unconquerable.[7]

98. But in the case of diseases consisting of periodical attacks
and intermissions, it was not thought advisable to employ the
medicament where the paroxysms recurred at short intervals,
but only where the intervals were longer. In diseases, however, which presented great and regular intermissions, it was
deemed expedient to commence the treatment a long time before the attack, but if the intermissions were short and irregular, the hellebore was to be had recourse to after the termination of an attack, especially in epilepsy.[8]

Preparatory treatment for helleborism.

99. When it was deemed necessary to employ the veratrum,
the patient was put on a regulated diet, which was in general,
according to the advice of Hippocrates,[9] for those who vomited
with difficulty that they should before taking the medicine have
their bodies moistened by plenty of nourishment and repose
(the pseudo-Hippocratic books, particularly the sixth book of
Epidemic diseases, add, " by the bath.") The doctrine of the
later physicians was—*that they should be made to practise artificial
vomiting.*

100. Even those who vomited *easily* were ordered to vomit
three times before they commenced the great medication; first,
after supper;[10] secondly, when their stomach was empty; and

---

[1] Rufus, l. c.—Pliny, l. c.

[2] Celsus, l. c., lib. iv., cap. 16.—Aretaeus, *Cur. diut.*, lib. 2, cap. 7.

[3] Rufus, l. c., p. 264.

[4] Celsus, lib. v., cap. 28, § 7.

[5] Rufus, l. c.

[6] Aëtius (quoting Antyllus and Posidonius), l. c., cap. 121: τό δὲ ἐξαριθμεῖν ἐφ'ὧν
πάθων εὐδόκιμος ἐστιν ὁ ἑλλέβορος, οὐ ῥᾴδιον διὰ το πλῆθος.

[7] Rufus, l. c., p. 264.

[8] Rufus, l c., p. 265.

[9] Sect. iv., aph. 13.—Also Celsus, libr. ii., cap. 15.

[10] After supper, and also when fasting or coming out of the bath, the patients pro-

lastly, after having partaken of radishes[1] (or origanum, or hyssop, or rue[2]).—Others ordered the patients to vomit three times immediately after supper;[3] and then to wait two or three days before drinking the hellebore.

101. But those who were known to vomit with difficulty, were prepared a long time previously, as long as three weeks,[4] and on repeated occasions (e. g. every third or fourth day) were subjected to vomiting,[5] in such a manner that the patient should be made to vomit more frequently the nearer the time approached for taking the medicine, attention being paid to the strength of the body in order that he should not be weakened more than necessary by these, for this treatment requires more than any other thing, strength on the part of the patient.[6]

102. Therefore betwixt the several vomitings three or four days were allowed to elapse, during which the body was refreshed by food easy of digestion, by repose, and by amusement of the mind.

103. After the last vomiting, one or two days[7] intervened before the patient took the veratrum, during which time the bowels were opened by means of a clyster,[8] baths were used, and a spare diet.

Mode of exhibiting the veratrum album for the purpose of inducing helleborism.

104. There were three general methods of administering veratrum; in infusion, in decoction, and in substance.

105. The kind that was preferred[9] was that in which the root

---

voked vomiting, either by tickling the fauces with their fingers, or with a feather dipped in oil.

[1] From a pound to a pound and a half of pungent radishes were eaten after a moderate meal with water for drink; the patient then waited a whole hour until nausea and eructations commenced; then by means of the finger or a feather introduced into the fauces he provoked vomiting, and this was called *vomiting from radishes*. Archigenes, cited by Oribasius, l. c., lib. viii., cap. i, p. 270.

[2] "Herbs lightly boiled should be eaten." Rufus quoted by Aëtius, lib. iii , cap. 119.

[3] Aëtius lib. iii., cap. 127.

[4] Archigenes, l. c., p. 267.

[5] To those that vomited with great difficulty, the most that used to be ordered was generally four vomitings after supper, and two after radishes. Archigenes, l. c., pp. 267—271.

[6] Rufus, l. c., p. 266.

[7] Archigenes, t. c., p. 268.

[8] Archigenes, l. c.—Aëtius, lib. iii., cap. 127.

[9] Rufus, l. c., p. 266.

was *cut with scissors*[1] into coarse particles, resembling our coarser kinds of groats (which the ancients called bruised polenta), or of the form and size of sesame-seeds.[2] The coarser particles were selected when it was wished to produce milder vomiting,[3] but care was taken that they should be of equal size, and not mixed up with the finer dust, lest the vomiting that ensued should occur at unequal periods.[4]

106. Some gave as the largest dose to robust patients two drachms and a half (= 180 of our grains) of this granulated preparation;[5] others only gave two drachms[6] (= 144 grains) as the largest dose, ten oboli (= 120 grains) as the moderate dose, and eight oboli (= 96 grains) as the smallest dose. It was given either in water, or in wine, or in raisin wine,[7] or in decoction of lentils; but to persons out of their mind it was given (in order that they might not be aware that they were taking it) in broth,[8] or in oxymel,[9] or in pills.[10]

107. This most simple preparation of veratrum album caused vomiting more rapidly than the others, and for the most part in less than two hours brought up the bile and the pituita without much disturbance,[11] then, after the medicine itself had been ejected by the vomiting, the evacuation ceased in from four to five hours.[12]

---

[1] In a passage in Antyllus preserved by Aëtius (lib. iii., cap. 128), this preparation of the root is termed ψιλιστὸν (*cut with scissors*). Oribasius quotes the same passage (*Collect.* i. 8, cap. 5, p. 277); but Rasarius renders it incorrectly, " in ramenta derasam."—Antyllus, a little further on (Aëtius, l. c., cap. 131), describes this operation more at length : τὰ κάρφη λαβὼν τέμνε ψαλίδι εἰς ἀλφιτῶδη(of the size of groated wheat) μεγέθη ἢ πιτυρώδη. He orders these *particles cut by the scissors to the size of groats* to be wiped with a cloth, in order to remove the small dust, and thus prevent suffocation. Archigenes (l. c. p. 272) recommends that the coarse fibres of the hellebore should have one or two longitudinal incisions made in them before being cut in pieces.

[2] Paulus Aegineta, lib. vii., cap. 10.

[3] Rufus, l. c., p. 266. These coarser particles offered fewer points of contact to the lining membrane of the stomach, so that the largest dose of this preparation was considered no more than equal to a smaller dose of the fine powder; moreover this larger size of the particles prevented their descent into the intestines, and the production of purging downwards.

[4] Archigenes, l. c., p. 272.

[5] Aëtius (quoting Antyllus and Posidonius), l. c., cap. 131.

[6] Archigenes, in Oribasius, lib. viii, cap. 2, p. 273.

[7] Wine prepared from the dried grapes.

[8] Archigenes, l. c.

[9] Composed of honey and vinegar.

[10] Archigenes, l. c., p. 275. The finest powder was employed for the pills.

[11] Ἄνευ πολλοῦ σπαραγμοῦ, Antyllus, in Aëtius, l. c., cap. 128.

[12] Antyllus in Oribas., l. c., p. 277, and in Aëtius, l c., cap. 128.

108. Another mode was to *bruise the root in a mortar*, and to separate the very fine dust by means of a very close sieve.[1] To the bolder patients the coarser powder[2] was given in the dose of a drachm and two oboli (= 96 grains). This preparation confessedly acted slower,[3] vomiting often occurring only after four or five hours, but it brought away all the bile and pituita, certainly not without the risk of causing spasms (cramps)[4] and too violent vomiting, on account of the too great abundance of the evacuation, but it was useful in various ways.

109. For the most part the fibres of the roots were bruised up along with the medulla, but sometimes the most fleshy fibres were moistened with a sponge, and the swollen bark split up longitudinally with a needle; after drying it again in the shade it was bruised, and thereby, it was thought, a more efficacious medicine was obtained.[5]

110. The *infusion* of veratrum album was also employed. Five drachms (= 310 gr.) of the cut particles of the root were macerated for the space of three days[6] in half a hemina (= 5 oz. 3 drs.)[7] of rain water; the liquor was then strained and administered warm to old persons, children,[8] and hectic subjects.[9]

111. Others considered the *decoction* the most certain preparation,[10] and they prepared it in the following way: one pound (= 14 4-5 oz.) of veratrum, cut into small pieces with scissors,[11]

---

[1] The finest powder being thus removed was made into pills with thickened honey (Aëtius, l. c., cap. 131); 96 grains of these pills were given when it was deemed requisite to employ this form.

[2] Aëtius, l. c., cap. 131.—To the insane this coarser powder was given generally in cakes or broth, in order to deceive them (Archigenes, l. c., p. 274).

[3] Aëtius, l. c., cap. 128.

[4] Συνολκῆς, Aëtius, l. c.

[5] Pliny, *Hist. nat.*, lib. xxv, sect. 21.—Archigenes, l. c., p. 272.

[6] This long maceration in water greatly diminished the power of the veratrum, for all parts of plants when mixed with water undergo fermentation, and the longer this maceration and infusion are continued the more are the medicinal powers weakened, unless spirituous fluids, obtained by the distillation of fermented vegetable substances, are added, which, however, the ancients were not possessed of. The root of veratrum album, unless thoroughly dried, is more prone to the decomposition of its constituent parts than the roots of other plants; its powder is particularly apt to become mouldy and to ferment, unless perfectly dried. Mouldiness very quickly destroys almost all the medicinal power of plants.

[7] Massarius, *De ponderibus et mensuris*, Tiguri, 8, 1584, lib. iii, cap. 14.

[8] Antyllus, in Oribasius, l. c., p. 277; in Aëtius, lib. iii, cap. 129.

[9] Aëtius, l. c.

[10] Herodotus, l. c., p. 275.

[11] Ἐψαλτισμένον, Aëtius, l. c., cap. 129.

was macerated for three days in six heminas (= 64 4-5 oz. of water, and then boiled down over a slow fire to one-third less; the root was then removed, and to the liquor two heminas (= 21 3-5 oz.) of honey[1] was added to thicken it,[2] so that it should not spoil,[3] or, according to Archigenes,[4] to make it of the consistence of an electuary. Archigenes gave to a person prepared for the helleborism a small mystrum[5] (= 260 to 288 of our grains) of this syrup for a dose; Herodotus gave to robust subjects one mystrum, but to those who did not require to be evacuated two spoonfuls (= 144 grains).[6] Others gave the decoction inspissated with a third of honey, in the dose of a large spoonful[7] (108 gr.), to be licked up by the patient, whereby they affirmed that the occurrence of spasms and of excessive evacuation was avoided.[8] Others formed the inspissated decoction into pills, which they gave principally to insane persons in order to deceive them.[9]

Substances that were mixed with the veratrum. Sesamoides.

112. But the ancient physicians did not always employ such a simple method of administering the veratrum album. Some added to the infusion origanum, or absinthum, or natrum, others mixed it with thapsia,[10] and others with the wild grape.[11]

113. But the principal thing that was mingled with the medicine white hellebore was a certain kind of seed called *sesamoides*, in consequence of their (oval) form bearing a resemblance to the seeds of the same;[12] they were also called *Anticyran hellebore* or *Anticyricon*, not because the plant that furnished the sesamoid

---

[1] Archigenes, 1 c., adds double the quantity of honey (= 43 1-5 oz)

[2] This long boiling and inspissation diminished not a little the strength of the medicine, so that the doses of this inspissated preparation, though not small in bulk were actually of but little strength.

[3] Herodotus, l. c., p. 275.

[4] In Oribasius, lib. viii, cap. 2.

[5] See Massarius, l. c., lib. iii, cap. 30, 31, compared with cap. 2.—The cotyle contained 15 3-5 of our ounces of honey; the *large* Attic *mystrum* contained an eighteenth part of the cotyle, the *small mystrum* on the other hand only a twenty-fourth part

[6] In Oribasius, l. c., p. 275.

[7] Massarius, l. c., cap. 38.

[8] Aëtius, l. c., cap. 130.

[9] Archigenes, l. c., p. 275.

[10] The root of the *Thapsia Asclepium*, Linn.

[11] The seed of the *Delphinium staphisagria*, Linn.

[12] "Granum sesamae (sc. simile)." Pliny, *Hist. nat.*, lib. xxii, sect. 64. Also Dioscorides, lib. iv, cap. 152: σπέρμα ὅμοιον σησάμῳ.

seed had any resemblance to the white hellebore, but partly
because this seed excited vomiting[1] like hellebore, partly because
to those undergoing helleborism[2] it was given at Anticyra in
Phocis,[3] in order to prevent the suffocation arising from the use
of the veratrum album,[4]—at least so the Anticyrans persuaded
themselves and others.

114. Anticyra in Phocis, was, as I have said, very celebrated
in ancient times for the treatment by hellebore, the best preparation of veratrum album for the production of helleborism being
made there, wherefore, as Strabo relates,[5] a large number of
persons resorted thither for the sake of the treatment. There
grew moreover in Phocis a remedy resembling sesame, with
which they prepared the hellebore of Oeta. Thus Pliny says:
"in Anticyra insula—ibi enim tutissime sumitur elleborus,
quoniam sesamoides admiscent."[6]

115. Sometimes, for the purpose of procuring vomiting, the
sesamoides were given alone, in the dose of one drachm (72
grains)[7], rubbed up with oxymel; when it was intended to cause
helleborism, one-third part of these seeds was added to the dose
of veratrum.[8]

116. In the earliest times,[9] this seed which it was usual to
mix with the veratrum album for the production of helleborism,

---

[1] Διὰ τὸ καθαίρειν αὐτοῦ τὸ σπέρμα παραπλησίως ἐλλεβόρῳ, Galen, *De simpl. med. fac.*,
lib. viii, cap. 18, § 11.

[2] Διὰ τὸ μίλυνσθαι ἐν ταῖς καθάρσεσι τῷ λευκῷ ἐλλεβόρῳ, Dioscorides, lib iv, cap. 152.

[3] Strabo, l. c.

[4] Σησαμοειδὲς—ξυμμίσγεται—ἐλλεβόροισιν, παὶ ἧσσον πνίγει. See the continuation of the
book *De victu acutorum* (*Opera Hippocrat. et Galeni*, edit. Chart., t. xi, p. 182.)

[5] Διὰ τοῦτο ἀπσδημεῖν δεῦρο πολλοὺς καθάρσεως καὶ θεραπείας χάριν· γίνεσθαι γάρ τι
σησαμοιδὲς φάρμακον ἐν τῇ φωκικῇ, μετ' οὐ σκευάζεσθαι τον εἰταῖον ἐλλίβορον. (*Geogr.*, lib.
ix. p. 640.)

[6] *Hist. nat.*, lib. xxv, sect. 21. Pliny is however wrong in here stating Phocian
Anticyra to be an *island*, for it was situated on the continent, half a mile from the
port. Pausanius (*Geogr.*, lib. x, p. 682, edit. Hanoviae, 1613) has lucidly described
its situation. Livy also testifies to the same when he says (lib. xxvi, cap. 26) "breve
terra iter eo (Anticyram)—ab Naupacto est."

[7] Pliny, lib. xxii, sect. 64.—The pseudo-Hippocratic continuer of the book *De Diaeta
acutorum* (edit. Chart. t. xi, p. 182) orders a large dose: σησαμοειδὶς ἄνω καθαίρει· ἡ
πόσις ἡμιώλιον δραχμῆς ὁ σταθμὸς (a drachm and a half) ἐς ὀξυμέλιτα τετριμμένον

[8] The same continuer of the book *De diaet. acut.*, loc. cit.—Dioscorides teaches a
more definite proportion (lib. iv, cap. 152): "As much of the seed as can be held
with three fingers, with an obolus and a half (= eighteen grains) of veratrum album
in hydromel."

[9] This word does not occur in the genuine writings of Hippocrates. The first that
mentions it is Diocles (who flourished twenty years after Hippocrates' death), see the
dictionary of Erotianus (*Op. Hipp. et Galeni*, edit. Chart. t. ii, p. 133).

was called by simple term *sesamoid*, but subsequently it was called *great sesamoid*, not on account of the size of the plant, but evidently because it was used in the *great cure* (helleborism), and because it was considered superior to another seed of the same name,[1] but chiefly in order to distinguish it from a certain white sesamoid, which was called the *small*[2] *sesomoid*.

117. It is not certainly known what plant this emetic seed sesamoid belonged to, which in those days was mixed with the veratrum album, chiefly at Anticyra[3] of Phocis, in order to diminish the suffocation. Theophrastus says: the seed of a small plant, *helleborine*, is to be mixed with hellebore when that is administered, in order to facilitate its emetic action.[4] The name *helleborine* was probably given to it because it resembled the hellebore in its emetic action, and its seed seems to have been the same as what was afterwards termed (great) sesamoid. The plant whence this was derived bore a great outward resemblance to erigeron or senecio,[5] with its white flowers, slender root and bitter seed.

118. We might, then, say with great plausibility, that this was the seed of some species of erigeron (acris? graveolens? viscosus?) seeing that our *erigeron acris* is highly emetic, as Stedman's observations[6] demonstrate, who saw violent vomiting ensue merely from the application of the recent plant to the skin. Cullen[7] also observes, that the common people make use of this plant as a powerful emetic. If this be so, how powerful the *seeds* must have been when taken in the form of potion and brought in contact with the nerves of the stomach, seeing that

---

[1] In the time of Theophrastus (*Hist. plant.* lib. x, cap. 11), the seed of the black hellebore also bore the name of sesamoid, and this, as Rufus (in Oribas. *Collect.*, lib. vii, cap. 27, p. 251) alleges, resembles the seed of the cnicus (carthamus) and taken in the dose of two drachms it *purges downwards* more violently than the root itself.— Dioscorides asserts the same thing: ὃν καὶ αὐτὸν (καρπον τοῦ ἐλλεβόρου' μέλανος) καλοῦσιν οἱ ἐν 'Αντικύρᾳ σησαμοειδῆ. (Lib. iv, cap. 151).

[2] The seed of an unknown plant, the dose of which, in order to produce purging downwards, Dioscorides (lib. iv, cap. 153) and Rufus (l. c, p. 255) fix at half an acetabulum (a measure that can hold nine of our drachms).

[3] Hence the reason why this sesamoid was termed *Anticyricon* (Pliny, l. c.), and at Anticyra itself it was even called *hellebore*, though this was an abuse of terms; by strangers it was termed *Anticyran hellebore*. See Galen, *De facult. simpl.*, lib. viii.

[4] Μίσγεται πρὸς τὴν πόσιν, ὅπως εὖ ἐμέσῃ, τὸ τῆς ἐλλεβορινῆς σπέρμα. *Hist. plant.*, lib. x, cap. 11.

[5] Rufus, l. c., p. 250.—Pliny. l. c., "caetera," he says, "simile erigeronti herbae." In like manner Dioscorides says (l. c., cap. 152): ἔοικεν ἡ πόα ἠριγέροντι.

[6] *Edinburgh Medical Essays*, vol. ii, art. 5.

[7] *Materia Medica*, vol. ii.

in general the whole power of the plant is concentrated in the seeds, as is seen, for instance, in the seeds of the conium maculatum, and of the helleborus niger.

Regimen to be employed to assist the emetic action of the veratrum album.

119. As soon as the patient had drunk the veratrum, cold water was given him to rinse his mouth, and perfumes were employed to remove and avert a premature nausea.[1]

120. If the strength admitted of it the patients were desired to remain seated; if they were weak they were made to lie down on a bed on the ground, for two or three hours, to smell perfumes, and to rinse their mouth with cold water. It was sought to amuse them with some entertaining story; their limbs were rubbed and ligatures were applied to them; they were advised to keep quiet, lest the medicine should be ejected by vomiting sooner than it ought.

121. After two or three hours they were placed in a suspended or elevated bed and swung about, and thus allowed to vomit.

122. At first, the patients in whom the emetic action went on properly, felt heat in the fauces and œsophagus; then the saliva flowed copiously into the mouth, and was often ejected by spitting. After the lapse of some time they vomited part of the food that had been taken before, and part of the medicine, along with pituita. This was repeated after some time; and after they had ejected the medicine and the food, they vomited first pituita with a small portion of bile, then pituita with a large proportion of bile, and finally, pure bile. During that time they had slight hiccough, very red face, swollen veins, small and quick pulse.

123. When the vomiting went on right, the countenance resumed its proper colour, the pulse became larger, the hiccough ceased. They now vomited gradually at longer intervals.[2] The bowels were frequently moved, although the evacuation in other respects might have been moderate.[3]

124. If the hiccough was excessively troublesome during the

---

[1] Vomiting which occurred *too soon* (before two hours) was generally considered to be inefficacious for the removal of the disease, and it was observed that where it occurred too late (commencing only after four or five hours) it produced great prostration of the strength and terrible symptoms.

[2] Antyllus, in Oribasius, *Collect.*, lib. viii, cap. 6, pp. 277 278.

[3] Aëtius, l. c.

evacuation, melicrat,[1] in which rue had been boiled, was given them to drink, and thereafter a little warm water, which they were made to vomit again.[2] The body was rubbed over with oil, and, after the lapse of two hours, they were made to take a bath and appropriate food was supplied to them.[3]

Remedies employed in cases where the vomiting did not take place properly.[4]

125. In order to remove the obstacles to the right performance of the vomiting, the following things were always in readiness : a high and swinging hammock and a bed with a soft mattress,[5] sponges, posca,[6] and melicrats prepared in various ways, one of which contained decoction of hyssop, another origanum, another rue, another thyme ; there were also oils, diluted infusion of veratrum album, cupping glasses, little wedges, a feather, glove fingers, clysters, fomentations, wine, &c.

126. *If the patients were seized with vomiting sooner than they ought,* and there was reason to fear lest the medicine should be rejected before any advantage could be derived from it, cold water was given to rinse their mouths with incessantly, and if this did not allay the premature vomiting, diluted vinegar was employed, the limbs were bound with ligatures, and frictions were applied to them ; they were directed to keep in their mouths something seasoned with kitchen salt, to keep silence, not to move, but to sit upright.

127. If by these means the inclination to vomit was not stopped, cupping-glasses well heated were applied to the back and scrobiculus cordis, and a small quantity of hot water was given the patients to drink occasionally ; if however this did not allay the desire to vomit, a small quantity of the juice or decoction of wormwood was given. Two or three of these remedies always sufficed to arrest this inclination to vomit and to overcome the aversion of the stomach.

128. On the other hand, *if the vomiting was too long delayed,* and the patients did not commence to evacuate at the proper time, some gave the patient to drink warm honey and water in

---

[1] Honied water.
[2] By putting the finger into the fauces.
[3] Antyllus, l. c.
[4] Chiefly from the instruction of Antyllus, in Oribasius, l. c.
[5] Aëtius, lib. ii, cap. 132.
[6] Vinegar diluted with water

which rue had been boiled, or oil mixed with water[1] (*hydrelaeum*), others placed the patient on an elevated couch, the head directed downwards, and made him put his finger into his mouth and irritate the uvula and tonsils, so as to excite vomiting. Moreover he was told to flex and extend alternately his back and legs as much as possible, and to beat with his fists on the abdomen.

129. If the evacuation could not be obtained by these means, the patient was placed in the suspended hammock and swung about,[2] he was at the same time exhorted or ordered to endeavour to vomit by introducing into his mouth his fingers covered with some nauseous oil or with a solution of scammony.

130. If even this would not do, eight or ten feathers from a goose's tail, dipped in some nauseous oil (oil of iris or of cypress[3]), or fingers of a glove made of soft leather, twelve finger-breadths long, stuffed in front with wool and smeared with some ointment, were introduced into the fauces,[4] and in this way nausea and vomiting were excited.

Treatment of the bad and serious symptoms occasioned by the action of veratrum.

131. Those who are in danger of *suffocation* after they have drunk veratrum, have a moderate flow of saliva, and, in spite of the most violent effort to vomit that arises, do not bring anything off their stomach; their face swells, the eyes project, the respiratory organs are constricted, with the greatest difficulty of breathing; in some the tongue is projected and the whole body covered with profuse perspiration; in others the jaws are closed, with chattering of the teeth, and the mind becomes affected.[5]

132. This feeling of strangulation, which usually occurs in those who vomit with difficulty, was allayed by the continual drinking of melicrat in which rue had been boiled or some other of those substances which have already been mentioned as useful in the irritation of the stomach.

---

[1] Aëtius, l. c., cap. 133, where Cornarius has erroneously translated the words χρονιζούσης καθάρσεως, by *perseverante vomitu*, in place of *cunctante vomitu*.

[2] Hippocrates forbids those who have taken veratrum to indulge in sleep or repose; he orders that they shall be made to move about continually.—'Επὴν πίη τις ἐλλέβορον, πρὸς μὲν τὰς κινήσιας τῶν σωμάτων μᾶλλον ἄγειν, πρὸς δὲ τοὺς ὕπνους καὶ μὴ κινήσιας, ἦσσον· ὀηλοῖ δὲ καὶ ἡ ναυτιλίη, ὅ τι κίνησις τὰ σώματα ταράσσει (sect. iv, aphor. 14). —'Επὴν βούλῃ μᾶλλον ἄγειν τὸν ἐλλέβορον, κίνει τὸ σῶμα (sect. iv, aphor. 15).

[3] Oil rendered very fragrant by boiling in it the buds of the cypress (an Egyptian tree).

[4] Antyllus, l. c., pp. 278—280

[5] Herodotus, in Oribas., l. c., p. 283.

133. If, however this affection was of a very urgent character, three or four cupfuls[1] of the diluted helleborine medicine[2] were given, which, possessing the same properties as the veratrum already taken would best procure the emetic action. Other substances called emetics were prohibited, as they are of a different quality, and only irritate the stomach without expelling the veratrum taken as first.[3]

134. If none of these remedies succeeded in removing the danger of impending suffocation, the bowels were acted on by a very acrid clyster, in order to give some relief to this symptom and to afford time to obtain other remedies. Then the patient was made to swallow three oboli (36 grains) of galbanum, or to drink three cupfuls of very old urine, these being considered useful for removing suffocation.[4]

135. But if this also failed to relieve the suffocation, a powerful sternutatory was applied to the nostrils, the patient was assiduously swung about in the suspended hammock, and his fauces irritated by the introduction of feathers.

136. *If there occurred loss of voice and consciousness*, the little wedges were introduced betwixt the teeth of the patient on both sides, and feathers or the glove-finger introduced into the fauces in order to excite vomiting and remove the affection. Sneezing was excited by means of the powder of veratrum itself (or of euphorbium); and it not unfrequently happened that on sneezing a mass of pituita was expelled, which in consequence of remaining too long in the stomach had caused the suffocation and loss of breath.

137. When this means failed, the patient was laid upon a linen cloth, which was held up by stout young men, and the patient at one time thrown up into the air, and at another swung from side to side. If all these commotions and succussions failed to restore him to consciousness, it was thought there was no other remedy for bringing him back to life.[6]

138. *The hiccough* that occurred to every one who took veratrum was not interfered with if it was slight and at long intervals; it was considered to be useful in exciting the stomach to

---

[1] The cup (cyathus) contained twelve drachmes (=14 2-5ths of our drachms), see Massarius, l. c., p. 43.

[2] The infusion or decoction of veratum album.

[3] An ingenious idea and mode of practice, and perfectly comformable to nature.

[4] Antyllus, l, c.

[5] Aëtius, lib. iii, cap. 132.

[6] A saturated infusion of coffee would be useful here.

action.[1] But when it was very severe, and if the mouth was affected with vibration and twitching, melicrat in which rue was mixed was prescribed to be drunk warm after every hiccough.

139. If this did no good, a sternutatory was employed, and if the affection still persisted, cupping-glasses were applied the whole length of the spine, ligatures were applied to the limbs, and they were heated either by fermentations or by putting them in warm water. It was endeavoured to frighten or insult the patient, or he was ordered to keep in his breath a long time, or to inspire and expire very slowly.[2]

140. For those symptoms that occurred as frequently as the hiccough, the *muscular contraction* and the *cramp*, chiefly in the legs, in the thighs, in the arms and muscles of mastication, also in the extremities of the feet and hands, if they were violent it was sought to allay them by plentiful inunctions, by the application of heat, by frictions and fomentations of the affected parts, by strongly compressing the muscles with the hands, and by giving castoreum internally.

141. Moreover if the vomiting was abundant, as it often was in many of those who laboured under cramp, this affection was usually removed by baths frequently repeated.[3]

142. *The vomiting, if excessive,* was allayed by the administration of the hottest drinks, by ligature of the limbs, and violent frictions, also by the application of cupping glasses now to the hypochondria, now to the back, and then tearing them forcibly away. It is stated that wormwood given in drink was excellent for stopping the vomiting. But if the vomiting persisted, medicines to cause sleep were employed, as it was believed that sleep had the power of stopping the excretions.[4]

143. For the *loss of strength* that ensued recourse was had to food and wine, and if the patient had been excessively evacuated he was revived by the administration of bread soaked in old wine diluted, or in omphacomel.[5]

---

[1] Antyllus, l. c, p. 281.

[2] Antyllus, l. c., pp. 281, 282.

[3] Antyllus, l. c., pp. 282, 283.

[4] Antyllus, l. c., and Aëtius, l. c., cap. 134. Hippocrates also (sect. iv, aph. 15.) advised repose and sleep, in order to arrest the evacuation caused by hellebore : ἐπὴι ἰὲ παῦσαι (βούλῃ, τον ἐλλέβοροον,) ὕπνον ποίει, καὶ μὴ κίνει.

[5] Honey, mixed with the juice of unripe grapes, was termed *omphacomel*.

39

Conclusion.

144. Such was the mode of producing helleborism employed by the ancients, which was more dangerous in appearance than in reality, as most of the earliest physicians assert. For besides the passage[1] in Aretaeus, a very distinguished physician, which I formerly[2] quoted as authoritative, we find the following in Rufus:[3] "The administration of hellebore seems to have been a very serious matter, wherefore it is that many medical men and patients eschewed the employment of this medicament; but he who is acquainted with the whole art and apparatus of helleborism, and administers veratrum, will find that there is nothing more convenient than this medicine, that it is an excellent remedy for procuring evacuations, and that it can scarcely do any harm." The testimony of Pliny agrees with this, where he speaks concerning his own time thus: "In former times it (veratrum) was considered a terrible remedy, but latterly it was so commonly used, that many engaged in study were in the habit of taking it frequently in order to facilitate their comprehension of their studies."[4]

145. It is not, however, my intention to recommend to my fellow-men that Herculean treatment by which, under the name of helleborism, the ancients attempted to remove so many and such serious diseases, by giving large doses of veratrum album, and whereby they often succeeded in doing so in a most miraculous manner, for I know not if it could be reconciled with our habits and modes of treatment. No one is better aware than myself of the force of habit and of its influence on the art of healing itself (which however from its very nature ought to be quite free). If it did not reign despotically over the medical art, it is very possible that the treatment with veratrum with some modifications might be now-a-days turned to great advantage in relieving some of the worst and most inveterate of the diseases to which man is liable.

146. This much is certain, that the same diseases may be eradicated with much milder and even with the very smallest doses of veratrum, provided the medicine is exactly suitable to the disease, nor could the ancients have cured by helleborism

---

[1] Ὑγιέας τοὺς κάμνοντας ποιέει καὶ ἐπ' ὀλίγῃ καθάρσι, καὶ ἐπὶ σμικρῇ ἐντάσι Chron. curat., ii, cap. 10.

[2] In § 71.

[3] In Oribasius, l. c., p. 263.

[4] Hist. nat., lib. xxv, sect. 21.

any other diseases besides those for which veratrum was gene
rally and, in any dose whatever (provided it were not too strong),
adapted.

147. This, indeed, is evident from this passage from the
ancients[1] "It is not the vomiting whereby the veratrum album
is of use in chronic diseases, for many have taken and digested
veratrum with hardly any purgation, and yet have experienced
not less benefit from its use than those who had been evacuated
by this medicine."

148. It is to be regretted, therefore, that all those chronic diseases for which this medicine is from its nature the most appropriate and, indeed, the only [2] remedy, should be left uncured by
modern physicians, owing to the aversion to employ veratrum,
which, however, may be given in such minute doses, that whilst
they are powerful enough for any disease, be it ever so chronic,
they are incapable of causing any bad effects worth mentioning
on the human body.

OF THE BLACK HELLEBORE.

149. This medicine is termed *black* on account of the black
colour of its roots externally, which in the veratrum (white hellebore) are extremely white. It remains for me to make a few
remarks upon it, partly on account of its name, partly because
the physicians of Anticyra who, as a rule, devoted themselves to
the practice of helleborism, were accustomed to employ the black
hellebore also as an auxiliary in the treatment of chronic diseases

150. In the time of Hippocrates the black hellebore was scarce
ly or not at all known, or at least not yet designated by this
name; for neither in his genuine writings nor in those of his
predecessors or of his grandfather (*Praenotiones Coacae*, and the
books *De Fracturis* and *De articulis*) is any mention whatever
made of this plant or of this name.

151. The only place where this name occurs (*De victu acut.*,
t. xi, p. 44), although no one has ever doubted that Hippocrates
was its author, is certainly not a genuine work of his.[3]

---

[1] Πολλοὶ λαβόντες τον ἐλλέβορον καὶ πέψαντες αὐτὸν ἐκαθαρθησαν μὲν οὐδὲν ὅλως, ὡψελήθησαν
δὲ οὐδὲν ἦττον τῶν καθαρθἑντων.—(Aëtius, quoting from Antyllus and Posidonicus, lib. iii.
cap. 122.

[2] For as every disease differs from every other in such a manner as to demand a
special medicine appropriate to its nature, to be selected carefully from the great
store of the most diverse medicines, by which alone it can be cured quickly, safely,
and permanently, so all the other remedies less adapted to the disease present, are
either useless, or contrary, or hurtful.

[3] It is more than probable that the book under the title of *De victus ratione in*

152. It follows of necessity, therefore, that this new plant (the black hellebore) which was employed as a purgative, was either discovered or named [1] some time after Hippocrates; for it is both mentioned in the pseudo-Hippocratic writings of those physicians who were his immediate successors, and is described by Theophrastus with the addition of the word "μέλας" to distinguish it from the original hellebore (veratrum album) which for so many ages, until the discovery of this new plant, had been the

morbis acutis, which has generally been alleged to be Hippocatic, was written by three or four different authors. The first part was by Hippocrates himself, and is called Liber de Ptisana (see Athenaei Dipnosoph., lib. ii. p. 57, also Caelius Aurelianus and Pliny) and it contained nothing except the use of ptisan ("nihil continabat nisi ptisanae usum"—see Plin., Hist. nat., lib. xviii, sect. 15, and lib. xxii, sect. 66). This book seems to have begun at the words: δοκέει δὲ μοὶ ἄξια γραφῆς εἶναι (l. c., p. 7) and to have gone on to the words: ἀκριβῶς Θεωρῶν, but no farther. What follows immediately, from the words: δὲ πλευροῦ (l. c., pp. 36—116) is doubtless an addition (in which the discourse concerning ptisan is suddenly broken off) apparently by the same author who wrote the prologue to the beginning of the book upon ptisan. This addition certainly contains many excellent observations respecting the diet in acute diseases, but it is plain they are of a more recent date; for here (l. c., p. 42) we observe a scrupulous selection of "the internal vein in the flexure of the elbow to be opened in pleurisy," and in that part of the text (p. 44) which particularly engages our attention at present, not only are black hellebore and peplium recommended as purgatives, and a subtle distinction made between the effects of each, but several aromatic seeds are added to the formula of the purgative medicine on account of their pleasant odour, an artificial luxury only met with in more recent times, as history teaches us. Moreover, in this place (p. 44, also p. 3) many other cathartics (ἄλλα πολλὰ τῶν ὑπηλάτων) are alluded to, which could not have been done before the time of the reign of the Ptolemies; for it was only then that in consequence of commerce having extended to near and distant nations, the number of medicines was increased, kings themselves having in those days (within 300 years before our era) devoted themselves to the study of medicine. As to the peplium which is alluded to here, it was not, if I am not mistaken, known to Theophrastus a hundred years after Hippocrates; and this spurious addition to the book on ptisan could not have been written at that time for this reason, that the peplium is mentioned along with the black hellebore. This is, moreover, confirmed by the resemblance this addition bears to the first book De mulierum morbis which is certainly pseudo-Hippocratic. The author of this book (probably the same person) expresses the same idea in the same words: πέπλιον φυσῶν εἶναι καταῤῥηκτικὸν.—Finally, they reproaches and vituperation addressed to other medical men, because the employed too few medicines, the acrimonious partizanship for a particular sect, the abstruse ratiocinations concerning the nature of things, the later dogmas respecting the artificial classification of diseases and their names, the scrupulcus selection of some particular vein to be opened in a certain disease,—all these things, which are vehemently discussed by the anonymous author of the afore-mentioned prologue and addition to the book on ptisan, are nowhere to be found in the genuine writings of Hippocrates.

[1] Perhaps Hippocrates himself had already begun to employ this plant (as seems to be implied towards the end of his book De vulneribus capitis, t. xii, p. 128: τοῦτον χρὴ τὴν κάτω κοιλίην ὑποκαθῆραι φαρμάκῳ, ὅ, τι χολὴν ἄγει,), but if so it had not yet received its distinctive appellation.

only evacuant medicine, and which therefore, as might be expected, was known by the simple name only.[1]

153. But it remains to be inquired whether or not the black hellebore of the ancients is the same as our helleborus niger. And this is a question of no small difficulty to decide if we stick to Sarrazin's text[2] of Dioscorides, which is that commonly followed; but if we bring to our aid the different readings of different manuscripts, and examine the thing critically, it appears from the text thus restored that it is the same plant as our own; it would then read thus: Ἔχει δὲ τὰ φύλλα χλωρὰ, πλατάνῳ προσεμφερῆ, ἐλάττονα δὲ[3]—καὶ πολυτχιδέστερα, καὶ μελάντερα καὶ ὑποτραχία· καυλὸς βραχὸς,[4] ἄνθη δὲ λευκὰ ἐμπόρφυρα, τῷ δὲ σχήματι ῥοδοειδῆ,[5] ἡαὶ ἐν αὐτῷ καρπὸς κνήκῳ ὅμοιος·—ῥίζαι δ᾽ ὕπεισι λεπταὶ, μέλαναι, οἱονεί ἀπό τινος κεφαλίου κρομμυώδους ἠρτημέναι, ὧν καὶ ἡ χρῆσις.——that is to say, "its leaves are green, like those of the plane-tree, but less, more divided, blacker, and slightly rough, the stalk short, the flowers white, purpled, like a rose; the seed resembles that of the carthamus;—the roots are small below, black, depending from a head like an onion, and these are the parts used in medicine."

154. With this restoration of the text it will be seen that Dioscorides' description of the plant corresponds pretty strongly to our helleborus niger. For our hellebore has also rosaceous flowers with white petals, the external surface of which is covered with red coloured spots, like little clouds, which grow pur-

---

[1] See above § 10—16.

[2] *Materia Med.*, lib. iv, cap. 151.

[3] The words πρὸσ τὰ τοῦ σφονδυλίου which exist in the ordinary text may be left out; they are not to be found in some manuscripts.

[4] Sarrazin's text has τραχὺς; but with Serapion (*De Simpl*) we may read βραχύς, for the stalk of hellebore, if it have any, is very short, but not rough.

[5] I have restored the word ῥοδοειδῆ, which is to be found in some manuscripts in place of βοτρυώδη, which we find in Sarrazin's text, but which has no sense. In this rendering, ῥοδοειδή, I am fully borne out by Avicenna's Arabic version of this passage, (lib. ii, *De medicamentis simpl.* Art. *Charbak Aswad:* يشبه ذي هتنة الول that is: "similar in its form to a rose." That the word βοτρυώδη, on the contrary was not to be found originally in the text, appears from this, that it does not exist in a certain edition of the book, as the marginal notes of Sarrazin attest; that it got into the text at a very early period (perhaps from some marginal correction which was intended to supply the word ῥοδοειδή that had been almost effaced by the injury of time) may be suspected from the same place in Avicenna, who immediately afterwards adds the version of this spurious word βοτρυώδη (which has no sense if it refer to the flowers), and renders it "the fruit of the botry," following some copy of Dioscorides which he employed, and which without doubt had received from the margin into the text, in place of the genuine ῥοδοειδή, that unmeaning substitute βοτρυώδη.

ple as the flowering advances. Bellon moreover asserts that he
has found on Mount Olympus the helleborus niger with reddish
flowers.

155. But Theophrastus of Eresus, describes this plant[2] still
better (according to Scaliger's and my own reading[3]), in these
words: Τῶ μελάνου μὲν καυλὸν—βραχὺν σφόδρα, φύλλον δὲ πλατύσχιστον,
μῆκος ἔχον εὐμηκες, εὐθὺς δὲ ἐκ τῆς ῥίζης ἠρτημένον τε καὶ ἐπιγειόφυλλον·
πολλύρριζον δ᾽ εὖ μάλα ταῖς λεπταῖς καὶ χρησίμοις. That is to say:
"the stalk is very short, the leaf rather large and divided into
broad lobes, attached to the root itself, and spread upon the
ground; the roots are numerous, small, and are the parts made
use of." Scaliger, however, in place of πλατύσχιστον, proposes
to read πλατανοσχιστον, probably following Pliny;[4] but he has no
reason for doing so, for it is quite right as it stands, and is analogous to the Greek compounds πλατύκαρπος, πλατύκαρφος, πλατόφυλλος,
&c., and the leaves of the black hellebore have in reality that
form.

156. Finally, that the plant of the ancients is indubitably the
same as our own is not less shewn by this, that Avicenna
describes the black hellebore of Dioscorides under the name of
خم بق اسود, and that Forskal, an eye witness, testifies that
in the East the helleborus niger goes by the same name to this
day.[5]

157. "It grows," says Dioscorides, "in rough, elevated and
dry places, and that which grows in those places is esteemed
the best; such is the case with the black hellebore of Anticyra,[6]
and it is the best."[7] He also praises that which grew in Helicon,
Parnassus, and Aetolia, but prefers the Heliconian. Theophrastus likewise prefers this to the others; he mentions that it grows
also in Boeotia, in Euboea, and in many other places. Rufus[7]

---

[1] Petri Bellonii, *Observat. sing. et memorab. rerum in Graecia, Asia, &c.*, per
Clusium, Antwerp, 1589-8.

[2] *Hist. plant.*, lib. x, cap. 11.

[3] See above where I have criticised the text of Theophrastus, in reference to
veratrum album, § 24—27.

[4] "Platano similia" says Pliny, *Hist. nat.*, lib. xxv, sect. 21.

[5] See *Mat. Med. Kahirina*, in the Appendix to *Descript. animalium in itinere
orientali*, p. 152.

[6] Such is the character of the country about Anticyra, as described by Pausanius
(*Graeciae descr.*, Hanoviae, 1613, p. 682): τὰ δὲ ὄρη τὰ ὑπὲρ 'Αντίκυραν πετρώδη τε
ἄγαν ἐστὶ, καὶ ἐν αὐτοῖς φύεται μάλιστα ὁ ἐλλέβορος· ὁ μὲν οὖν μέλας ἐστὶ γαστρὶ παθάρσιον,
&c. Among us it also grows in places similar to those described by Dioscorides and
Pausanius.

[7] In Oribasius, l. c., p. 249.

also commends that which grew in Lycestes, and above the Ascanian marsh.

158. According to Dioscorides, the preferable roots are those which have swollen and fleshy fibres, a small medulla, and an acrid burning taste.

159. The ancients believed that it purged by stool without difficulty the black and the yellow bile, as also the pituita,[1] and that it was also useful in intermittent fevers.[2] They gave it in chronic and hemicranial headache, in mania,[3] in melancholia,[4] in dropsy without fever,[5] in epilepsy,[6] in paralysis,[7] in long-standing gout,[8] in diseases of the joints,[9] in inflammation of the liver,[10] in chronic jaundice,[11] in old affections of the trachea.[12] Aretaeus[13] gave black hellebore in oxymel at the commencement of lethargy, in order to cause moderate purging.

160. If they wished to purge strongly, they administered a drachm (=72 gr.) of the root, if mildly, three oboli,[14] (=thirty six gr. or four oboli (=forty-eight gr.) either in melicrat or in decoction of lentils, or in broth. They mingled with it scammony or salt.[15] Others gave two drachms of the powder of the dry root by itself, in sweet wine, or in oxymel, or in decoction of lentils, or in ptisan,[16] or in chicken broth, if they wished to purge gently; but if they wished to cause a severe purgation, they gave one drachm of the root mixed with three oboli of scammony.[17]

161. It was used externally in obscuration of the eyes;[18] in difficulty of hearing it was introduced into the ears and kept there for two or three days;[19] it was applied to swellings on the

---

[1] Aëtius, lib. iii, cap. 27. Freind (*Histoire de la médecine*, ii, p. 167) is wrong in saying that Johannes Actuarius was the first to allege that the hellebore (the *black* one, for it is this that Actuarius is speaking of in the place referred to) acts without difficulty; for none of the ancient physicians (if except that insignificant Arabian author, Avenzoar) considered it dangerous.

[2] Aëtius, l. c.

[3] Rufus, l. c., p. 251—Aëtius, l. c.

[4] Dioscorides, lib. iv, cap. 151.—Celsus, lib. ii, cap. 12: "veratrum nigrum aut atra bile vexatis, aut cum tristatia insanientibus, aut iis, quorum nervi parte aliqua resoluti sunt."

[5] Pliny, l. c., lib. xxv. sect. 22.—Actuarius, *Method. medend.* lib. v, cap. 8.

[6] Dioscor., l. c.

[7] Dioscor., l. c.—Pliny, l. c.

[8] Pliny, l. c.

[9] Dioscor., l. c.—Pliny, l. c.

[10] Corn Celsus, l. c., lib. iv, cap. 8.

[11] Aëtius l. c.

[12] Paulus Aegineta, lib. vii, cap. 4.

[13] *Curat. Acut.*, lib. i, cap. 2.

[14] Dioscor., l. c.

[15] Pliny, l. c.

[16] Decoction of pearl-barley.

[17] Rufus, l. c., p. 251.

[18] Pliny, l. c.

[19] Dioscor., l. c.

neck;[1] it entered into the composition of an ointment, with which the parts affected with scabies were covered;[2] it was applied, mixed with vinegar, to vitiligo, impetigo, and lepra;[3] it was boiled with vinegar to make a gargle for toothache;[4] it was applied to the abdomen of dropsical persons, made up with flour and wine,[5] and finally it was used externally for callous fistulous openings for two or three days.[6]

162. The seed, which is a more violent purgative than the root (and went by the name of *sesamoides*)[7] was given for the same purposes, but in a smaller dose than two drachms, in melicrat.[8]

163. The black hellebore, with which the ancient physicians cured many chronic diseases, has also fallen into disuse in our times (or other plants have been substituted for it), although it is certain that it is an excellent and highly estimable medicine, if it be exactly suitable and appropriate to the disease for which it is administered.

ANALYSIS
OF THE ESSAY ON
THE HELLEBORISM OF THE ANCIENTS.

---

[1] Pliny, l. c.

[2] Dioscor., l. c.

[3] Dioscor., l. c.

[4] Dioscor., l. c.—Pliny l. c.—Galen, *De Simpl. med. fac.*, lib. vi.

[5] Dioscor., l. c.

[6] Dioscor., l. c.—Galen, l. c.

[7] See above, note to § 116.

[8] Rufus, l. c., p. 251.

SPIRIT OF THE HOMŒOPATHIC DOCTRINE OF MEDICINE. [1]

It is impossible to divine the internal essential nature of diseases and the changes they effect in the hidden parts of the body, and it is absurd to frame a system of treatment on such hypothetical surmises and assumptions : it is impossible to divine the medicinal properties of remedies from any chemical theories or from their smell, colour or taste, and it is absurd to attempt, from such hypothetical surmises and assumptions, to apply to the treatment of diseases these substances, which are so hurtful when wrongly administered. And even were such practice ever so customary and ever so generally in use, were it even the only one in vogue for thousands of years, it would nevertheless continue to be a senseless and pernicious practice to found on empty surmises an idea of the morbid condition of the interior, and to attempt to combat this with equally imaginary properties of medicines.

Appreciable, distinctly appreciable to our senses must that be, which is to be removed in each disease in order to transform it into health, and right clearly must each remedy express what it can positively cure, if medical art shall cease to be a wanton game of hazard with human life, and shall commence to be the sure deliverer from diseases.

I shall show what there is undeniably curable in diseases, and how the curative properties of medicines are to be distinctly perceived and applied to treatment.

     *   *   *   *

What life is can only be known empirically from its phenomena and manifestations, but no conception of it can be formed by any metaphysical speculations *a priori;* what life is, in its actual essential nature, can never be ascertained nor even guessed at, by mortals.

---

[1] This essay appeared in a journal twenty years ago, in those momentous days (March 1813) when the Germans had no leisure to read and still less to reflect upon scientific matters. The consequence of this was that these words were not listened to. It may now have more chance of being perused, particularly in its present less imperfect form. (*Reine Arzneimittellehre,* 2ter Thl. 1833.)

To the explanation of human life, as also its two-fold conditions, health and disease, the principles by which we explain other phenomena are quite inapplicable. With nought in the world can we compare it save with itself alone ; neither with a piece of clockwork nor with an hydraulic machine, nor with chemical processes, nor with decompositions and recompositions of gases, nor yet with a galvanic battery, in short with nothing destitute of life. Human life is *in no respect* regulated by purely physical laws, which only obtain among inorganic substances. The material substances of which the human organism is composed no longer follow, in this vital combination, the laws to which material substances in the inanimate condition are subject ; they are regulated by the laws peculiar to vitality alone, they are themselves animated just as the whole system is animated. Here a nameless fundamental power reigns omnipotent, which suspends all the tendency of the component parts of the body to obey the laws of gravitation, of momentum, of the *vis inertiæ*, of fermentation, of putrefaction, &c., and brings them under the wonderful laws of life alone,—in other words, maintains them in the condition of *sensibility* and *activity* necessary to the preservation of the living whole, a condition almost spiritually dynamic.

Now as the condition of the organism and its healthy state depend solely on the state of the life which animates it, in like manner it follows that the altered state, which we term disease, consists in a condition altered originally only in its vital sensibilities and functions, irrespective of all chemical or mechanical principles ; in short it must consist in an altered dynamical condition, a changed mode of being, whereby a change in the properties of the material component parts of the body is afterwards effected, which is a necessary consequence of the morbidly altered condition of the living whole in every individual case.

Moreover the influence of morbific injurious agencies, which for the most part excite from without the various maladies in us, is generally so invisible and so immaterial, [1] that it is impossible that it can *immediately* either mechanically disturb or derange the component parts of our body in their arrangement and substance, or infuse any pernicious acrid fluid into our blood-vessels whereby the mass of our humours can be chemically altered and destroyed—an inadmissible, improbable, gross in-

---

[1] With the exception of a few surgical affections and the disagreeable effects produced by indigestible foreign substances, which sometimes find their way into the intestinal canal.

vention of mechanical minds. The exciting causes of disease rather act by means of their special properties on the state of our life (on our health), only in a dynamic manner, very similar to a spiritual manner, and inasmuch as they first derange the organs of the higher rank and of the vital force, there occurs from this state of derangement, from this dynamic alteration of the living whole, an altered sensation (uneasiness, pains) and an altered activity (abnormal functions) of each individual organ and of all of them collectively, whereby there must also of necessity secondarily occur alteration of the juices in our vessels and secretion of abnormal matters, the inevitable consequence of the altered vital character, which now differs from the healthy state.

These abnormal matters that shew themselves in diseases are consequently merely products of the disease itself, which, as long as the malady retains its present character, must of necessity be secreted, and thus constitute a portion of the morbid signs (symptoms); they are merely effects, and therefore manifestations of the existing internal ill-health, and they do certainly not react (although they often contain the infecting principle for other, healthy individuals) upon the diseased body that produced them, as disease-exciting or maintaining substances, that is, as material morbific causes,[1] just as a person cannot infect other parts of his own body at the same time with the virus from his own chancre or with the gonorrhœal matter from his own urethra, or increase his disease therewith, or as a viper cannot inflict on itself a fatal bite with its own poison.[2]

Hence it is obvious that the diseases excited by the dynamic and special influence of morbific injurious agents can be originally only dynamical (caused almost solely by a spiritual process) derangements of the vital character of our organism.[3]

[1] Hence by clearing away and mechanically removing these abnormal matters acridities and morbid organizations, their source, the disease itself, can just as little be cured as a coryza can be shortened or cured by blowing the nose frequently, as frequently as possible; it lasts not a day longer than its proper course, although the nose should not be cleansed by blowing it at all.

[2] [These statements are not strictly correct, at least as regards the chancrous and gonorrhœal matters, for it is well known that chancres may be produced on different parts of the body of an individual by inoculation from his own chancre, and the gonorrhœal process may be excited in the eye by the incautious application of the discharge to that organ by the patient himself.]

[3] [Unfortunately for this vital or dynamic theory of Hahnemann, the examples he has cited absolutely disprove his position in regard to dynamic or spiritual causes of disease. Since this essay was written, Ricord has immortalized himself by demonstrating that the virus of chancres and the matter of gonorrhœas, are both capable of

We readily perceive that these dynamic derangements of the vital character of our organism which we term diseases, since they are nothing else than altered sensations and functions, can also express themselves by nothing but by an aggregate of symptoms, and only as such are they cognizable to our observing powers.

Now as in a profession of such importance to human life as medicine is, nothing but the state of the diseased body plainly cognizable by our perceptive faculties can be recognized as the object to be cured, and ought to guide our steps (to chose conjectures and undemonstrable hypotheses as our guide would be dangerous folly, nay, crime and treason against humanity), it follows, that since diseases, as dynamic derangements of the vital character, express themselves *solely* by alterations of the sensations and functions of our organism, that is, *solely* by an aggregate of cognizable symptoms, this alone can be the object of treatment in every case of disease. *For on the removal of all morbid symptoms nothing remains but health.*

Now because diseases are only dynamic derangements of our health and vital character, they cannot be removed by man otherwise than by means of agents and powers which also are capable of producing dynamical derangements of the human health, that is to say, diseases are cured virtually and dynamically by medicines.[1]

---

reacting, and of reproducing these diseases upon the bodies from whence they are taken. It is now a general practice among surgeons, when a suspicious ulcer is presented to them, to innoculate another part of the same individual with the matter, for the purpose of ascertaining whether a chancre can be reproduced. This test is now deemed conclusive. In these instances, surely no dynamic or spiritual influences can be recognized as causes of the maladies under consideration, but manifestly the *actual contact* of morbid material substances with other healthy material structures. We cannot, therefore, with any degree of propriety term these causes or their effects upon the organism, either dynamic or vital. Hahnemann labours under a similar error, in regard to the bites of vipers, as it is well known at present, that when very much enraged, certain reptiles destroy themselves by their own bites.] *Am. P.*

[1] Not by means of the pretended solvent or mechanically dispersing, clearing-out, and expulsive powers of medicinal substances, not by means of a (blood-purifying, humour-correcting) power they possess of electively excreting fancied morbific principles, not by means of any antiseptic power they contain (as is effected in dead, putrifying flesh), not by any chemical or physical action of any other imaginable sort, as happens in dead material things, as has hitherto been falsely imagined and dreamt by the various medical schools.

The more modern schools have indeed begun in some degree to regard diseases as dynamic derangements, and also intended in a certain manner to remove them dynamically by medicines, but inasmuch as they have failed to perceive that the sensible, irritable and reproductive activity of life is *in modo et qualitate* susceptible of an infi-

These active substances and powers (medicines) which we have at our service, effect the cure of diseases by means of the same dynamic power of altering the actual state of health, by means of the same power of deranging the vital character of our organism in respect of its sensations and functions, by which they are able to effect also the healthy individual, to produce in him dynamic changes and certain morbid symptoms, the knowledge of which, as we shall see, affords us the most trustworthy information concerning the morbid states that can be most certainly cured by each particular medicine. Hence nothing in the world can accomplish a cure, no substance, no power effect a change in the human organism of such a character as that the disease shall yield to it, except an agent capable of absolutely (dynamically) deranging the human health, consequently also of morbidly altering its healthy state.[1]

On the other hand, however, there is also no agent, no power in nature capable of morbidly affecting the healthy individual, which does not at the same time possess the faculty of curing certain morbid states.

Now, as the power of curing diseases, as also of morbidly affecting the healthy, is met with in inseparable combination in all medicines, and as both these properties evidently spring from one and the same source, namely from their power of dynamically deranging human health, and as it is hence impossible that they can act according to a different inherent natural law in the sick to that according to which they act on the healthy, it follows that it must be the same power of the medicine that cures the disease in the sick as gives rise to the morbid symptoms in the healthy.[2]

Hence also we shall find that the curative potency of medicines, and that which each of them is able to effect in diseases, expresses itself in the other mode in the world so surely and palpably, and cannot be ascertained by us by any purer and

---

nity of changes, and to regard the innumerable varieties of morbid signs that (infinity of internal alterations only cognizable by us in their reflex) for what they actually are, the only undeceptive object for treatment, but as they only hypothetically recognize an abnormal increase and decrease of their dimensions *quoad quantitatem*, and *in an equally arbitrary manner* confide to the medicines they employ the task of changing to the normal state this one-sided increase and decrease, and thereby curing them; they thus have before their view nothing but chimeras, both of the object to be cured and of the action of the medicine.

[1] Consequently no substance, for example, that is purely nutritious.

[2] The different result in those two cases is owing solely to the difference of the object that has to be altered.

more perfect manner than by the morbid phenomena and symptoms (the kinds of artificial diseases) which the medicines develop in the healthy individuals. For if we only have before us a register of the peculiar (artificial) morbid symptoms produced by the various medicines on healthy individuals, we only require a series of pure experiments to decide what medicinal symptoms will always rapidly and permanently cure and remove certain symptoms of disease, in order to know, in every case beforehand, which of all the different medicines known and thoroughly tested as to their peculiar symptoms must be the most certain remedy in every case of disease.[1]

---

[1] Simple, true and natural as this maxim is, so much so that one would have imagined it would long since have been adopted as the rule for ascertaining the curative powers of drugs, it is yet a fact that it has hitherto been far from being recognized. During the many thousands of years over which history extends, no one fell upon this natural method of ascertaining the curative powers of medicine *a priori* and before their application to diseases. In all ages up to the present times it was imagined that the curative powers of medicines could be learned in no other way than from the result of their employment in diseases themselves (*ab usu in morbis*); it was sought to learn them from those cases where a certain medicine (more frequently a combination of various medicines) had been found serviceable in a particular case of disease. But even from the efficacious result of one single medicine given in an accurately described case of disease (which was rarely done), we never can know the case in which that medicine would again prove serviceable, because (with the exception of diseases caused by miasms of a fixed character, as small-pox, measles, syphilis, itch, &c., and those arising from various injurious agencies that always remain the same, as *rheumatic gout*, &c.), all other cases of disease are mere individualities, that is to say, all present themselves in nature with different combinations of symptoms, have never before occurred, and can never again occur in exactly the same manner; consequently a remedy in one case can never allow us to infer its efficacy in another (different) case. The forced arrangement of these cases of disease (which nature in her wisdom produces in endless variety) under certain nosological heads, as is arbitrarily done by pathology, is a human performance without reality, which leads to constant fallacies and to the confounding together of very different states.

Equally deceptive and untrustworthy, although in all ages generally introduced, is the determination of the general (curative) actions of medicines from special effects in diseases, where in the materia medica—when, for example, here and there, in some cases of disease *during* the use of a medicine (generally mixed up with others) there occurred a more copious secretion of urine, perspiration, the irruption of the catamenia, cessation of convulsions, a kind of sleep, expectoration, &c.,—the medicine (on which was conferred the honour of having ascribed to it more than to the others in the mixture the effect produced) was instantly elevated to the rank of a diuretic, a diaphoretic, an emmenagogue, an antispasmodic, a soporific, an expectorant, and thereby not only was a fallacium causæ committed by confounding the word *during* with *by*, but quite a false conclusion was drawn *a particulari ad universale*, in opposition to all the laws of reason, and indeed the conditional was made unconditional. For a substance that does not in every case of disease promote urine and perspiration, that does not in every instance bring on the catamenia and sleep, that does not subdue all convulsions, and cause every cough to come to expectoration, cannot

If then we ask experience what artificial diseases (observed to be produced by medicines) can be beneficially employed against certain natural morbid states; if we ask it whether the change to health (cure) may be expected to ensue most certainly and in the most permanent manner :

1. by the use of such medicines as are capable of producing in the healthy body a *different* (allopathic) affection from that exhibited by the disease to be cured,

2. or by the employment of such as are capable of exciting in the healthy individual an *opposite* (enantiopathic, antipathic) state to that of the case to be cured,

3. or by the adminstration of such medicines as can cause a *similar* (homœopathic) state to the natural disease before us (for these are the only three possible modes of employing them), experience speaks indubitably for the last method.

But it is moreover self-evident that medicines which act *heterogeneously* and *allopathically*, which tend to develop in the healthy subject different symptoms from those presented by the disease to be cured, from the very nature of things can never be suitable and efficacious in this case, but they must act awry, otherwise every disease must necessarily be cured in a rapid, certain and permanent manner by any medicine whatsoever, be its action ever so different. Now as every medicine possesses an action different from that of every other, and as, according to eternal natural laws, every disease causes a derangement of the human health different from that caused by all other diseases, this proposition contains a self-evident contradiction (*contradictio in adjecto*), and is self-demonstrative of the impossibility or a good result, since every given change can only be effected by an adequate cause, but not *per quamlibet causam*. And daily experience also proves that the ordinary practice of prescribing complex recipes containing a variety of unknown medicines in diseases, does indeed do many things, but very rarely cures.

The *second mode* of treating diseases by medicines is the employment of an agent capable of altering the existing derangement of the health (the disease, or most prominent morbid

---

be said by a person of sound reason to be unconditionally and absolutely diuretic diaphoretic, emmenagogue, soporific, antispasmodic, and expectorant ? Indeed it is impossible that in the complex phenomena of our health, in the multifarious combinations of different symptoms presented by the innumerable varieties of human diseases, the employment of a remedy can exhibit its pure, original medicinal effect, and exactly those derangements of our health that we might expect from it. These can only b shewn by medicines given to persons in health.

symptom) in an *enantiopathic, antipathic,* or *contrary* manner (a medicine employed *palliatively*). Such an employment, as will be readily seen, cannot affect a permanent cure of the disease, because the malady must soon afterwards recur, and that in an aggravated degree. The process that takes place is as follows: According to a wonderful provision of nature, organized living beings are not regulated by the laws of unorganized (dead), physical matter, they do not receive the influence of external agents, like the latter, in a passive manner, but strive to oppose a contrary action to them.[1] The living human body does indeed allow itself to be in the first instance changed by the action of physical agents; but this change is not in it as in inorganic substances, permanent (—as it ought necessarily to be if the medicinal agent acting in a *contrary manner* to the disease should have a *permanent* effect, and be of *durable* benefit—): on the contrary, the living human organism strives to develop by antagonism,[2] the exact opposite of the affection first produced in it from without,—as for instance, a hand kept long enough in ice-cold water, after being withdrawn does not remain cold, nor

---

[1] The expressed, green juice of plants, which is in that state no longer living, when spread upon linen cloth and exposed to the sun's light, soon loses its colour and becomes completely decomposed, whereas the living plant that has been kept in a cellar deprived of light and thereby blenched, soon recovers its full green colour when exposed to the same sun's light. A root dug up and dried (dead), if buried in a warm and damp soil, rapidly undergoes complete decomposition and destruction, whilst a living root in the same warm damp soil sends forth gay sprouts—Foaming malt-beer in full fermentation rapidly turns to vinegar when exposed to a temperature of 96° Fahr. in a vessel, but in the healthy human stomach at the same temperature the fermentation ceases, and it soon becomes converted into a mild nutritious juice.—Half-decomposed and strong-smelling game, as also beef and other flesh meat, partaken of by a healthy individual, furnish excrement with the least amount of odour; whereas cinchona-bark, which is calculated powerfully to check decomposition in lifeless animal substances, is acted against by the intestines in such a manner that the most fetid flatus is developed.—Mild carbonate of lime removes all acids from inorganic matter, but when taken into the healthy stomach sour perspiration usually ensues.—Whilst the dead animal fibre is preserved by nothing more certainly and powerfully than by tannin, clean ulcers in a living individual, when they are frequently dressed with tannin, become unclean, green and putrid. A hand plunged into warm water becomes subsequently colder than the hand that has not been so treated, and it becomes colder in proportion as the water was hotter.

[2] This is the law of nature, in obedience to which, the employment of every medicine produces at first certain dynamic changes and morbid symptoms in the living human body (*primary* or *first action of the medicines*), but on the other hand, by means of a peculiar antagonism (which may in many instances be termed the self-sustaining effort), produces a state the very opposite of the first (the *secondary* or *after action*), as for instance, in the case of narcotic substances, insensibility is produced in the primary action, sensitiveness to pain in the secondary.

merely assume the temperature of the surrounding atmosphere, as a stone (dead) ball would do, or even resume the temperature of the rest of the body, no! the colder the water of the bath was, and the longer it acted on the healthy skin of the hand, the more *inflamed* and hotter does the latter afterwards become.

Therefore it cannot but happen that a medicine having an action opposite to the symptoms of the disease, will reverse the morbid symptoms for but a very short time,[1] but must soon give place to the antagonism pervading the living body, which produces an opposite state, that is to say, a state the direct contrary of that transient delusive state of the health effected by the palliative (one corresponding to the original malady), which constitutes an actual addition to the now recurring, uneradicated, primary affection, and is consequently an increased degree of the original disease. And thus the malady is always *certainly* aggravated after the palliative—the medicine that acts in an opposite and enantiopathic manner—has exhausted its action.[2]

In chronic diseases,—the true touch-stone of a genuine healing art,—the injurious character of the antagonistically-acting (palliative) remedy often displays itself in a high degree, since from its repeated exhibition in order that it should merely produce its delusive effect (a very transient semblance of health) it must be administered in larger and ever larger doses, which are often productive of serious danger to life, or even of actual death.[3]

There remains therefore, only a *third* mode of employing medicines in order to effect a really beneficial result, to wit, by

---

[1] As a burnt hand remains cold and painless not much longer than whilst it remains in the cold water, but afterwards feels the pain of the burn much more severely.

[2] Thus the pain of a burnt hand is subdued by cold water quickly, it is true, but only for a few minutes, afterwards however, the pain of the burn and the inflammation become worse than they were previously (the inflammation or secondary action of the cold water makes an addition to the original inflammation of the burn, which is not to be eradicated by cold water). The troublesome fulness of the abdomen in cases of habitual constipation, appears to be removed, as if magically, by the action of a purgative, but the very next day the painful fulness returns together with the constipation, and becomes worse afterwards than before. The stupified sleep caused by opium is succeeded by a more sleepless night than ever.—But that the state that subsequently occurs is a true aggravation, is rendered evident by this, that if we design again to employ the palliative (*e. g.* opium for habitual sleeplessness or chronic looseness of the bowels), it must be given in a stronger dose, *as if for a more severe disease*, in order that it should produce its delusive amelioration for even as short a period as before.

[3] As for instance, where opium is repeated in always stronger doses for the suppression of urgent symptoms of a chronic disease.

40

employing in every case such a one as tends to excite of itself an artificial, morbid affection in the organism *similar* (homœopathic), best if *very similar*, to the actual case of disease.

That this mode of employing medicines is and must of necessity be the only best method, can easily be proved by reasoning, as it has also already been confirmed both by innumerable experiences of physicians who practise according to my doctrines, and by ordinary experience.[1]

It will, therefore, not be difficult to perceive what are the laws of nature according to which the only appropriate cure of diseases, the homœopathic, takes place, and must necessarily take place.

---

[1] I may adduce merely a few examples from daily experience; thus, the burning pain produced by the contact of boiling water on the skin, is overpowered and destroyed, as in the case of cooks by approaching the moderately burnt hand to the fire, or by bathing it uninterruptedly with heated alcohol (or turpentine), which causes a still more intense burning sensation. This infallible mode of treatment is practised and found to be corroborated by varnishers and others engaged in similar occupations. The burning pain produced by these strong spirits and their elevated temperature, then remains *alone* present, and that for but a few minutes, whilst the organism, homœopathically freed by them from the inflammation occasioned by the burn, soon restores the injury of the skin and forms a new epidermis through which the spirit can no longer penetrate. And thus, *in the course of a few hours,* the injury caused by the burn is cured by a remedy that occasions a similar burning pain (heated alcohol or turpentine), whereas if treated with the ordinary cooling palliative remedies and salves, it is transformed into a bad ulcer and usually continues to suppurate for many weeks or months with great pain. Practised dancers know from old experience that those who are extremely heated by dancing are very much relieved for the first moment by stripping themselves and drinking very cold water, but thereafter infallibly incur a fatal disease, and they do not allow persons excessively heated to cool themselves by exposure to the open air or by taking off their clothes, but wisely administer a liquor whose nature is to heat the blood, such as punch or hot tea mixed with rum or arrack, and in this manner, walking at the same time gently up and down the room, they rapidly lose the violent febrile state induced by the dance. In like manner no old experienced reaper, after inordinate exertion in the heat of the sun, would drink anything in order to cool himself but a glass of brandy; and before an hour has elapsed, his thirst and heat are gone and he feels quite well. No experienced person would put a frost-bitten limb into warm water, or seek to restore it by approaching it to the fire or a heated stove; applying to it snow, or rubbing it with ice-cold water, is the well-known homœopathic remedy for it. The illness occasioned by excessive joy (fantastic gaiety, trembling restlessness and uneasiness, palpitation of the heart, sleeplessness) is rapidly and permanently removed by coffee, which causes a similar morbid affection in persons unaccustomed to its use. And in like manner there are many daily-occurring confirmations of the great truth, that nature intends that men should be cured of their long-standing diseases by means of similar affections of short duration. Nations, for centuries sunk in listless apathy and serfdom, raised their spirit, felt their dignity as men, and again became free, after having been ignominiously trodden in the dust by the western tyrant.

The first of these unmistakeable laws of nature is: *the living organism is incomparably less capable of being affected by natural diseases, than by medicines.*

A multitude of disease-exciting causes act daily and hourly upon us, but they are incapable of deranging the equilibrium of the health, or of making the healthy sick; the activity of the life-sustaining power within us usually withstands the most of them, the individual remains healthy. It is only when these external inimical agencies assail us in a very aggravated degree, and we are especially exposed to their influence, that we get ill, but even then we only become seriously ill when our organism has a particularly affectable, weak side (predisposition), that makes it more disposed to be affected by the (simple or compound) morbific cause in question, and to be deranged in its health.

If the inimical agents in nature that are partly physical and partly psychical, which are termed morbific injurious agents, possessed an unconditional power of deranging the human health, they would, as they are universally distributed, not leave any one in good health; every one would become ill, and we should never be able to obtain an idea of health. But as, taken on the whole, diseases are only exceptional states of the human health, and it is necessary that such a number of circumstances and conditions, both as regards the morbific agents and the individual to be affected with disease, should conjoin before a disease is produced by its exciting causes, it follows, *that the individual is so little liable to be affected by such injurious agencies, that they can never unconditionally make him ill, and that the human organism is capable of being deranged to disease by them only by means of a particular predisposition.*[1]

But it is far otherwise with the artificial dynamic agents which we term medicines. Every true medicine, namely, acts at *all* times, under *all* circumstances, on every living, animated body, and excites in it the symptoms peculiar to it (even in a perceptible form if the dose be large enough) so that evidently *every living human organism must always and inevitably be affected by the medicinal disease and infected so to speak,* which, as is well known, is not the case with respect to medicines.[2]

---

[1] [Innumerable facts, of daily occurrence, establish the truth of this important remark.]—*Am. P.*

[2] Even the pestilential diseases do not effect every one unconditionally, and the other diseases leave many more individuals unaffected, even when all are exposed to

All experience proves incontestably, that the human body is much more apt and disposed to be affected by medicinal agents and to have its health deranged by them, than by the morbific injurious agencies and contagious miasms, or, what is the same thing, that the medicinal powers possess an absolute power of deranging human health, whereas the morbific agencies possess only a very conditional power, vastly inferior to the former.

To this circumstance is owing the possibility of the cure of diseases by medicines generally (that is to say, we see, that in the diseased organism the morbid affection may be effaced, if it be subjected to the appropriate alteration by means of medicine); but in order that the cure should take place, the *second* natural law should also be fulfilled, to wit, *a stronger dynamic affection permanently extinguishes the weaker in the living organism, provided the former be similar in kind to the latter ;* for the dynamic alteration of the health to be anticipated from the medicine should, as I think I have proved, neither *differ in kind* from or be *allopathic* to the morbid derangement, in order that, as happens in the ordinary mode of practice, a still greater derangement may not ensue, nor should it be *opposite* to it, in order that a merely palliative delusive amelioration may not ensue, to be followed by an inevitable aggravation of the original malady, but the medicine must have been proved by observations to possess the tendency to develop of itself a state of health *similar* to the disease (be able to excite similar symptoms in the healthy body), in order to be a remedy of permanent efficacy.

Now, as the dynamic affections of the organism (caused by disease or by medicine) are only cognizable by the phenomena of altered function and altered sensation, and consequently the similarity of its dynamic affections to one another can only express themselves by similarity of symptoms ; but as the organism (as being much more liable to be deranged by medicine than by disease) must be more susceptible to the medicinal affection, that is to say, must be more disposed to allow itself to be influenced and deranged by medicine than by the similar morbid affection, it follows undeniably, that it will be freed from the morbid affection if we allow a medicine to act on it, which, while differ-ing[1] in its nature from the disease, resembles it very closely in

---

changes of the weather, the seasons, and to the influences of many other injurious impressions.

[1] Without this difference in the nature of the morbid affection from that of the medicinal affection, a cure were impossible; if the two were not merely of a similar.

similarity of symptoms, that is to say, is homœopathic; for the organism, as a living, individual unity, cannot receive two similar dynamic affections at the same time, without the weaker yielding to the stronger similar one, consequently, as it is more disposed to be more strongly affected by the one (the medicinal affection), the other, similar, weaker one (the morbid affection) must necessarily give way, whereupon it is cured.

Let it not be imagined that the living organism, if a new similar affection be communited to it when diseased by a dose of homœopathic medicine, will be thereby more seriously deranged, that is, burdened with an addition to its sufferings, just as a leaden plate already pressed upon by an iron weight is still more severely bruised by placing a stone in addition upon it, or a piece of copper heated by friction must become still hotter by pouring on it water at a more elevated temperature. No, our living organism does not behave passively, it is not regulated by the laws that govern dead matter; it reacts by vital antagonism, so as to surrender itself as an individual living whole to its morbid derangement, and to allow that to be extinguished within it, when a stronger affection of a similar kind, produced in it by homœopathic medicine, takes possession of it.

Such a spiritually reacting being is our living, human organism, which with automatic power expels from itself a weaker derangement (disease), whenever the stronger power of the homœopathic medicine produces in it another but very similar affection, or in other words, which, on account of the unity of its life, cannot suffer at the same time from two similar general derangements, but must discard the primary dynamic affection (disease), whenever it is acted on by a second dynamic power (medicine) more capable of deranging it, that has a great resemblance to the former in its power of affecting the health (its symptoms). Something similar takes place in the human mind.[1]

but of the same nature, consequently identical, then no result (or only an aggravation of the malady) would ensue; as for example, if we were to touch a chancre with other chancrous poison, a cure would never result therefrom.

[1] For example: a girl plunged into grief by the death of her companion, if taken to see a family where the poor, half-naked children have just lost their father, their sole support, does not become more sorrowful from witnessing this touching scene, but is thereby consoled for her own smaller misfortune; she is cured of her grief for her friend, because the unity of her mind cannot be affected by two similar passions at once, and the one passion must be extinguished when a *similar* but stronger passion takes possession of her mind, and acts as a homœopathic remedy in extinguishing the first. But the girl would not be tranquillized and cured of her grief for the loss of her companion, if her mother were angrily to scold her (*heterogenous, allopathic*

But as the human organism even in health is more capable of being affected by medicine than by disease, as I have shewn above, so when it is diseased, it is beyond comparison more affectable by homœopathic medicine than by any other (whether allopathic or enantiopathic), and indeed it is *affectable in the highest degree*, since, as it is already disposed and excited by the disease to certain symptoms, it must now be more liable to be deranged to similar symptoms (by the homœopathic medicine) —just as similar mental affections render the mind much more sensitive to similar emotions—; hence only the *smallest dose* of them is *necessary* and *useful* for their cure, for altering the diseased organism into the similar medicinal disease, and *a greater one is not necessary* on this account also, because the spiritual power of the medicine does not in this instance accomplish its object by means of quantity, but by potentiality and quality (dynamic fitness, homœopathy),—and *it is not useful that it should be greater*, but on the contrary *injurious*, because whilst the larger dose, on the one hand, does not dynamically overpower the morbid affection more certainly than the smallest dose of the most appropriate medicine, on the other hand it imposes a complex medicinal disease in its place, which is always a malady, though it runs its course in a shorter time.

Hence the organism will be powerfully affected and possessed by the potency of even a very small dose of a medicinal substance, which, by its tendency to excite similar symptoms, can outweigh and extinguish the totality of the symptoms of the disease; it becomes, as I have said, free from the morbid affection at the very instant that it is taken possession of by the medicinal affection, by which it is immeasurably more liable to be altered.

Now as medicinal agents do of themselves, even in larger doses, only keep the healthy organism for a few days under their influence, it will readily be conceived that a small dose,

---

agency), but on the contrary, her mind would be still more distressed by this attack of grief of another kind; and in like manner the sorrowing girl, if we were to cause an apparent but only *palliative* alleviation of her grief, by means of a gay entertainment, would subsequently in her solitude sink into still more profound sadness, and would weep much more intensely than previously for the death of her friend (because this affection would here be only of an *opposite, enantiopathic* character).

And as it is here in psychical life, so it is in the former case in organic life. The unity of our life cannot occupy itself with, and take in two general dynamic affections of the same kind at once; for if the second be a similar one, the first is displaced by it, whenever the organism is more affected by the last.

and in acute diseases a very small dose of them (such as they must evidently be in homœopathic treatment), can only affect the system for a short time, the smallest doses however, in acute diseases, only for a few hours, for then the medicinal affection substituted for the disease passes unobservedly and very rapidly into pure health.

The nature of living organisms seems not to act otherwise in the permanent cure of diseases by means of medicines than in accordance with these, its manifest laws, and thus indeed it acts, if we may use the expression, according to mathematical laws. *There is no case of dynamic disease in the world* (excepting the death struggle, and when it comes under this category, extreme old age and the destruction of some indispensable viscus or member), *whose symptoms can be met with in great similarity among the positive effects of a medicine, which will not be rapidly and permanently cured by this medicine.* The diseased individual can be freed from his malady in no more easy, rapid, certain, reliable and permanent manner, by any conceivable mode of treatment,[1] than by means of the homœopathic medicine in a small dose.

TREATMENT OF THE TYPHUS OR HOSPITAL FEVER AT PRESENT PREVAILING.[2]

As all ordinary modes of treatment with emetics, blood-letting, acetate ·of ammonia, elder-flower tea, juniper juice, cold and warm baths, naphtha, musk, opium, camphor and cinchona bark did so much havoc in this disease, and the somewhat more appropriate remedies, chamomile, serpentaria, valerian, and muriatic acid were but indifferent comforters, moved by purely

----

[1] Even those striking cures occurring in rare instances in ordinary practice take place only by means of a homœopathically appropriate medicine, which forms the chief agent in the receipt, into which it may have been *accidentally* introduced. Physicians hitherto could not have *chosen* the medicines homœopathically for diseases, as the positive effects of the medicines (those resulting from their administration to healthy persons) have not been investigated by them, and accordingly remain unknown to them ; and even those which have been known otherwise than by my writings, were not regarded by them as serviceable for treatment,—and moreover, the relation of the effects of medicines to the symptoms of the disease they resemble (the homœopathic law of cure), which is requisite in order to effect radical cures, was unknown to them.

[2] From the *Allgem. Anzeig. der Deutschen*, No. 6, 1814.

philanthropic motives, I here propose an efficacious mode of treatment, in order to preserve perhaps from death by this pestilence the remaining victims, if ordinary prejudices do not prevent its employment.

This fever has two principal stages. *In the first period* (which is all the shorter the worse the disease is to be) there are present, full, increased sensation of the pains usually present, with intolerable bad humour, sensation of heat in the body, and especially in the head, dry feeling or actual dryness in the mouth, causing constant thirst, bruised feeling in the limbs, restlessness, &c.; but *in the second period*, that of the delirium (a metastasis of the whole disease upon the mental organs) no complaint is made of all those symptoms—the patient is hot, does not desire to drink, he knows not whether to take this or that, he does not know those about him, or he abuses them, he makes irrelevant answers, talks nonsense with his eyes open, does foolish things, wishes to run away, cries aloud or whines, without being able to say why he does so, has a rattling in the throat, the countenance is distorted, the eyes squinting, he plays with his hands, behaves like a madman, passes the excrements unconsciously, &c.

In the first period of the pains and consciousness, two vegetable substances are of use and generally quite remove the disease at its commencement—the *bryonia alba* and the *rhus toxicodendron.*

We take a drachm of the powdered root of bryona, shake it up with ten drachms of alcohol and allow it to stand for six hours so as to extract all its medicinal power. In the meantime we pour six drachms of the strongest pure alcohol into each of twelve bottles, which should be of such a size that this quantity does not fill them completely, and then we number them. Into the first of these bottles, marked No. 1, we drop a single drop of the tincture prepared as above, and shake it strongly for three minutes; then from this bottle No. 1, we drop a single drop into bottle No. 2, and shake it strongly for the same length of time; then again, from this we drop a single drop into bottle No. 3, and thus we go on until each bottle has received a drop from the preceding one, so that bottle No. 12, is impregnated with a drop from No. 11, and thereafter, like all the preceding ones, is strongly shaken for three minutes.

It is this last bottle, No. 12, which contains the bryonia tincture in the suitable dilution, and which may be successfully employed in the first stage of the disease.

If, for instance, the patient complains of dizziness, *shooting* (or jerking-tearing) *pains* in the head, throat, chest, abdomen, &c., which are felt *particularly on moving the part*—in addition to the other symptoms, the hemorrhages, the vomiting, the heat, the thirst, the nocturnal restlessness, &c., we give him on a piece of sugar a single drop from bottle No. 12, in the morning, in preference to any other time, for the fever tends to increase towards night. Improvement takes place in the course of four and twenty hours, and as long as the improvement goes on, we give him no other medicine, nor even repeat the same one ; for none of the medicines here recommended can be used oftener than once (in the dose of a drop)—seldom can they be given a second time with advantage.

In this interval, until it is time for giving the second medicine, we may, in order to satisfy the desire of the patient for medicine and to quiet his mind, give him something innocuous, *e. g.* a few tea-spoonfuls of raspberry juice in the course of the day, or a few powders of milk-sugar.

If now, the amendment produced by the single dose of bryonia goes off in the course of two, three, or four days, that is to say, if the patient then complains of *shooting pains in one or other part of the body, whilst the part is at rest;* if the prostration and anorexia are greater, if there is harassing cough or such a debility of certain parts as to threaten paralysis, we give a single drop of the tincture of rhus toxicodendron, prepared in the same way as the above and diluted to the same degree, so that *one* drop of the tincture prepared with a drachm of the powder of the leaves and ten drachms of alcohol, is added to a bottle containing six drachms of strong alcohol and mixed by being shaken strongly, and from this one drop is added to a second bottle and so on, until the last of the twelve bottles has been impregnated by a drop from No. 11, and, like all the previous ones, has been strongly shaken, just as was the case in preparing the diluted tincture of bryonia.

Of this highly diluted tincture of rhus toxicodendron we give in the last-mentioned case, or if the symptoms I have described occur at the very commencement of the attack, we give, *at its very commencement,* a single drop from bottle No. 12, on sugar, and no more, nor any other medicine as long as the improvement is manifest and continued, unless it be (on the days when he is getting no medicine) some of the above mentioned innocuous substances.

Neither of the medicines can be used in a lower dilution or in a larger dose; they are too strong.

No domestic remedies of any kind, perfumes, pure wine, herb-teas, clysters, fomentations or the like should be used any more than other medicines, if we wish the case to turn out success-fully. We should only put upon the patient the amount of bed-clothes he feels agreeable, and keep him neither too warm nor too cool, and we should let him drink or eat what he has a fancy for; he never wishes for anything that will not do him good.

The whole disease will generally be removed by a single drop of the second or of the first medicine (according as the one or the other is indicated, without the addition of any other). *But rhus is suitable more frequently than bryonia, and hence can be more frequently used at first and alone.*

If, notwithstanding, the disease should pass into the above-described stage of delirium and mania, then *hyoscyamus niger* meets all the indications of the case.

A tincture from the leaves of this plant should be prepared, (the extracts of it are generally of indefinite strength or quite powerless) and diluted in the above-described manner, but only through eight bottles, and a single drop from the last bottle, No. 8, given upon sugar, and during the following days of ameliora-tion only the above-described innocuous things given instead of medicine, for then reason, strength, tranquillity, appetite, &c. usually return completely, although they might have seemed to be almost entirely lost, and the patient an inevitable prey of death.

This medicine also should not be given oftener than one single time; a single drop of the tincture diluted in this manner almost always suffices.

Nothing particular need be administered for local inflamma-tions or swellings, nor yet for eruptions, twitchings, long-con-tinued constipation, diarrhœa, anorexia, vomiting, hemorrhages or cough that occur in this disease. Those symptoms which arise from the main disease also go off simultaneously with its disappearance, under the use of the remedies I have directed to be given.

But there sometimes occurs a *third state*, a sort of lethargy of the internal common sensorium, a kind of half-paralysis of the mental organs. The patient remains indolently lying, without sleeping or speaking; he scarcely answers whatever we may do to induce him to do so, he appears to hear without understanding what is said or without allowing it to make any impression on him (the few words he says he whispered but not irrelevant) ; he appears to feel almost nothing, and to be almost immoveable, and yet not quite paralysed.

In this case a remedy is useful that previously used to be employed in large doses for purposes not very clearly defined; I mean the *sweet spirit of nitre*. It must be so old, that is to say, so thoroughly sweetened that it no longer reddens the cork of the bottle. (It then contains in a concrete form, nitrous oxide, respecting whose power the experiments of Dr. Beddoes give us important hints).

One drop of this is to be shaken up with an ounce of water, and given by tea-spoonfuls so as to be consumed in the four and twenty hours. In the course of a few days this state passes into health and activity.[1]

ON THE TREATMENT OF BURNS.[2]

It is to be regretted that Professor Dzondi, of Halle, should have recommended as the only sure, efficacious and best remedy for burns, a means of the injurious nature of which all who have much to do with fire are perfectly convinced. Has he then instituted comparative experiments with all remedies recommended for this purpose, that he can now with any degree of truth vaunt his cold water as being the only sure, the best remedy ? In such injuries the question is, not what shall give relief for the first few moments, but what shall most speedily render the burnt skin entirely destitute of pain and heal it. This can only be determined by comparative experiments, not by speculation. But it has already been settled by observations, which may easily be repeated, that it is *exactly the opposite of cold water*

---

[1] [In the introduction of the proving of *rhus toxicodendron* (R. A. M. L., pt. ii, p. 358), Hahnemann refers with satisfaction to his success in the treatment of this epidemic of typhus.—" Of 183 patients whom I treated for this affection in Leipzic, I did not lose one, which excited a great sensation among the members of the Russian Government then occupying Dresden, but was taken no notice of by the medical authorities."]

[2] From the *Allg. Anz. d. D.*, No. 156, 1816. In reply to Professor Dzondi's recommendation of cold water in the same journal, No. 104.

that heals burns most rapidly. For with the true physicion the object should be *to heal*, not to *relieve* for a few moments.

Slight burns—for example, when a hand has been scalded with hot-water of from 180° to 190° Fahr.—heal without any application, in the course of from twenty-four to forty-eight hours; but they take a somewhat longer time to do so if we employ cold water in order to give relief at first. For such slight injuries hardly any remedy is requisite, least of all one like cold water, which delays the cure. But for large severe burns, the best remedies are not so generally known, and the public requires some instruction on that subject; it is in these that cold water especially shews itself to be the most wretched palliative and in some cases the most dangerous remedy that can be conceived. Comparative experiments and observations will, I repeat, convince every one most conclusively, that the exact opposite of cold water is the best remedy for severe burns Thus the experienced cook, who from the nature of his occupation must so often happen to burn himself, and must consequently have learned by experience the remedy for burns, never puts his hand that he has burnt with boiling soup or grease into a jug of cold water (he knows from experience the bad consequences of so doing), no, he holds the burnt spot so near to the hot glow of the incandescent coals, that the burning pain is thereby at first increased, and he holds it for some time in this situation, until, namely, the burning pain becomes considerably diminished and almost entirely removed in this high temperature. He knows, if he does so, that the epidermis will not even rise and form a blister, not to speak of the skin suppurating, but that, on the contrary, after thus bringing his hand near the fire, the redness of the burnt spot, together with the pain, will often disappear in a quarter of an hour; it is healed all at once, quickly and without any after-sufferings, though the remedy was at first disagreeable. To this method he gives decidedly the preference, because he knows from experience that the use of cold water, which at first procures for him a delusive alleviation, will be followed by blisters and suppuration of the part, lasting for days and weeks.

The maker of lackered ware and other workmen who use in their business alcohol and etherial oils, and who have to do with boiling linseed oil, know from experience that the most rapid and permanent way to cure the most severe burns and to get rid of the pain, is to apply to them the best alcohol and oil of turpentine, substances which on a sensitive skin (as that of the mouth, the nose, the eyes) cause a pain of burning like fire, but in cases of burning of the skin (the slightest, more severe, and even the most serious ones) act as a most incomparable[1] remedy. True, they know not the rationale of this cure—they only say, "One bad thing must drive out another"; but this they know from multiplied experience,—that nothing will make the burnt spot painless and cause it to heal without suppurating, except rectified alcohol and oil of turpentine.

Does Professor Dzondi imagine that it would never have oc-curred to these workmen to use cold water as a palliative reme-dy immediately after burning themselves? Any child who had burnt itself would in its alarm fly to cold water; it would not require any advice to do so; but the workman has repeatedly tried it to his own injury, and experience, which in such cases is always purchased at the expense of one's own suffering, has taught and convinced him that the very opposite of cold water is the surest, quickest and truest remedy for even the worst burns: he has been rendered wise by experience, and in all cases he greatly prefers the remedy which at first causes pain (alcohol, oil of turpentine) to that which deludes by instanta-neous relief to the pain (cold water).

Let Professor Dzondi only make upon himself, as he offers to do, one pure comparative experiment, and he will be convinced that he has made a grievous mistake in recommending cold wa-ter as the only sure and best remedy for burns.

Let him plunge both his healthy hands at the same instant into a vessel full of boiling water, and retain them there for from two to three seconds only, and withdraw them both at the same time: they will, as may easily be imagined, be both equal-ly severely scalded, and as the hands belong to one and the same body, if one hand be treated with cold water and the other with alcohol or oil of turpentine, the experiment will furnish a pure comparison and convincing result. This case will not ad-mit of the excuse offered in that of the burns of two different individuals, where the bad consequences that always result when the hand is treated by cold water are sought to be ascribed to impure humours, bad constitution, or some other difference in the one so treated to the one that has been much more easily cured by alcohol. No, let one and the same individual (best of all the professor himself, in order to convince him), scald both

---

[1] Homœopathic.

his hands in the most equal manner before competent witnesses, and then plunge one hand (which we shall call A) into his cold water as often and as long as he pleases, but let him hold the other hand (which we shall call B) uninterruptedly in a vessel full of warmed alcohol, keeping the (covered) vessel constantly warm. In this the burning pain of the hand B rises in a few seconds to double its intensity, but thereafter it will go on diminishing, and in three, six, twelve, or at most twenty-four hours (according to the degree of the burn) it will be completely and for ever removed, but the hand, without the production of any blister, far less of suppuration, will become covered with a brown, hard, painless epidermis, which peels off in a few days, and appears fresh and healthy, clad in its new skin.

But the hand A, which the Professor plunges into cold water as often and as long as he pleases, does not experience the primary increase of pain felt by the hand B; on the contrary, the first instant it is as if in heaven; all the pain of the burn is as if vanished, but—after a few minutes it recommences and increases, and soon becomes intolerably severe, if cold water be not again used for it, when the pains are likewise in the first instants as if extinguished; this amelioration, however, also lasts but a few minutes; they then return even in this colder water, and in a short time increase to greater and greater intensity. If he now puts his severely burnt hand into the coldest snow water, he runs the risk of sphacelus, and yet after a few hours he can find no relief from the pains in water that is less cold. If he now withdraws his ill-treated hand from the water, the pain, instead of being less than it was immediately after the scald, is four and six times greater than it was at first; the hand becomes excessively inflamed, and swells up to a great extent with blisters, and he may now apply cold water, or saturnine lotion, lead ointment, hemp-seed oil, or any other of the ordinary remedies he likes; the hand A, treated in this manner, inevitably turns into a suppurating ulcer, which, treated with these ordinary so-called cooling and soothing remedies, at length heals up, after many weeks or even months (solely by the natural powers of his body), with hideously deformed cicatrices and tedious, agonizing pains.

This is what experience teaches us with respect to burns of any severity.

If Professor Dzondi imagines he knows better than is here stated, if he believes he is certain of the sole curative power of cold water, which he lauds so much, *in all degrees of burns*, then he may confidently undertake to institute the above decisive, purely comparative experiment before competent witnesses. It is only by such an experiment that truth will be brought to light. What risk does he run if his cold water will procure as rapid relief for the hand A as the warm alcohol will for the hand B?

But no! I pity the poor hand; I know very well how it would be! Let the Professor, if he is not quite so sure of the efficacy of cold water in severe burns, perform but a small portion of this experiment, let him dip only two fingers of each hand into boiling water for two or three seconds, and let him treat the fingers of hand A and those of hand B in the way above described, and this little comparative experiment will teach him how wrong he was to recommend to the public as the only, best and efficacious remedy in all degrees of burns, cold water, an agent which, though it is uncommonly soothing in the commencement, is subsequently so treacherous, so extremely noxious. For severe burns he could not advise any thing more injurious than cold water (except perhaps the ointments and oils ordinarily used for burns), and in slighter cases where no blister would rise if left alone, blisters come on when they are treated with the palliative cold water.

In the meantime, before Professor Dzondi can make known the result of this decisive experiment upon himself, it may be useful for the public to know, that one of the greatest surgeons of our times, Benjamin Bell[1] of England, instituted a similar experiment for the instruction of the world, which was almost as pure as the one I have proposed. He made a lady who had scalded both arms, apply to the one oil of turpentine, and plunge the other into cold water. The first arm was well in an hour—but the other continued painful for six hours; if she withdrew it an instant from the water she experienced in it more intense pain, and it required a much longer time for its cure than the first.[2] He therefore recommends, as A. H. Richter[3] had already done, the application of brandy,[4] he also advises

---

[1] Heister already knew and had recommended the treatment of burns by oil of turpentine, which has recently created so much sensation in England: "expeditum quoque hic esse solet terebinthinae oleum; siquidem opportune ac saepius corpori illinatur."

[2] See *Physisch-Medic. Journal*, herausgegeben von Kühn, Leipzig, 1801, Jun., s. 428.

[3] *Ansfangsgr. d. Wundarz.*, Bd. i.

[4] The strongest alcohol heated is much more excellent in burns of various parts,

that the part be kept constantly moistened with it.[1] Kentish[2] also greatly prefers, and that very properly, the spirituous remedies to all others. I shall not adduce the experience confirmatory to this I have myself had.

From all this it appears that Professor Dzondi has made a mistake, and that cold water, far from being a curative agent, is, on the contrary, an obstacle to the cure of slight burns, and occasions a great aggravation of more serious ones, that in the highest degree of such lesions, it even exposes the part to the risk of sphacelus, if the temperature of the water applied be very low (just as warm applications are apt to cause mortification of frost-bitten limbs), and that on the other hand, warm alcohol and oil of turpentine are inestimable, wonderfully rapid, perfectly efficacious, and *genuine remedies* for burns, just as snow is for frost-bitten limbs.

The adherents of the old system of medicine ought not longer to strive against the irresistible efforts towards improvement and perfection that characterizes the spirit of the age. They must see that it is of no use doing so. The accumulated lumber of their eternal palliatives, with their bad results, stands revealed in its nothingness before the light of truth and pure experience.

I know very well that the doctor insinuates himself uncommonly into the affections of his patient, if he procures him a momentary heavenly relief by plunging the seriously burnt part into cold water, unmindful of the evil consequences resulting therefrom, but his conscience would give him a much higher reward than such a deluded patient ever can, if he would give the preference to the treatment with heated alcohol (or oil of turpentine), which is only painful in the first moments, over all traditional pernicious palliatives (cold water, saturnine lotions, burn salves, oils, &c.); if he could be taught by experience and pure comparative experiments, that by the former means alone is all danger of mortification guarded against, and that the patient is thereby cured and relieved of all his sufferings, *often in*

---

even where the epidermis has come off; but in scalds of the whole body (from which no one ever recovered under the usual mode of treatment with cold water, saturnine lotions, burn-salves, or oils, all died generally within four days), we must content ourselves with ordinary spirits made very warm, or at least commence the treatment for the first hours with this, and constantly renew this warm application, keeping the patient warmly wrapped up in bed. Of all conceivable modes of treatment this is the best.

[1] Benjamin Bell's *System of Surgery*, Vol. v.
[2] On *Burns*, London, 1797.

less than a hundredth part of the time required for the cure by cold water, saturnine lotions, salves and oils.

So also the girl heated by dancing to the highest degree of fever, and tormented by uncontrollable thirst, finds the greater refreshment for the first few moments from exposure to a draught of air, and from drinking a glass of ice cold water, until she is taught by the speedy occurrence of a dangerous or even fatal illness, that it is not what affords us the greatest gratification for the first few moments that is for our real welfare, but that, like the pleasant cup of sin, it is fraught with evil, often with ruin and death.

ADDITION TO THE FOREGOING ARTICLE.[1]

When ancient errors that should justly sink into oblivion are attempted to be palmed off upon the world anew, he who knows better ought not to neglect to publish his convictions, and thereby to consign the pernicious error to its proper ignominious place, and to exalt the true and the salutary to its right position for the welfare of mankind. It was this idea that guided me in No. 156 of this Journal,[2] where I displayed the inestimable advantages of warm spirituous fluids for the rapid and permanent healing of *extensive burns*, over cold water, which only alleviates for an instant, but whose results are extremely pernicious.

The most convincing tests of the relative value of these two opposite methods, viz., the *curative* (the really healing) method, (the employment of warm spirituous fluids, such as alcohol or oil of turpentine), and the *palliative* (alleviating) method, (the use of cold water, &c.), are furnished *firstly*, by pure comparative experiments, where burns of two limbs of the same body are simultaneously treated, the one by the one method, the other by the other; *secondly*, by the expressed convictions of the most unprejudiced and honourable physicians. One single such authority, who, knowing the worthlessness as facts of the favourite pre-conceived notions of the age, dispossesses his mind of them, and, rejecting the old pernicious errors from genuine conviction, is not afraid to claim for truth its merited station, is worth thousands of prejudiced upholders and combatants for the opposite.

Thousands of over hasty advocates of the pernicious employ-

---

[1] From the *Allgem. Anzeiger der Deutschen.* No. 204. 1816.
[2] [See above.]

ment of cold water in serious burns, must hold their peace before the expressed convictions of that most upright of practical physicians, Thomas Sydenham, who despising the prejudiced opinion that has prevailed universally from Galen's time till now, *morbi contrariis curentur* (therefore cold water for burns), and influenced by his convictions and by truth alone, thus expresses himself:[1] *As an application in burns, alcohol bears the bell from all other remedies that have ever been discovered,* for it effects a most rapid cure. Lint dipped in alcohol and applied, immediately after the injury, to any part of the body that shall have been scalded with hot water or singed by gunpowder, will do this, provided that as long as the pain lasts the spirit be renewed; after that, only twice a-day will suffice." Let him who can prove this to be false come forward!

Or, who can contradict one of the best and most enlightened practical surgeons of our time, Benjamin Bell, when from his extensive experience he alleges:[2] "*One of the best applications to every burn of this kind is strong brandy,* or any other ardent spirit; it seems to induce a momentary additional pain, but this soon subsides and is succeeded by an agreeable soothing sensation. It proves most effectual when the parts can be kept immersed in it; but where this cannot be done, they should be kept constantly moist with pieces of old linen soaked in spirits."

Kentish, who, as a practitioner in Newcastle, had to treat the workmen who were often fearfully burnt in the coal pits, considers very carefully in his book[3] all the claims preferred in favour of cold water and all other cooling remedies for burns, and he finds as the result of all his experience, contrary to the great prejudice he felt in favour of these long used things, that under their use no single person who had got a severe burn on a great part of his body ever recovered, but that all were cured who

---

[1] *Opera.* Lipsiae, 1695, p. 343, (Edit. Syd. Soc. p. 255). "Ambustis extus (admovendus), quo casu omnibus remediis, quotquot adhuc inventa fuere, hic liquor (spiritus vini) facile palmam praeripit, cum curationem quam cito absolvat;—nempe si lintea spiritu vini imbuta partibus ab aqua fervente, pulvere pyris, vel simili laesis, quam primum hoc infligitur malum, applicentur, eademque dicto spiritu madefacta subinde repetantur, donec dolor ab igne penitus evanuerit, et postea solum bis in die." That cold external applications to burnt parts render them liable to increase of pains, that such parts soon become altogether painless from the application of external heat as he had often witnessed, is testified by the great observer, John Hunter, in his work *On the blood and inflammation,* p. 218.

[2] *System of Surgery,* 3rd Edit. Vol. v.

[3] *On Burns,* London and Newcastle, 1797, two Essays

were treated by the speediest possible application and frequent renewal of hot turpentine.

But no proof for the truth of this can be so strong as that which is afforded by comparative experiments performed simultaneously on one and the same body. In my former paper I cited the case of a lady who got both her arms burnt, one of which was treated by Bell with cold water, but the other was kept covered with oil of turpentine; in the first the pains persisted for a much longer time and a much greater period was required for the cure than in the last, which was treated with the volatile oil.

Another experiment of not less convincing character is related by John Anderson.[1] A lady scalded her face and right arm with boiling grease; the face was very red, very much scalded, and the seat of violent pains; the arm she had plunged into a jug full of cold water. In the course of a few minutes oil of turpentine was applied to the face. For her arm she desired to continue the use of the cold water for some hours, because it had formerly been of service to her in burns (she could not say whether those had been more severe or less so than the present one). In the course of seven hours her face looked much better and was relieved. In the meantime she had often renewed the cold water for the arm, but whenever she withdrew it she complained of much pain, and *in truth the inflammation in it had increased. The following morning I found that she had suffered great pain in the arm during the night; the inflammation had extended above the elbow, several large blisters had risen, and thick eschars had formed on the arm and hand. The face on the contrary was completely free from pain, had no blisters,* and only a little of the epidermis had become detached. The arm had to be dressed *for a fortnight* with emollient remedies before it was cured."

Who can read these honest observations of illustrious men without being satisfied of the much superior healing power of the application of spirituous fluids to that of cold water, which affords a delusive alleviation, but delays the cure?

I shall not, therefore, adduce my own very extensive experience to the same effect. Were I even to add a hundred such comparative observations, could they prove more plainly, strongly, and convincingly than is done by these two cases, that (warm) spirituous fluids possess an inestimable advantage over the transiently alleviating cold water in the case of severe burns?

---

[1] *Kentish's second essay on burns,* p. 43.

How instructing and consoling, then, for mankind is the truth that is to be deduced from these facts: *that for serious and for the most severe injuries from burning, though cold water is very hurtful for them, spirituous applications (warm alcohol or oil of turpentine) are highly beneficial and capable of saving many lives.*

These proofs will serve to guide the great numbers of mankind who require help, to the only effectual method, to the only health bringing (*sanative*) remedy, without which, in the case of extensive burns (that is where the greater part of the surface of the body has been scalded or burnt), delivery from death and recovery is perfectly impossible, and has never been witnessed.

This one single, and, as I have imagined, not unworthy object of my essay, was evidently not perceived by Professor Dzondi, as is proved by his violent letters to me; he only perceives in my remarks an attack upon his opinion. It is a matter of very little interest to me to find that cold water which has already been recommended ninety-nine times by others for burns, from a predilection in favour of this palliative whose effects are so injurious, is now served up to us again for the hundredth time, and I should feel ashamed to make use of a Journal so useful in promoting the happiness of the people as this is, for the purposes of merely personal recrimination and discussion. Moreover, as in the article I allude to I advised him to convince himself of the truth of my assertions by an experiment upon himself, my object was thereby to inform every one of the conditions necessary to be observed in order to constitute a really convincing pure experiment of this kind.

I avail myself of this opportunity to expose the disadvantage of cold water (and other ordinary palliatives) in the treatment of *serious* burns, and call the attention of the public to the only effectual remedies, warm spirituous fluids, in order that they may avail themselves of them in the hour of need. This is not any mere idea of my own, but it has been clearly *proved* and irrefragably demonstrated by the observations of the most honourable and illustrious men of our profession (Sydenham, Heister, B. Bell, J. Hunter, Kentish), and especially by the convincing comparative experiments of Bell and Anderson.

I shall only observe further, that the burnt parts must be kept moistened *uninterruptedly* with the warm spirituous fluid, *e. g.* warm alcohol, for which end the linen rags soaked in it should first be simply laid upon the injured parts, and then, in order to prevent evaporation, and to keep all warm, covered with pieces of woollen cloth or sheepskin. If a very large portion of the surface of the body is burnt, then some one will be obliged to devote himself entirely and constantly to the external care of the patient, removing the pieces of cloth or skin one by one, and pouring with a spoon warm alcohol (or oil of turpentine) over the linen rags upon the skin (without removing them), then as soon as they are dry, covering up the part and going on to others, so that when the last part has been moistened and covered up, it is time to commence again with the first part, which, in the case of such a volatile fluid as warm alcohol, has in the meantime generally become dry. This process must be continued day and night unremittingly, for which purpose the person engaged in performing it must be changed every two hours for a fresh one. The chief benefit, especially in severe and very serious injuries from burns, depends on what is done within the first twenty-four hours, or in the worst cases, the first forty-eight hours, that is, until all trace of the pain of the burn is permanently removed. A basin should be at hand containing very hot water, which should be frequently renewed, in which some vessels full of alcohol should stand, of which the attendant takes out the warmest for the purpose of wetting the rags, whilst the rest stand in the basin in order to remain sufficiently warm, so that there never shall be a want of warm alcohol for the purpose of pouring on the rags. If the parts of the body on which the patient is obliged to lie are also burnt, the rags, dipped in warm alcohol, should be applied to them at the commencement, and a layer of water-proof cloth spread underneath; these parts can subsequently be wetted from above without being removed. If the greater part of the body is burnt, the first application must only consist of warm brandy, in order to spare the first shock to the patient, which is the worst, the second wetting should be performed with stronger alcohol, and afterwards the very strongest alcohol may be used. And as this operation must be continued uninterruptedly during the night, the precaution must be used of keeping the candle (or lantern) at a good distance, otherwise the warm spirituous vapour rising from the skin might readily catch fire, and prove destructive to the patient.

If the burn has been effected with gunpowder, the small black particles should not be picked out of the skin before all traces of the pain of the burn are permanently removed.

ON THE VENEREAL DISEASE AND ITS ORDINARY IMPROPER TREATMENT.[1]

As long as the defects of the constitutions of countries put difficulties in the way of matrimony, as long as celibacy shall be considered fashionable and marriage as a political yoke, in place of being regarded as the most honourable connexion of the two sexes for their mutual moral and physical perfection, but especially for the development of the really human and of the divine and immortal in them; as long as the notable difference of both sexes shall be viewed merely as an object of sensuality, and nothing more dignified is seen in a union with the opposite sex than a mere animal copulation, and not a mutual communication and fusion of the excellencies of both to constitute a more noble whole, so long will the all-powerful and sexual passion thus unnaturally separated from moral duty seek its gratification in the arms of common prostitution, and as a necessary consequence not fail to contract the destructive lues, and so long is the extinction of such a communicable virus not to be thought of.

It is the duty of the physician to cure patients ill of this disease who trust themselves to his care, as the object of medicine (like that of legislation) is not so much the prevention of the evils incident to humanity as the correction of those which exist. Medicine should therefore prove itself to be really the helpful art it professes to be in this disgraceful and destructive malady, if it would act up to its pretensions. Its services should be rendered with all the more facility and certainty in this case, as the venereal disease is one of those happy few that remain always the same with respect both to their origin and nature (and consequently cannot be mistaken at its commencement), and the specific remedy for which (*mercury*) was discovered by a lucky hit in domestic practice shortly after the invasion of the disease, now 323 years ago. We might therefore have expected that physicians would at all events in this disease have acted judiciously, and in this long period of time have learned the way to cure this disease radically, easily and permanently, although their treatment of all other diseases might have remained, as indeed it has, mere subjective and objective delusion; which might to a certain extent be excused, since almost all

---

[1] From the *Allgem. Anz. d. D.*, No. 211, 1816.

other diseases differ so widely from each other and among themselves, and the appropriate remedy for each several case remained an eternal problem until homœopathy solved it.

But no! physicians have mistaken even this so easily cognizable venereal disease, and a fallacious and pernicious treatment of it is the consequence of this mistake. Up to this hour almost all the physicians of the habitable globe, in Pekin as in Paris and Philadelphia, in London as in Vienna, in Petersburg as in Berlin, have bungled the venereal disease from its commencement, and *have regarded the local removal of the chancre as the main point of the treatment of syphilis, and the simultaneous employment of mercury as a mere accessory;* and it is publicly taught that if the chancre have existed but for a few days, its mere local destruction is all the treatment required.[1] And yet there can be nothing more inappropriate, nothing more pernicious than this procedure.

I shall in the first place show its inappropriateness. The analogy with other miasmatic exanthematous diseases would lead us to infer that the venereal disease arises only by infection by means of corporeal contact. Now all infectious diseases have this character in common, that on the part of the body where the virus was first applied, at first no alteration is perceptible, although the inoculation may have taken place. If we scrape off the epidermis on a child's arm till we come to the sensitive cutis vera, and rub thereon either the matter of small-pox or the lymph of cow-pox, for the first five days there will be no change at all perceptible on this spot; it is only after the fourth day in the case of cow-pox inoculation, and much later in that of small-pox inoculation, that a change begins to appear on the inoculated spot, and it is only on the seventh day that the perfect cow-pox vesicle is formed on this spot, amid febrile symptoms, and the small-pox pustule on the twelfth or fourteenth day. *Neither of them appears before the internal infection and*

---

[1] The boldest propounders of this erroneous doctrine were Girtanner and A. F. Hecker. The former says (*Treatise on the venereal disease*, Göttingen, 1803, p. 215), "Recent chancres must be only locally cured, burnt or driven off. The poison must be destroyed at the commencement on its seat, for then it has not yet had time to be absorbed"(?)—and Hecker roundly asserts (*On the venereal disease*, 2d edition p. 67), "In the chancre the poison lies as it were out of the system," "therefore it yields (p. 180) to a mere external treatment (by desiccative and corrosive remedies) *without any ill effects*" (?), and if it date from not more than twelve days (p. 182), it must "only be treated with external, local means." Almost all other authors incline to the same opinion, though they do not express themselves so distinctly—Hunter, Bell, Schwediaur, &c.

development of this disease is completed in the system. So it is with the measles and other acute exanthematous diseases: namely, the part whereon the infecting virus was first brought does not produce the eruption peculiar to each disease, before the whole organism has undergone a change and is completely infected. And on the other hand, the perfect production of the specific eruption is an infallible proof of the completed internal infection and development of the miasmatic disease in every case. The cow-pox prevails throughout the body as soon as the cow-pox vesicle is produced in its perfect form with its red, hard areola, at the part where it was first introduced, and so it is with other inoculable diseases. But from the moment when the miasm has taken, and the whole living organism has become aware of (has perceived) the presence of its action, the poison is no longer only local at the point of inoculation; a complete infection would still occur, even though the seat of inoculation should be cut out. At the very moment when the inoculation has taken, the first general attack on the system has occurred, and the full development of the disease is in all probability not to be avoided by the destruction of the inoculated part.

In the case of the bite of the mad dog, where the system was predisposed to be affected by the miasm,[1] we possess undeniable observations to show that even cutting out[2] and removing the bitten part does not afford any protection from the occurrence of hydrophobia.

Small-pox would still be developed, even though at the moment the inoculation was effected the inoculated part were cut out.

So far is the miasm from remaining local when once it has been inoculated in the body. When that has taken place, the complete infection of the whole system and the gradual development of the miasmatic disease in the interior cannot be prevented by any local treatment.

But the disease can only be considered as completely de-

---

[1] For in many of those bitten by the rabid dog the poison does not infect; of twenty persons bitten, usually from eighteen to nineteen escape without injury, even though they do not use any antidote whatever. Hence the undeserved recommendation of so many pretended preventitive remedies; they may all easily protect, if the poison has not taken in those bitten, as is so often the case.

[2] A girl of eight years old, in Scotland, was bit by a mad dog on the 21st of March, 1792; a surgeon immediately cut the piece clean out (kept it suppurating and gave mercury till slight salivation was produced), and, notwithstanding, hydrophobia broke out, and death followed the fortieth day after the bite.—The new London Medical Journal, Vol. ii.

veloped in the whole organism when the perfect pock has appeared on the seat of inoculation.

Thus the miasmatic exanthematous diseases indicate their completion in the interior by the occurrence of one or more shut boils of smaller or greater size.

Thus the pustula maligna appears on the part that has been touched (some four days previously) by the blood of a cow which has died of malignant anthrax, and in like manner the cow-pock or small-pock appears generally and primarily on the part inoculated or its vicinity, and the same is the case with the itch of wool-manufacturers.

The last-named disease belongs to the chronic exanthematous diseases (like the venereal disease), and in it nature also produces the itch vesicles, at first in the neighbourhood of the part that was originally touched by the itch-virus, *e. g.*, betwixt the fingers and on the wrist, if the hands (palms) were first infected. As soon as the itch vesicles have made their appearance this is a sign that the internal itch-disease is already fully developed. For at first there is actually no morbid change observable on the infected part, no itching, no itch-vesicles. Usually from nine to twelve or fourteen days after the application of the itch-virus there occurs, along with a slight fever, which is not noticed by many persons, the eruption of the first itch vesicle—nature requires this time, in order to complete the full infection, that is to say, the development of the itch-disease in the interior throughout the organism. The itch-vesicles that now appear are hence no mere local malady, but a proof of the completion of the internal disease. The itch-miasm, as soon as it has contaminated the hand, remains no longer local the instant it has caused inoculation, but proceeds to alter the interior of the organism and to develop itself into this peculiar disease until the entire infection is accomplished, and then only (after several days) does the eruption produced by the internal malady appear on the skin, and that at first in the vicinity of the original point of infection. These itch-vesicles are an abnormal organ produced by the inner organism upon the skin, designed by nature to be the external substitute of the internal disease, to take the latter upon itself, to absorb it as it were, and so to keep it subdued, slumbering and latent. That this is the case is evident from this, that so long as the vesicles remain on the skin and continue to itch and discharge, the internal disease cannot make its appearance, and from this also, that whenever it is partially destroyed on the skin, without any previous cure being effected of the internal itch disease (especially if it be of somewhat long standing and have attained to any extent) by means of the internal employment of its specific remedy, *sulphur*, this internal disease then bursts forth rapidly, often in a frightful manner, in the form of phthisis, asthma, insanity, dropsy, apoplexy, amaurosis, paralysis, and it not unfrequently occasions sudden death.

A very similar process is observed in the case of the *venereal disease*. On the spot where the venereal virus was first rubbed in (*e. g.* during an impure coitus), for the first days, in like manner, nothing morbid is observable. The virus has indeed first come in contact with the living fibres at that part, but at the moment that the inoculation has taken place, that is, when the living body has felt (perceived) the presence and action of the poison, that same moment it is no longer only local, it is already the property of the whole organism. From that instant the specific (venereal) alteration in the interior advances onwards until the venereal disease has completely developed itself in the interior, and it is only then, that nature, oppressed by the internal malady, produces the abnormal organ, *the chancre*, which it has formed for the purpose of keeping in subjection the internal disease, in the neighbourhood of the part primarily infected.[1] In the neighbourhood, I say, for it does not always arise on the seat of the primary application of the virus, it sometimes appears on the scrotum, &c., sometimes, though more rarely, only in the groin, in the form of inguinal bubo, which is also a kind of chancre.

In order to subdue and form a substitute for the internal venereal constitutional disease, nature produces the chancre; for as I have seen, chancres remaining untouched for as long as two or three years (certainly enlarging gradually in that time), do not permit the more general venereal disease to break out. As long as the chancre remains uninterfered with, no venereal affection, no symptoms of syphilis are to be met with on any other part of the body.

It is very probable that the infection during impure coitus takes place in the first seconds, and then no washing or cleansing of the genitals is of any avail, nature from that time proceeds uninterruptedly in her course, altering the whole internal organism in the manner peculiar to this disease. But from the

---

[1] At first as a vesicle, which increases in a few hours and grows into an ulcer with a hard base.

moment of the primary local infection, nature requires in our days, several, usually seven, ten or fourteen days, not unfrequently three weeks, there are even some instances of its requiring five, six, seven or eight weeks before it has completed the development of the venereal malady in the interior, and it is only then, as a sign of the completed internal general venereal disease, that the chancre appears on the skin, and this chancre, the evidence of the now internal affection, is designed by nature to assume, as it were, the palliative office of substitution, relieving and keeping in subjection the latter.

For the first thirty or forty years after the occurrence of the venereal disease, that is, from the year 1493 until the first third of the following century, this infecting virus was much worse than it is now; nature then strove much longer before it allowed the completion of the general internal disease in the organism; often several months elapsed after the local infection before the chancre then burst forth. At that time too, the opposing action of the body and the general ill state of health before its appearance, as the signs of the development of the venereal disease going on in the interior, were much more distinct and striking[1] than now-a-days, when the infecting virus is much milder. The venereal disease pursues the same course even yet, for since that period it has only decreased in violence, but its nature is not altered. Even at the present day there is, immediately after the infection, absolutely nothing abnormal to be perceived on the spot: the change only goes on in the interior, and a general feeling of illness is felt by sensitive individuals for some days or weeks, until the thorough alteration of the organism is effected by the venereal poison, and it is only after this that the chancre is produced by nature on the suitable spot, and is the infallible sign of the perfect development of the venereal disease in the entire organism, and the silencer of the internal malady. After the breaking out of the chancre the previous feelings of debility and fatigue, the dulness of the sensorium

---

[1] Passing over the testimony of several physicians of that time, such as C. Torella, N. Massa, A. Ferro, P. Hanschard, I would merely refer to the description in *Luisini Collectio script. de morbo gallico*, Venet. 1566, t. i, given by H. Frascatorius at p. 163 and 173, and by Fallopius at p. 667, of the sufferings of those then infected before the outbreak of the chancre (then called *caries*), and it is astonishing to find how generally ill and miserable the infected crawled about for months, without the slightest change being observable on their genital organs, until at length after the internal development of the venereal disease was completed, the chancre burst forth in full fury, and the general state of ill health moderated, and, as it were, retired.

commune, the depression ot the spirits, the earthy complexion with blue borders round the eyes, &c., go off. The internal venereal disease then remains as it were enchained (latent) and concealed, and can never break out as syphilis, as long as its external substitute and silencer remains uninterfered with on its seat; but when the in-dwelling venereal disease is completely destroyed and cured by the sole internal employment of the best mercurial preparation, then the chancre heals up of itself without the aid of the slightest external remedy; if however it is driven off by external means, without curing the internal malady, the latter inevitably bursts forth in the form of syphilis.

From a consideration of this mode of the production and of this nature of the venereal disease, and of this true signification of the chancre, which are founded on incontrovertible observations, what plan of treatment of this disease would suggest itself to any person endowed with common sense? Certainly none other—for I have a high idea of sound unprejudiced common sense—than the following: "*Treat the venereal affection of the whole system by the best internal remedy until it is completely eradicated, that is to say, until the thoroughly cured organism no longer requires any virulent chancre, any external silencer and substitute for the now annihilated internal venereal disease, and from the period of the completed internal cure, it must become a healthy ulcer, without any assistance from without, and rapidly heal up of its own accord, without leaving behind the slightest trace of its previous existence.*"[1]

Thus, I imagined, plain common sense would advise and carefully warn against meddling with the chancre by any local application, either before or during the internal treatment, that might cause its premature disappearance, for it is the only certain sign of the indwelling venereal disease, and it only can, by its persistence, infallibly demonstrate to the patient and to the physician, that the cure of the disease throughout the organism is not completed, whilst on the other hand, by its perfect spontaneous healing under the internal exhibition of mercury (without the employment of any sort of external remedy), it gives the most irrefragable proof that the cure is completed, and that nature

---

[1] It is worthy of remark that any chancre burnt off without the preliminary cure of the internal disease, always leaves behind it a certain amount of redness and hardness as long as the virus in the interior is not destroyed; a bubo must then occur in its stead, which assumes the office of substitution, and keeps the internal affection in abeyance.

no longer requires this substitutive organ for an in-dwelling venereal malady, since it has been completely healed and annihilated by the medicine given internally.

But as experience moreover incontrovertibly teaches us, that when the chancre is driven off by local means, and nature is thus deprived of the silencer and substitute of the internal venereal disease by external desiccative or corrosive applications, it then *invariably* happens that either an inguinal bubo soon occurs, or after a few months the general venereal disease (syphilis) breaks out; we might have imagined, that physicians would have had the sense to perceive the importance of preserving the chancre inviolate, and without disturbing it by any external remedy whatsoever, have made it their duty to employ only internal treatment, with the best antivenereal medicine, until the system was completely cured of this disease.

But no!—In spite of all these loud speaking facts, proving the true nature and signification of the chancre, almost all the physicians and surgeons of the habitable globe have gone on regarding it as a purely local and at first insignificant ulcer confined to the outer surface of the skin, and have exerted themselves to dry it up and destroy it by local means as rapidly as possible, and have even considered this destruction of the chancre as the chief object of their treatment, just as though the venereal disease proceeded from it (the chancre) as its source, just as if the chancre were the originator and producer of the venereal disease; whereas it is only an evidence of the fully developed internal malady, which they might have inferred from this, that the consequence of the local destruction of a chancre [1] performed ever so early, and even on the very first day of its appearance, was always a subsequent breaking out of syphilis; and they might also have learned this from the incontrovertible experience, that not a single patient escapes syphilis if his chancre have been only locally destroyed.[2]

---

[1] John Hunter's *Treatise on the venereal disease,* p. 551—553 (Leipzic edition).

[2] Hunter, op. cit., 531. "Not one patient out of fifty will escape syphilis if the chancre be only locally destroyed."—So says Fabre also (*Lettres, supplement à son traité des maladies veneriennes,* Paris, 1786)—"A chancre always causes syphilis if it be only treated with external remedies." Let it not be supposed that these local irritating corrosive remedies caused a recession of the virus from the chancre into the interior of the body, and thus produced the syphilis. No! a chancre destroyed locally without employing any irritant remedies, produces the same result. "Petit (so says Fabre, loc. cit.) excised a portion of the nymphæ of a woman on which some chancres had existed for some days; the wound healed, it is true, but the syphilis

Now, as the in-dwelling venereal malady can never break out as long as the chancre, undisturbed by external applications, remains on its seat (however long it remains there) and as the venereal disease at every period, whether it has broken out as syphilis or betrays its hidden existence merely by the presence of the chancre (or the bubo) can *only* be radically cured [1] by the use of (the best preparation of) mercury (when the chancre heals up spontaneously without the aid of external remedies) I would ask if it be not very foolish, nay, sinful, to destroy the chancre by external desiccative and corrosive applications, seeing that thereby, not only is no part of the venereal disease removed, but we deprive ourselves of this conclusive sign of a perfect or imperfect cure, which should be our guide during an internal mercurial treatment: nay, more, what is much worse, we even cause the outbreak of the syphilis, which had hitherto continued to lie latent and enchained in the interior, and as long as the chancre existed could never burst forth, but would have been for ever healed and destroyed had we medicinally treated the disease solely by the use of the internal remedy, whilst the chancre still existed until its cure was completed, that is to say, until the chancre had disappeared without the aid of an external remedy !

"But," say these medical men, "we give mercury internally whilst we dry up or burn off the chancre." [2]

I would ask—in a sufficient or insufficient manner? (It must have been insufficient if the syphilis, as usually happens, breaks out afterwards.)

"Oh, we give it in a sufficient manner," they reply.

Possibly: but how can they tell during their treatment whether their internally administered mercury sufficed for the cure, as it is only the healing of the chancre that has remained untouched, under the influence of internal remedies alone, that can give us the sole certain proof thereof; but the chancre has been burnt off by them before or during the treatment.

---

broke out notwithstanding." And this might naturally have been expected, as the venereal disease exists completely in the body before the chancre appears, and is only prevented bursting forth by the presence of the chancre on the skin.

[1] Fritze *On the venereal disease*, Berlin, 1790, and Sam. Hahnemann, *Instruction for surgeons respecting venereal diseases.* Leipzig, 1789, § 273—284, 290—293, 614, 635, [vide antea, p. 72, et seq.] wherewith, although they contradict themselves, the other better writers agree, as Schwediaur, Hunter, Bell.

[2] The worst kind of physicians advise nothing more to be done than destroying the chancre, *e. g.* Girtanner, *Treatise on the venereal disease.* Göttingen, 1803, p. 215, and Hecker, *On the venereal disease.* 2d edit. pp. 67, 180, 182.

Had their employment of mercury sufficed for the perfect cure of the internal venereal disease, they had not needed to burn off the chancre, this would and must have disappeared [1] at the same time that the internal malady was eradicated without the simultaneous employment of any external remedy whatever!

But it is just because they know that their internal treatment does not suffice for the extirpation of the internal malady, consequently also not for the spontaneous healing of the chancre; it is just for this reason, that they burn off the chancre to give their treatment the superficial appearance of having cured everything (the poor patient is deceived; he cannot help believing himself to be cured); they give at the same time—if they wish to do the thing thoroughly—mercury internally without knowing (since the chancre, the guiding sign, is gone) how much or how long they require to give it, [2] and this they do under the idea that even though the patient may not be thereby thoroughly cured, they have at least advanced the treatment of the disease as far as it will go.

But this is a mere delusion. For they torment the patient by burning off his chancre, which is of no use, but is of the greatest injury, as it is certainly followed by the breaking out of syphilis, and they at the same time harass him by giving him an indefinite quantity of mercury by the mouth without avail. For the venereal disease cannot be half or three quarters cured; it must either be quite cured (and in that case not a trace of it is left), or it is not at all cured; even though it be treated until it is almost cured (but not perfectly eradicated) it is *not at all* cured; what has been done for it is equivalent to nothing, for in the course of time it infallibly spreads round about again and reaches

---

[1] See Fritze and Hahnemann, *op. cit.*

[2] They often attempt to justify themselves by saying that they pushed the internal administration of mercury until the appearance of the mercurial fever, whereby they obtained a certainty of cure being effected. But what do they usually call mercurial fever? Something that is not the least like it, and that affords no proof whatever of an internal cure; looseness and falling out of the teeth, ulceration of the mouth, swelling of the cheek and neck, violent pains in the belly, salivation? No! not every violent assault with useless mercurial preparations as is now the fashion (calomel with or without opium) can deserve that appellation; these remedies very seldom produce that peculiar febrile state which can still serve as the sign of the internal cure, when some mischievous hand has burnt off the still more convincing chancre. It is only the purest, most perfect, and hence most efficacious sesquioxyde of mercury that produces it in venereal diseases, whereby the chancre (if it be still present) spontaneously heals without the aid of an external remedy, shewing that the internal disease has been completely eradicated.

the same extent and again plants itself just as firmly as if nothing at all had been done for it.

Therefore what is the certain consequence of this local drying-up and often very tedious, often very painful burning off of the chancre, whereby a portion of the genital organ is destroyed, and of the blind employment of internal mercurial remedies? That the patient is deceived into believing himself cured, and that his lesser evil (chancre with latent internal venereal disease) is changed into a greater! Now, either a bubo (a now much more troublesome substitute for the indwelling venereal disease) or (where no bubo has appeared, or if it have, has been driven off again) after a few (3, 4, 6, 9) months syphilis breaks forth.

And if, after it has broken out, (as it inevitably must if the patients were not assailed with unhelpful mercurial preparations so violently that there was a struggle betwixt life and death, when if they did not go the way of all flesh, some few of them were thereby freed from their venereal disease) the physician be asked if the ulcers on the tonsils, the bluish pimples on the face, extending even into the hairy scalp, the round copper-coloured spots on the skin, &c. be not remains of the venereal disease that was thought to be cured, he usually seeks to get out of the scrape by alleging: "That he certainly had thoroughly cured him on the former occasion, there was then nothing more to be seen about him" (he had burnt off the chancre and removed from sight the proof of the existence of the indwelling disease; this he calls a cure)—"the patient must certainly have caught a fresh infection during these four, six, or nine months, whence this venereal ulceration of the throat, &c. has arisen."

Thus the poor betrayed sufferers must, in addition to their misfortune, bear the doctor's disgrace, because they knew not how syphilis can and must arise.

It can only proceed from the uncured indwelling venereal disease, whose external substitute and suppresser (the chancre, which, as long as it exists undisturbed, prevents the outbreak of the syphilis) has been destroyed locally by the physician, and can consequently no longer hinder its outbreak; and even though our patient may be conscious of having had several suspicious connexions since the removal of his former chancre, but got no chancre therefrom, yet he has not been infected anew, and the syphilis that has broken out must be derived indisputably from the chancre that was formerly burnt off, consequently from the bad treatment of his former venereal disease. For it has never occurred that syphilis has been produced without a previous (destroyed) chancre, [1] there is no authentic instance on record of such a case having happened.

Did the patients, whose syphilitic symptoms the physician attributes to a new infection, know this, they having in the meantime contracted no fresh chancre (which has been driven away), they would know how to reply to the physician when he tries to transfer his disgrace upon them, whose treatment he has bungled.

But as patients are ignorant on this subject, they alone have to bear the injury and the disgrace; the doctor subjects them to a new course of mercury, and if this be not pushed by him to a much more violent and serious extent than the former one during the destruction of the chancre was—if, I say, the patient be not assailed until his life is endangered with the ordinary un-serviceable mercurial preparations, a radical cure of the disease will not be effected even with this second course; the patient gets rid of his ulcers in the throat for example (for each of the primary symptoms of syphilis is easily removed even by small quantities of a bad mercurial remedy, whereby the disease is not radically cured) but after a few, or after many months, a new syphilitic symptom appears in their stead—and after a third and a fourth similar, imperfect mercurial treatment, a third and a fourth affection appear in succession, and at length the affections of the joints and the agonizing nocturnal pains in the bones, for which the useless mercurials, decoctions of woods and baths are no longer of any avail; and the patient is left in the lurch, that is to say, to suffer his tortures.

Thus, from an insignificant primary malady (for the original venereal disease still accompanied by chancre may be readily cured by the internal use of the best mercurial preparations), there arises a sucession of sufferings and morbid alterations of many years' duration, often on account of the health-destroying treatments attended with danger to life, and all this—*from the original local destruction of the chancre* which was designed by the beneficent Creator to be the constant preventive of the breaking forth of the syphilitic malady and the sure monitor of the physician as to whether the internal treatment is complete (if it heals up of itself), or the disease is not yet radically cured (if it remains unaltered on its seat).

---

[1] Hunter, op. cit. p. 487, says: " Probably not in one case out of 5 0," *i. e.* in no case.

42

It is only by the discretion of the patients themselves that physicians can ultimately be improved. Let every one that is infected immediately dismiss the physician who wishes to commence the distructive plan with him, of treating the chancre by local remedies, though he bestow on the remedy he would employ externally the mildest and most seductive of names, even though he should call it cooling, sedative, alleviating, emollient, relaxing, descutient, purifying or healing; all these fine appellations serve but to disguise the enemy. The chancre, being the most important witness of what takes place within, must on no account be touched or treated with any kind of external remedies by whatevernames they may be called.[1] The patient ought only to be allowed to wash the genitals occasionally with tepid river-water or warm cow's milk.

On the contrary, let him choose a physician, who, fully alive to the extreme importance of the chancre, leaves this quite alone, and understands how to conduct the internal treatment alone in a masterly way; that is to say, eradicate it by means of the best mercurial preparation that is capable of doing so, given internally without the production of salivation, in such a manner that the chancre heals up of its own accord, without the aid of the slightest external remedy.

Then and then only can the patient be sure that his disease is cured.

The best mercurial preparation for effecting this, is the dark-coloured pure sesquioxide of mercury, of which a small portion rubbed with a drop of water on the palm of the hand by means of the point of the finger, runs into minute globules of metallic mercury which are observable either with the naked eye or with a lens. My mode of preparing it will be found in many books. This only is the most innocuous and most powerful preparation wherewith the venereal disease of all degrees may be cured,

---

[1] And should the patent have allowed himself to be seduced and have permitted the external driving off of his chancre, and should there arise, as usually happens, in the place of it a bubo, let him remember that this has the same significance as the chancre, and is a substitute for the internal malady, and that if allowed to stay there undisturbed it also prevents the outbreak of the syphilis. Therefore he should not allow this at least to be driven off by external remedies (inunctions of the blue ointment beneath the bubo, called *frictions*, and the application of many other things which physicians term *resolving* the bubo), for after a few months the syphilis follows inevitably; but he should rather let himself be only treated by the best mercurial preparation, only inwardly, until the bubo, without the aid of external remedies and without frictions, disappears spontaneously when the internal malady is cured; and it is only thus that be can be certain of his complete recovery.

witnout salivation, if the general state of the patient's health be not very much broken up and weakened.

If, however, the patient have been mistreated by a physician by having his chancre or the subsequent bubo driven off by external remedies, and the syphilis have consequently broken out; if it be already present, after several long-continued, fruitless treatments with bad mercurial preparations, in a high degree, the general health that has been ruined by such violent treatment must first be restored, and the accesssory ailments usually present must first be removed before the master in his art can employ even the best mercurial preparation to effect the perfect cure.

In such master-pieces of treatment, where the malady has taken such deep roots, and the chancre having been previously driven off serves no more as a loadstar; there is nothing to shew that the treatment has accomplished a perfect cure, but the closest observation for the arrival of the period, when, after the complete restoration of the patient, some fresh symptoms present themselves that are only peculiar to the action of mercury, but which are quite new to the patient in the course of his venereal complaint, and have scarcely ever been experienced before, but among which neither salivation, nor toothache, nor ulcers of the mouth, nor pains in the bowels, nor diarrhœa are to be found.

NOTA BENE FOR MY REVIEWERS.[1]

I have read several false criticisms on the second part of my *Pure Materia Medica*, especially on the essay at the beginning of it, entitled "Spirit of the Homœopathic[2] Medical Doctrine."

---

[1] From the 3d Part of the *Reine Arzneimittellehre*, dated February, 1817.

[2] What an immense amount of learning do not my critics display! I shall only allude to those who write and print *homopathic* and *homopathy* in a place of *homœopathic* and *homœopathy*, thereby betraying that they are not aware of the immense difference betwixt ὁμὸν and ὅμοιον, but consider the two to be synonymous. Did they then never hear a word about what the whole world knows, how the infinite difference betwixt ὁμοούσιος and ὁμοιούσιος once split the whole Christian Church into two parts, impossible to be re-united? Do they not understand enough Greek to know that (alone and in combination) ὁμὸν means *common, identical, the same* (e. g. εἰς ὁμὸν λέχος εἰσαναβαίνοι, Iliad 9.) but that ὅμοιον only means *similar, resembling the object, but never reaching it in regard to nature and kind, never becoming identical with it?* The homœopathic doctrine never pretended to cure a disease by the *same*, the

Now I could easily settle them here after the traditional man
ner of writers, and expose them in all their nakedness. But I
shall not do so. I do not wish to burden myself with the sin
of immortalizing these follies and their perpetrators, and prefer
not to reveal the weaknesses of my contemporaries to an
assuredly more discerning posterity.

I shall only say this much in a general way.

Perversions of words and sense, incomprehensible palaver,
which is meant to appear learned, abuse and theoretical sceptical shakings of the head, instead of *practical* demonstrations of
the contrary, seem to me to be weapons of too absurd a character
to use against a fact such as homœopathy is; they remind me
of the little figures which mischievous boys make with gunpowder and set on fire in order to tease people—the things can
only fizz and splutter, but are not very effective, are on the
whole very miserable affairs.

By such tricks, the pitiful character of which recoils on their
authors, homœopathy cannot be blown up.

My respected brethren on the opposition benches, I can give
you better advice as to how you should set about overthrowing,
if possible, this doctrine, which threatens to stifle your art, that
is founded on mere assumption, and to bring ruin upon all your
therapeutic lumber. Listen to me!

Your attempts against the systematic exposition of the
doctrine, entitled the "Spirit of the Homœopathic Medical
Doctrine," have as you perceive, proved unsuccessful. You had
better leave it alone! Spirits such as this is, are no subjects for
joking with. It is said there are spirits whose appearance has
left behind a life-long disquiet in the conscience of the wicked
and of those who act contrary to their knowledge of what is
right and which nightly torment them, for their neglect of

---

identical power by which the disease was produced—this has been impressed upon
the unreasonable opponents often enough, but, as it seems, in vain ;—no! it *only* cures
in the mode most consonant to nature, by means of a power never exactly corres
ponding to, never the *same* as the cause of the disease, but by means of a medicine
that possesses the peculiar power of being able to produce a *similar* morbid state
(ἱμοιον πάθος.)

Cannot those persons feel the difference betwixt "*identical*," (the same) and
"*similar?*" Are they all *homopathically* labouring under the same malady of stupidity! *Should not any one who ventures to step forward as a reviewer of the* "Spirit
of the Homœopathic Medical Doctrine" *have at least a rudimentary idea of the
meaning of the word* " Homœopathy."

acknowledged and yet neglected duties! Mark this; otherwise you may not be able to silence the judge within you, which has wakened to speak to you in unmistakeable accents!

No! there is another and an infallible method of overthrowing this doctrine, if that is possible to be done.

This doctrine appeals not only chiefly, but solely to the verdict of experience—"repeat the experiments," it cries aloud, "repeat them carefully and accurately, and you will find the doctrine confirmed at every step"—and it does what no medical doctrine, no system of physic, no so-called therapeutics ever did or could do, it *insists* upon being "judged by the result."

Here, then, we have homœopathy just where we wished to have it; here we can (come on, dear gentlemen, all will go on nicely) give it the death blow from this side.

Take one case of disease after another, note it down according to the directions given in the Organon, specially in respect of all its discernible symptoms, in so exact a manner that the founder of homœopathy himself shall be unable to find fault with the minuteness of the report (of course any case selected must be one for which a homœopathic medicine is to be found amongst those medicines whose peculiar symptoms are known) and administer the most appropriate homœopathic medicinal substance that can be discovered, pure and unmixed, for the case of disease in question, in a dose as small as this doctrine directs; but, as is expressly insisted on, *taking care to remove all other kinds of medicinal influences from the patient*, and if it do not give relief, speedy, mild and permanent relief, then, by a publication of the duly attested history of the treatment *according to the principles of the homœopathic system strictly followed out*, you will be able to give a public refutation of this doctrine which so seriously threatens the old darkness.

But I pray you to beware of playing false in the matter!—all roguery comes to light and leaves an unfavourable stigma behind it as a warning.[1]

If then, following your conscientious example, every other equally conscientious and careful medical experimentalist meets

---

[1] As a warning example in point, I would refer to the notorious (exquisitely recorded) history of a disease which Kotzebue was said to have had, and of which he was said to be miraculously cured by means of the excitement theory method. It was, however, as was soon shewn a pure invention; invented in order to serve the purposes of the excitement-theory of that time, and the disgrace of the deception is still and will ever be attached to the name of its author.

with the same result—*if all that the homœopathic doctrine promises from being faithfully followed out does not take place*—then homœopathy is as good as lost, it is all up with homœopathy if it does not shew itself efficacious, remarkably efficacious.

Or, gentlemen on the opposition corporation benches, do you know any other and more potent method for suppressing this accursed doctrine, with its truths[1] that cut into the very soul of the dogmatists of ancient and modern times, well-armed though they be—*ignea inest illis vis et coelestis origo*—which, as it is asserted for certain, only needs to appeal to impartiality and sound human reason, in order to find an entrance into the uncorrupted understanding, and can point to the infallibly beneficial effects that result from a faithful following out of its precepts, and is thus enabled to triumph certainly over all obduracy;—

---

[1] The truth of this, the only rational doctrine of medicine, must seize upon the convictions of these gentlemen if they possessed but a spark of reason, and it did so to a certain extent, as we may observe here and there in their writings, from the piteous lamentations caused by their apprehension of the speedy overthrow of the antiquated edifice of their corporation.

But, see, they feel their brains so stuffed full of the hundred thousand fanciful ideas, insane maxims, systems and dogmas and the load of everlasting practical trash, they are no longer capable of laying aside this useless furniture, in order then, with freedom of mind to practise impartially a system so simple as homœopathy is, for the benefit of mankind. They feel themselves, I say, so incapable of doing this, that the ill-humour this causes distorts not only their mind, but also their features, and can only find vent in impotent abuse of the better way that they can never attain.

I am almost sorry for them; for the old falsehoods so often paraded before them as truths hover incessantly before their memory as though they still were truths; the fictions presented to them as articles of faith, and testified to by illustrious and great names, have been so often dunned as important and proper things into their ears, that they continue still to resound there; the illusory doctrinal maxims and the suppositions, *a priori* explanations, definitions and distinctions of the schools, offered to them as axioms, have been so often read by them again and again in print, and custom has habituated their whole mode of operations to such an easy-going routine readiness, that they are unable any longer to resist the pressure of those accustomed things that have become their second nature, and they must, in spite of themselves, continue to think and act in the same way—(at the very first view of the patient some particular anatomical seat in the body occurs to them as the undoubted seat of the disease, some nosological name for the disease presses itself upon them, they already feel at their finger ends the elegant compound prescription, which they will dash off upon the nearest piece of paper)—so that even if they wished seriously to reform and lead a new medical life in simplicity and in truth, worthy of the Allseeing Maker of our mind that he has created to enable us to administer to the relief of sick and suffering humanity, *they are now incapable of doing so.*

Such is the character of the self-styled critics of the reformed system of medicine and their aiders and abettors; how can their criticisms be other than they are? God have mercy on their poor souls!

do you, gentlemen, I repeat, know any more effectual mode o
suppressing this doctrine?

Yes! apparently you think you do.

Continue then to exalt the common-place twaddle of your
school to the very heavens with the most fulsome praise, and to
pervert and ridicule with your evil mind what your ignorance
does not pervert; continue to calumniate, to abuse, to revile:—
and the unprejudiced will be able plainly to comprehend on
whose side truth lies.

The improved (homœopathic) medical doctrine will stand out
in more prominent relief and appear to greater advantage
against the foil of this nonsense, and (—for who can entertain a
doubt respecting the feeling for truth inherent in the better part
of mankind?—) will dispel the nocturnal darkness of antiquated
stupidities, for it teaches how to afford *certain* benefit in diseases,
where hitherto mere incomprehensible learned palaver, at the
bed-side of the late lamented, sought in vain to hide the damage
done by pint and quart bottles full of unsuitable mixtures o:
unknown, life-destroying drugs.

And what do you say when you see the author and firs
teacher of homœopathy, together with his genuine disciples,
cure without suffering and permanently, a *much greater* proportion of patients, and such as are suffering from the worst, the
most tedious complaints, with few, mild tasteless medicines?
Can your so-called art do the like? Does not such a result
laugh to scorn your miserable theoretical scepticism, and the
impotent routine of your cut-and-dry system?

If you really wish to do as well, imitate the homœopathic
practice rationally and honestly!

If you do not wish this—well then, harp away—we will not
prevent you—harp away on your comfortless path of blind and
servile obedience in the dark midnight of fanciful systems, seduced hither and thither by the will-o'-the-wisps of your venerated authorities, who, when you really stand in need of aid,
leave you in the lurch—dazzle your sight and disappear.

And if your unfortunate practice, from which that which you
intended, wished and promised, does *not* occur, accumulates
within you a store of spiteful bile, which seeks to dissipate itself
in calumniating your betters—well then, continue to call the
grapes up yonder, which party-pride, confusion of intellect,
weakness or indolence prevents your reaching, sour, and leave
them to be gathered by more worthy persons.

Continue, if it pleases you, enviously to slander the sublime art, but know that envy gnaws in vain at adamantine truth, and only consumes the marrow of the bones of its possessor.[1]

EXAMINATION OF THE SOURCES OF THE COMMON MATERIA MEDICA.[2]

Next to a knowledge of what there is to cure in each particular case which presents itself for treatment, there can be no more necessary knowledge for a practical physician, than an acquaintance with the *curative implements*, to know, namely, what each of the remedies can certainly cure.

Twenty-three centuries have been spent in fruitless labour to discover the way by which the end of this knowledge may be reached; and not a step has been gained by all the efforts.

Had the millions of physicians who during this long space of time occupied themselves with the subject, only discovered the way *to the knowledge of how this end* (the discovery of the healing properties of each medicine) *was to be attained*, then had much, almost everything been accomplished; for then would this way have been capable of being pursued, and the zeal and exertions of the better class of physicians must have soon won a considerable territory of knowledge, so that what still remained to be investigated would also soon have been within our grasp.

But observe, that *not one*, as yet, ever trod the path that surely and certainly leads to this end. All the paths hitherto trodden were, consequently, as one century was forced to say of those of another, mere ways of error. These we shall examine somewhat more closely.

The *first source* of the Materia Medica hitherto extant is *mere guess work and fiction*, which attempts to set forth the *general therapeutic virtues* of drugs.

Exactly as the text ran in Dioscorides, seventeen centuries ago: this or that substance is *resolving, dissipating, diueretic, diaphoretic, emmenagogue, antispasmodic, cathartic*, &c.,—so runs it now in most recent works on Materia Medica. The same description of the general virtues of particular drugs, *which do not turn out true;* the same general assertions, *which did not hold*

---

[1] Αἰῶνα βρ͵τοῖς, Aeschyl., *Eumen.*, 329.
[2] From the *Reine Arzneimittellehre*, part iii.

good when put to the trial at the sick-bed. Experience declares, that such a medicine very seldom performs, in the human body, what these books allege respecting its general therapeutic virtues; and that when it does, this happens either from other causes, or it is a merely palliative passing effect (primary action), which is certainly followed by the opposite, to the greater detriment of the patient.

If a medicine prized for its diuretic, diaphoretic, or emmenagogue qualities, when given by itself alone, had, *in special circumstances, and in one out of many cases,* seemed to have had this effect, should it, on this account, be pronounced as absolutely possessing these qualities, that is, would it deserve the title of an unconditional diaphoretic, emmenagogue, or diuretic? In that case, we should dignify with the name of an honest man, one who only occasionally acted honestly; and on one who only lied on rare occasions, we should bestow the honourable name of a truthful man, a man of his word!

Are our conceptions to be thus perverted and reversed?

But these rare instances do not prove that a certain effect will take place even in rare cases ; for not in one case out of a hundred were the substances given alone, but almost always in combination with other medicines.

How few physicians are there who have given a patient but one single simple substance at a time, and waited for its sole operation, avoiding altogether the concomitant use of all other medicinal substances! It is nothing but a mixture of various medicines that ordinary practitioners employ! And if they ever give a simple substance, for example, in powder, they are sure to order also some herbal infusion (another kind of medicine), or medicated clyster, or embrocation, or fomentation of some other kind of herbs, to be used along with it. They never act otherwise. *This inherent vice clings like pitch to the ordinary practitioner, so that he never can rid himself of it.* He is in straits before and behind, and he cannot rest, and is not at ease, if this and that, and a score of other drugs, are not prescribed into the bargain.

And for this they have plenty of excuses.

They maintain that this or that medicine (of the peculiar and pure effects of which, however, they know nothing) is the principal ingredient of their compound prescription, and that all the effects must be attributed to it. The other substances were added for different objects, some to aid their principal ingredient, some to correct it, others to direct it to this or that part of the body, or to give it the necessary instructions on its passage (their own peculiar operation being all the time unknown); as if the drugs were intelligent beings, endowed with well-disposed wills and complaisant obedience, so that they would produce just that effect in the body which the doctor ordered them, and not a particle more!

But do these accessory substances cease, on your command, to confuse and to counteract, with their own peculiar and unknown medicinal influence, the action of your principal, and to produce, in accordance with the eternal laws of their own inherent nature, effects which cannot be surmised or predicted, and can only be discovered and brought to our knowledge by pure experiment?

Is it not foolish to estimate the effect of *one* force, while other forces of another kind were in action, which often contributed mainly, though in common with the rest, to produce the result?

It would not be more absurd if some one were to try to persuade us that he had discovered a good article of nutriment in kitchen salt; that he had ordered it to a man half-starved, and that he had no sooner eaten of it than he was invigorated, satiated, and strengthened, as if by miracle; that the ounce of common salt was the basis and chief ingredient of the nutritious receipt prescribed by him, which he had caused to be dissolved, *lege artis, in quantum satis* of boiling water as the excipient and vehicle, then he had added as a corrective, a good lump of butter, and, as an adjuvant, a pound of fine cut rye-bread. This mixture (soup), after being properly stirred, he caused to be taken at once by the famished patient, and by it his hunger was completely appeased;—all the latter ingredients were merely accessaries in the prescription, the chief ingredient was the ounce of salt. This was prescribed by him as the basis of the whole receipt; and see!—in his hands it had, when prepared accurately according to these directions, always exhibited the most beneficial results.

If, in the *kitchen* Materia Medica, the virtues of *saturans, analepticum, restaurans, reficiens, nutriens* should, from these circumstances, be ascribed to the article *Sal culinare*, it would not be more childish and absurd than the conduct of the physician who should arbitrarily ordain one substance to be the basis of his diuretic, then add two, three, or four other powerful (unknown) medicinal substances (with the sage object,

forsooth, of serving as *corrigens, dirigens, adjuvans, excipiens*),
and order the patient to walk up and down the room while
taking the mixture, drinking in the meantime largely of warm
sack-whey, made of Rhine-wine well sweetened with sugar, and
then publish triumphantly the extraordinary success of the basis
he had prescribed: " The patient has passed more urine than
usual." In his eyes the added substances and the regimen are
mere unimportant accessaries, and innocent of the result, in
order that he may be able to ascribe to the substance which he
has constituted the chief ingredient in the receipt, and in which
(he knows not why) he takes the deepest interest, and whose
fame he wishes to extend, the sole honour of the effects produced.
Thus it naturally happens, when, by such arbitrary and wilful
praise of a medicine which some one has taken a fancy to, and
to which he was determined to attribute some definite curative
property, the undeserved and surreptitious attributes of *diuretic,
emmenagogue, resolvent, sudorific, expectorant, antispasmodic*, are
inscribed in the willing Materia Medica, where they afterwards
figure as truths, deluding those that trust to it.

Thus this rare effect must be attributed to the action of all
these medicines which were used at once! How small a part of
the uncertain credit of being a diuretic, diaphoretic or emmenagogue, or any other sort of medicine, falls to the share of each
individual ingredient in the receipt!

Consequently, the general theraputic virtues of drugs ascribed
to them by Dioscorides, and re-echoed by his successors, which
occupy the greatest share in Materia Medicas even of our own
day, as, for instance, that this or that medicine was diuretic, diaphoretic, purgative, expectorant, or a purifier of the blood and
humours, are quite unfounded.[1]

The assertion that this or that medicine is resolvent, discutient,
an exalter or depresser of sensibility, irritability, or the repro-

---

[1] When no other virtue could be attributed to a medicine, it must be at least an
evacuant: evacuant in some way or other; for, without an evacuation—without an
evacuation of the morbific matter which their grossly material conceptions of disease
led them to seek in all diseases, they could not imagine that a medicine could affect
a cure. Since, then, the generation and existence of a disease was due to this hypothetical morbific matter, they bethought themselves of all the conceivable exits from
the body by which this desperate matter could be driven out by medicines ; and the
medicine had to do them the favour, to take upon itself the office of expelling this
imaginary morbid matter from the numerous vessels and fluids, and of clearing it
away by means of the urine, sweat, expectoration, or alvine discharge. These were
the principal effects they hoped and expected from their remedies: this was the part
all the medicines in the Materia Medica had to play.

ductive function, rests upon baseless hypothetical assumptions alone. It was in itself a false and hypothetical assumption, destitute of proof and of reality, that it was necessary *directly* to perform these operations in diseases at all. How then, in the name of reason, could it be ventured to ascribe these in themselves nugatory virtues to individual medicines, without proof, irrespective altogether of the fact they were almost never prescribed singly, but almost always only in combination with others? Thus every such assertion is a palpable lie.

What was ever seen *dissolved* or *resolved* in the interior of the human body by medicines? By what facts was such a power of dissolving *living* parts of the organism proved to be possible by drugs? Why is irrefragable evidence of the manifestation of this power by some substance not brought forward? Or why, since it is impossible to observe such *mechanical* and *chemical effects* of a drug in the undiscovered and undiscoverable penetralia of the organism, has not a sense of shame restrained men from publishing such inventions as truths and dogmas, and, with unblushing brow, falsely ascribing such actions to medicines, since error in the most serious and important of all earthly vocations, the healing of the sick, must have the most grievous consequences; and falsehood here is the greatest crime, being nothing less than high treason against humanity?

And what is there, even in the hidden internal parts of the living body, to dissolve or dissipate, which the human organism, when acted on by medicine proper for its recovery, cannot itself, when necessary, dissolve?

Is there anything actually present in the body to be dissolved from without, as the opinion implies? Has not our Sömmering proved that the swollen glands, which had always hitherto been considered to be obstructed, had, on the contrary their vessels greatly dilated. Has it not been established by experiment on healthy peasants, that by the persevering use of Kämpf's clysters there may be produced in and evacuated from their bowels the same abominable evacuations which Kämpf, on hypothetical grounds, assumed to exist in the body of almost all patients affected by chronic disease, in the form of stoppage, infarctus, and accumulations; although he had at first, by his compound herbal decoction, administered in the form of several hundred clysters, brought on the unnatural condition of the bowels which produced these secretions, and then got them evacuated, to the horror of all beholders; and, unfortunately, the rest of the profession were almost without exception his followers, and in their mind's eye they now saw in almost all patients nothing but obstructions of the smallest vessels of the abdomen, infarctus and accumulations, took the senseless herb-mixture of Kämpf to be really dissolving and dissipating, and clystered the poor patients, for the sake of an hypothesis, with the greatest vigour and perseverence, almost to death, so much so that it was a sin and a shame.

Now, supposing that these imaginary cases were indeed real, and that there could be something to dissolve and dissipate in the diseased human body, who has ever seen this dissolution or dissipation effected by the direct action of the medicine when the patient recovers, so that the vital force, which before presided over all the operations of the organism, had remained, in this instance, a passive spectator, and had allowed the medicine to work, unaided, upon the supposed obstructed and indurated parts, as a tanner operates on his hides?

By means of calomel, according to the history of a case,[1] a chronic vomiting that occurred after meals was removed. The cause of this vomiting was represented as nothing less than an induration of the stomach and pylorus; this the narrator of the case avers with the greatest effrontery, without adducing the slightest evidence in support of his position, only that he might attribute in this manner an unconditional resolvent power to calomel, and assume the honour to himself of curing a disease which is as rare as it is incurable. Another writer,[2] rants in the same imaginative strain about pressure on the stomach, cramps in the stomach, eructation and vomiting in his patient being due to some organic disease of the stomach, scirrhus, indurations and tumours, and believes that as these were removed by drinking for a length of time decoction of *triticum repens* (and at the same time preserving a well-regulated diet and regimen?), that he has fully established that this herb can cure scirrhus of the stomach, of the existence of which in his case there was not the slightest proof. But pressure of the stomach, eructation, and vomiting after meals, even when of long standing, are by no means rare maladies, and are often easily curable by an improved diet and regimen, and, alone, afford no proof of induration or scirrhus of the stomach or pylorus. This disease is ac-

---

[1] *Hufeland's Journal*, 1815, Dec., p. 121.
[2] In *Hufeland's Journal*, 1813, p. 63.

companied by *much more serious* symptoms than pressure, eructation, and mere vomiting are.

This is however the highly commendable way in which a medicine is raised to the undeserved honour of being a resolving, dissipating, &c. remedy, namely, by blind conjecture and bold assumption of the presence of an important internal malady, never seen or capable of being proved to be there.

The *second source* of the virtues of drugs, as ascribed to them in the materia medica, has, it is alleged, a sure foundation, viz., *their sensible properties*, from which their action may be inferred. We shall see, however, what a turbid source this is.

I shall spare the ordinary medical school the humiliation of reminding it of the folly of those ancient physicians who, determining the medicinal powers of crude drugs from their *signature*, that is, from their colour and form, gave the testicle-shaped Orchis-root in order to restore manly vigour; the *phallus impudicus*, to strengthen weak erections; ascribed to the yellow tumeric the power of curing jaundice, and considered *hypericum perforatum*, whose yellow flowers on being crushed yield a red juice (*St. John's blood*) useful in hæmorrhages and wounds, &c.; but I shall refrain from taunting the physicians of the present day with these absurdities, although traces of them are to be met with in the most modern treatises on materia medica.

I shall only allude to what is scarcely less foolish, to wit, the attempts, even of those of our own times, to guess the powers of medicines from their *smell* and *taste*.

They pretended, by dint of tasting and smelling at drugs, to find out what effect they would have on the human body; and for this they invented some general therapeutical expressions.

All plants that had a *bitter* taste should and must (so they decreed) have one and the same action, solely because *they tasted bitter*.

But what a variety even of bitter tastes there are! Does this variety not indicate a corresponding variety of action.

But how does the bitter taste obtain the honour awarded to it by the Materia Medica and practical physicians, that it is a *proof of the so-called stomachic and tonic powers of drugs, and an evidence of their similar and identical action*, so that, according to this arbitrary axiom, all the *amara* possess *no other medicinal action but this alone?*

Although some of them have, besides, the peculiar power of producing nausea, disgust, oppression of the stomach and eruc-

tations in healthy individuals, and consequently of curing, homœopathically, an affection of a similar nature, yet each of them
possesses peculiar medicinal powers quite different from these,
which have hitherto been unnoticed, but which are often more
important than those ascribed to them, and whereby they differ
extremely from each other. Hence, to prescribe bitter-tasted
things without any distinction, the one in place of the other, as
if they all acted in the same manner, or thoughtlessly to mix
them together in one prescription, and under the name of bitters
(*extracta amara*) to administer them, as if they were indubitably
identical medicines, having only the power of strengthening and
improving the stomach, betrays the most wretched, rudest
routinism!

And if, as this dictatorial maxim of the authorities in materia
medica and therapeutics would have us believe, the bitterness
alone is sufficient to prove that everything that tastes bitter
(*amara!*) is absolutely and solely strengthening, and improves
the digestion, then must *colocynth*, *squills*, *boletus laricis*, the
thick-barked, much-abused *angustura*, *eupatorium*, *saponaria*,
myrica gale, *lupina*, *lactuca virosa*, *prussic acid*, and *upas-poison*,
all be entitled, as bitters, to rank among the tonic, stomachic
medicines.

From this any one may easily see how irrational and arbitrary
the maxims of the ordinary materia medica are, how near they
are to downright falsehoods! And to make falsehoods the basis
of our system of treating the sick—what a crime!

Cinchona was found to have a bitter and astringent taste.
This was quite enough for them in order to judge of its inward
powers; but now all bitter and astringent tasting substances and
barks must possess *the same* medicinal powers as cinchona bark.
Thus was the action of medicines on the human frame determined, in the materia medica, in the most unthinking and hasty
manner from their taste alone! And yet it must and ever will
be false, that willow-bark, or a mixture of aloes and gall-nuts,
have the same medicinal properties as cinchona bark. How
many such *Chinæ factitiæ*, which were to answer all the purposes
of the true cinchona bark, have been publicly recommended by
celebrated physicians, manufactured and sold, and administered
with the greatest confidence to their patients by other physicians!

Thus, the life and health of human beings were made dependent on the opinion of a few blockheads, and whatever entered
their precious brains went to swell the materia medica.

In the same manner a number of inconceivably dissimilar smells were jumbled together in *one* category, and all christened *aromatics*, in order that under this name a similar medicinal action might *conveniently* be invented for them. Thus they were, without the slightest hesitation or consideration, one and all pronounced to be *exalters of the forces* (excitants), *strengtheners of the nerves*, deobstruents, &c.

Thus the most imperfect, the most deceptive of all the senses of civilized man, that of smell,[1] which admits of the expression by words of so few perceptions of sensible differences—this should suffice to determine the dynamic properties of a medicine in the human organism, whilst all our senses together, employed with the utmost care, in the examination of a medicinal substance *with regard to its external properties*, do not give us any, not even the slightest information respecting this most important of all secrets, the internal immaterial power possessed by natural substances to alter the health of human beings; in other words, respecting their true medicinal and healing power, which is so extremely different in every active substance, from that of every other, and which can only be observed when it is taken internally, and acts upon the vital functions of the organism!

Must mayflower, mint, angelica, arnica, sassafras, serpentaria, sandal, coriander, chamomile, rosemary, necessarily have the same medicinal action, because forsooth, it pleases the olfactory organ of the respectable teachers of materia medica to discover that they all have an aromatic smell?

Can a materia medica composed of such a jumble of dissimilar medicines, all highly important, from the very variety of their action, shew aught else than intemperate presumption and dishonest, ignorant self-complacency?

No art, be it ever so mean, has been guilty of such wanton fictions with respect to the uses and powers of its materials and tools. The agent to be employed was, at all events, always tried upon smaller parts of the object it was intended to work upon, in order to ascertain what alterations it was capable of effecting, before it was employed on a large scale in the precious work, where an error might be productive of serious injury. The cotton bleacher tried the effects of chlorine, which is so destructive to vegetable matters, in the first instance on a small portion

---

[1] Precisely the most powerful medicines, belladonna, digitalis, tartar emetic, arsenic, &c., have little or no smell.

of cloth, and thereby avoided exposing all his stock of goods to danger. The shoemaker had previously convinced himself of the properties of the hempen thread, that it was stronger in the fibre, that when it was exposed to damp, it filled the holes in the leather by its expansion more completely, and resisted putrefaction more powerfully than flax, before he preferred it to the latter for stitching all his shoes: and that, after all, was but cobbler's work !

But in the arrogant medicine of the common stamp, the medicines—the tools of the healing art—are employed without the least hesitation in the most important work which one man can perform for his brother man—a work whereon life and death, nay, sometimes the weal or wo of whole families and their descendants depends, namely, the treatment of disease; and the acquaintance with these remedies being derived solely from their deceptive outward appearance, and from the preconceived notions and desultory classifications of teachers of materia medica, there is the greatest danger of deception, of error, and of falsehood. But even then, as if to conceal the effect of each individual one, several remedies are given mixed together in one prescription, with no anxiety as to the inevitable result !

So much for the unfounded allegations respecting the general therapeutic virtues of the several medicines in the materia medica, which are all elevated to dogmas, on a foundation of blind guess-work, preconceived ideas, extraordinary notions and presumptuous fiction. So much for this *second* impure source of the materia medica, as it is called, hitherto in use !

Chemistry, also, has taken upon itself to disclose a source at which the general therapeutic properties of drugs are to be ascertained. But we shall soon see the impurity of this *third source* of the ordinary materia medica.

Attempts were made a century ago by Geoffrey, but still more frequent have such attempts been made since medicine became an art, to discover, by means of chemistry, the properties of remedies which could not be known in any other way.

I shall say nothing about the merely theoretical fallacies of Baume, Steffens, and Burdach, whereby the medicinal properties of medicines were *arbitrarily* declared to reside in their gaseous and certain other chemical constituents alone, and at the same time it was assumed, without the slightest grounds, *on mere conjecture*, that these hypothetical elementary constituents possessed

43

certain medicinal powers; so that it was really amusing to see the facility and rapidity with which those gentlemen could create the medicinal properties of every remedy out of nothing. As nature, trials on the living human organism, observations and experience were all despised, and mere fancy, expert fingers and overweening confidence were alone employed, it is easy to conceive that the whole affair was very soon settled.

No! I allude to the earnest aspirations, and the honest exertions of those of the present day, to arrive, by means of vegetable and animal chemistry, at a knowledge of the real pure action of medicines on the human frame, in which, as was deeply felt, the materia medica up to that period was miserably deficient.

True it is that Chemistry—that art which reveals to us such astonishing miracles, appeared to be a much more *likely* source for obtaining information with respect to the properties of drugs, than all the idle dreams, and learned *salti mortali* of ancient and modern times, which we have just been considering; and many were infatuated with this expectation, yet, chiefly such as either did not understand chemistry (and sought much more from it than it could give or possessed), or knew nothing about medicine and its requirements, or were ignorant of both the one and the other.

Animal chemistry can merely separate from animal substances such inanimate matters as shew a different chemical action with chemical re-agents. But it is not these component parts of animal tissues, separated by animal chemistry, on which the medicines act when they derange the health, or cure the diseases of the living organism, either through their elementary parts, as the chemist would have us believe, or directly upon them. The fibrine, coagulable lymph, gelatine, organic acids, salts and earths, separated from muscular substances by chemical operations, differ *toto cœlo* from the living muscle, endowed with irritability in its perfect organized state in the healthy and diseased individual; the matters separated from it have not the most distant resemblance to the living muscle. What information respecting the nature of the living organism, or the changes which the different medicines are capable of effecting on it when alive, can be derived from these separated inanimate portions? Or is the process of digestion (that wonderful transmutation of the most dissimilar kinds of food for the purpose of promoting the perfect development of the living individual in all the variety of his organs and humours) rendered in the slightest degree *comprehensible* from the discovery of a little soda and phosphatic salt in the gastric juice? Can even the material, not to speak of the dynamic, cause of a morbid digestion or nutrition be understood by what chemistry finds in the gastric juice, so that a sure method of treatment could be founded thereon? Nothing could be more futile than any expectation of this kind.

In like manner, in the chemical constituents shewn by vegetable chemistry to exist in plants, even in such as possess the most powerful medicinal properties, there is nothing either to smell or taste which can express or reveal those so varied actions, which, experience shews us, each of these medicinal substances is capable of performing, in altering the state of an individual, whether in health or disease.

The water or oil, distilled from the plant, or the resin obtained from it, is certainly not its active principle; this only resided, invisible to the eye, in those parts now extracted from it—the resin, the oil, the distilled water; and is *in itself* perfectly imperceptible to our senses. Its effects are manifested to our senses only when this distilled water, this oil, this resin, or, still better, the plant itself, is taken by the living individual, and when they act dynamically on the susceptible spiritual-animal organism, in a spiritual manner.

Moreover, what medicinal action do the other parts which chemistry extracts from plants indicate, the vegetable fibrine, the earths, the salts, the gums, the albumen, &c., which, with few exceptions, are found almost uniformly in all plants, even those most opposite in their medicinal effects? Will the small quantity of oxalate of lime which chemistry shews us to exist in rhubarb-root, account for this medicine producing in healthy individuals such a morbidly altered sleep, and such a curious heat of the body without thirst, and for its curing similar morbid states?

What information can all these parts, though analysed ever so carefully by chemistry, give us, relative to the power of each individual plant, virtually to alter the health of the living human organism in the most peculiar and various manners?

The chemist, Gren, who knew nothing about medicine, in his Pharmacology, which is full of the most reckless assertions, thus holds forth to physicians: " The knowledge of the principles contained in medicines, which chemistry gives us, can alone determine the efficacy of remedies."

Knowledge indeed! And what *knowledge* does chemistry give us with respect to the inanimate, speechless, component parts of medicines? Answer: It merely teaches their chemical signification, it teaches us that they act so and so with chemical re-agents, and hence are called gum, resin, albumen, mucus, earths and salts of one kind or another;—matters of vastly little importance to the physician. These appellations tell us nothing of the changes in the sensations of the living man which may be effected by the plant or mineral, each differing from the other in its peculiar invisible, internal, essential nature; and yet, forsooth, the whole healing art depends *on this alone!* The manifestations of the active spirit of each individual remedial agent during its medicinal employment on human beings, can alone inform the physician of the sphere of action of the medicine, as regards its curative power. The name of each of its chemical constituents, which in most plants are almost identical, teaches him nothing on this point.

That calomel, for example, consists of from six to eight parts of mercury, united by sublimation to one of muriatic acid—that when rubbed up with lime-water, it becomes black, chemistry can teach us; but that this preparation can cause in the human being the well-known salivation with its peculiar odour, of this chemistry, as chemistry, knows nothing; this no chemistry can teach us. This dynamic relation of calomel to the human organism can only be learned from experience, derived from its medicinal employment, and from its internal administration, when it acts dynamically and specifically on the living organism: and thus it is only actual experiment and observation relative to the action of medicinal substances on the living human subject that can determine their dynamical relation to the organism, in other words, their medicinal properties; but this chemistry, in whose operations merely inorganic substances are brought to act upon one another, can never do.

Chemistry can indeed give us the useless information, that the leaves of belladonna are very similar in their chemical composition to cabbage and to a great many other vegetables, as they contain albumen, gelatine, extractive matter, green resin, vegetable acid, potash, calcareous and siliceous earths, &c.; but if, as Gren asserts, the knowledge of the principal constituents, so far as they are known to chemistry by means of its re-agents, that is, chemically, suffices to determine the medicinal properties of substances, it follows that a dish of belladonna must be just as wholesome and innocent an article food as one of cabbage. Is that what the chemist means? And yet the chemistry which presumes to determine the medicinal properties of natural substances from their chemical composition, cannot avoid asserting that the same medicinal powers are possessed by substances which are proved by analysis to consist of the same constituents; it cannot consequently help declaring cabbage and belladonna to be equally innocent vegetables, or equally poisonous plants; thereby shewing, as clear as day, the absurdity of its presumption, and its incompetence to judge of the medicinal powers of natural substances.

Do Gren and his followers not perceive that chemistry can only give chemical information with respect to the presence of this or that material component part of any physical body, and that these are consequently *to chemistry* merely chemical substances? Chemical analysis can tell us their action with chemical re-agents, and this in its proper domain; but it can shew us neither in its dissolving nor digesting alembics, neither in its retorts nor yet in its receivers, what dynamical changes any single medicine, when brought in contact with the living organism, can produce.

Each science can only judge and throw light on subjects within its own department; it is folly to expect from one science information upon matters belonging to other sciences.

The science of hydrostatics enables us to determine with precision the specific gravity of fine silver in comparison with that of fine gold; but it presumes not to fix the different commercial value of the one in comparison with that of the other. Whether gold have twelve, thirteen, or fourteen times the value of its weight of silver in Europe or in China, hydrostatics can never tell; it is only the scarcity of and the demand for the one or the other, that can determine their relative mercantile value.

In like manner, indispensable as *a knowledge of the particular form of plants* is to the true farmer, *and the power of distinguishing them by their external appearance,* which constitutes *botany,* yet botany will never teach him whether a given plant is suitable or the reverse as for his sheep or swine, nor will it inform him what grain or what root is best for making his horse strong, or for fattening his ox; the botanical systems of neither Tournefort, nor Haller, nor Linnæus, nor Jussieu, can tell him this; pure, careful, comparative trials and experiments on the different animals themselves can alone give him the requisite information.

Each science can decide on such matters only as are within its own province.

What does chemistry find in the native magnet and the artificial magnetic rod? In the former it discovers nothing but a rich iron ore, intimately combined with silica, and a small quantity of manganese; in the latter, nothing but pure iron. No chemical re-agent can discover, by the most minute chemical analysis, the slightest trace of the mighty magnetic power in either the one or the other.

But another science, natural philosophy, shews in its experiments the presence of this wonderful power in the native magnet and magnetized steel, as also its physical relation to the external world, its power of attracting iron (nickel, cobalt), the direction of one end of the magnetic needle towards the north, its deviation from the north pole in different decenniums and in different regions of the globe, at one time towards the west, at another towards the east, and the variety in its dip in different degrees of latitude.

The science of natural philosophy, then, is capable of telling something more respecting the magnet, and of discovering more of its powers, than chemistry can, namely, its magnetic power in a natural philosophical point of view.

But the knowlege of what is worth knowing about the magnet, is not exhausted by chemistry and natural philosophy; neither of these two sciences can detect anything in it beyond what belongs to their own province. Neither the range of the chemical nor that of the physical sciences can inform us, what mighty, what peculiar, what characteristic effects the magnetic power is capable of producing on the health of the human body, when brought into contact with it, and what curative powers peculiar to itself it possesses in diseases in which it is suitable; of this chemistry and natural philosophy are equally ignorant; this subject they must both abandon to the experiments and observations of the physician

Now, as no science can pretend to that which can only be explained by another science, without rendering itself ridiculous, I hope that medical men will gradually have the sense to see that the proper province of chemistry is merely to separate the chemical constituents of substances from each other, and to combine them together again, (*thus affording technical aid to pharmacy*); I hope that they will commence to see that medicines do not exist for chemistry as medicines (*i. e.*, powers capable of dynamically altering the health of an individual), but merely in so far as they are chemical substances (*i. e.*, in so far as their component parts are to be regarded in a chemical light); that chemistry, consequently, can only give chemical information with respect to medicinal substances, but cannot tell what spiritual, dynamical changes they are capable of effecting in the health of the human being, nor what medicinal and curative powers each particular drug possesses, and is capable of exercising in the living organism.

Finally, from the *fourth impure source* flowed the *clinical* and *special therapeutic indications for employment* (*ab usu in morbis*), into the ordinary materia medica.

This, the most common of all the sources of the materia medica, whence a knowledge of the curative powers of medicines was sought to be obtained, is what is termed the practice of physic, namely, *the employment of medicines in actual diseases,* whereby it was imagined that information would be obtained with respect to the diseases in which this and those in which that remedy was efficacious.

This source has been resorted to from the very beginning of the medical art, but has, from time to time, been relinquished, in order to try and hit upon some more profitable mine for the knowledge required but it was always had recourse to again, as it *appeared* the most natural method of learning the action of medicines, and their exact uses.

Let us grant, for a moment, that this were the true way to discover their curative virtues; one would, at least, have expected that these experiments at the sick-bed would have been made with single, simple drugs only; because, by mixing several together, it would never be known to which among them the result was to be ascribed. But in the records of medicine, we meet with few or no cases in which this so natural idea was ever carried into execution, viz., to give only one medicine at once in a disease, in order to be certain whether it could produce a perfect cure in that disease.

It accordingly happened, that, in almost every instance, a *mixture of medicines* was employed in diseases; and thus it could never be ascertained *for certain*, when the treatment was successful, to which ingredient of the mixture the favourable result was due; in a word, *nothing at all* was learned. If, on the contrary, this medicinal mixture proved of no avail, or, as usually happened, did harm, just as little could it be learned, from this result, to which of all the medicines the bad result was attributable.

I know not whether it was an affectation of learning which induced physicians always to administer medicines mixed together in prescriptions as they are called, or whether it was their anxiety which made them fancy that a single remedy was too powerless and was not sufficient to cure the disease. Be this as it may, the folly of prescribing several remedies together has prevailed from the remotest antiquity; and immediately after Hippocrates' time diseases were treated with a mixture of medicines, instead of with one single medicine. Among the many writings falsely attributed to Hippocrates, of which the greater part were written under his name, shortly after his death, principally by his two sons, Draco and Thessalus, as also by their sons, Hippocrates the third and fourth, and among those works fabricated by the Alexandrians Artemidorus Capiton and his kinsman Dioscorides, in the name of Hippocrates, there is not one practical treatise in which the prescriptions for diseases do not consist of several medicines, just as in the prescriptions of their immediate followers, those of more modern times, and those of the physicians of the present day.

But that from the employment of mixed prescriptions, it cannot be ascertained what each individual remedy is capable of effecting in diseases, consequently, that no materia medica can be founded thereon, was first commenced to be perceived by physicians of later times, whereon several zealously set about prescribing in a simple manner, in order to ascertain experimentally in what diseases this or that medicine was efficacious. They also published cures which were said to have been effected by a single simple remedy.

But how was the execution of this apparently rational idea carried out? We shall see.

In order to do so, I shall just run over what is to be found on this subject in the three volumes of Hufeland's Journal for 1813, 1814 and 1815, and shall shew that the power of curing such and such diseases has merely been attributed to single drugs, without their having been employed simply and alone.[1]

---

[1] It is true one single individual in all these three volumes, Ebers, instituted experiments with one single remedy only, in various diseases (*Hufeland's Journal*, September and October 1813.)—With arsenic alone. But what sort of experiments? Such as could throw no light on the curative powers of this substance. In the first place, the cases of intermittent fever in which he employed arsenic were not minutely described, and then the dose was such that it must have done much more harm than

Consequently, this is a new piece of fallacy in the place of the old one with its acknowledged composite prescriptions.

That ulceration of the lungs has been cured by *phellandrium aquaticum* is pretended to be shewn in the history of a case (*Hufeland's Journal*, August, 1813), whereby it appears (p. 110) that *tussaligo*, *senega* and *Iceland moss* were used at the same time. With what right can the advocate for this mode of treatment (which was so complex) exclaim, in conclusion:—" I am *convinced* that the man owes the recovery of his health to this remedy *alone*"?

Such was the sort of convictions that were produced by the impure source of the virtues ascribed to simple medicinal substances in the materia medica!

In like manner (*ibid.*, February, 1813), a case of inveterate syphilis, which would not yield to various mercurial preparations, (it was, in fact, a mercurial disease!) was cured in four weeks by *ammonia*, along with which nothing, actually nothing, was employed--except *camphor* and *opium!*--Is that nothing?

An *epilepsy* (*ibid.*, 1813, March) was cured in 14 months by *valerian* alone, nothing else being used at the same time—but *oleum tartari per deliquium*, *tinctura colocynthidis*, and baths of *acorus calamus*, *mint*, and other *aromatic* substances (pp. 52, 53). *Is that nothing?*

In another case of epilepsy (*ibid.*, p. 57) *velerian* alone effected a cure, but there were employed, besides, an ounce and a half of *pomegranate leaves*. *Is that nothing?*

---

good. However, his candid acknowledgment of the harm it did is infinitely more praiseworthy than the many alleged cases of cure recorded by others, in which arsenic in the largest doses *is said* to have done nothing but good, and never the least harm. Ebers affirms that the doses he administered were so small, that, in most cases, they did not amount to one grain. To one patient he only gave 2-9ths of a grain within the 24 hours (p. 55), and her life was put in danger, whereby it may be perceived that even this minute dose is capable of producing the most fearful effects. *Honestly*-observing physicians have long known this; but Ebers, led astray by the materia medica, fancied that 2-9ths of a grain in 24 hours was a very small dose of arsenic. Pure experience tells us it is *a monstrous, a most unjustifiable dose in diseases!* When was it ever shewn that arsenic should be employed in doses of a grain, or even of a tenth of a grain, *in diseases?* Many experiments with small and still smaller doses (more and more diluted solutions) have shewn, that *one* drop which contains the decillionth of a grain of arsenic in solution, is, in many cases, *much too strong* a dose, even when arsenic is exactly suited for the case of disease. Had he known this he would not have been astonished that his 2-9ths of a grain put his patient's life in peril. Thus, from these trials, which are otherwise evidently very honest, nothing can be learnt, not even what arsenic *cannot cure;* for the monstrous doses effectually prevented any good effect from taking place.

Madness, with *nymphomania*, is said to have been cured by *drinking cold water alone* (*ibid.*, 1814, Jan). But *infusion of valerian* and *tinctura chinœ Whyttii* (p 12) were very prudently administered along with it, in order that the action of the cold water should be so completely masked as to be unrecognisable; and the same happened in the case of another patient, who used these powerful adjuvants only *less* frequently (p. 16).

Tymon (*ibid.*, 1814, Aug. p. 38) professes to have found *bleeding to syncope* a specific in *hydrophobia*. But, see! he gives at the same time 300 *drops of laudanum*, in clysters, *every two hours*, and rubs in a *drachm of mercurial ointment every three hours. Does this prove venesection to be the only true remedy for hydrophobia ?*

In like manner (*ibid.*, 1814, April) a venesection, followed by an hour of syncope, is said to have cured, solely and specifically, a case of hydrophobia; at the same time (p. 102), however, there were *only* administered *strong doses of opium, James's powder*, and *calomel till salivation was produced*. Is that nothing?

If the case (*ibid.*, 1815, July, p. 8—16) is to be a proof of the efficacy of bleeding to syncope in already developed hydrophobia, as the author would have it, *cantharides* should not have applied, and still less should *mercurial ointment have been rubbed in every two hours*, and *large doses of calomel* and *opium* given until *violent salivation* supervened. It is ludicrous when the author adds (p. 20) that "the *calomel* was scarcely necessary."

This art of surreptitiously obtaining for a favourite remedy the merit of a cure, when the other equally powerful drugs employed might at all events claim a share, is an established custom with ordinary physicians; it being particularly requested that the courteous reader will shut his eyes, and allow the author to designate all the secondary means employed *inactive*.

A case of tetanus is reported (*ibid.*, 1814, Sept., p. 119) to have been cured *by cold water effusion alone*. It is true *opium* was *at the same time* employed; "*as, however, the patient himself attributed the amendment to the effusion alone, to the effusion should the cure be ascribed.*" This is what I call a pure source at which to learn the virtues of drugs!

In a similar manner (*ibid.*, 1815, Sept., p. 128) the healing power of *potash* in *croup* is established;[1] but along with it were

---

[1] One case, in which potash is said to have been efficacious when administered alone was that of a child in the country, *which the author did not see*, and which, from the description alone, he *suspected* to be this disease.

used other very powerful substances; for example, at the commencement of the (supposed?) disease two children were relieved by salt of tartar *in an infusion of senega root.* Is what properly pertains to two substances to be ascribed to the action of but one, the potash? According to what hitherto unheard-of system of logic?

In like manner, *graphites* (*ibid.*, 1815, Nov., p. 40) is said to have cured a large number of *old fistulous ulcers,* and yet *corrosive sublimate was in the mixture!* The explanation in the note, that sublimate had already been tried in vain, is of no avail here: *it was not given alone,* but in combination with opium, a quantity of *decoctions of various woods,* and the favourite *china factitia;* it was consequently greatly or completely destroyed by the astringent parts of these accessory medicines, just as other metallic salts are thereby destroyed and decomposed, and consequently it could not develop its curative powers in such a mixture. Still less can the apology, in the same note, for the addition of the mercurial to the graphites be received, "that the sublimate was merely to serve as an adjuvant here." Were this the fact, then must medicines act agreeably to the commands of the prescribing physician, not according to their natural powers, no! they must do exactly neither more nor less than what the physician commanded and permitted them to do. Can arrogance and presumption be carried farther than this? What man of sound intellect can attribute such slavish obedience to medicinal substances, which act according to eternal laws? Did the author wish to see whether graphites could prove efficacious by itself and to convince his readers of this, he ought to have given it *alone:* but if he add to the graphites corrosive sublimate, this must perform what corrosive sublimate can and from its very nature *must,* not what the prescribing physician pleases that it shall or shall not do. Here again we have a case from which nothing can be learnt. Graphites is represented as having alone proved serviceable, and yet that tremendously powerful medicinal substance, corrosive sublimate, was used along with it.

The cure of a case of florid pulmonary consumption by means of charcoal powder is, if possible, still more unfounded. Here the limewood charcoal was *never* employed *alone,* but always *in conjunction with foxglove.* So then the foxglove in the mixture has no action? None at all? and yet a medicine of such mighty power! Do the authors of such observations deceive themselves, or do they mean to make game of us?

Angelica root is said (*ibid.*, 1815, April, p. 19) to have cured a *dropsy*, properly speaking an unknown case of disease with swelling. (*The quid-pro-quo*-giving pathology collects together all diseases having the most distant resemblance in this respect under the name of "*dropsy*.") But no! *tincture of opium, œther*, and, finally, *calamus*, were used in addition to the tincture of angelica. Can any rational man lay to the account of the angelica alone the issue of this case?

No one will deny that the mineral water of Driburg has great medicinal powers; but when the cures related in *Hufeland's Journal*, 1815, April, pp. 75, 80, 82, are ascribed to it alone, we must declare these statements to be false, *as so many other strong medicines were used along with it*; nor can the pretended cure of a case of cramp in the stomach with frequent vomiting by this water (p. 85 to 93), nor that of hypochondriasis and hysteria (p. 94 to 97), prove anything in favour of the Driburg water, partly on account of the ambiguity and vagueness of these two names of diseases, but principally on account of the constant employment of other medicines at the same time. Were we to receive these cases as proofs of the efficacy of the mineral water, we might, with equal justice, give to a single man the credit of having alone lifted a large rock, without reckoning his many active co-operators and the helpful machines employed. It would be ridiculous to ascribe to one only that which was done by all in conjunction.

These are a few samples from among the multitude I might adduce from the writings of the more modern physicians, samples of nominally simple treatment of diseases, each of which was said to have been cured with one single remedy—in order to obtain at last a knowledge of its true powers,—but along with which there was always employed some medicine or other more powerful than itself; and although the physician should protest ever so vehemently that "that one medicine" to which he would fain attach all the glory of the cure, "*alone did it, he firmly believes*," "the patient himself ascribed the good effects to this remedy alone," "to it *alone he entrusted the cure.*" "he *only* employed the second medicine as an adjuvant," or, "it had once before been employed without effect;" yet all these shufflings will not avail to persuade a rational man that the cure was owing to that medicine *alone* to which the partiality of the physician would award the honour of the cure, if any other—even one single other remedy—have been used in the treatment. It must ever remain untrue that the cure is due to this remedy alone; and the materia medica which shall ascribe such a curative power to this remedy, on the authority of such an impure observer as this, propagates falsehoods which must inevitably be fraught with the most unhappy consequences to humanity.

I will not deny that the cures of which I have just adduced examples did *approach* towards simplicity. They certainly came *nearer, much nearer* to the treatment of a disease with one single remedy (without which mode of proceeding we can never be sure that the medicine was the real instrument in effecting the cure), than those of ordinary routine practitioners, who make it a glory to adminster to their patients several complex prescriptions, one after the other, or even to prescribe daily one or two fresh mixtures.

But to have approached *merely nearer* to the adminstration of single remedies implies that the true mark has been actually and completely *missed.* Were it not so, then might we congratulate a person on his good fortune whose number in the lottery differed by a single cipher from that which won the highest prize; or a sportsman whose shot has gone within a hair's breath of his game; or a shipwrecked mariner who would have escaped shipwreck had he been a single finger's breadth farther from the fatal rock.

What credence do the assertions in the ordinary materia medica deserve with respect to the virtues of drugs *ab usu in morbis?* What shall we say to the alleged powers of drugs in this or that disease, when we know that the materia medica has obtained its information thereupon from such observations; sometimes indeed merely from the titles of the recorded observations of physicians who scarcely ever treated with one single remedy, but generally with a mixture of drugs, whereby as much uncertainty existed as to which among them the result was to be ascribed to, as if, like the routine practitioner, they had prescribed a great hotch-potch of medicines? What shall we say to the curative powers ascribed with so much confidence by the materia medica to simple medicinal substances, seeing that these were almost never employed singly? We can say naught but this : among a thousand such allegations and commendations, scarcely one deserves credence, whether they refer to general therapeutical, or to clinical or special therapeutical matters. Hence it is undeniable, that *to ascribe any powers to a medicinal substance which was never tested purely, that is, unless along with others, consequently might as well have been never tested at all, is to be guilty of deception and falsehood.*

" What if all physicians were to agree from this time hence-forth to turn over a new leaf, and to prescribe in every disease, only one single simple medicine ? Would we not, by this means, ascertain what each medicine is capable of curing ?"

This will never happen as long as a Hufeland lives, who con-siders the statements of the ordinary materia medica though derived from the impurest sources, to be truths, and seriously defends the employment of a mixture of many medicines in dis-eases, imagining that " one medicine cannot suffice for all the indications in a disease; several must be given at once, in order to meet the several indications."

This statement, as pernicious as it is well meant, rests upon two perfectly erroneous premises, *the first*, whereby it is taken for granted " that the baseless declarations with respect to the virtues of simple drugs in practical works, and in the materia medica compiled from them, are well founded; and consequently, that they were *really* capable of meeting the indications presented by the case in which they were prescribed," (which, as we have shewn, and shall again shew, is false);—*the second*, " that several medicines should be prescribed at once in order to satisfy the several indications in a disease, for this reason, because a single medicine can do little more than respond to a single indication, but not to several or many."

But what does the ordinary materia medica know about the vast sphere of action of a simple medicinal substance, that ma-teria medica which, from impure observations of the result of the employment of *several medicines* in one disease, attributes to a drug whatever powers it has pleased the physician to ascribe to a simple ingredient of the mixture; which never subjected the powers of a simple medicinal substance to a pure trial, that is, on a healthy individual not affected with any symptoms of disease ? Does that mixture of falsehood and truth which the materia medica has scraped together from prescribers of com-pound medicines, in diseases of which merely the pathological name, but no accurate description is given,—does this comprise the whole extent of the sphere of action which the Almighty has bestowed on his instruments of cure ? No ! He has im-planted in his healing instruments undiscovered (but certainly discoverable) miracles of his wisdom and goodness, in order that they may prove beneficial and helpful to his beloved children of mankind, in a far greater measure than was ever dreamt of by the short-sighted materia medica of the old school.

But though it is certain that a single medicine at once is always sufficient for the rational and appropriate treatment of a disease, I am far from advising the medical world, *on that account*, to prescr... imply, that is, a single medicine in each disease, *in order to ascertain what medicine is useful in this, what in that, disease*, so that thereupon a materia medica, or treatise on the virtues of drugs *ab usu in morbis*, should be formed.

Far be it from me to advise anything of the kind, notwithstanding that this idea might seem, and has seemed, to ordinary physicians, to promise the best results.

No! not the slightest useful addition can be either now or ever made to our knowledge of the powers of drugs, with regard to their *usus in morbus*, from observations on cases of disease even with single medicines.

This were just as foul a source as all the others above mentioned, hitherto employed. No useful truth, with respect to the curative powers of each individual medicine, could flow from it.

I shall explain myself.

Such a mode of testing medicines in diseases were only possible in two ways. Either a single drug must be tried in all diseases, in order to ascertain in which of them it is efficacious; or all drugs must be tried in a particular disease, in order to ascertain which remedy can cure it most certainly and most perfectly.

And, first, with regard to the latter of these ways; and from it may be inferred what reliance can be placed on the former.

By an infinite number of trials of all imaginable simple substances used in domestic practice, in a *well-defined disease, which shall constantly present the same characters*, a true, certainly efficacious, specific remedy for the greater number of individuals and their friends suffering from the *same* disease *might* certainly be discovered, though only *casu fortuito*.

But who knows how many centuries the inhabitants of deep valleys were forced to suffer from their goîtres before accident, after thousands of drugs and domestic nostrums had been tried in vain, put it into the head of an individual, that *roasted sponge* was the best thing for it; at all events it was not until the thirteenth century that Arnault of Villeneuve notices its *power of curing goître*.

It is well known that for many years after its first invasion, the *venereal disease* was treated in a most unsuccessful manner by the physicians of the schools, by starvation, by purgatives, and other useless remedies, which had been employed to combat the Arabian leprosy, until at last, after many attempts and repeated trials of an innumerable multitude of things by empirical physicians on many thousands of patients who sought their aid, *mercury* was hit upon, and proved itself specific in this dreadful scourge, in spite of all the violent theoretical opposition of the pedantic physicians of the Arabian school.

The intermittent fever endemic in the marshy regions of South America, which has a great resemblance to our own *marsh ague*, had long been treated by the Peruvians, probably after innumerable trials of other drugs, with *cinchona bark*, which they found to be the most efficacious remedy, and which was first made known by them as a febrifuge to Europeans in the year 1638.

The bad consequences resulting from blows, falls, bruises and strains were long endured, ere chance revealed to the labouring classes who principally suffered from such accidents, the specific virtues of *arnica* in such cases; at least Franz Joel was the first who, in the sixteenth century, makes mention of its virtues, and, in the eighteenth century, they were more particularly described by J. M. Fehr and J. D. Gohl, after they had become generally recognised.

Thus, after thousands upon thousands of blind trials with innumerable substances upon, perhaps, millions of individuals, the suitable, the specific remedy is at last discovered *by accident*. In order to discover the remedies for the few maladies mentioned above, there was no necessity for the employment on the part of indolent man, of that reason and mature knowledge which the Almighty has given to him, in order to enable him to free himself from those inevitable natural and other evils involving his health—the vast multitude of diseases;—in fact, no true medical knowledge at all was required. *Mere experimenting* with all imaginable substances which might come into the head or hands was undoubtedly *sufficient* (to be sure after the lapse of perhaps hundreds of years) to enable him to discover, by accident, a suitable remedy, which never afterwards belied its specific power.

These few specifics in these few diseases constitute all the truth which is contained in the voluminous materia medica in common use;

and these are, for the most part, I may say, almost entirely, derived from domestic practice.

"But if specific remedies, which were always serviceable in the above diseases, were discovered in this way, why could not some remedies against all the remaining innumerable diseases be discovered by similar experiments?"

Because all other diseases only present themselves as individual cases of disease differing from each other, or as epidemics which have never been seen before, and will never be seen again in exactly the same form. The constant specific remedies in these few diseases were capable of being discovered by means of trying every imaginable medicinal substance, only because the thing to be cured, *the disease*, was of a *constant character ;*— they are diseases which always remain the same; some are *produced by a miasm which continues the same* through all generations, such as the venereal disease; others have *the same exciting causes*, as the ague of marshy districts, the goitre of the inhabitants of deep valleys and their outlets, and the bruises caused by falls and blows.

Had it been possible, by blind trials of all imaginable substances, to discover accidentally the suitable (specific) remedy for each of the innumerable other diseases, then must they all have been as *constant* in their nature, have appeared always in the same manner and in the same form, have shewn themselves to be always as identical in their character, as those few diseases we have mentioned.

Only for a want of a constant character can we suppose a supply of a constant character.

That it was requisite, in order to find out empirically the proper remedy, that all diseases, for which the specific was sought should be identical and preserve an invariable fixed character, appears not only to have been surmised, but to have been deeply felt by the medical community of the old school. They imagined that they must represent to themselves the various diseases of humanity in certain fixed forms, before they could hope to discover for each a suitable, trustworthy remedy, and this (as they knew no other better—scientific—way of finding the fitting medicine in diseases) by means of experimenting on them with all possible drugs,—a method which had succeeded so well in the few fixed diseases above alluded to.

This undertaking, to arrange all other diseases in a certain

44

fixed classification, appeared to them at first certainly very plausible and practicable.

In order to set about it, they conceived the idea of considering all those from among the vast array of diseases, which bore any resemblance to each other, as one and the same disease; and having provided them with a name, and given them a place in their nosological works, they were not deterred, by the constantly occurring differences in their appearance, from declaring them to be definite forms of disease, which they must always have before them, in order thereby to be able to discover, as they flattered themselves, a particular remedy for this disease.

Thus they collected the infinite variety of diseases into a few arbitrarily formed classes of diseases, without reflecting that nature is immutable, whatever false notions men may form of her. In like manner, the polyhedrical kaleidoscope held before the eye arranges in one illusory picture a number of external very different objects, but if we look behind it into nature, we discover a great variety of dissimilar elements.

It is no excuse to say that this arbitrary and unnatural amalgamation of diseases of nominally constant character was framed with the good intention of thus discovering for each separately a sure remedy, by means of trying on them the large number of known drugs, or by accident. *As was to have been expected*, there were found in this way no sure remedial agents for these artificially classified diseases; for we cannot imagine any real weapons to combat figments and phantoms of the imagination!

All the uses and virtues, therefore, which the materia medica ascribes to different medicines, in these surreptitious and fictitious kinds of diseases, cannot make the slightest pretence to certainty.

What advantage has been gained in so many centuries, with all the host of new and old medicines, over the artificial nosological classes of diseases, and names of diseases? What remedies have been found that can be relied on? It is not now as it was long ago,—2300 years ago,—that by the employment of all the various drugs in the innumerable cases of disease which occur in nature, some are, it is true, much altered, generally, however, for the worse, and but few are cured by them? And was it possible, even in this enormous space of time, that it could be otherwise, that it could be improved, as long as the old system remained as it was, with its *imaginary thing to be cured, and imaginary virtues of the instruments for effecting the cure, and its ignorance of their true, pure action?* How could really useful truths spring from the employment of the latter against the former?

Let it not be alleged, "that not unfrequently many a severe disease—which some called by one, others by a different pathological name—was cured as if by miracle, by a simple domestic remedy, or by some medicine or prescription which accidentally fell into the hands of the physician."

No doubt this sometimes happened; no well-informed man would deny it. But from this we can learn nothing but what we all know already, "that medicines can cure diseases;" but from these *casus fortuiti* nothing is to be learnt; as yet they occupy an isolated position in history, altogether useless for practice.

Our congratulations must only be bestowed on the sufferer who reaped advantage from this rare godsend, and was cured quickly (and lastingly?) by this *accidental* remedy. But from this wonderful cure nothing at all is learned; not the slightest addition has thereby been made to the resources of the healing art.

On the contrary, these very chance cases of accidental cures, when they have occurred to physicians, have done most to fill the materia medica with false seductive declarations respecting the curative actions of particular medicines ab usu in morbis.

For, as the ordinary physician seldom or never describes the case of disease correctly, and, indeed, considers the circumstantial description of a case of disease in all its symptoms as useless, if he cannot bestow on it a pathological name (the illusory representation of a disease above alluded to), so he does not fail to apply some illusory pathological name to his chance case, which, together with his prescription, or the single remedy in the mixture to which alone he ascribes the cure, straightway finds its way into the materia medica, which, moreover, is incapable of making use of anything but mere pathological names of diseases in its account of the uses of medicines.

He who, thereafter, is inclined to regard a case occurring to himself as the same pathological species of disease (and why should he not? the schools teach him to do so), has nothing to do but to resort immediately to this magnificent receipt, this splendid specific, at the bidding of its first recommender, or by the advice of the materia medica. But he certainly has, under the same illusory pathological name, a case before him vastly different in the detail of its symptoms, and hence happens what was inevitable, the medicine does no good; it does harm, as might have been anticipated.

This is the impure, this is the unhallowed source of all the declarations respecting the curative virtues of medicines ab usu in morbis in the ordinary materia medica, whereby every imitator is led astray.

Had the so-called observers—what they almost never did—communicated to the world those cases of lucky chance cures, *only describing minutely* the case of disease, *with all its symptoms*, and mentioning the remedy employed, they had at least written truth; and the materia medica (finding no pathological name attached) had not been able to glean any lies from them.   They had, I say, written truth, which, however, would only have been useful in one single way, namely, to teach every future physician the exact case of disease beyond which the remedy, in order to prove useful, should not be employed; and thus no false, and consequently unsuccessful, imitation would have occurred. From such an accurate description it would have been evident to all future physicians that the same, *the exact same*, case of disease *never recurs* in nature, consequently could never again be cured miraculously.

Thus we would have been spared all the many hundred delusive accounts of the curative actions of particular drugs in the ordinary materia medica, *whose truthfulness and honesty has hitherto consisted, and still consists, in this, that it has faithfully re-echoed whatever authors have chosen to invent with respect to the general therapeutical virtues of drugs, and has accepted, as genuine coin, their alleged special therapeutic powers ab usu in morbis, ascertained from accidental cases of cure,* by associating the specific pathological name of a disease bestowed on his case by the so-called observer, with, as the curative power, the presumed single medicine to which, among all the drugs employed in the compound prescription, the physician chose principally, if not entirely, *to entrust and ascribe* the successful result.

So turbid and impure are the sources of the ordinary materia medica, and so null and void its contents!

What a healing art, with such ill-understood medicines!

From the circumstance that constant remedies have already been discovered for those diseases, few though they be,[1] which have a constant character, one might infer, that for all diseases

---

[1] To be sure this was only effected by blind trials of all imaginable drugs; for hitherto a scientific mode of making such discoveries has been entirely wanting in medicine.

of a constant character, constant (specific) remedies might be found.

And accordingly, since the only trustworthy way, the homœopathic, has been pursued with honesty and zeal, the specific remedies for several of the other constant diseases have already been discovered.[1]

In order to treat successfully the other cases of disease occurring in man, and which, be they acute or chronic, differ so vastly among each other, if they cannot be referred to some primary disease which is constant in its character, they must each be regarded as peculiar diseases, and a medicine which in its pure

---

[1] In this homœopathic way, from a consideration of the symptoms of the smooth *scarlet-fever*, with bright erysipelatous redness of the skin, which formerly prevailed in Europe from time to time, as a contagious epidemic (but has been almost totally supplanted by the *purpura miliaris*, which, in 1800, came from the Netherlands into our country, and has been improperly confounded with *scarlet-fever*, by physicians, who knew not the latter disease), I found the specific curative and prophylactic remedy for this true, smooth scarlet-fever in the smallest doses of *belladonna*, which has the power of producing a very similar fever, with a similar lobster-red colour of the skin.

So, also, from a thorough consideration of the symptoms presented by the *purpura miliaris* just mentioned, in the particular character of its purely inflammatory fever with agonizing anxiety and restlessness, I found that *aconite* must be the specific remedy (occasionally alternately with raw coffee); and experience has confirmed the truth of the remark.

The symptoms of *croup* are to be found in the pure materia medica, among the symptoms produced by *burnt sponge* and *hepar sulphuris*; and see! these two alternately, and in the smallest dose, cure this frightful disease of children, as I first discovered.

No known medicine is so capable of producing a state similar to that of the epidemic *hooping-cough* as the *sundew*; and this disease, which, notwithstanding all the exertions of allopathic physicians, either becomes chronic or terminates fatally, is cured in a few days in a certain and safe manner, as I first shewed, by the smallest portion of a drop of the decillionth dilution of the juice of *drosera rotundifolia*.

What physician before me, and before the publication of the " *Pure Materia Medica*," was able to cure radically the constitutional and local sycosic condylomatous disease? They were content with removing the morbid growths by the cautery, the knife, or the ligature, as often as they appeared externally, but none succeeded in *curing* the disease. The symptoms of *thuja occidentalis* taught me, however, that it must cure this disease; and, behold! a very small dose of its highly diluted juice actually cures the internal disease, so that the external growths vanish also, shewing the cure to be radical.

With an infinity of empirically chosen drugs the allopathist attacks the autumnal dysentery, but with what miserable success! The symptoms of *corrosive sublimate*, however (*vide* the " *Pure Materia Medica*"), resemble so closely those of this disease, that this medicine must be its specific remedy; and experience convinced me, many years since, that a single dose, consisting of a small portion of a drop of the trillionth dilution of *mercurius sublimatus corrosivus* is sufficient to produce a rapid and complete cure.

effects on the healthy body shews symptoms similar to those of the case before us, must be administered.

This improved healing art, *i. e.*, the homœopathic, draws not its knowledge from those *impure sources of the materia medica hitherto in use*, pursues not that antiquated, dreamy, false path we have just pointed out, but follows the way consonant with nature. It administers *no* medicines to combat the diseases of mankind *before* testing their pure effects; that is, observing what changes they can produce in the health of a healthy man—this is pure *materia medica*.

Thus alone can the power of medicines on the human health be known; thus alone can their true importance, the peculiar action of each drug, be exhibited clearly and manifestly, without any fallacy, any deception, independent of all speculation; in their symptoms thus ascertained, all their curative elements lie disclosed; and among them may be found a signalization of all the cases of disease which each fitting (specific) remedy is capable of curing.

According to this improved system of medicine, cases of disease, in all their endless variety of appearance (if they cannot be traced back to some more profoundly rooted primary disease of constant character), must be regarded in every instance as new, and never before seen; they must be noted, exactly as they present themselves, with all the symptoms, accidents and altered sensations discoverable in them; and a remedy must be selected which, as has been shewn by previous experiments of its action on perfect health, is capable of producing symptoms, accidents, and altered sensations most similar to those of the case under treatment; and such a medicine, given in a very small dose, cures, as experience teaches, much better and more perfectly than any other method of treatment.

This doctrine of the pure effects of medicines promises no delusive, fabulous remedies for names of diseases, imagines no general therapeutic virtues of drugs, but unostentatiously possesses the elements of cure for diseases accurately known (that is, investigated in all their symptoms; and he who will take the trouble to choose the remedy for a disease by the rule of the most perfect similarity will ever find in it a pure inexhaustible source whence he may derive the means for saving the lives of his fellow-men.

LEIPZIG, *April*, 1817; and
CÖTHEN, *January*, 1825.

ON

THE UNCHARITABLENESS TOWARDS SUICIDES.[1]

The propensity to self-destruction always depends upon a disease which is to a certain extent endemic in England, but in many other countries it prevailed epidemically, so to speak, more some time since than now, but it by no means affected the very worst characters, but often otherwise honest, well-conducted individuals. It is generally the friends of the individual —who do not pay attention to his corporeal disease, that often passes rapidly into this mental disease—and his medical attendants, who know not how to cure the suicidal-malady, that are to blame for the catastrophe.

By their unsteady, shy, anxious look, by the despondency they display in their words and deeds, by their restlessness, that increases at certain times of the day, by their avoidance of things that were formerly most agreeable to them, and sometimes by their inconsolable lamentations over some slight corporeal ailments, the patients betray their internal malady. This most unnatural of all human purposes, this disorder of the mind that renders them weary of life, might always be with certainty cured if the medicinal powers of pure *gold* for the cure of this sad condition were known. The smallest dose of pulverized gold attenuated to the billionth degree, or the smallest part of a drop of an equally diluted solution of pure gold, which may be mixed in his drink without his knowledge, immediately and permanently removes this fearful state of the (body and) mind, and the unfortunate being is saved.

ON

THE TREATMENT OF THE PURPURA MILIARIS.[2]

Almost all of those, without exception, who are affected by the *red miliary fever* (falsely called *scarlet-fever*) that is often so fatal, will not only be rescued from death, but also cured in a few

---

[1] From the *Allgem. Anzeig der Deutschen*, No. 144. 1819.

[2] From the *Allgem. Anzeig. der Deutschen*, No. 26. 1821

days by *aconite* given alternately with tincture of *raw coffee.* The expressed juice of the fresh aconite-plant should be mixed with equal parts of alcohol, and diluted with a hundred times its quantity of alcohol, until the last dilution is in the octillionth degree. Of this a small portion of a drop is to be given for a dose when there is *increasing restlessness, anxiety and heat of the body,* all acids being carefully avoided; and *when there are increasing pains* (in the head, throat, &c.) combined *with a disposition to weep,* a small portion of a drop of the tincture of raw coffee diluted to the millionth degree.

The one will usually be necessary when the other has acted for from sixteen to twenty-four hours.[1] Not oftener.

Besides this nothing should be done or given to the patient— no venesection, no leeches, no calomel, no purgative, no cooling or diaphoretic medicine or herb-tea, no water compresses, no baths, no clysters, no gargles, no vesicatories or sinapisms.

The patients should be kept in a moderately warm room, and allowed to adapt their bed coverings to their own feelings, and to drink whatever they like, warm or cold, only nothing acid during the action of aconite.

* * * *

But even should these remedies be prepared and administered as directed, where is the practitioner who would refrain from giving something or another from his routine system, thus rendering the treatment nugatory?

ON THE

PREPARATION AND DISPENSING OF MEDICINES BY THE HOMŒOPATHIC PHYSICIAN.

I. REPRESENTATION TO A PERSON HIGH IN AUTHORITY.[2]

"Non debet cui plus licet quod minus est non licere."
Ulpian, lib. 27, *ad Sabinum.*

The complaint of the Leipzic apothecaries that by dispensing my medicines I encroach upon their privileges," is untenable for the following reasons.

---

[1] ["Every twelve, sixteen or twenty-four hours, according as the one or the other is indicated." (R. A. M. L., *Introd. to Bell.,* pt. i, p. 15.)]

[2] Written in 1820, first published in Stapf's collection in 1829. [The subject of this and the two following essays is not of so much interest to the English homœopathist, as his right to prepare and dispense his own medicines has never yet been

My system of medicine has nothing in common with the ordinary medical art, but is in every respect its exact opposite. It is a *novum quid*, to which the standard of measurement hitherto applicable to the dispensing of medicines is completely unsuitable.

The old system makes use of *complex mixtures of medicines, each containing several ingredients in considerable quantity.* The compounding of these prescriptions, which in general consist of several medicinal substances, demands skilful, often laborious work and time, neither of which the ordinary practitioner can devote to this purpose, as he is occupied with visiting his patients, and does not possess the skill required for compounding these various, often heterogeneous, substances, and therefore must be glad to have at hand an assistant in the apothecary, who relieves him of the toilsome, time-wasting preparation of the medicines; in a word, who undertakes for him the *dispensing* business. For where the laws relative to medical affairs speak of *preparing the medicines*[1] and of *dispensing*, they always and invariably imply thereby *the compounding of several medicinal substances in one formula or prescription.* Nor can the state medicinal regulations imply anything else thereby, for hitherto all the prescriptions of doctors for their patients have been as a rule compound recipes, that is, consisting of several medicinal ingredients mixed together; and up to the present day *the treatment of patients*, as taught in our universities, colleges and hospitals, *consists solely in writing prescriptions*, which are directions to the apothecary relative to the different medicines he is to bring together in one formula, for hitherto patients as a rule have only been treated with compound prescriptions, the compounding and mixture of which was entirely left to the apothecary.

This right to prepare compound medicinal formulas for the physician was conceded to the privileged apothecary by the laws relating to medicine solely on this account, that none unconversant with this work or having a bad stock of medicines might make a bungle of the prescriptions, because the physician who

questioned, but the papers themselves are well worth perusal, and could not have been with propriety omitted from this collection. The first is a remonstrance addressed to the chief magistrate, in reply to an accusation, brought against him by the Leipzic apothecaries, of dispensing his own medicines.]

[1] When the medicinal laws speak of simple remedies, they make use of the words *simplicia* and *species*, and by the expression, *medicines* and *medicaments*, they always mean *compound* medicines.

is engaged in practice would have often neither the skill to make
these often elaborate mixtures himself, nor the great time often
requisite to devote to their preparation.

All the royal mandates of this kind refer to this dispensing
and preparation of drugs (*compound medicinal formulas*) which
exclusively appertains to the privileged apothecaries.

But their exclusive privilege is entirely limited to this, but does
not refer to the sale of the *simplicia* (simple drugs) otherwise
there could exist no druggists in the kingdom, for they are not
prevented by any law at present from selling *simples* to every
one.

The only right and privilege belonging to the apothecary,
*exclusively to make up the mixtures ordered in prescriptions contain-
ing several medicinal ingredients* is *not in the slightest degree* interfered with by the new method of treatment called homœopathy,
the exact opposite of the ordinary medical art hitherto practised,
for this new system has no prescriptions that it could give to
the apothecary, has no compound remedies, but gives for every
case of disease only one single, simple medicinal substance, in
an unmedicinal vehicle, therefore it does not *compound,* and
consequently, does not *dispense.* Its practice is, therefore, not
included in the prohibition to dispense contained in the laws
regarding medicine.

Now, as every art admits of improvements in the course of
ages, which must be welcome to every civilized state, the medical
art also can and must advance farther on the way to perfection.
If, then, by the ordination by an All-wise Providence there
arise the art of curing diseases (more easily, surely and permanently) without compound remedies, without mixtures of medicines, and if there be now physicians who know how to treat
every disease efficaciously by means of one single, simple remedy
(simplex), this cannot be prevented by any privilege referring
to the preparation of compound prescriptions; the new healing
art advancing nearer to perfection cannot thereby be obstructed
in its beneficent progress, for it is open to the physician for the
purpose of curing diseases to make use of every simple power
in nature which is best adapted to this end; for example, the
employment by himself of electricity, of galvanism, of the
magnet, and so likewise of every kind of simple agent; and in
this the scientific physician has never yet been, and can never
be, fettered by any regulations of medical police.

For where is a syllable to be found in all the royal ordinances relating to medicine that distinctly forbids physicians to administer *simplicia* with their own hands to the patients?

And as long as no such distinct prohibition for the practitioner exists in the laws, as long as no privilege granted to the apothecaries refers to their exclusive administration of the *simplicia*, as long as it is allowed to the ignorant dealers in roots and herbs in the weekly market to sell for money to those who seek their aid, *simplicia*, medicinal roots and herbs, so long must it be allowed to the scientific physician skilled in all the knowledge of nature, its forms, and its phenomena, and entrusted with the care of human maladies, to administer *gratuitously* to his patient the simple remedy which he considers will prove most efficacious for the disease, *for this*, as I shall shew, *cannot be done by the apothecary.*

Such is exactly the case with the new method of treatment of which I am the founder, which is something quite different from the ordinary mode of treatment. In my treatise upon the homœopathic system, *all prescriptions, all compound medicinal mixtures* are prescribed, and I inculcate that only one single, simple medicine at a time is to be given in every case of disease,[1] and I never treat a patient in any other way than this.

According to this improved method of treatment, I require for the cure of even severe diseases, that have hitherto been considered incurable, only the smallest possible doses of simple substances, either solutions of some minerals and metals in pure alcohol without the addition of any acid (preparations that are known to me alone, but not to any chemists, consequently, not to any apothecary) or equally small doses of vegetable and animal substances—always only one dose of a single, simple medicament—doses which are so small that they are quite undetectable by the senses, and by every conceivable chemical analysis, in their ordinary unmedicinal vehicle (sugar of milk).

This inconceivable minuteness of the doses of simple medicinal substances in this new system of medicine quite sets aside all possible suspicion of a hurtful size of the dose of simple medicine given to the patient.

Incapable of being taught that the great curative power of such small doses of simple medicines, that shews itself in the beneficial effects of their administration, depends upon a plan of

---

[1] See the *Organon of Medicine*, 2d edit. 1819, § 297, 298, 299—[*vide* fifth edition, 272, 273, 274.]

selection for the cases of disease for which they are adapted hitherto unknown and peculiar to the homœopathic art, whereof the ordinary system of medicine never dreams, the apothecary ridicules the nullity of such small doses, since all his senses, as well as the best chemical analysis, cannot enable him to detect any medicinal substance in the vehicle (sugar of milk).

If, then, even the apothecary, with all his jealous animosity against the new healing art, cannot detect anything medicinal or poisonous in the remedies of the genuine homœopathic physician, nor anything that could appear medicinal, not to mention too strong or injurious, how completely satisfied may the government which is concerned for the welfare and health of the community be with respect to the effects of such efficacious remedies given in such small, such inconceivable doses, as those homœopathy administers to its patients! It may be infinitely more satisfied than with respect to the trade of the apothecary, where the *very same medicines* which the homœopathic physician employs in such inconceivably small doses are unhesitatingly sold by the apothecary in quantities upwards of a million times greater, to every one (citizen or peasant), to persons who do not know what damage these things may do when employed improperly; his only limitation being that he shall not sell arsenic, corrosive sublimate, opium, and a few other things, to strangers.

I take leave to draw the attention of the medical police of the state to this subject.

Moreover, the homœopathic physician cannot employ the apothecary as an assistant in the practice of his new art. The medicinal doses of such a physician are so minute, so imperceptible, that if the apothecary had to put it into the vehicle alluded to according to the directions of the physician (which the physician himself can do in a minute without waste of time), the homœopathic physician, if he did not himself see the operation performed, could not, either by the aid of his senses or by that of chemistry, determine whether the apothecary gave the medicine he ordered, or some other, or none at all.

This impossibility on the part of the homœopathic physician, to exercise control over such an act of the apothecary, renders it impossible for the physician of the new school to avail himself in his treatment of an assistant, be he who he may. In this case he can trust to himself only; he alone can know what he has himself done.

And yet this uncommon minuteness of the dose of all dynamically-acting medicines is indispensably necessary in this new art, which is *excellent* for the treatment of every disease, but which is *indispensable* for the cure of the serious chronic diseases which have hitherto been abandoned as incurable, and it is *so* indispensahly necessary, that the cure of these diseases is impossible without that minuteness of dose.

Now if the spirit of the laws relating to medicine is really directed chiefly and before everything else to the *salus publica*, and if the diseases most worthy of commiseration and hitherto abandoned as incurable can only be transformed into health by means of this new method, as, for instance, the cases I have cured testify, which have roused to bitterness the envy of many of the ordinary practitioners, then it surely cannot be doubted that the sanitary police will prefer the welfare of the suffering public to all unfounded private claims, and will afford its protection to the new efficacious healing art, but that it will not force upon the new system as its assistant the art of the apothecary, which was originally instituted for preparing the *medicinal mixtures* of the ordinary system, from prescriptions containing many strong ingredients; such an act could only be obstructive and never advantageous to homœopathy.

I am correct in saying, "unfounded private claims," and I add that these claims are "insignificant and unmeaning." For how much would an apothecary be entitled to if (as the homœopathic physician himself does without waste of time) to the vehicle of three grains of sugar of milk he were to add, for example, one drop of an alcoholic solution of a grain of tin, rhubarb or cinchona bark, diluted to more than the millionth degree? According to all scales of apothecaries' charges hitherto framed, which are all calculated only according to the weight of the ingredients of the ordinary formulas, and the trouble (which does not exist in the new system) of compounding the ingredients, for making up any such homœopathic prescription, I say, he is entitled to just—nothing.

If then for the preparation of homœopathic medicine he were entitled to nothing, it is to be feared that if the Leipzic apothecaries still persist with their untenable proposition, there may be some secret motive at work which determines them to force their services, contrary to their interests, on the homœopathic physician. I would fain hope that this is not done with the intention of throwing an insuperable obstacle in the way of the recently developed and highly important new healing art, for which nothing can be a substitute, as some of the practitioners who are envious of its success would seem to wish.

The true homœopathic physician, moreover, does not in the least infringe on the rights of the apothecary as a dealer in drugs, for he cannot charge the patient anything for such an inconceivably small dose of the simple medicine which no chemical analysis can detect in the vehicle ; he can only, as is proper, be paid for the trouble he expends in investigating the morbid state, and in choosing the most efficacious remedy, which is much greater in this new beneficent system of medicine than under the old system.

Now, as the new system has nothing in common with the method of treatment hitherto practised, which consists in the giving of compound prescriptions, for the preparation of which the apothecaries are alone privileged ; as the new system bears no resemblance to this, seeing that it never treats with mixtures of ponderous, massive doses of medicines, but with inexpressibly small and subtle doses of always simple medicines prepared in a manner which is in some respects not attainable by the apothecaries, regarding which, consequently, the art of the apothecary with its old privileges, can have no privilege ;[1] I therefore make the following suggestion with all respect, but with a thorough conviction of its justice :

" To keep the Leipzic apothecaries within the limits of their privileges, and to notify to them that their rights do not extend to a new method of treatment which has never before been practiced, which, far from dispensing, that is, making up prescriptions of the ordinary kind composed of several powerful medicines (the preparation of which belongs of right to the apothecary), or requiring them for its treatment, on the contrary, only requires inexpressibly small doses of simple medicines (which the apothecary laughs at), consequently, only *simplicia*, which no ruler ever yet forbade scientific physicians to administer to their patients, and which consequently are, as we may naturally suppose, not prohibited in any regulations of medical police."

---

[1] Pure human reason is the voice of God! No government ever yet permitted the sock-mill to extend its right of monopoly to the person who can extract—what the mill cannot do—pure starch from wheat without the employment of any machine (the starch-maker) ; no government ever allowed the old privileges of the art of printing to interfere with the development of divine lithography, which also multiplies a thousand fold thoughts upon paper, and does this much more rapidly and easily but without the artificial composition of massive types.

This concession I look forward to with all the more confidence and tranquillity, seeing that this new system has, on account of its immense importance, already gained a public character, and already in all countries where German is spoken, men are arising who know how to estimate it as a great benefit for suffering humanity.

Finally, as regards what relates to my disciples,[1] I must state that I am in no way connected with them, and as the subject is quite irrelevant I shall refrain from touching on it. I do not consider any as my followers, who, in addition to leading an irreproachable, perfectly moral life, does not practise the new art in such a manner, that the remedy he administers to the patient in a non-medicinal vehicle (sugar of milk or diluted alcohol) contains such a small subtle dose of the medicine, that neither the senses nor chemical analysis can detect the smallest absolutely hurtful medicinal substance, indeed not the slightest trace of any thing medicinal at all, which pre-supposes a minuteness of dose that must indubitably dispel all anxiety from all officers of state who have to do with medical police.[2]

II.—THE HOMŒOPATHIC PHYSICIAN IS PREVENTED BY NO EXISTING LAWS RELATING TO MEDICINE FROM HIMSELF ADMINISTERING HIS MEDICINES TO HIS PATIENTS.[3]

No homœopathic physician dispenses; according to the principles of his art it is impossible for him to dispense.

To dispense means to mix together and to compound several medicinal substances, as the apothecary does.

At the period when the word "*dispense*" was first used in a medical sense, the pharmacopœias under the name of *dispensatoria*, contained only compound medicinal formulas, as, for example, the first *dispensatorium* that appeared in Germany, published at Nürnberg in 1551

----

[1] ["In the very bitter] and abusive complaint of the apothecaries, which was drawn up by a Leipzig advocate," says Stapf, "malicious insinuations were made regarding Hahnemann's disciples."]

[2] ["And what," exclaims Stapf," "was the result of this representation which Hahnemann addressed to a high personage in the state, in consequence of a complaint made against him, by the Leipzig apothecaries regarding the dispensing his own medicines?—The fatherland lost thereby one of its most illustrious sons!"

[3] Sent to the Authorities of State in 1821, first published in Stapf's Collection in 1829.

At the same time, the laws regarding medical affairs ordered that the apothecary alone, and no one else, should compound the various kinds of medicine according to the formulas of such a book (*dispensatorium*), or, according to the prescription of the physician, into a uniform mixture (to dispense) for the treatment of the sick.

In that alone consisted, and still consists, the apothecaries' privilege, and no apothecary has any other privilege.

The laws regulating medicine give to these mixtures of medicines the names of *medicines*, *medicaments*, and *composita*, but the several medicinal substances and ingredients they do not term either *medicines* or *medicaments*, but *simplicia* and *species*.

When therefore, the medicinal regulations forbid the physician to administer himself *medicines* and *medicaments* to his patients, in other words, to *dispense*, they cannot thereby mean any thing else than to prevent him compounding medicinal mixtures from various medicinal ingredients; but they nowhere forbid him giving *simplicia* to his patients.

They also forbid the apothecaries to dispense of themselves, or to make up and give out medicinal mixtures (medicaments) for patients, *without the physician's prescription*. Hence the apothecary dare not prepare for patients without the doctor's prescription any *medicines* (composita, medicinal mixtures, medicaments), but he is permitted to sell to any one simple medicinal substances (excepting those that act too violently in large dose), without the doctor's prescription; whence we perceive that the giving the *simplicia* cannot constitute dispensing, otherwise the apothecary would not be permitted to sell the *simplicia*.

But it is only *permitted* to the apothecary to sell simple medicinal substances; he has no *privilege* for this sale; otherwise there would be no druggists, who, also sell simple medicinal substances to every one.

Therefore the apothecary is not justified in preventing the physician from administering, himself, a simple medicinal substance to his patients.

The medicinal regulations never call the common sale by the apothecary *dispensing*, consequently it cannot be said of the physician who administers a simple medicinal susbtance for the relief of his patients, that he *dispenses*, because he does not compound for them any so-called *medicines* and *medicaments*, in the legal sense, that is, any *composita* consisting of several ingredients. In his unprivileged sale the apothecary gives to any one for money not only the crude simple medicinal substance, but also the simple preparations therefrom : he gives the buyers tincture of rhubarb, anise sugar, peppermint lozenges, &c., without let or hindrance, rightly taking for granted that the alcohol used in preparing the tincture and the sugar in the lozenges are not to be looked upon as medicinal substances, but as unmedicinal vehicles, in the former case for the rhubarb, in the latter for the anise or peppermint oil, consequently, that these simple preparations are not to be regarded as medicinal mixtures, nor their sale as dispensing.

But to be consistent, he must allow that when the physician gives a simple medicinal substance mixed with sugar to his patients, this also cannot be considered dispensing.

Hitherto, however, this has almost never been the case.

From the most remote periods physicians were *traditionally* directed by their teachers, by their colleges for instruction in the art of prescribing, in their hospitals, and by their medical authorities, to treat their patients by prescribing *medicines* (composita) in receipts from the apothecary's shop, and the apothecaries were directed to compound those medicinal mixtures called *medicines* and *medicaments par excellence*, from a variety of ingredients in considerable quantities, which was called dispensing.

But there unexpectedly arose—since all that is imperfect in the world gradually advances inevitably towards its perfection—an entirely new system of medicine, called by its founder *Homœopathy*, and taught in the book entitled *Organon of Medicine*. This system of medicine, which, as the book teaches, is much more consonant to nature, and as its results shew, is much more successful, is the direct opposite of the ordinary treatment. According to this new system, medicinal substances are employed for diseases in which the ordinary method gave exactly the opposite, but these were never given as in the ordinary method, in mixtures, but a single medicinal substance (simplex) *only* was *always* given for each case of disease, and that in such an extremely small dose, that the ordinary physician of the old school and the apothecary regard it as an unimportant nothing, for the former was accustomed to employ in treatment only large doses of medicine, but with entirely opposite aims, which could not do much good ; and the latter was accustomed to compound only large doses of several medicinal ingredients, and to transform them into medicaments. Whilst, for instance, the ordinary

45

physician employs the tincture of rhubarb in drachm doses, introduced into a formula along with other medicines, for the purpose of causing *purging*, the homœopathic physician gives a small part of a drop of the quadrillionth dilution, and for the very opposite object, namely for the *cure* of morbid *diarrhœas*, for which the old-school physician prescribes large doses of opium, often in vain, whilst the homœopathic physician employs this same tincture of opium more appropriately for the opposite state, and permanently removes continued *constipation* with a small part of a drop of the billionth dilution.

With this new, much more beneficent healing art, the homœopathic physician does not interfere with any apothecary's privilege, nor does he break any existing medicinal regulation.

No medicinal law has ever alleged that the physician must not give to his patient a single medicinal substance.

No privilege gives to the apothecary the exclusive right that *he alone* shall sell, unhindered, to every one, simple medicinal substances in large quantities, at hap-hazard (often to the great injury of the patient), whilst the physician dare *not* give to his patients, with a scientific purpose, *the same* simple medicinal substances in such small doses that the patient can only pay for the physician's skill, not for the remedy, because the latter, on account of its minuteness, has no commercial value, but on account of this incredible minuteness, must be given by the physician himself, and cannot be left to any assistant.

According to the principles of his art, which prove the employment of any mixture of medicines whatever for the cure of disease as *contrary to sound reason*,[1] it is impossible that the homœopathic physician can ever administer a medicinal mixture to his patients, consequently it is impossible that he can dispense, and so encroach upon the apothecary's privilege.

III.—How may homœopathy be most certainly eradicated ?[2]

In no way more certainly than by the authoritive commandment, " *Thou shalt not dispense.*" I have only a few observations to make on this subject. Although it were undoubtedly desirable that there was a method of more certainly curing the sick than can be done by the ordinary system of treatment, yet homœopa-

---

[1] *Organon of Medicine*, § 297-299, [*vide* last edition, § 272. 274].

[2] From the *Allgem. Anzeig. der Deutschen*, No. 227. 1825.

thy granting it fulfilled this desirable end, could not be tolerated,—

First, because from its practice the apothecaries would suffer so much ;

Second, because the large number of physicians instructed according to the old system would see themselves too strikingly placed in the shade if homœopathic treatment in their neighbourhood did much more than the prevailing system of medicine, was able to do.

These two classes of professional men endangered by homœopathy, the apothecaries and the physicians who practise and teach the old system of medicine, have consequently done all they could in order to prejudice the public against this treatment; they have tried to ridicule it, to malign it, and publicly to insult its practitioners in every way.

But as the fame of several remarkable homœopathic cures of diseases, hitherto incurable, spread among the public, and the latter, as it always does, paid more attention to the facts than to the calumnies respecting the new art by its opponents, a different plan was had recourse to. Those who sought relief for their maladies at length no longer paid any attention to the invectives and pasquils, anonymous and otherwise, that appeared in the journals that lent themselves to this purpose, they did not regard the bitter attacks in Jörg's *Critische Hefte*, nor Heinroth's theoretical sophisms in his *Anti-organon*, nor Kieser's nor Sprengel's writings—they looked to what had actually been effected here and there, and in many places, and embraced with increasing fervour the new healing art that did such great things.

All these manœuvres did homœopathy no harm; they were unable to effect its suppression in the slightest degree. It raises its head more joyfully than ever. Accordingly some persons gifted with a greater amount of worldly wisdom have already abandoned these useless counter-mines, and have hit upon the happier expedient *of endeavouring to obtain its suppression by the laws of the land, in order thereby to annihilate it.*

It is a main point for the homœopathic physician, in order that he may undertake and accomplish the cure of serious diseases with certainty, that he should himself select his remedies, prepare them himself, and administer them to the patient with his own hand, otherwise he is as little able to effect anything certain and excellent of its kind as the caligrapher would be if he were not allowed to select his own quills and cut them himself, or the painter if he were forbidden to prepare his own colours, and was obliged to get every tint he used prepared by a colour-mixing institution established by government.

As little would the homœopathic physician be able to perform a masterpiece of a cure, indeed he would not be able to cure at all, if he were prevented preparing his own curative agents, the preparation of which demands so much care and such extreme delicacy, but must let them be made by the apothecary, whose chief endeavour is and must be to annihilate a system of treatment that is exciting such attention, which not only is unprofitable to him, but as it undeniably demands infinitely fewer drugs for the accomplishment of the greatest cures, must one day open the eyes of the world, and render his business, which is only profitable by the amount of drugs disposed of to patients, useless.

Thus the homœopathist would naturally not be able to do any good with his medicines prepared by the apothecary, heaven only knows how! for no supervision can be exercised over him (seeing that one white powder of sugar of milk looks, tastes, smells and reacts chemically exactly like another, whether it contain nothing or whether it contain the minute homœopathic medicine or some medicine quite different), and he must naturally cease to be a homœopathic practitioner if he were to be prohibited and forbidden by law to prepare his own remedies.

This it is that the institute of apothecaries and those physicians brought up in the old system who are not able to equal the homœopathists in their cures, so earnestly desire for the new school, in order to destroy the practice of the homœopathists, consequently homœopathy itself, and they are, as we hear, attaining their object, inasmuch as they prosecute legally the homœopathists who give their own medicines to their patients, on the strength of the laws that forbid the physician to dispense his own medicines ; they avail themselves of the worldly arm of the judge to paralyse for ever the hand of the homœopathist. In this they were an dare successful, for the judge, as a man not belonging to the profession, acting upon the maxim *cuilibet in arte sua credendum*, imagines he must listen to the opinion of the medical authorities on the subject, and make their reasons and deliverances *his own*. It is only a pity that in this case he does not hear the calm, well-weighed allegations of impartiality, but only the embittered, fiery zeal of the *adverse* medical authorities, consisting of doctors deeply imbued with the learning of the past, whose traditional high position, together with that of their antiquated school, must, as they are aware, decline if homœo-pathists be at liberty to exercise their art freely.   This adverse party will undoubtedly win the day if the judge does not per-ceive partizanship in their so-called estimation of homœopathy, or if he attends to the interested insinuations of his family phy-sician, who as a physician of the old school trembling for the renown of the time-honoured faculty, takes great pains to join in the cry of the complainants and of the medical authorities, "Crucify him, crucify him!"

If the judge, I repeat, do not estimate all this partizan talk at its true value, and do not himself fulfil the sacred duty of a wise impartial *applicatio legis ad facta*, do not himself examine the law and its exact meaning with impartiality, then it is all up with the poor homœopathists,—he will be condemned, as a dis-penser, of having infringed upon the apothecaries' privilege, and he will be compelled to abandon his profession.   Such a verdict is as laudable as that of the town magistrate, who, when his friends the inn-keepers of the place, endowed with the ex-clusive right to feed guests with dishes made in their kitchens, brought an accusation against a man, "that he had encroached upon their privilege and *fed* persons," condemned the latter to punishment and the costs, in spite of all the representations of this benefactor to the effect, "that there was a great difference betwixt the way he *fed* and that in which the inn-keepers fed, and that though the latter might have the exclusive right to dispense their composite dishes, and to set them before their guests for money, yet that he had merely, during a period of general scarcity, distributed gratuitously to those who required it only simple articles of food, namely, bread to him who stood in need of bread, meat to him who wanted meat, or uncooked vegetables to him for whom they were suitable."

The homœopathic physician is in the position of this benefac-tor.   In the midst of the dearth of relief for diseases, where allopathy is of no use, he administers simple things, to cure one thing this, to cure another that, whatever is most suitable for each, and this he does *gratuitously*.

On the other hand the apothecaries' privilege runs as follows: "that no one shall prepare *medicines* or *medicaments*, that is, *dispense* them, except the apothecary, from the prescription of the physician—therefore that the physician shall not dispense medicines, nor the apothecary prepare (dispense) medicine of his own accord for patients, without the prescription of a legally qualified physician."

But the words *medicine* and *medicament* are *never* employed in any laws relative to medicine, except as signifying *a medicinal mixture composed of several medicinal ingredients, and the preparation of this alone* is exclusively entrusted to the privileged apothecary, who is to prepare it according to the prescription of a legitimate physician, that is, to dispense; and in like manner the physician of the old school is enjoined to prescribe *several* medicinal ingredients in his recipe which are to be mixed together by the apothecary. Thus Professor Gruner in the preface to his *Art of prescribing*, says expressly, that a prescription *must* consist of several medicinal ingredients to be united together, for a single medicinal substance written down does not constitute a prescription,—and for this reason every candidate for a medical degree must shew by his certificates that he has attended the lectures of a professor on the *art of prescribing*, and in order to shew that he is thorough master of it, so as to be able to write prescriptions for a patient to be made up at the laboratory, he must at the bidding of the examiner write extempore prescriptions for any diseases named to him; otherwise (and if he gives expression to his thought that diseases may also be cured with simple things) he will be rejected, *as has happened more than once.*

Thus it is certain that *according to law* the prescription must direct *several* medicinal ingredients to be united together, *so as that they shall constitute one medicament,* in the dispensing of which the apothecary's privilege solely and alone consists.

On the other hand, the homœopathic physician gives his patient *nothing but one simple substance, he never mixes several together,* nor can he do so consistently with his doctrine and his conviction, consequently he cannot employ in treatment any mixed by the apothecary. *It is therefore impossible that he can encroach on the business of compounding medicines, in which alone the apothecary's privilege consists, if he always gives his patient only a simple medicinal substance.* Then who could accuse the homœopathic physician of interfering with the right appertaining to the apothecary exclusively of preparing medicinal mixtures (*medicines, medicaments*), seeing that he has no medicinal ingredients to mix, and that he mixes none himself, consequently he does not dispense?

Simple medicinal substances (*species, simplicia*) are *not* termed *medicines* or *medicaments* by the medicinal laws of any land, on the contrary these terms are used in contradistinction to one another. *Medicines* or *medicaments* are, in the letter and spirit of these laws, *only compounds and mixtures of several medicinal ingredients prepared from the physician's prescription by the apothecary, and mingled together into a composite whole* (called by the laws *medicine* and *medicament*), which is sufficiently obvious from this, that the same medicinal laws that confer his *privilegium exclusivum* on the apothecary, whereby he obtains the right to prepare medicinal mixtures according to the physician's prescription, that is, *to dispense medicines* (*medicaments*), and whereby he is at the same time forbidden to dispense *medicines* without the physician's prescription, that is, to prepare of his own accord mixtures of several medicinal ingredients for the public—that the same medicinal laws, I say, allow him to deal in simple medicinal substances, to sell to any one that asks for them—rhubarb, cinchona bark, jalap, aloes, castor, asafœtida, valerian, and all other *simplicia* and *species* that are not dangerous in small quantities—whence it is obvious that the laws which forbid the apothecary to dispense medicines of his own accord, do not understand by the term "*medicines*" (*medicaments*), simple substances, and do not consider that *the giving of simple medicinal things* should be regarded as dispensing medicines; otherwise they would not have allowed the apothecary to sell them. They, however, universally allow the apothecary to do this as a regular retail seller of drugs, just as they appoint the druggist a wholesale dealer in drugs.

But if, in order to suppress the homœopathic physician, persecuted as he is by the old school of medicine and the apothecaries—seeing that he cannot be accused of practising the apothecaries' business of mixing medicines (dispensing)—it is sought to indict him as a *seller of simplicia*—an accusation that could not be brought under the category of the prohibited dispensing (compounding simplicia into a medicament)—be it known that the homœopathic physician *does not get paid* by the patient for his simple remedy (for *medicines* and *medicaments* in the sense of the medicinal laws they are not, as we have shewn), nor can he be paid for them, as they are so minute, so inconceivably delicate, that it is impossible to attach a commercial value to them on account of their incalculable minuteness! No! *he does not get paid for them*, he can only justly demand for his skill and trouble the fee that cannot be refused to any legitimate physician.

But in order to prevent his escape if possible, the apothecaries and allopathic physicians sophistically allege, "that the homœopath also makes up mixtures, and thereby encroaches on the apothecary's privilege, seeing that he unites his medicinal substance (simple though it be) with sugar of milk." But sugar of milk is not a medicinal ingredient, it is a mere vehicle and recipient for the simple medicinal substance of the homœopathic practitioner, just like the cane sugar in peppermint lozenges, in anise-sugar, in sugared worm-seeds and many other similar nonmedicinal things prepared and sold by the apothecary to the public, which no medicinal regulations forbid him to sell on the ground of their being mixtures of medicines or their sale coming under the head of dispensing, and which, in spite of the sugar in them as a vehicle, remain simple things (*simplicia.*)

Or shall the apothecary alone be allowed to give to the public a medicinal substance mingled with sugar, but when the scientific physician does the same for the purpose of curing disease, shall it be forbidden, not allowed, punishable? Is there a judge who could pronounce such a sentence?

And is there a judge, who, after a careful consideration of the above truthful representation, could, with the slightest semblance of justice, so misapprehend and distort our medicinal regulations that lay down so clearly and so accurately the definition of dispensing medicines, as to interpret them to condemn the homœopathic physician, who gives his simple substance (never any mixtures) *gratuitously* in order to relieve his patient, of dispensing and infringing on the apothecaries' privilege (which only refers to the compounding of medicaments consisting of several ingredients)? Could any impartial judge help acquitting him according to the letter of these plain and unanimous laws?

Let any one point out to us a single passage in any code of medicinal laws which forbids the legitimate physician to administer a simple medicinal substance in order to relieve his patient!

CONTRAST OF THE OLD AND THE NEW SYSTEMS OF MEDICINE.[1]

As long as accurate observation, unwearied research, and careful comparison have failed to demonstrate really constant original types of disease for the amazing number of morbid phenomena and cases of disease occurring in the human subject, which nature appears to produce in endless variety and very

---

[1] From the *Reine Arzneimittellehre*, part iv. 2d edit. 1825.

dissimilar to one another, so long will it be manifest that every single morbid phenomenon must be homœopathically treated, just as it presents itself, according to the array of symptoms that shew themselves in every case, by which means however they will all be infinitely better removed than by all the routine treatment that has hitherto prevailed in ordinary practice.

The adherents of the old school of medicine imagined that they would best succeed with the treatment of that great variety of morbid phenomena, if they arbitrarily drew up upon paper a list of types of disease, which should represent and include within them all the cases of disease that were met with at the sick-bed. They gave the name of *pathology* to this work of theirs.

Seeing the impossibility of efficaciously treating every case of disease according to its individuality, they imagined that their business was to select from the apparently infinite variety of different morbid phenomena which nature displays, a number of diseased states, all resembling each other in having some particular prominent symptom in common, as fundamental forms, and, having assigned to them general symptoms that were of not unfrequent occurrence in diseases and bestowed on them special names, to give them out for constant, distinct diseases, that always remained the same. The collection of these forms of disease manufactured by themselves, they asserted to constitute the whole range of the world of disease, in other words, *pathology, in order that they might be able to lay down special modes of treatment for these their imaginary morbid pictures,* and this constituted the science of *therapeutics.*

Thus they made a virtue of necessity, but they did not consider the evil that must arise from this perversion of nature, they did not reflect that this arbitrary procedure that did violence to nature, after having grown old by being propagated through thousands of years, would at length come to be regarded as a symbolical, unimprovable work.[1]

The physician who was called in to a case, to determine, as the rules of his art enjoined, the nosological name of the disease

---

[1] It is only a pity that this fond dream is dispelled when we look at the various systems of pathology with their different names and dissimilar descriptions of disease, when we look at the hundred and fifty definitions of fever, and the very various modes of treatment in the many works on therapeutics, which all lay equal claim to infallibility. Which of all of them is right? Is not the unnatural, unreal, apocryphal character of all apparent?

his patient laboured under, must take for granted, in reference to some symptoms that the pathological works describe as belonging to this form of disease, that they are merely accidentally absent in his patient, that they *might* very well be there, *although they are not*—the remaining often very numerous and serious sufferings and symptoms which the patient was really affected with, but which do not occur in the definition of the nosological name in the pathological work, he must, so the rules of his art required, regard as unessential, as accidental, as unimportant, as wild, exuberant offshoots, so to speak,—symptoms of symptoms—which he need not pay attention to.

It was only by such extraordinary capricious adding-to the actual morbid state, and equally capricious paring-down of it, that the adherent of the arbitrary old school succeeded in concocting the list of diseases, recorded in nosological works, and in practice demonstrating that his patient laboured under one of the diseases in this nosological system, of which nature never thought when she made him ill.

"What do we care," say the medical teachers and their books, "what do we care about the presence of many other diverse symptoms that are observable in the case of disease before us, or the absence of those that are wanting? The physician should pay no attention to such empirical trifles; his practical tact, the penetrating glance of his mental eye[1] into the hidden nature of the malady, enables him to determine at the very first sight of the patient what is the matter with him, what pathological form of disease he has to do with, and what name he has to give it, and his therapeutic knowledge teaches him what prescription he must order for it."

Thus then were prepared from that human piece of manufacture termed pathology those deceptive pictures of disease which were transferred *lege artis* to the patient, and falsely attributed to him, and this it was that rendered it so easy for the physician to recal to his memory without hesitation a couple of prescriptions which the clinical therapeutics (of the prescription pocketbook) had in readiness for this name.

---

[1] What honest man not endowed with clairvoyance could boast of possessing a mental eye which should enable him to penetrate through flesh and bone into that hidden essential nature of things that the Creator of mankind alone understands, of which mortal man would have no conception, for which he would have no words, if it were laid open to him? Does not such pretension reach the climax of boastful charlatanery and mendacious delusion?

But how did the prescriptions for these names of diseases originate? Were they communicated by some divine revelation?

My dear sir, they are either formulas prescribed by some celebrated practitioner for some case or other of disease to which he has arbitrarily given this nosological name, which formulas consist of a variety of ingredients, *known to him no doubt by name*, that came into his head and were put by him into an elegant form by the aid of that important art which is called *the art of prescribing* (*ars formulas concinnandi recteque concipiendi*), whereby the requirements of chemical skill and pharmaceutical observance were attended to, if not the welfare of the patient; —one or several receipts of this kind for the given case, under the use of which the patient at least did not die, but—thanks to heaven and his good constitution!—gradually recovered. These are therefore receipts taken from the writings of illustrious practitioners; or they are formulas which, at the request of some publisher who well knew how capitally prescription-manuals sell, were fabricated in a garret, off-hand, for the pathological names, by some willing soul in his pay, who was well skilled in the *ars formulas concinnandi*, and who was guided in his labour by the account of the virtues that the lying works on Materia Medica have liberally attributed to the several medicinal substances.

But if the physician found the disease in his patient too unlike any of the pathological forms of disease to permit him to give it a definite name of this sort, it was admissible for him, according to his books, to assume for the malady a more remote and concealed origin, in order to establish a treatment thereupon (on this assumption). Thus, supposing the patient at some former period had suffered from pain (no matter what kind) in the back, his disease was instantly ascribed to concealed or suppressed hemorrhoids—if he had had a tense abdomen, mucuous excrements, anorexia alternating with bulimia, or even only itching in the nose, his disease was called a worm disease; or if he had occasionally had pains (no matter what kind) in the limbs, his disease was pronounced to be concealed or immature gout, and against this fancied internal morbific cause the treatment was directed. If there were attacks of pain in the abdomen, spasm must be to blame for them; if there were frequent determination of blood to the face, or if the nose bled, the patient was decidedly too full-blooded; if the patient grew very thin during the treatment, as he naturally would, marasmus had to be combatted; if he was at the same time of a very sensitive disposition, nervous weakness was the enemy to be attacked; if he suffered from cough, then concealed catarrh or a tendency to phthisis was in the back ground; if the patient sometimes felt pains in the right side of the abdomen, or even only in the right shoulder, it was undoubtedly concealed inflammation or hidden in- duration of the liver that was to be taken into considera- tion. An old cutaneous disease or an ulcer on the leg must, in order that the treatment should be directed against it, be at- tributed either to some herpetic humour or to some scrofulous virus, and a chronic prosopalgia must of course be ascribed to the cancerous virus. After having in vain treated first this then the other fancied hidden morbid state according to the directions of the clinical books, and after all the mineral waters, *which are said to be useful in some indefinite manner for every thing,* had been visited, nothing else remained but to view the case as one of infarctus of the abdomen and obstruction of the minute vessels of that part according to the idea of the formerly cele- brated Kämpf, and torture the patient, in Kämpf's fashion, with injections into the colon of hundreds of his absurd mixtures of vegetable decoctions, until he had got enough of them.

In consequence of the ease with which conclusions relative to the essential nature of diseases were come to, there could, thank heaven! never be any lack of plans of treatment whereby the days of suffering of the patient might be fully occupied (for there are prescriptions in plenty for all names of diseases), as long as his purse, his patience, or his life lasted.

"But no! we can go to work in a more learned and sagacious manner, and investigate and conjecture upon the maladies that afflict mankind in the depths and concealment of abstract views of life, as to whether, in the case before us, the arterial, the venous or the nervous system, the sensibility, the irritability or the reproductive function suffer *quantitively more or less* (for we purposely avoid considering the infinite variety of *qualitive* affections from which these three expressions of vitality may suffer, in order not to burthen ourselves to a still greater ex- tent with the labour of research and conjecture); we merely *make a guess* as to whether these three expressions of vitality are in a state either of excessive depression or excessive exaltation. If we are of opinion that the first, second or third of them is suf- fering from one or other of these states of *too high* or *too low,* we may boldly proceed to manœuvre against it, according to the plan of the new iatro-chemical sect, which found out, 'that nitrogen, hydrogen and carbon alone constituted the souls of medicines, that is, the only active and curative thing in them; that, moreover, carbon, nitrogen and hydrogen could at pleasure regulate and screw up or screw down (potentize and depotentize) the irritability, the sensibility and the reproductive function, consequently (if the premises are correct) the whole vitality, and therefore they were capable of curing all diseases.'—'Tis only a pity that they are not yet agreed as to whether external agents act by means of their *similarity* or their *contrariety* to the compotent parts of our organism!"

But in order that medicines should really contain these elementary principles, which, as far as was known, they had not hitherto possessed, they were one holiday evening formally ascribed to them at the desk, and, in a system of materia medica specially created for this purpose, it was decreed how much carbon, nitrogen and hydrogen each medicinal substance should henceforth contain.

Could medical caprice go farther, or trifle more sinfully with human life?

But how long shall this irresponsible playing with human life still last?

After three and twenty centuries of such a criminal mode of procedure, now that the whole human race seems to be awaking in order powerfully to vindicate its rights, shall not the day begin to dawn for the deliverance of suffering humanity which has hitherto been racked with diseases, and in addition tortured with medicines administered without rhyme or reason, and without limit as to number and quantity, for phantoms of diseases, in conformity with the wildest notions of physicians proud of the antiquity of their sect?

Shall the pernicious jugglery of routine treatment still continue to exist?

Shall the entreaty of the patient, to listen to the account of his sufferings, vainly resound through the air unheard by his brethren of mankind, without exciting the helpful attention of any human heart?

Or can the so remarkably different complaints and sufferings of each single patient indicate anything else than the peculiarity of his disease? If not, what can this distinct voice of nature, which expresses itself in terms so appropriate to the various symptoms of the patient, what can it mean if not to render his morbid state as cognizable as possible to the sympathizing and attentive physician, in order to enable him to distinguish the very minutest shades of difference of this case from every other?

Would beneficient nature, that makes such efforts for our preservation, by her extremely wise, simple, and wonderful arrangement for enabling the patient to reveal to the observer, by words and signs, the great variety of his altered sensations and morbid actions, have enabled him to do this so utterly in vain and without object, and not in order to furnish a clear and accurate description of his morbid state in the only conceivable manner so as not to lead the practitioner astray? The disease, being but a peculiar condition, cannot speak, cannot tell its own story; the patient suffering from it can alone render an account of his disease by the various signs of his disordered health, the ailments he feels, the symptoms he can complain of, and by the alterations in him that are perceptible to the senses. But the pseudo-wisdom of the ordinary physicians thinks all this scarcely worth listening to; and even if they listen to it, they allege that it is of no importance, that it is empirical and expressed in a very unlearned manner by nature, that it does not coincide with what their pathological books teach them and is, therefore, not available for their purpose, but in place thereof they put forward a figment of their learned reveries as the picture of the internal (never ascertainable) state of the disease, in their folly substitute this delusive pathological picture for the individual state of each case of disease as nature faithfully delineates it, and direct their medicinal weapons against this trumped-up phantom of their imagination, the production of what they call their practical tact.

And what are these weapons of theirs? Large doses of medicines; that is, be it observed, powerful substances, which, where they do no good, must and really do injure the patient (seeing that the peculiar and sole nature of all medicines in the world consists in their capability, when brought in contact with the living sensitive body, of morbidly deranging it, each in its own peculiar way), which must accordingly make the patient worse, if they have not been selected for remedial purposes with the utmost care that their peculiar properties shall be adapted to the morbid state! These medicinal substances, which *in themselves are injurious, often very injurious* (and only useful in the cases for which they are suitable) and which are unknown in regard to their peculiar, true action, were so blindly resorted to, or in obedience to the mandates of the mendacious book called materia medica, mingled together (if the mixture was not taken ready-made from the receipt-book) as though they were drawn at hap-hazard from the wheel of fortune or rather misfortune, *with no correct knowledge or rather no knowledge at all of their true, peculiar effects,* and they served but to increase the tortures of the patient already suffering from his disease, with this barbarous olla-podrida full of disgusting smells and tastes (one spoonful to be taken every hour!). Was such a procedure beneficial to him? oh God! no, prejudicial to him. The usual result of such an unnatural and false mode of treatment pursued during every hour of the day, must be visible aggravation of his state, aggravation which the ignorant patient is made to believe is the malignant nature of his disease. Poor, unhappy wretch! what else than to make bad worse can be done by such powerful noxious substances raked together, according to the whims of the prevalent medical school, taken at blind hazard and administered in an inappropriate place?

And in this homicidal manner have practitioners gone on acting in despite of the truth that speaks trumpet-tongued for our information, because, since the remotest times, it has been the habit with their profession to torture methodically suffering humanity in this unnatural manner for their money—to their injury!

What human heart in whom the smallest spark of the God-implanted monitor, conscience, still exists, but must shudder at such abominable behaviour?

In vain, in vain dost thou seek to silence the audible, terrible voice of the incorruptible judge in thy conscience, of that sacred tribunal of God's justice that holds its seat in thy bosom, by the miserable excuse that others do so likewise, and that such has been the practice since the most remote ages; in vain dost thou seek to stifle its still small voice by atheistical ridicule, wild pleasures, and goblets of reason-obscuring, intoxicating drinks. The Holy One, the Almighty lives, and eternal unchangeable justice lives with him.

* * * *

Now, as the internal operations and processes of the living human organism cannot be inspected, and, as long as we are merely men and not God, cannot be perfectly known to us, either in the healthy or yet in the diseased state, and on that very account all deductions from the exterior respecting the interior are deceptive, and as the knowledge of disease can be neither a metaphysical problem nor the product of fantastic speculation, but is an affair of pure experience by the senses, because disease as a manifestation can only be apprehended by observation; therefore every unprejudiced person must at once perceive that, as careful observation finds every individual case of disease to differ from every other,[1] no name borrowed from a pathological system of man's fabrication which falsely alleges diseases to possess constant unvarying characters, should be attached to morbid states, which in reality differ so much among themselves, and that there can scarcely be any hypothetical representation which we can form to ourselves respecting any one disease, that shall not be imaginary, delusive and untrue.

Diseases are nothing more than alterations of the healthy, regular state of health, and as an alteration of this sort consists merely in the occurrence of many accidents, morbid symptoms and perceptible divergences from the former healthy state, seeing that after the removal of all these accidents and symptoms nothing but health can remain; so there can be for the physician no other true view of diseases which shall enable him to discover what should be the aim of his treatment, and what there is to be cured, save and except what is perceived by the senses of the observable alterations of health in the patient.

The honest physician, therefore, whose conscience forbids him with superficial haste to invent a delusive picture of the malady to be cured, or to consider it as one of the forms of disease already existing in pathological works; whose earnest desire it is, in one word, to investigate the peculiar character of the disease before him, in order to be able to restore the patient with certainty,—the honest physician, I say, will observe his patient minutely, with all his senses, will make the patient and his attendants detail all his sufferings and symptoms, and will carefully note them down without adding anything to or taking anything from them; he will thus have a faithful genuine picture of the disease, and along with that an accurate knowledge of all there is in it to be cured and removed; he will then have a true knowledge of the disease.

Now as diseases can be nothing more than alterations of the healthy, regular state of health, and as every alteration of the health of a healthy person is disease, therefore cure can be no-

---

[1] With the exception of such diseases as are caused by a miasm of constant character, or by an always identical cause.

thing than transformation of the irregular state of health into the regular and healthy state.

If, then, as cannot be denied, medicines are the agents for curing diseases, they must possess the power of effecting an alteration in the state of health.

Now as there can be no other alteration of the sound state of health than this, that the healthy person shall become sick, therefore medicines, inasmuch as they possess the power of healing, consequently of altering the health of man, the healthy as well as the sick, must, in their action upon the healthy, produce many symptoms, morbid sufferings, and divergences from the healthy state.

Now admitting, what likewise cannot be denied, that, in order to cure, the main business of the physician consists in knowing beforehand the medicine from which a cure is most certainly to be expected, he must, seeing that a cure by medicines takes place *only* by reason of an alteration effected in the state of the health, above all things know beforehand, what alterations in man's health the several medicines can effect, before he selects one of them for administration, if he do not wish to be guilty of a criminal inconsiderateness, and an unpardonable attack upon human life;—for if every powerful medicine can make the healthy sick, an ignorantly selected, consequently an unsuitable, medicine must necessarily render the patient worse than he was.

The most zealous efforts of one who devotes himself to the cure of diseases (a physician), must hence before all things, be directed to obtain a foreknowledge of those properties and actions of medicines by means of which he may effect the cure or amelioration of every individual case of disease with the greatest certainty, that is to say, he must, before commencing the practice of physic, have previously obtained a thorough knowledge of the peculiar alterations in the health of man the several medicines are capable of effecting, in order to be able to select, in every case of disease, the health-altering medicine most suitable for effecting a cure.

Now it is impossible that the alterations in man's health which medicines are capable of producing, can be known and observed more purely, certainly and completely, by any other method in the world, than by the action of medicines upon healthy individuals; indeed there is no other way besides this conceivable, in which it were possible to obtain experience that shall be at all of an accurate character respecting the real alterations they are

46

capable of effecting in man's health. For the action they shew with chemical re-agents, reveals only chemical properties, which are no clue to their power over the living human organism. The alterations they produce when given to animals, only teach what they can do to them each according to its nature, but not what they would effect on man, endowed as he is with an organization of a perfectly different character, and with very different powers both of mind and body. Even when given in human diseases in order to ascertain their effects, the peculiar symptoms which were solely due to the medicine can never be distinctly recognised, never accurately distinguished, amid the tumult of the morbid symptoms already present, so as to admit, of our ascertaining which of the changes effected were owing to the medicine, which to the disease. Hence not the slightest claim to a knowledge of the true, pure action of the various medicines can be made by the ordinary materia medica, which has scraped together its fables respecting the virtues of drugs, from the confused use of *mixed medicaments* in diseases, its descriptions of which are often not more lucid than the pathological names bestowed upon them.

The simple natural way alone remains for us, in order to ascertain clearly, purely and with certainty, the powers of medicines upon man, that is, the alterations they are capable of effecting on his health—the only genuine and simple natural way, viz., to administer the medicines to healthy individuals who are attentive enough to notice upon themselves what each individual medicine is capable of producing in and on them of a peculiar morbid and altered character, and to make a careful record of the complaints, symptoms and alterations in their corporeal and mental state produced by its administration, as the peculiar alterations of man's health this medicine may henceforth be expected to produce; for whilst the action of a medicine lasts (provided violent moral emotions and other injurious influences from without do not intervene) all the symptoms that occur in a healthy individual must be the effects of the medicine, seeing that its influence alone dominates over our state of health at that period.

The physician must possess the most perfect knowledge possible of the pure alterations in the health produced on the healthy human body by the greatest possible number of single medicines, before he ventures to undertake the most important of all vocations, namely, the administration of medicines to a sick person for his disease, to a suffering fellow-creature who appeals to our most sacred sense of duty to relieve him, who demands all our compassion and all our zeal, to enable us to rescue him, for these medicines if given improperly are frightful substances, and are attended with injurious effects, and not unfrequently with danger to life.

In this way alone will the upright physician act in the most important matter of conscience that can be, in gaining a knowledge of the pure effects of medicines, and in investigating the case of disease committed to his care, according to the distinct indication and obvious requirements of nature, and in this way alone will he act in accordance with the dictates of nature and conscience, even though he know not as yet what morbid symptoms, artificially produced by medicine on the healthy individual, nature has destined for the eradication of any given symptom in natural diseases.

This problem he cannot solve by any speculative *a priori* research, nor by any fantastic reveries—no! he can only solve this problem also, by experiment, observation, and experience.

Now it is not merely one single observation, but *all* experiments and observations carefully conducted demonstrate in the most convincing manner (to every sensible individual who *will* be convinced) that among medicines tested as to their pure effects, that one alone, which can produce in the healthy individual a *similar* morbid state, is capable of transforming a given case of disease, rapidly, gently, and permanently into health, *indeed, that such a medicine will never fail to cure the disease.* The place of the natural disease in the organism is occupied by the artificial somewhat stronger medicinal disease, which now alone occupies the vitality, and in consequence of the minuteness of the dose of the medicine which produced it, runs but a brief course before being extinguished, and the body is then left without disease, that is, quite well and (homœopathically) cured.

If then, beneficent nature shews us, in the homœopathic method of treatment, the only sure and infallible way by which we can remove easily and permanently the totality of the symptoms in a patient, that is, his whole morbid state,[1] and by which we are able to make him well at will; if every instance of treatment conducted on this plan shews us the most unfailing cure; who could remain so perverse, and neglect to such a degree the good of himself and of humanity, as to refuse to tread in this

---

[1] After the removal of all his ailments, symptoms and the morbid changes in his feelings, can anything besides health remain !

path of truth and nature, but stick to the indefensible, antiquated, purely imaginary phantoms of diseases and modes of treatment, to the ruination of the sick?

I know full well that it requires heroic courage in order to cure ourselves of prejudices grown almost into mental infirmities, which have become sacred to us on account of their hoary age, and that it demands a very uncommon strength of mind to eradicate from our memory all the absurdities that have been imprinted upon our youthful susceptibilities as oracular deliverances, and to exchange them for new truths.

But the oak-garland with which a consciousness of acting right crowns us, rewards these victories over ourselves a thousand-fold!

Do old, antiquated untruths become anything better—do they become truths—by reason of their hoary antiquity? Is not truth eternal, though it may have been discovered only an hour ago? Does the novelty of its discovery render it an untruth? Was there ever a discovery or a truth that was not at first novel?

THE MEDICAL OBSERVER.[1]

(A FRAGMENT.)

In order to be able to observe well, the medical practitioner requires to possess, what is not to be met with among ordinary physicians even in a moderate degree, the capacity and habit of noticing carefully and correctly the phenomena that take place in natural diseases, as well as those that occur in the morbid states artificially excited by medicines, when they are tested upon the healthy body, and the ability to describe them in the most appropriate and natural expressions.

In order accurately to perceive what is to be observed in patients, we should direct all our thoughts upon the matter we have in hand, come out of ourselves, as it were, and attach ourselves, so to speak, with all our powers of concentration upon it, in order that nothing that is actually present, that has to do

---

[1] From the *Reine Arzneimittellehre*, pt. iv, 2nd edit. 1825.

with the subject, and that can be ascertained by the senses, may escape us.

Poetic fancy, fantastic wit and speculation, must for a while be suspended, and all overstrained reasoning, forced interpretation and tendency to explain away things, must be suppressed. The duty of the observer is then only to take notice of the phenomena and their course; his attention should be on the watch, not only that nothing actually present escape his observation, but that also what he observes be understood exactly as it is.

This capability of observing accurately is never quite an innate faculty; it must be chiefly acquired by practice, by refining and regulating the perceptions of the senses, that is to say, by exercising a severe criticism in regard to the rapid impressions we obtain of external objects, and at the same time the necessary coolness, calmness and firmness of judgment must be preserved, together with a constant distrust of our own powers of apprehension.

The vast importance of our subject should make us direct the energies of our body and mind towards the observation; and great patience, supported by the power of the will, must sustain us in this direction until the completion of the observation.

To educate us for the acquirement of this faculty, an acquaintance with the best writings of the Greeks and Romans is useful, in order to enable us to attain directness in thinking and in feeling, as also appropriateness and simplicity of expressing our sensations; the art of drawing from nature is also useful, as it sharpens and practises our eye, and thereby also our other senses, teaching us to form a true conception of objects, and to represent what we observe, truly and purely, without any addition from the fancy. A knowledge of mathematics also gives us the requisite severity in forming a judgment.

Thus equipped, the medical observer cannot fail to accomplish his object, especially if he has constantly before his eyes the exalted dignity of his calling—as the representative of the all-bountiful Father and Preserver, to minister to His beloved human creatures, by renovating their systems when ravaged by disease. He knows that observations of medical subjects must be made in a sincere and holy spirit, as if under the eye of the all-seeing God, the Judge of our secret thoughts, and must be recorded so as to satisfy an upright conscience, in order that they may be communicated to the world, in the consciousness that no earthly good is more worthy of our zealous exertions than the preservation of the life and health of our fellow-creatures.

The best opportunity for exercising and perfecting our observing faculty, is afforded by instituting experiments with medicines upon ourselves. Whilst avoiding all foreign medicinal influences and disturbing mental impressions in this important operation, the experimenter, after he has taken the medicine, has all his attention strained towards all the alterations of health that take place on and within him, in order to observe and correctly to record them, with ever-wakeful feelings, and his senses ever on the watch.

By continuing this careful investigation of all the changes that occur within and upon himself, the experimenter attains the capability of observing all the sensations, be they ever so complex, that he experiences from the medicine he is testing, and all, even the finest shades of alteration of his health, and of recording in suitable and adequate expressions his distinct conception of them.

Here alone is it possible for the beginner to make pure, correct and undisturbed observations, for he knows that he will not deceive himself, there is no one to tell him aught that is untrue, and he himself feels, sees and notices what takes place in and upon him. He will thus acquire practice to enable him to make equally accurate observations on others also.

By means of these pure and accurate investigations, we shall be made aware that all the symptomatology hitherto existing in the ordinary system of medicine, was only a very superficial affair, and that nature is wont to disorder man in his health and in all his sensations and functions by disease or medicine in such infinitely various and dissimilar manners, that a single word or a general expression is totally inadequate to describe the morbid sensations and symptoms which are often of such a complex character, if we wish to portray really, truly, and perfectly the alterations in the health we meet with.

No portrait painter was ever so careless as to pay no attention to the marked peculiarity in the features of the person he wished to make a likeness of, or to consider it sufficient to make any sort of a pair of round holes below the forehead by way of eyes, between them to draw a long-shaped thing directed downwards, always of the same shape, by way of a nose, and beneath this to put a slit going across the face, that should stand for the mouth of this or of any other person; no painter, I say, ever went about delineating human faces in such a rude and slovenly manner; no naturalist ever went to work in this fashion in describing any natural production; such was never the way in which any zoologist, botanist, or mineralogist acted.

It was only the semiology of ordinary medicine that went to work in such a manner, when describing morbid phenomena. The sensations that differ so vastly among each other, and the innumerable varieties of the sufferings of the many different kinds of patients, were so far from being described according to their divergences and varieties, according to their peculiarities, the complexity of the pains composed of various kinds of sensations, their degrees and shades, so far was the description from being accurate or complete, that we find all these infinite varieties of sufferings huddled together under a few bare, unmeaning, general terms, such as *perspiration, heat, fever, headache, sore-throat, croup, asthma, cough, chest-complaints, stitch in the side, belly-ache, want of appetite, dyspepsia, back-ache, coxalgia, hœmorrhoidal sufferings, urinary disorders, pains in the limbs,* (called according to fancy, *gouty* or *rheumatic*), *skin diseases, spasms, convulsoins,* &c. With such superficial expressions, the innumerable varieties of sufferings of patients were knocked off in the so-called observations, so that—with the exception of some one or other severe, striking symptom in this or that case of disease—almost every disease pretended to be described is as like another as the spots on a die, or as the various pictures of the dauber resemble one another in flatness and want of character.

The most important of all human vocations, I mean *the observation of the sick, and of the infinite varieties of their disordered state of health,* can only be pursued in such a superficial and careless manner *by those who despise mankind,* for in this way there is no question either of distinguishing the peculiarities of the morbid states, nor of selecting the only appropriate remedy for the special circumstances of the case.

The conscientious physician who earnestly endeavours to apprehend in its peculiarity the disease to be cured, in order to be able to oppose to it the appropriate remedy, will go much more carefully to work in his endeavour to distinguish what there is to be observed; language will scarcely suffice to enable him to express by appropriate words the innumerable varieties of the symptoms in the morbid state; no sensation, be it ever so peculiar, will escape him, which was occasioned in his feelings by the medicine he tested on himself; he will endeavour to convey an idea of it in language by the most appropriate expression, in order to be able in his practice to match the accurate delineation of the morbid picture with the similarly acting medicine, whereby alone, as he knows, can a cure be effected.

So true it is that the careful observer alone can become a true healer of diseases.

HOW CAN SMALL DOSES OF SUCH VERY ATTENUATED MEDICINE AS HOMŒOPATHY EMPLOYS STILL POSSESS GREAT POWER ?[1]

This question is asked not only by the ordinary allopathic physician, who thinks he cannot go far enough with the huge quantities of medicines he prescribes, but the beginner in homœopathy also ignorantly puts the same question.

To doubt, if it be possible that they can have the requisite power, seems to be of itself very foolish, because they are actually seen to act so powerfully, and manifestly to compass the object intended, and this they may be seen to do daily.

And what *actually takes place* must at least be possible!

But even when the hostile scoffers can no longer deny the effect that lies before their very eyes, they seek, by means of false analogies, to represent what is actually occurring, if not as impossible, at least as ridiculous.

" If a drop of such highly attenuated medicine," so they talk, " can still act, then the water of the lake of Geneva, into which a drop of some strong medicine has fallen, must display as much curative power in each of its separate drops, indeed much more, seeing that in the homœopathic attenuations a much greater proportion of attenuating fluid is used."

The answer to this is, that in the preparation of the homœopathic medicinal attenuations, a small portion of medicine is not merely added to an enormous quantity of non-medicinal fluid, or only slightly mingled with it, as in the above comparison, which has been devised in order to bring ridicule upon the affair, but, by the *succussion* and *trituration*, there ensues not

---

[1] From the *Reine Arzneimittellehre*, pt. vi., 1st. edit. 1827.

only the most intimate mixture, but at the same time—and this is the most important circumstance—there ensues such a great, and hitherto unknown and undreamt of change, by the developement and liberation of the dynamic powers of the medicinal substance so treated, as to excite astonishment.

In the above thoughtlessly adduced comparison, however, by the dropping of one drop of medicine into such a great lake, there can be no question of even its superficial admixture with all parts of a body of water of such extent, so as that every part shall contain an equal portion of the drop of medicine.

There is not the slightest question of an intimate mixture in such a case.

Even only a moderately large quantity of water, for instance, a hogshead of water, if we attempted to impregnate it *in its entirety, in a mass*, with a drop of medicine, could never, after any length of time, or by any imaginable stirring about, be equally mixed—not to mention that the constant internal changes and uninterrupted chemical decomposition of the component parts of the water, would have destroyed and annihilated the medicinal power of a drop of vegetable tincture in the course of a few hours.

In like manner, a hundred weight of flour taken *as one whole mass*, can by no mechanical contrivance be mixed so equally with a grain of medicine as that each grain of flour shall obtain an equal portion of the medicinal powder.

In the homœopathic pharmaceutical operations, on the contrary, (admitting they consisted merely of a common mixture, which they do not), as *only a small quantity* of the attenuating fluid is taken at a time (a drop of medicinal tincture shaken up along with 100 drops of alcohol), there ensues a union and equal distribution in a few seconds.

But the mode of attenuating practised in homœopathy effects not only an equal distribution of the medicinal drop throughout a great proportional quantity of unmedicinal fluid (which is out of the question in the above absurd comparison), but it also happens—and this is of infinitely greater importance—that by the *succussion* and *trituration* employed, a change is effected in the mixture, which is so incredibly great and so inconceivably curative, that this development of the spiritual power of medicines to such a height by means of the multiplied and continued *trituration* and *succussion* of a small portion of medicinal substance with ever more and more dry or fluid unmedicinal substances, deserves incontestably to be reckoned *among the greatest discoveries* of this age.

The *physical* changes and development of power that may be produced by *trituration* from substances in nature, which we call matter, have hitherto only been surmised from some circumstances—but the extraordinary effects in the way of developing and exciting the dynamic forces of medicines it can produce, have never been dreamt of.

Now with respect to the development of physical forces from material substances by *trituration*, this is a very wonderful subject.[1]

It is only the ignorant vulgar that still look upon matter as a dead mass, for from its interior can be elicited incredible and hitherto unsuspected powers.

All new discoveries of this sort are usually met by denial and incredulity from the great mass of mankind, who have neither adequate acquaintance with physical phenomena nor with the causes of these phenomena, nor the capacity to observe for themselves, and to reflect upon what they perceive. They see, for example, that when a piece of steel is strongly and rapidly rubbed against a hard stone (agate, flint), an operation that is termed striking fire, incandescent sparks fly off (and kindle the tinder or punk they fall on): but how few among them have carefully observed and reflected upon what really takes place there. All of them, or at least almost all, go on thoughtlessly lighting their tinder, and almost no one perceives, what a miracle, what a great natural phenomenon thereby takes place. When sparks are thus struck with sufficient force, and caught on a sheet of white paper, then we may see, either with the naked eye or by means of a lens, usually small pellets of steel lying there, which have been detached in a state of fusion from the surface of the steel by the smart collision with the flint, and have fallen in an incandescent state, like small fire balls, in the form of sparks, upon the paper, where they cooled.

How! can the violent friction of the flint and steel (in the operation of striking fire) cause such a degree of heat as to fuse steel into little balls. Does it not require a heat of at least

[1] [What follows appeared in 1825, in the *Allg. Anz. d. D.*, No. 194, and was intended as a reply to a correspondent of that Journal, who endeavoured to show the nothingness of homœopathy by some of those calculations respecting the minuteness of the dose, which to this day constitute the stereotyped arguments, of the opponents of the system. In the *R. A. M. L.* this is abridged, I have restored it to its original form.]

3000° of Fahrenheit's thermometer in order to melt steel? Whence comes this tremendous heat? Not out of the air, for this phenomenon takes place just as well in the vacuum of the air-pump! therefore it must come from the substances that are rubbed together; which is the fact.

But does the ordinary individual really believe that the cold steel which he draws thoughtlessly from his pocket to light his tinder, contains hidden within it (in a latent, confined, undeveloped state) an inexhaustible store of caloric, which the blow only develops, and as it were, wakes into activity? No, he does not believe it, he has never reflected, *and never will reflect*, upon the phenomena of nature. And yet it is so. And yet his steel, which when at rest is cold, contains—whether he believe it or no—an inexhaustible store of caloric, which can only be released by *friction*. An inexhaustible store of caloric, I repeat, which is not calculable by the cyphers of any of those arithmeticians who seek to limit nature and render her contemptible, by applying their multiplication table to the phenomena of her illimitable forces. The great natural philosopher, Count Rumford,[1] teaches us how to heat our rooms solely by the rapid motion of two plates of metal rubbing against one another, without the employment of any ordinary combustible material whatever. No further proof is required to convince the reflective that natural bodies, and especially metals, contain an inexhaustible store of caloric concealed within them, which however can be called into life *only by means of friction*.

The effect of *friction* is so great, that not only the physical properties, such as caloric, odour,[2] &c., are thereby called into life and developed by it, but also the dynamic medicinal powers of natural substances are thereby developed to an incredible degree, *a fact that has hitherto escaped observation.* The founder of the homœopathic system was the first who made this great, this extraordinary discovery, that the properties of crude medicinal substances gain, when they are fluid by repeated *succussion* with unmedicinal fluids, and when they are dry by frequent continued *trituration* with unmedicinal powders, such an increase of medicinal power, that when these processes are carried very far,

---

[1] Count Rumford's treatise on caloric fills the first division of the 4th Vol. of his works, which have been published by the Weimar *Industrie-Comptoir.*

[2] Horn, ivory, bone, the calcareous stone impregnated with petroleum, &c., have of themselves no smell, but when filed or *rubbed* they not only emit an odour but an extremely fetid one, hence the last-mentioned substance has obtained the name of *Stinkstone,* though when not rubbed it has no smell.

even substances in which for centuries no medicinal power has been observed in their crude state, display under this manipulation a power of acting on the health of man that is quite astonishing.

Thus pure gold, silver and platina have no action on the human health in their solid state—and the same is the case with vegetable charcoal in its crude state. Several grains of gold leaf, silver leaf or charcoal may be taken by the most sensitive person without his perceiving any medicinal action from it. All these substances present themselves to us in a state of suspended animation as far as regards their medicinal action. But if a grain of gold leaf be triturated strongly for an hour in a porcelain mortar with one hundred grains of sugar of milk, the powder that results (the first trituration) possesses a considerable amount of medicinal power. If a grain of this powder be triturated as strongly and as long with another hundred grains of sugar of milk, the preparation attains a much greater medicinal power, and if this process be continued, and a grain of the previous trituration be rubbed up as strongly and for as long a time, each time with a fresh hundred grains of sugar of milk until, after fifteen such triturations, the quintillionth attenuation of the original grain of gold leaf is obtained, then the last attenuations do not display a weaker, but on the contrary, the most penetrating, the greatest medicinal power of the whole of the attenuations. A single grain of the last (quintillionth) attenuation put into a small, clean phial, will restore a morbidly desponding individual, with a constant inclination to commit suicide, in less than an hour to a peaceful state of mind, to love of life, to happiness, and horror of his contemplated act, if he perform but a single olfaction in the phial, or put on his tongue a quantity of this powder no bigger than a grain of sand.[1]

---

[1] [In connexion with this subject I may be permitted to adduce a few points bearing on the question of the dose of *gold*. In the first place we learn from the 4th part of the *R. A. M. L.* and the *Chr. Kr.* that this substance was proved upon healthy individuals in doses of from 100 to 200 grains of the first trituration (one to two grains of pure gold). Then, with respect to the doses to be administered in disease, we find it stated in the introduction to *gold* in the second edition of both these works (published respectively in 1825 and 1835, probably a repetition of what appeared in the 1st edition of the *R. A. M. L.*, published about 1820) that Hahnemann had cured several (*mehre*) individuals suffering from suicidal melancholia with from 3-100ths to 9-100ths of a grain of gold for the whole treatment. He also mentions in these places that he had found a smaller quantity, viz: 1-10000th part of a grain of gold not less powerful, especially in caries of the nasal and palatial bones, from the abuse of mercurials. In the essay of which our text is a translation (published in 1825) he

From this we perceive that the preparations of medicinal substances of *trituration*, the farther the development of their powers is thereby brought and the more perfectly capable they are thereby rendered for displaying their power, become capable of answering the homœopathic purpose in proportionately smaller quantities and doses.

Medicinal substances are not dead masses in the ordinary sense of the term, on the contrary, their true essential nature is only dynamically spiritual—is pure force, which may be increased in potency by that most wonderful process of *trituration* (and *succussion*) according to the homœopathic method, almost to an infinite degree.

In the same way liquid medicines do not become by their greater and greater attenuation, weaker in power but always more potent and penetrating. For homœopathic purposes this dilution is performed by well shaking a drop of the medicine with a hundred drops of a non-medicinal fluid; from the bottle so shaken a drop is taken and shaken up in the same manner with another hundred drops of unmedicinal fluid, and so on. This result, so incomprehensible to the man of figures, goes so far that we must set bounds to the succussion process, in order that the degree of attenuation be not over-balanced by the increased potency of the medicine, and in that way the highest attenuations become too active. If we wish, for example, to attenuate a drop of the juice of *sundew*[1] to the decillionth, but shake each of the bottles with twenty or more succussions from a powerful arm, in the hand of which the bottle is held, in that case this medicine, which I have discovered to be the specific remedy for the frightful epidemic *hooping-cough* of children, will have become so powerful in the fifteenth attenuation (spiritualization) that a drop of it given in a tea-spoonful of water would endanger the life of such a child; whereas if each dilution-bot-

states that a quintillionth (15th dilution) was the preparation he then generally used; in the same essay as it appears in the 6th part of the *R. A. M. L.*, (published in 1827), and in the introduction to *gold* in the *R. A. M. L.*, (published in 1825), he recommends a quadrillionth of a grain (12th dilution) for a dose. In the *Chr. Kr.*, (published in 1835) he of course advises the decillionth (30th dilution) to be given in every case. The following, then, was the state of Hahnemann's practice in reference to the dose of this remedy at different periods. About 1820, 1st or 2d attenuation; in 1825, 12th or 15th attenuation; in 1827, 12th attenuation; in 1835, 30th attenuation.]

[1] *Drosera rotundifolia*, a plant, which, along with its various species, grows on moist meadow-ground, and is very noxious to sheep.

tle were shaken but twice (with two strokes of the arm) and prepared in this manner up to the decillionth attenuation, a sugar globule the size of a poppy seed moistened with the last attenuation cures this terrible disease with this single dose without endangering the health of the child in the slightest degree.[1]

But these homœopathic medicinal attenuations (—pity there is no more appropriate word in any language to express what takes place in the process, as this phenomenon was never heard of before its discovery—) these attenuations are so far from being diminutions of the medicinal power of this grain or drop of the crude medicinal substance keeping pace with its extreme fractional diminution as expressed by figures, that, on the contrary, experience shews them to be rather an actual exaltation of the medicinal power, a real spiritualization of the dynamic property, a true, astonishing unveiling and vivifying of the medicinal spirit.

But there are various reasons why the sceptic ridicules these homœopathic attenuations. *First*, because he is ignorant that by means of such triturations the internal medicinal power is wonderfully developed, and is as it were liberated from its material bonds, so as to enable it to operate more penetratingly and more freely upon the human organism; *secondly*, because his purely arithmetical mind believes that it sees here only an instance of enormous subdivision, *a mere material division and diminution*, wherein every part must be less than the whole—as every child knows; but he does not observe, that in these spiritualizations of the internal medicinal power, the material receptacle of these natural forces, the palpable ponderable matter, is not to be taken into consideration at all; *thirdly*, because the sceptic has no experience relative to the action of preparations of such exalted medicinal power.

If, then, he who pretends to be a seeker after truth will not search for it where it is to be found, namely, in *experience*, he will certainly fail to discover it; he will never find it by arithmetical calculations.

---

[1] [In the version of this passage as it stands in the *R. A. M. L.*, the decillionth attenuation prepared with twenty succussions to each bottle is spoken of as endangering the life of the hooping-cough patient, and from this circumstance and the fact that it is not stated that such a preparation *did* endanger the life of any patient, but only that it *would* (*würde*) endanger it, we are, I think, justified in inferring that Hahnemann did not actually observe any such case, but that he merely supposed that it would occur, which his theory of the increase of potency in homœopathic medicaments by the processes of trituration and succussion would lead him to do.]

ON THE IMPREGNATION OF THE GLOBULES WITH MEDICINE.[1]

If we add to the mode of procedure recommended by the esteemed author of this letter, that the globules, from 5 to 600 of which should be in each little bottle, and fill it only about half full, should be moistened with from three to four drops of the alcoholic medicinal dilution, and not shaken in the corked up bottle, but rather stirred about in it with a silver or glass pin, and the bottle kept uncorked until by the evaporation of the alcohol they become dry and no longer adhere to each other, so that each globule may be taken out separately; in this way the homœopathist possesses indisputably the most convenient process for having his medicines always of the same good quality and ready for immediate use.

The medicated alcohol that evaporates whilst the globules are thus stirred for about an hour, is no loss for the globules that that are thus dried in the bottle, seeing that, strictly speaking, for the purpose of moistening 600 of the smallest globules a single drop would suffice, and consequently in this desiccation by the evaporation of the superfluous medicated alcohol, they do not undergo any diminution whatsoever of their medicinal power, as I have been superabundantly convinced by employing them in practice.

With this little alteration the process recommended by my esteemed and patriotic correspondent deserves the thanks of every homœopathic practitioner, for it is the most perfect that has been proposed, as my own experience convinces me.

It is only in this form that the homœopathic medicines can be sent to the most distant parts without any alteration of their powers, which is impossible to be done in their fluid form; for in that case the medicinal fluid, which has already been sufficiently potentized during their preparation (by two successions at each dilution), receives an enormous number of additional

[1] From the *Archiv der hom. Heilk.*, Vol. viii, pt. 2, p. 162. 1829. [This article appears as a note appended to a communication from M. Korsakoff, a Russian homœopathic dilettante, suggesting the use of little tubes for holding the globules ready made, such as those at present in almost universal use for pocket cases. He proposed that the globules should be saturated by pouring upon them two or three drops of the medicinal dilution, and shaking the bottle several times strongly.]

successions during the transport, and they are so highly potentized during a long journey, that on their arrival they are scarcely fit for use, at least not for susceptible patients, on account of their excessive strength, as many observations go to prove.

The manufacture of little bottles from glass tubes by means of the blow-pipe, as our author directs, is a real improvement, as they can be prepared in this way much more easily, neatly and completely (with scarcely any constriction of the neck) than they can be obtained in ordinary glass manufactories.[1]

ALLOPATHY:
A WORD OF WARNING TO ALL SICK PERSONS.[2]

Allopathy, or the method of treatment of the old school·of medicine, boasts, that for two and a half milleniums it has possessed the art *of removing the cause of the diseases* entrusted to it, and thus—in opposition to homœopathy, which cannot do this— *that it alone effects cures of the cause,* and *heals in a rational manner.*

If, however, the allopathists would remove the cause of chronic diseases, which constitute much the greater number of all diseases, it must previously be known to them. But it has in all ages been *completely unknown* to them, and they went almost beside themselves, when the new discoveries of homœopathy shewed them that all chronic diseases depend solely and alone upon three chronic miasms, whereof the whole of the old school of medicine had not hitherto the most distant idea.

---

[1] [Hahnemann, as we learn from his writings, used globules of various sizes. Those for administration by the mouth he usually describes as of the size of a poppyseed; he states them to be of the weight of 300 (*Introd. to Belladonna* and *to Aconite, R. A. M. L.,* pt. i.) or 200 (*Chr. Kr.* pt. i, p. 188) to the grain, and he says that 1000, many more than 1000 (*R. A. M. L.,* loc. cit.) or 300 (*Organon,* § cclxxxv, note) of them are sufficiently moistened by one drop of alcohol. Those for olfaction he usually states to be of the size of a mustard seed (*Organon,* p. 9, note) ; and he elsewhere (*Organon,* § cclxxxviii, note) states that 10, 20, or 100 may weigh a grain These globules were to be made by the confectioner of sugar (*Organon,* § cclxxxv. note, *Chr. Kr.,* pt. i, p. 187), and his latest mode of moistening them was to put them into a small glass or porcelain cup, to pour upon them a few drops of the medicinal dilution, to let them stand thus a minute, and then to empty them out on blotting paper, so as to dry them before putting them into a bottle for future use.]

[2] Published as a pamphlet. Leipzic, 1831.

Now, as during all this long period they knew not the originating cause of all chronic diseases, it follows that hitherto they have treated away at an unreal cause, that therefore they could not remove the fundamental cause which was unknown to them, and consequently, that they could not really cure chronic diseases.

The *result* also proved this; for if we except the diseases derived solely from the venereal chancre-miasm, in which mercury, which had been empirically discovered by non-medical persons, was no doubt efficacious, the whole array of physicians of the old school, with all their medicinal apparatus, could certainly aggravate all other chronic maladies, and make them incurable, but they were incompetent to restore *to health* one chronic patient. For, by the force of medicine to transfer the patient from one chronic disease into another and worse malady of different appearance, and then, as is usually done, to imagine that this took place accidentally, and that the physician was perfectly innocent of the appearance of this new sad state, is to delude one's self, and cannot be termed curing, nor restoring to health, but deceiving and ruining the patient.

The physician of the old school erroneously alleged the various, often purely imaginary, characters and phenomena of chronic diseases, to be their *cause* (whereas they are but the products and expressions of that cause), and they treated now for a chill, catarrh and rheumatism, anon for the gout, congestion in the portal system, hæmorrhoids, obstructions in the lymphatic vessels, indurations, morbid matters in the juices, impurities, excess of pituita in the primæ viæ, weakness of the stomach and digestive organs, nervous debility, spasm, plethora, chronic inflammation, swelling, and so on. They imagined these conditions to be the cause (causa) of the chronic diseases, which had to be removed, and the diminution or suppression of these by means of the treatment hitherto prevalent to be cures of the cause.

But when by the force of their medicines they succeeded in diminishing or dispelling one of these characters or states, there naturally always came in its stead another morbid phenomenon (another product of the original cause). How then could the first state have been the fundamental cause when its removal was followed by no true cure, no restoration of health—when in place of the one that had been driven away, another morbid phenomenon and that always of a worse kind, made its appear-

47

ance? Whence was *originally* derived the apparent morbid character and its attendant phenomena? whence proceeded the patient's liability to get cold, catarrh, rheumatism, gout, congestion of the portal system, hæmorrhoids, obstruction in the lymphatic vessels, indurations, mucosities and impurities in the primæ viæ, the apparent acridity in the blood, the weakness of the stomach and digestive organs, the febrile state, the nervous debility, spasm, plethora, chronic inflammation, swelling, and so forth? Whence did these actually and *originally* come, since they are nothing more than single glimpses of the probable character of the disease, and only single expressions (symptoms) of the undwelling malady, the combatting of a single one of which (under the false title of *cause*) with medicines, is truly nothing else than (blameworthy) *symptomatic treatment*, which these gentlemen with unwarrantable pretension allege to be rational *treatment of the cause?* But what, then, was the proper and real *original cause* of these varying, secondary maladies and phenomena, whose removal would constitute a *true causal treatment, a radical, permanent cure, a real rational mode of practice?* Of all the many thousands of physicians of the old school, none knew it, nor will they now deign to learn[1] it from homœopathy, but yet to this day they assert that their bungling treatment which never conduces to the advantage, but invariably to the aggravation of the chronic diseases, is rational treatment.

A more ludicrous pretension, and, as the universal, inevitable result teaches, one more fraught with injurious consequences to humanity, there never has been! In the first place, as regards their treatment of diseases of a rapid course (acute diseases), experience shews, that patients affected with such maladies, who, without any allopathic interference, were left entirely to their unaided vital force, recovered on an average much sooner and much more certainly than when they gave themselves up to the treatment of the old school of medicine, under which many died who, without its unhelpful operations, would have lived, and after which many long remained in a wretched state, and usually at last died miserably of the consequences of the fine treatment, who without these medicinal onslaughts on their lives, would much sooner have recovered and would much more certainly have been preserved.

The reason of this was, that allopathy attributed a false

---

[1] Is it much less shameful not to know a thing, than to refuse to learn it!

character to the acute diseases it had to cure, in order that they might conform to the plan of treatment once adopted for them. Thus we see that in inflammations of the lungs and acute pleurisy, the allopathists pre-supposed an excess of blood (plethora), of inflammatory blood, as the fundamental cause, and they did nothing but draw off blood, and go on drawing off blood, from the veins, when—as homœopathy teaches and practises—they ought merely to have removed the morbid irritation of the arterial system by means of the few internal medicines suited for allaying it (and eradicating all the inflammatory character of the blood), in order to extinguish the entire, seemingly fatal disease in a few hours, without it being at all requisite, according to their old destructive routine treatment, by venesections and leeches, to rob the patient of this innocent, indispensable life's-juice, and, consequently, of all his strength, which after this mistreatment he could either, as was most usual, never regain, or only after a long indisposition.

It is incomprehensible how the allopaths can consider it a great sin, if, in inflammatory diseases, e. g., pleurisy and inflammation of the lungs, blood be not drawn off, and that repeatedly and in large quantity, as they most injuriously, according to their stiff observances and agreeably to their art which has grown grey in gross material notions, make it an invariable rule to do, and would wish to make it the same for better physicians.

But if this is an efficacious sort of method, how can they reconcile it with the fact that of all that die in a year, a sixth part of the whole number dies under them of inflammatory affections, as their own tables prove! Not one twelfth of these would have died had they not fallen into such sanguinary hands, *had they been but left to nature*, and kept away from that old pernicious art.

Hundreds and thousands more die miserably every year—the most promising youths of the country, in the bloom of their age —of wasting, consumption and suppuration of the lungs! You have their death on your consciences! for is there one among you that has not laid the seeds for it by your fine mode of treatment, by your senseless bloodletting and your antiphlogistic appliances in a previous inflammation of the lungs, which must thereby infallibly turn into pulmonary consumption, and prove fatal? This irrational, antipathic, barbarous mode of treating inflammation of the lungs by numerous venesections, leeches and debilitating substances (termed by you antiphlogistics), yearly sends thousands to the grave, by fever from deprivation of the forces (nervous fever), general swelling (dropsy), and suppuration of the lungs! Truly an excellent, privileged mode of covertly destroying wholesale the flower of mankind!

Can that be called curing, curing rationally, treatment of the cause?

On the other hand, no patient cured by homœopathy (often with wonderful rapidity) from even the most severe inflammation of the lungs will be found who died thereafter of wasting and suppuration of the lungs, for it cures the seemingly most fatal inflammations of the lungs in this way only, by removing the dangerous morbid commotion of the circulating system, together with the accompanying pains, by means of a few mild but appropriate internal medicinal agents, often within the twenty-four hours, and allows the patient's strength to remain unaffected by avoiding all evacuations of blood and all debilitating antiphlogistic remedies; for it knows what the physicians of the ancient school do not yet know, and, alas! do not wish to know, that violent acute inflammations of the chest (and of other parts) are nothing but explosions of an exanthematous miasm (psora) that lies hid in the interior (no one free from psora ever gets inflammation of the lungs!) and it knows how that, after subduing the inflammatory excitement of the circulation, it has to take care that the psora be cured without loss of time by means of appropriate antipsoric medicines, so that it shall not establish its seat in the lungs which it can so easily destroy; and this the homœopathic curer of the acute pulmonary inflammation may all the more readily accomplish, since he has not wasted the vital forces (so indispensable for producing the re-action to the antipsoric remedy to be employed) by tapping off the blood and by antipathic cooling remedies, *as is invariably done by the allopathist.*

Moreover the allopathist does not treat the other diseases of rapid course (acute) according to their several peculiarities, as the homœopathist does, but he treats them according to the pathological denomination introduced in the old school, upon one and the same plan of treatment that has once been laid down in the book. Thus all epidemic intermittent fevers, differ they ever so much among each other, are not cured by him with the medicine specifically adapted for each individual intermittent fever, but are invariably merely *suppressed* by strong, the very strongest doses of cinchona bark, repeated often for weeks together; *the patient, however, does not get well;* by this process he indeed loses all the alternations of rigour and heat (this they call getting well), but he becomes more ill, in another way than he was while he still had the fever, with the insidious bark disease which has been forced upon him, and which often lasts for years.

And in like manner these physicians, who arrogate to themselves the title of rational practitioners, have in their books ready-made, fixed names for the acute diseases that attack mankind, either singly (sporadic) or generally prevalent (epidemic) or infectious (contagious), and for each name they are pleased to bestow on the prevailing disease they have also a certain defined plan of treatment (only varied from time to time to suit the fashion), which this fever, that is often quite unknown or that has never appeared in the same form, must be content with, whether it do good or harm. Those whom a giant's constitution does not help through must infallibly succumb under such treatment.

Very differently does the homœopathist act: he judges of the prevailing disease according to its peculiarities and phenomena (its individuality) without suffering himself to be led astray to a wrong mode of treatment by any pathological systematic nomenclature, and by attention to the present state, complaints and ailments of the patient, he generally, by means of the suitable (specific) remedy, brings about the desired recovery.

But I must return to the immeasurably more numerous, long-lasting (chronic) diseases of mankind, which, under the old system of physic, have hitherto made the world a very vale of tears, in order to shew how infinitely inferior, in such diseases also, the injurious Allopathy is to the beneficent Homœopathy.

Without knowing (from the earliest time till now) the true and only cause of chronic diseases, Allopathy violently attacks the patients with a number of medicines given in large doses in rapid succession, often continued for a long time, in order—agreeably to the misapplied saying of the common people, "much helps much"—to conquer the disease by physical force. And by the power of what medicines do they seek to accomplish this? By such as (although the old school physicians alas! know it not) invariably have powers of quite a different kind, and produce effects on the human health of quite another character than what are suitable for the cure of the disease.

Hence the medicines they usually employ in these diseases are appropriately termed *allopathic* (ἀλλοῖα, *aliena, ad rem non pertinentia, unsuitable*), and their mode of treatment is justly denominated *Allopathy*.

But how did it happen that they could make use of such *inappropriate* (ἀλλοῖα) medicines, to the injury of they patients? Evidently from no evil design, but from *ignorance !* They employ them because they know not their real properties and real effects upon the human body; and moreover, because it is a custom introduced among them to administer them in such diseases, because it stands so printed in their books, and because when they were students it was long so taught them *ex cathedra*.

But how did it happen that in the employment of these medicines among patients during the many centuries that this system of medicine has existed, they should not gradually have noted in these medicinal substances what peculiarities each individually possessed, and what were the effects of each upon the health of man, so that at length they might have so gathered what each was adapted to as a curative agent?

To this it will suffice to reply, that these physicians of the old school possessed and do still possess a most approved method of guarding and preserving themselves from the knowledge of the peculiar mode of action of each individual medicine, and thereby rendering it imperceptible to their eyes and observation.

Every one of their young physicians, namely, on undergoing his examination for the high degree of Doctor of their art, must prove by the certificates of the professors that he has diligently attended the lectures on *the art of prescribing*, and must by the extempore writing of prescriptions, that is to say, of *recipes composed of several different medicinal substances* for the names of diseases given him by the examiner (like *conti finti*), demonstrate that he is perfect master of the *noble* art, essential to allopathy, of *always prescribing* for the patient, *lege artis, several medicinal ingredients, mingled in one prescription*, and, consequently, of carefully and entirely eschewing the employment of a single simple medicinal substance.

Thus even to this day every prescription composed of several different medicinal substances, betrays the prescriber to be without dispute an allopathist, one of the many thousands belonging to the unimprovable old school of physic !

Here I would ask my readers on their consciences to tell me, how it were possible that these physicians, although during these many centuries their numbers must amount to millions, could detect and learn the peculiar properties of each of the single medicinal substances while constantly using such mixtures of drugs?

If we should give one of the mixtures according to their prescription even to a quite healthy person, quite free from all morbid symptoms, would we from the effects that result from such a mixture, even though it should consist but of two [1] different ingredients, ever be able to decide with certainty which of the effects that ensue are to be attributed to the one, which to the other ingredient? Never!—in all eternity, never!

Now, as even in trying a mixture of only two different medicinal substances *upon a healthy person*, we can never satisfactorily observe the special effects of a single one of the two upon the human health—since the mixture can only manifest a middle action of both the two together; how, I should like to know, can it be otherwise than quite impossible to distinguish the peculiar powers and special action of each of the several ingredients in an artistic prescription, when it is given to patients, that is to say, to persons already suffering from a number of alterations of health?

Who can fail to perceive from all this, that, besides that the physicians of the old school never seriously set about making experiments with simple medicines on healthy individuals—who can fail to perceive, I say, *that they all, from the remotest times until now*, must remain up to *the present day perfectly and thoroughly ignorant of the countless, special, pure, real effects and powers of each individual medicine, consequently of all medicinal substances* (if we except the few most palpable phenomena of many medicines, that they display even when mixed, and that cannot remain

---

[1] According to that old so-called art of medicine, so repugnant to common sense, there should be more than two, at least three, different things in an artistical prescription; apparently, in order that the physician who prescribes *lege artis*, from the use of such prescriptions for diseases, may be deprived of all chance of ascertaining which of the different ingredients was useful or which did harm, and may also never see or be taught by experience what particular effects each of the several ingredients of the prescription, each simple medicinal substance therein produces on the human health, in order to be able to employ it with certainty in diseases. Thus a bad job always betrays itself by this, that its author seeks to keep us in the dark. When, however, now and then the conscience of the good gentlemen was troublesome, when of late a ray of the homœopathic truth struck upon their eyes, we have seen them put but two ingredients in their prescriptions, while they asserted that they now prescribed *quite simply*; just as if a compound could ever make a simple!—In all eternity, never!

concealed even from ordinary persons, *e. g.*, that senna-leaves purge, opium stupifies, mercury causes salivation, ipecacuanha excites vomiting, cinchona bark suppresses the type of intermittent fevers, and a few more of the same kind.)

This, therefore, is an art the professors of which have and wish to have no knowledge of all their tools!

Among the very meanest of arts there does not exist one such as this! The medical art of the old school alone gives an unheard of example of the kind!

And yet these gentlemen boast so loudly, notwithstanding their incredible irrationality, of being the only rational physicians, and, in complete ignorance of the original cause of all the innumerable chronic diseases not of a venereal character, of alone being able to perform cures of the cause! Perform them —with what? With tools whose pure actions are quite unknown to them, with medicinal substances (prescribed in mixtures), from a special knowledge of which they have introduced into their system, as I have shewn, the most effectual arrangements for preserving themselves?

Was there ever a more ridiculous pretension? a more recherché piece of stupidity? a more complete negation of a curative system?

Of this stamp, dear sick people, are all the ordinary physicians. Of such alone do the medical authorities of all civilized lands consist. These alone sit on the medical judgment-seat, and condemn all that is better, which, whatever advantage it may be of to mankind, is opposed to their antiquated system![1] These alone are the superintendents and directors of the countless hospitals and infirmaries, filled with hundreds and thousands of patients pining in vain for health! Of such alone are the body physicians of princes and ministers of state. Of such only are the ordinary professors of medicine in all universities! With such routine practitioners alone, of great and small degree, do our towns swarm, from the celebrities who knock up two pairs of horses daily in swift-rolling gilded chariots in order to pay visits a couple of minutes' duration to sixty, eighty, or more patients, down to the crowd of low practitioners, who, in worn-

---

[1] What wonder is it that they, with insolent pride in their principles transmitted to them from the dark middle ages, zealously strive to suppress, by the worldly arm of the lawgiver whose favoured house-physicians they are, the new medical art, which by its deeds of cure surpasses all their medical promises, and leaves their antiquated system of treatment far behind!

out clothes, must exert their legs to pester their patients with frequent visits and numerous prescriptions, with but scanty renumeration for their fruitless and hurtful efforts, which are certainly much better paid in the case of the high and mighty ones of their tribe.

If this innumerable host of doctors of the old school were merely useless, and merely not profitable to their patients, even that would be bad enough; but they are unspeakably hurtful and ruinous to sick mankind. Without knowing it, without for an instant dreaming of it—without even willing it, they produce incalculable mischief (although in chronic diseases this is not so obvious) by their furious assaults upon the patients with large doses of powerful, almost invariably unsuitable drugs, which they continue often for a great length of time, repeating them daily (often, indeed, several times a-day), and when this naturally does no good, they continue them in increasing quantities, and thus they not unfrequently punish the patient without cessation for years, now with this and now with that powerful medicinal mixture, unless they procure for him (and for themselves too) a kind of respite in the fine season, which they term the bath-season) by sending him to some mineral water or other, or still better to two in succession, which may just then happen to be the most fashionable, ordering him either to swallow daily no inconsiderable quantity, or to take daily at least one bath of several minutes' duration, for weeks together. And yet each draught of a mineral water, and each bath of it that is taken is a strong dose of a strong medicine !

What will the reflecting public say when they learn that the physicians of the old school of medicine have never in twenty-five centuries learned to know, that every medicinal substance, almost without exception, taken in one single dose, requires *several days*, sometimes even weeks to expend its full action on the human body, as innumerable careful observations, experiences, and experiments have taught and satisfactorily proved to the accurate observer of nature, the homœopathic physician ? What will the hitherto deluded world say to this, that the physicians of the old school, as a proof that they yet know nothing respecting this most indispensable truth, still go on to this day, giving their drugs to patients day after day in several doses a-day, each dose of which is disturbed in its action by the one that speedily follows it, so that from their ignorance no dose is allowed one hundredth part of the time required for the comple-

tion of its action—an over-loading of the body outside and in
with the same medicinal mixture, wherefrom only injury to the
health can be effected, but never anything good, appropriate,
beneficial!

The reflective, unprejudiced reader will find a difficulty in
solving the riddle of how in all the world the great crowd of
physicians could for so many centuries stick to such a disastrous
treatment of chronic patients?

The ordinary hurtful mode of treatment of the old school
physicians here alluded to would be incredible, did it not with
them depend on the grossest ignorance of the true process of
nature, I mean of what experience shews to be the relation between the substances called medicines and the human body, that
is to say, did it not depend even at the present day on the
wretched indefensible superstition of these men (called physicians), *that drugs, even in large, oft-repeated and increased doses, are
one and all per se and absolutely in all cases wholesome things.*

The smallest approach to accuracy in observation, had they
been capable of it, would have convinced them that this was
radically false, and that the reverse of it only was true, namely:
*that all things that can be termed medicinal are, per se, hurtful
substances, injurious in general to the health of man, which can only
become wholesome where each exactly corresponds in its injurious
power to the case of disease specially adapted for it, and where it is
given in appropriate dose and at the proper time.*

This truth, so indispensable to enable us to cure, I was the
first to declare to the world. The allopathists, taken by surprise,
seemed at first to admit it, just as if they had long been familiar
with it; but the result shewed that they still remained enchained
in their own blindness, and that this heaven-born truth could
find no entrance into their mechanical heads.

Had it been otherwise, it had been impossible that they could
persist to the present day in their quackish treatment of chronic
diseases, without endeavouring to ascertain the peculiar powers
of each several medicine in altering man's health, in cramming
their chronic patients, to their destruction, with a variety of
these unknown drugs in admixture, in giving large, frequent
and generally increasing doses of these important substances,
continued for a great length of time, happen what might, if they
had known or appreciated and kept in view this incontrovertible
truth: that medicines are in themselves hurtful substances, injurious in general to the health of man, and can only prove

beneficial where each exactly corresponds in its injurious effects to a case of disease specially adapted to it, and where they are given in appropriate dose and at the right time.

The mischievous effects to chronic patients that lie in this their blind treatment, in this overloading of them with strong unknown drugs, will be perfectly obvious to every reflecting, unprejudiced person, who knows *that every medicine is a disease-creating substance, consequently* every powerful medicine taken day after day in several and increasing doses will infallibly make any, *even healthy* persons, ill,—at first obviously and perceptibly so, but when longer continued their hurtful action is less apparent,[1] *but all the more profoundly penetrating*, and productive of permanent injury, in this way, because the ever active-life-sustaining power silently endeavours to ward off the injury with which these frequent assaults threaten life itself, by internal counter-operations by means of the construction of invisible protections and barriers against the life-invading medicinal enemy, —by the formation of morbid alterations in the organs, in order to exalt the function of one, and render it intolerably sensitive and hence painful, and the others again insensible and even indurated, whilst it deprives the other parts (that in their healthy state were easily excited to action) of their irritability, or even paralyses them; in short it brings about as many corporeal and mental morbid alterations as were requisite for warding off the danger to life from the hostile attacks of the constantly reiterated medicinal doses; that is to say, it effects in secret innumerable disorganizations and abnormal organizations, so that a persistent *permanent* derangement of the health of the body and mind is the consequence,—for which there cannot be a more appropriate appellation than chronic *medicinal disease*—an internal and external crippling of the health, whereby, if the powerful drug have only been used some months, the nature of the individual is so permanently altered that even should all medicine thereafter be discontinued, and the system be subjected to no further loss of humours and forces, yet this morbid metamorphosis in the interior cannot be again removed nor re-transformed into health and the normal condition by the vital force under two or three years.

---

[1] Least of all perceptible if the doses be not increased, in which case the allopathic physician seeks to persuade himself and his patient by saying, "his nature has become habituated to this medicine, therefore the dose of it must be increased,"—a radically wrong notion, leading to the patient's ruin!

Thus, for instance, the vital force of our organism, that is always exercising a preservative function, protects the sensitive parts of the palm of the hand of the pavier (as also of the worker among fire, the glassblower and the like) against the scratching and lacerating sharp angles and points of the paving stones, with a hard, horny covering, to protect the skin with its nerves, blood-vessels and muscles, from being wounded or destoyed. But should the man from this time forth cease to handle rough stones, and take nothing but soft things in his hands, at least a year must elapse ere the vital force (for no surgical or other art can do this) brings about the removal of this horny skin, which was formerly constructed by it on the workman's hands, for their protection against the continued action of the rough stones.

Equally protective does our preservative power exert itself to rescue life at least, if it can do no more, by the formation of organic and dynamic barriers in the interior, against the injurious and inimical assaults of long-continued doses of strong allopathic medicines, that is, by the establishment of permanent alterations of our organisms, which always form a persistent medicinal disease that often lasts for years, that is not capable of being cured and removed by any human art, and that can only be changed back again to the normal state in several years by the vital force itself, provided all medicines are discontinued and the requisite strength of constitution still remains.

If, therefore, a psoric patient suffering from chronic non-venereal affections, in place of being cured homœopathically in a gentle, rapid and permanent manner, is assailed by physicians of the old school by the long-continued use of a variety of strong drugs, incapable of removing the chronic miasm, as the allopathic medicines are, and, as usually happens, given in increasing doses during a long period, as is the case in all their ordinary modes of treatment, we may readily conceive into what a sad and at length incurable state he must fall by such senseless attacks on his system, and how relentlessly he must be assailed in order that, without the very slightest diminution of his original psoric malady, permanent organic malformations and changes of the finest, most delicate parts of the organism, of those parts most indispensible for life and well-being, may be developed, and, as a consequence of them, new, permanent bark, opium, mercurial, iodine, prussic-acid, arsenical, valerian, foxglove, and other nameless chronic medicinal diseases, which all unite and become fused (complicated) into one many-headed, intolerable monster of disease, for which there is and can be no remedy on earth, no antidote, no restorative medicines in nature.

If, in addition to such bungling treatment to which the name of rational is applied, powerful debilitating practices are employ- ed, as is usually the case when the old school physician ima- gines the disease to lie in some corruption of the blood (dyscra- sia) that must be removed, or in full-bloodedness (plethora), (such treatment he terms *treatment of the cause*), and he hence from time to time taps off the blood (wherein the life of man chiefly resides) by venesections and leeches, or reduces the sys- tem by repeated warm baths, or when he, in his efforts for years to expel an imaginary morbific substance (the favourite matter of the material mind of allopathic physicians), robs the diseased body and utterly wastes its most nutritive juices with so-called mild, blood-purifying (?) laxatives, then these insidious medi- cinal diseases produced *secundum artem* by such admirable modes of treatment, become, on account of this pitiless robbery of the vital force, so *incurable*, that recovery is not to be thought of, and a miserable death can alone release the patient from the maltreatment of his physicians and from his nameless torments.

Be not too anxious, I advise you, to insist on the dissection of the corpses of those you have done to death! You would not do it did you know what you thereby revealed to him who knows the truth! Besides some rare congenital malformations, and perchance some results of the deceased's dissipation, what of an abnormal character do you encounter, that is not chiefly the product of your injurious operations, of your medical igno- rance and your therapeutic sins of omission and commission ? There is displayed *not what was present before your treatment*, as you would fain persuade the relatives, *but what was produced by your treatment—the incurability of the deceased was not before* but *after* your treatment. It avails you nothing, that you thereby gladly take the opportunity of making a display of your subtle anatomical terminological learning, neither can it be concealed from those who have any knowledge, that this is no test of abili- ty to cure. The result of such autopsies is not the enriching of pathological anatomy, but the revelation of hideous therapeutic anatomy, to your disgrace—in spite of all your plausible sophis- tries!

But even should these last mentioned debilitating processes in the treatment of chronic (psoric) diseases have been avoided, yet the most perfect imaginable healing art **can never** remove these chronic medicinal diseases produced from bad treatment by the long-continued use of large doses of strong medicines unsuitable for the disease, nor indeed those that are developed by a single simple medicament employed for a length of time in frequent, large doses; for where are remedies to be found that can undo the organic mischief that has been affected? But still less can antidotes be thought of for persistent (chronic) maladies, the consequence of medicinal mixtures. It is manifestly impossible for the very best healing art to remove such vital injuries, for as certainly as the preservative power alone can produce in us organic permanent malformations and alterations for our protection and delivery, be it from the chronic miasms[1] or the inimical attacks of large, long-continued doses of the strong, unsuitable medicines of the allopathists, so certain is it that this life-preserving power alone can again remove these malformations and alterations in our internal parts that were first produced by itself, and restore again the normal state, but it can only do this after years, and provided the vital forces still suffice.

It only in the case of a very robust, undebilitated, youthful constitution, and under other favourable circumstances, that it is possible for the vital force (alone), gradually (in two, three, four years) to remove the organic degenerations which itself toilsomely erected to ward off the attacks of inimical medicinal forces, and to restore the healthy state, provided the psora that still remains at the root of the evil be at the same time homœopathically cured, for this can never be overcome, never extinguished by our vital force alone, and still less by the senseless bungling treatment of allopathy that plumes itself upon its superlative wisdom.

But if the patient be already advanced in years, if his spirits be depressed by sorrow, vexation, fear or want, or if in addition he has been weakened by venesections, leechings, purgations and the like, he can look for nothing with certainty but the sure advance of death—the inevitable lot of those who can boast of having employed many of the most distinguished physicians of the old school and a variety of the mineral waters, foolishly prescribed for them; none can ever help them more.

---

[1] Those internal malformations, abnormal organizations and disorganizations produced by nature for our protection against the violence of chronic miasmatic disease (psora), it can most rapidly remove and reconstruct with the assistance of the cure of the psora by homœopathy, but those caused by the injurious misuse of medicines, it has much more difficulty in curing.

Subjectively it may be a more cruel deed to stab one's enemy in the back from revenge, but objectively it is more cruel to undermine the system of a patient who sought our aid, and who might easily and certainly have been relieved from his natural disease by the appropriate remedies, so that life at length becomes intolerable to him, by secret instruments of destruction (wrong medicines, in scarcely legible prescriptions, forced upon him for half or whole years together, in several, often increasing, doses daily), so that he must hopelessly and irremediably drag out his wretched existence in constant misery, without having the power to die, and envying the poniarded Corsican his rapid death.

At the contemplation of this heart-breaking fact, of how difficult is it for a patient to escape from the destructive hands of those quacks who foolishly pride themselves on their old false art, and make a mighty display of incomprehensible pedantry, who lie in wait for customers in order to entice them into their toils by all manner of quackish expedients, I cannot forbear from affectionately beseeching my modest colleagues, the important, philanthrophic homœopathists (*O! multa mecum pejoraque passi durate et vosmet rebus servate secundis!*) to suffer for a short time the unmerited pressure from above, but in the meantime not to waste our divine art, so infallibly serviceable in natural unspoiled diseases, on those irremedial patients who have been destroyed to their very inmost marrow, not to receive at any price those patients who have been injured to the verge of incurability by the allopathic exterminating art, nor, by undertaking such impossibilities, to expose themselves to the scornful laughter of the renowned physicians of the old school, who have already taken the greatest pains to make them utterly incurable for hard cash. First let them be again restored by these high-titled destroyers of health to the former state of natural disease they were in before these medical onslaughts on their life were perpetrated, if they are able to do it!

On the contrary I beseech my homœopathic colleagues to be contented for the present with patients who have not been destroyed by the physicians of the old school, even though they be the poorest among the people, and laden with the most severe, chronic, natural diseases, and to be satisfied with the smallest remuneration for their labour, if these poor people can prove to them that their poverty has prevented them applying to other allopathic) physicians, and consequently being ruined by improper drugs. Though their income may be small they will yet have the unspeakable joy of certainly and rapidly re-establishing their patients' health, and thus putting flaunting allopathy to shame, which is incapable of curing, but can only aggravate diseases and render them incurable with a wilderness of drugs— as a warning to the befooled public. The homœopathic medical art can alone transform into health, as if by magic, all natural diseases not ruined by allopathic art, provided there remain a tolerable amount of vital force, and this it does without prating about *rationality* and *treatment of the cause*.

Before homœopathy, that gentle, safe healing art so consonant with nature, was discovered, no well disposed and honest philanthropist could forbear pitying the innumerable crowd of the old-school physicians, as they groped about in midnight darkness with their dreadfully learned ignorance, whilst their zeal in treating natural diseases, in place of serving to benefit them or bringing about the desired cure, only ruined them or rendered them incurable. For who among them could unravel the confusion of so many (wouldbe profoundly learned) baseless hypothetical doctrines and unnatural therapeutic maxims and modes of treatment with drugs whose peculiar action was unknown, given in senseless mixtures and repeated large doses ?— who among them could separate the false from the true, and reduce their mode of practice to a method of treatment that should be consonant with nature, and lastingly beneficial ? They were then fully as much to be pitied as those patients whom they injured and continue to injure to an infinite degree with their antiquated unimproved method. But since the light of the doctrine that is alone consonant with nature, of restoring health and well-being rapidly and certainly in unspoiled, natural diseases by small quantities of properly prepared, mild specific medicines, has appeared, and has shone throughout Europe in marvellous deeds, those who paid no regard to it but condemned and persecuted it are not to be pitied ; they deserve for their obstinate adherence to their antiquated homicidal mode of treatment naught but contempt and abhorrence, and unprejudiced history will brand their names with a stigma on account of their scornful rejection of the real aid which they might have afforded their much-to-be-pitied patients, had they not impiously closed their eyes and ears against the beneficent truth !

CAUSE AND PREVENTION OF THE ASIATIC CHOLERA.[1]

Preliminary.

A receipt has been given to the world, which proved so efficacious in Dünaburg in the Asiatic cholera, that of ten patients but one died. The chief ingredient is *camphor*, which is in ten times the proportion of the other ingredients. But not a tenth—nay, not one in a hundred of the patients would have died had the other ingredients, which were but injurious and obstructing, and the venesection been left out, and the *camphor* been given alone, and always at the *very commencement of the disease, for it is only when given alone, and at the first invasion of the disease that it is so marvellously useful.* But if physicians come, as usual, too late to the patient, when the favourable time for employing the *camphor* is past, and the second stage has already set in, when *camphor* is useless, then they may use it in vain; their patients will die under its employment. Hence every one, the instant any of his friends take ill of cholera, must himself immediately treat them with *camphor*, and not wait for medical aid, which, even if it were good, would generally come too late. I have received many communications from Hungary from non-medical persons, who have restored their friends, as if by magic, by giving *camphor the instant they became ill.*

Where the cholera first appears, it usually comes on in the commencement in its first stage (with tonic spasmodic character); the strength of the patient suddenly sinks, he cannot stand upright, his expression is altered, the eyes sunk in, the face bluish and icy cold, as also the hands, with coldness of the rest of the body; hopeless discouragement and anxiety, with dread of suffocation, is visible in his looks; half stupified and insensible, he moans or cries in a hollow, hoarse tone of voice, without making any distinct complaints, except when asked; burning in the stomach and gullet, and cramp-pain in the calves and other muscles; on touching the precordial region he cries out; he has no thirst, no sickness, no vomiting or purging.

In the first stage *camphor* gives rapid relief, but the patient's friends must themselves employ it, as this stage soon ends either in death or in the second stage, which is more difficult to be

---

[1] From the *Archiv. f. hom. Heilk.*, vol. xi, 1831.

48

cured, and not with *camphor*. In the first stage accordingly, the patient must get, as often as possible (at least every five minutes) a drop of spirit of camphor (made with one ounce of camphor to twelve of alcohol), on a lump of sugar or in a spoonful of water. Some spirit of camphor must be taken in the hollow of the hand and rubbed into the skin of the arms, legs, and chest of the patient; he may also get a clyster of half a-pint of warm water, mingled with two full teaspoonfuls of spirit of camphor, and from time to time some camphor may be allowed to evaporate on a hot iron, so that if the mouth should be closed by trismus, and he can swallow nothing, he may draw in enough of camphor vapour with his breath.

The quicker all this is done at the first onset of the first stage of the disease, the more rapidly and certainly will the patient recover; often in a couple of hours,[1] warmth, strength, consciousness, rest and sleep return, and he is saved.

If this period of the commencement of the disease, so favourable to recovery and speedy cure, by the above indicated employment of camphor, has been neglected, then things look worse; then camphor is no longer serviceable. There are moreover cases of cholera, especially in northern regions, where this first stage, with its tonic spasmodic character, is hardly observable, and the disease passes instantly into the second stage of clonic spasmodic character; frequent evacuation of watery fluid, mixed with whitish, yellowish, or reddish flakes, and, along with insatiable thirst and loud rumbling in the belly, violent vomiting of large quantities of the same fluid, with increased agitation, groaning and yawning, icy coldness of the whole body, even of the tongue, and marbled blue appearance of the arms, hands and face, with fixed sunken eyes, diminution of all the senses, slow pulse, excessively painful cramp in the calves, and spasms of the limbs. In such cases the administration of a drop of camphor spirit every five minutes, must only be continued so long as *decided* benefit is observable (which with a remedy of such rapid action as camphor, manifests itself within a quarter of an hour). If in such cases decided benefit is not soon perceived, then no time must be lost in administering the remedy for the second stage.

---

[1] There were cases of patients for whom camphor had not been employed, who had apparently died in the first stage and were laid out for dead, in whom a finger was seen to move; in these some camphor-spirit mixed with oil and introduced into the mouth, recalled the apparently dead again to life.

The patient is to get one or two globules of the finest prepa ration of *copper*[1] (prepared from metallic copper in the mode described in the second part of my work on Chronic Diseases), thus *cuprum* 0,00 X, moistened with water, and introduced into his mouth every hour or every half-hour, until the vomiting and purging diminish, and warmth and rest are restored. But noth ing else at all must be given beside; no other medicine, no herb tea, no baths, no blisters, no fumigation, no venesection, &c., otherwise the remedy will be of no avail. Similar good effects result from the administration of as small a portion of white hellebore (*veratrum album*, 0,00 X); but the preparation of copper is much to be preferred, and is more serviceable, and sometimes a single dose is sufficient, which is allowed to act without a second being given, as long as the patient's state goes on improving.[2]

The wishes of the patient of all kinds are only to be indulged in moderation. Sometimes, when aid is delayed many hours, or other and improper remedies have been administered, the pa tient falls into a sort of typhoid state, with delirium. In this case, *bryonia* 00 X, alternately with *rhus tox.* 00 X, proves of eminent service.

The above preparation of copper, together with good and moderate diet, and proper attention to cleanliness, is the most certain preventive and protective remedy; those in health should take, once every week, a small globule of it (*cupr.* 0 X) in the morning fasting, and not drink anything immediately after- wards, but this should not be done until the cholera is in the locality itself, or in the neighbourhood. The health of the indi vidual will not be in the least disturbed by this dose. I shall not, but any other homœopathic practitioner may, tell where the above medicines may be procured, excepting the camphor, which, like the alcohol, may be had at every chemist's shop.

Camphor cannot preserve those in health from cholera, but

---

[1] If the dear and scarce (frequently falsified) cajeput oil be actually so serviceable in the Asiatic cholera that out of ten scarcely one died, it must owe this quality to its camphor-like property (it may almost be regarded as a fluid camphor) and to the circumstance, that from the copper vessels in which it is imported from the East Indies, it takes up some portion of copper, and hence, in its unpurified state, it is of a blue-greenish colour. It has, moreover, been found in Hungary, that those who wore next the skin of their body a plate of copper, were exempt from infection; as trustworthy intelligence from that country informs me.

[2] Similar affections resulting from immoderate repletions of the stomach, with indigestible nutriment, are best removed by a few cups of strong coffee

only the above preparation of copper; but when the latter is taken the vapour of camphor must be avoided, as it suspends the action of the copper.[1]

COETHEN, 10th September, 1831.

THE MODE OF PROPAGATION OF THE ASIATIC CHOLERA.[2]

Two opinions, exactly opposed to each other prevail on this subject. One party considers the pestilence as only epidemic, of atmospheric-telluric nature, just as though it were merely spread through the air, from which there would in that case be no protection. The other party denies this, and holds it to be communicable by contagion only, and propagated from one individual to another.

Of these two opinions one only can be the right one, and that which is found to be the correct one will, like all truths, exercise a great influence on the welfare of mankind.

The first has the most obstinate defenders, who adduce the fact that when the cholera has broken out at one extremity of the town, it may the very next morning be raging at the other extremity, consequently the infection can only be present in the air; and that they (the physicians) are in their own persons proofs of the non-contagious character of cholera, seeing that they generally remain unaffected by it and in good health, although they are daily in personal communication with those dying of cholera, and have even tasted the matter they ejected and the blood out of their veins, lain down in their beds, and

----

[1] [In the first Vol. of the *Bibl. Homœopathique* we find the following extract of a letter from Hahnemann to the Editor:

"*Cuprum* as a prophylactic against cholera, has generally shewn itself efficacious wherever it has been employed, and where its action has not been disturbed by gross dietetic faults, or by the smell of camphor (which is its antidote). The best homœopathic practitioners have also found it indispensible in the second stage of the fully developed disease, alternated, if the symptoms indicate this, with *veratrum album* X. I have also advised the alternation of these two substances from week to week as a preventive against the disease.

"I learn from authentic sources that at Vienna, Berlin and Magdeburg, thousands of families by following my instructions respecting the treatment by camphor, have cured, often in less than a quarter of an hour, those of their members who were attacked by the epidemic, and that so effectually, that their neighbours knew nothing about it, and still less their medical attendants, who oppose with all their might this treatment, so simple, so rapid, and *so constantly certain in its effects.*"]

[2] Published as a pamphlet. Leipzic, 1831.

so forth. This foolhardy, disgusting procedure they allege to be the *experimentum crucis*, that is to say, an incontrovertible proof of the non-contagious nature of cholera, that it is not propagated by contact, but is present in the atmosphere, and for this reason attacks individuals in widely distant places.

A fearfully pernicious and totally false assertion !

Were it the fact that this pestilential disease was uniformly distributed throughout the atmosphere, like the influenza that recently spread over all Europe, then the many cases reported by all the public journals would be quite inexplicable, where small towns and villages in the vicinity of the murderously prevalent cholera, which, by the unanimous efforts of all their inhabitants, kept themselves strictly isolated, like a besieged fortress, and which refused to admit a single person from without —inexplicable, I repeat, would be the perfect exemption of such places from the ravages of the cholera. This plague raged fiercely over an extensive tract on the banks of the Volga, but in the very middle of it, Sarepta, which had strictly and undeviatingly kept itself secluded, remained perfectly free from the cholera, and up to a recent period none of the villages around Vienna, where the plague daily carries off a large number of victims, were invaded by cholera, the peasants of these villages having all sworn to kill any one who ventured near them, and even to refuse to permit any of the inhabitants who had gone out of the villages to re-enter them. How could their exemption have been possible had the cholera been distributed throughout the atmosphere ! And how easy it is to comprehend their freedom from it, seeing that they held aloof from contact with infected individuals.

The course followed by the cholera in every place it traversed was almost uniformly this : that its fury shewed itself most virulently and most rapidly fatal at the commencement of its invasion (evidently solely because at that time the miasm encountered none but unprepared systems, for which even the slightest cholera miasm was something quite novel, never before experienced, and consequently extremely infectious); hence it then infected persons most frequently and most fatally.

Thereafter the cases increased, and with them at the same time, by the communication of the inhabitants among each other, the quantity of diluted miasm, whereby a kind of local sphere of cholera-miasm exhalation was formed in the town, to which the more or less robust individuals had an opportunity of becoming gradually accustomed and hardened against it, so that by degrees always fewer inhabitants were attacked by it and could be severely affected by it (the cholera was then said to take on a milder character), until at last all the inhabitants were almost uniformly indurated against it, and thus the epidemic was extinguished in this town.

Did the miasm only exist in the general atmosphere, the cases could not be less numerous at last than they were at the commencement, for the same cause (said to be the general atmospheric constitution) must have remained identical in its effects.

The *only* fact brought forward by Hufeland against my proofs (viz., that on board an English ship in the open sea, about the latitude of Riga, that had had no (?) communication with the town, two sailors were suddenly seized with the cholera) proves nothing, for it is not known how near the ship came to the infected town, Riga, so that the sphere of the miasm-exhalation from the town, although diluted, might yet have reached and infected the sailors, who were still unused to the miasm, especially if they, as is often the case, were rendered more susceptible to it from intemperance.

The most striking examples of infection and rapid spread of cholera take place, as is well known, and as the public journals likewise inform us, in this way : On board ships—in those confined spaces, filled with mouldy watery vapours, the cholera-miasm finds a favourable element for its multiplication, and grows into an enormously increased brood of those excessively minute, invisible, living creatures, so inimical to human life, of which the contagious matter of the cholera most probably consists—on board these ships, I say, this concentrated aggravated miasm kills several of the crew; the others, however, being frequently exposed to the danger of infection and thus gradually habituated to it, at length become fortified against it, and no longer liable to be infected. These individuals, apparently in good health, go ashore, and are received by the inhabitants without hesitation into their cottages, and ere they have time to give an account of those who have died of the pestilence on board the ship, those who have approached nearest to them are suddenly carried off by the cholera. The cause of this is undoubtedly the invisible cloud that hovers closely around the sailors who have remained free from the disease, and which is composed of probably millions of those miasmatic animated beings, which, at first developed on the broad marshy banks of the tepid Ganges, always searching out in preference the human being to his destruction and attaching themselves closely to him, when transferred to distant and even colder regions become habituated to these also, without any diminution either of their unhappy fertility or of their fatal destructiveness.

Closely but invisibly environed by this pestiferous, infectious matter, against which, however, as has been observed, his own individual system is, as it were, fortified by the long resistance of his vital force to its action, and by being gradually habituated to the inimical influence surrounding him, such a sailor (flying from the corpses of his companions on board) has often gone ashore apparently innocuous and well, and behold! the inhabitants who hospitably entertained him, and first of all those who came into immediate contact with him, quite unused to the miasm, are first most rapidly and most certainly attacked without any warning, and killed by the cholera, whilst of those who are more remote, such only as are unnerved by their bad habits of life are liable to take the infection. Those who are not debilitated, and who have kept at some distance from the stranger who is surrounded by the cholera miasm, suffered only a slight attack from the miasmatic exhalation hovering about in a more diluted form; their vital force could easily ward off the weaker attack and master it, and when they subsequently came nearer it their system had by this time become somewhat habituated to the miasm, retained the mastery over it, and even when these persons at length approached nearer or quite close to the infected stranger, their vital force had thus gradually become so fortified against it, that they could hold intercourse with him with perfect impunity, having now become completely uninfectable by the contagious principle of the cholera. It is a wonderfully benevolent arrangement of God that has made it possible for man to fortify himself against, and render himself unsusceptable to, the most deadly distempers, and especially the most fatal of them all, the infectious principal of cholera, if he gradually approaches it ever nearer and nearer, allowing intervals of time to elapse in order to recover himself, provided always he have an undebilitated body.

When first called to a cholera patient, the physician, somewhat timid as yet, as is but reasonable, either tarries at first in the antechamber (in the weaker atmosphere of the miasmatic exhalation) or if he enter the patient's room prefers keeping at some distance, or standing at the door, orders the nurse in

attendance to do this or the other to the patient, he then prudently soon takes his departure promising to return again shortly;
in the meantime he either goes about a little in the open air, or
goes home and has some refreshment. His vital force, which
at the first short visit at some distance from the patient, was
only moderately assailed by the diluted miasm, recovers itself
completely in the meantime by this recreation, and when he
again comes into the patient's room and approaches somewhat
nearer to the patient, it soon by practice comes to resist more
powerfully the more concentrated infectious atmosphere that
exists closer to the patient, until at length, from frequent visits
and a nearer approach to the patient, it attains a mastery over
the assaults of the miasm, so that at last the physician is completely hardened against even the most poisonous cholera
miasm at the bedside, and rendered quite uninfectable by this
pestilence ; and the same is the case with the nurse who goes as
cautiously and gradually to work.

Both the one and the other then boast, because they can come
into immediate contact with the patient without any fear and
without any ill consequences, that they know better than to call
the disease contagious; it is not, they say, the least catching.
This presumptuous, inconsiderate, and perfectly untrue assertion
has already cost thousands their lives, who in their ignorance, and
quite unprepared, either approached the cholera patient suddenly
or came in contact with these cholera physicians (who do not treat
with camphor) or the nurses. For such physicians and nurses,
fortified in this manner against the miasm, now take away with
them in their clothes, in their skin, in their hair, probably also
in their breath, the invisible (probably animated) and perpetually reproductive contagious matter surrounding the cholera
patient they have just visited, and this contagious matter they
unconsciously and unsuspectingly carry along with them throughout the town and to their acquaintances, whom it unexpectedly
and infallibly infects, without the slightest suspicion on their
part of its source.

*Thus the cholera physicians and nurses are the most certain and
frequent propagators and communicators of contagion far and
wide;* and yet amazement is expressed, even in the public journals,
how the infection can spread so rapidly the very first day, from
the first cholera patient at the one end of the town to persons
at the other end of the town, who had not come near the
patient!

And thus the flame for the sacrifice of innocent persons breaks out in all corners and ends of the town, lighted up by the sparks of the black death scattered in every direction by physicians and their assistants! Every one readily opens the door to these plague-propagators; allows them to sit down beside him, putting implicit faith in their confidently declared assurance: " that it is ridiculous to call the cholera contagious, as the cholera pestilence is only diffused epidemically through the air, and cannot, therefore, be infectious"—and see! the poor cajoled creatures are rewarded for their hospitality with the most miserable death.

To the very highest people of the town and of the court the cholera angel of death obtains access, in the person of the physician who gives this evil counsel, enveloped by the fresh miasm; and no one detects the concealed, invisible, but, for that reason, all the more dangerous enemy.

Wherever such physicians and such nurses go (for what all-seeing eye could perceive this invisible danger on these healthy miasm-bearers?)—wherever they go, their presence communicates the spark, and mortal sickness bursts forth everywhere, and the pestilence depopulates whole towns and countries!

If physicians would but take warning, and, rendered uninfectable by taking a few drops of camphorated spirit, approach (ever so quickly) the cholera patient, in order to treat him at the commencement of his sickening with this medicine (*pure*, *unadulterated camphorated spirit*) which alone is efficacious, and which most certainly destroys the miasm about the patient, by giving him, as I have taught,[1] every five minutes one drop of it, and in the interval assiduously rubbing him on the head, neck, chest, and abdomen with the same medicine poured into the hollow of the hand, until all his giddy faint powerlessness, his suffocative anxiety, and the icy-coldness of his body has disappeared, and given place to reviving animation, tranquillity of mind, and complete return of the vital warmth—if they would but do this, then *every* patient would not only be *infallibly* restored within a couple of hours (as the most undeniable facts and instances prove), but by the cure of the disease with pure camphor, they would at the same time eradicate and annihilate the miasm (that probably consists of innumerable, invisible living beings) in and about the patient, about themselves, even in the clothes, the linen, the bed of the patient (for these all

Cure and Prevention of the Asiatic Cholera.—[See preceding article.]

would be penetrated by the vapour of the camphor if it were employed in this way) in the very furniture and walls of the apartment also, and they themselves (the physicians and nurses) would then carry off none of the contagious principle with them, and could no longer infect persons throughout the town.[1]

But these physicians, as we see, despise this; they prefer going on killing their patients in crowds by pouring into them large quantities of aqua-fortis and opium, by blood-letting, and so forth, or giving the camphor mixed with so many obstructing and injurious matters, that it can scarcely do any good, solely to avoid giving the simple, pure (efficacious) solution of camphor, because the reformer of the old injurious system of treatment (the only one they know), *because I*, from conviction, recommended it in the most urgent manner in all countries of Europe. They seem to prefer delivering over all mankind to the grave-digger, to listening to the good counsel of the new purified healing art.

But who can prevent them acting so, as they alone possess the power in the state to suppress what is good?

However, bountiful Providence has provided a beneficent remedy for this state of things (for these physicians are protected, even in their ill-deeds, by antiquated injurious laws).

Thus, the cholera is most surely and easily and almost miraculously curable, but only in the first couple of hours from the commencement of the sickening, by means of the employment of pure camphor, and that before the physicians in larger towns that are summoned can attend. But on their arrival they may even then, by the employment of unadulterated camphor-spirit, if not cure the cholera completely (for the lapse of a few hours generally makes it too late to do so) yet annihilate the whole of the contagious principle of this pestilence on and about the patient, and adhering to themselves and the bystanders, and cease to convey the miasm with them to other parts of the town. Hence the families of non-medical persons, by means of this employment of camphor, cure the members of their families by thousands in secret (the higher classes alone, must, *on account of their station*, be under the necessity of calling in the physician,

---

[1] The sprinkling of suspected strangers on their arrival, and of suspected goods and letters with camphor spirit, would most certainly destroy the cholera miasm in them. Not a single fact goes to prove that chlorine annihilates the miasm of cholera; it can only destroy odorous effluvia. But the contagious matter of the Asiatic cholera is far from being an odorous effluvium. What good then do the fumigations with chlorine, which is here perfectly useless, and only hurtful to man's health!

who, in defiance of the philanthropic reformer of the healing art, and his efficacious system of treatment, not unfrequently, with his improper remedies, dispatches them to Orcus).

It is members of a family alone that can most certainly and easily mutually cure each other with camphor spirit, because they are able instantaneously to aid those taken ill.

Will physicians ever come to comprehend what is essential, and what will at once put a stop to the devastation and depopulation of two quarters of the globe?

Dixi et salvavi animam!

Cöthen, the 24th October, 1831.

REMARKS ON THE EXTREME ATTENUATION OF HOMŒO-PATHIC MEDICINES.[1]

I. The essay of this intelligent and unwearied and honourable investigator and promoter of our art, incontestably corroborates the following truths that some observations of my own had already hinted at, viz., 1, that the development of the powers of medicinal substances by the process peculiar to homœopathy, may be assumed to be *almost illimitable ;* 2, that the higher their dynamization (dematerialization) is carried, the more penetrating and rapid does their operation become; 3, that, however, their effects pass off so much the more speedily.

All this is in strict accordance with my own experiments, though I have not carried them so far; one of them I may only allude to, namely, that once having prepared a dynamized attenuation of sulphur up to XXX (90th dilution), I administered a drop of it on sugar to an aged, unmarried lady, who was subject to rare epileptic attacks (one every 9, 12, 14 months), and

------

[1] [These remarks occur in the form of postscripts appended to a paper by Graf von Korsakoff, published in the 11th and again in the 12th Vol. of the *Archiv. f. hom. Heilk.* In this paper the author mentions that he had diluted medicines up to the 150th, 1000th and 1500th attenuation, and that he had found them even at that degree of dilution quite efficacious. He starts the idea that possibly the material division of the medicinal substance attains its limit at the third or sixth dilution, and that the subsequent attenuations obtain their medicinal properties by a kind of infection or communication of the medicinal power, after the manner of contagious diseases, to the non-medicinal vehicle; and in corroboration of this notion he relates several experiments, in which he says he communicated medicinal properties to large quantities of unmedicated globules, by shaking them up with one dry medicated globule. He likewise remarks that by diluting medicines highly, and by employing such infected globules, the force of the primary action of the medicines, or their tendency to produce homœopathic aggravations, declines, whilst the reaction of the organism, or the curative action of the medicine, continually increases.]

within an hour afterwards she had an epileptic fit, and since then she has remained quite free from them.

The opponents of homœopathy, obstinately attached to their old system, who seem to have made a resolution not to allow themselves to be convinced of this wonderful development of the powers of crude medicinal substances, which however manifests itself to every unprejudiced person who honestly puts the matter to the test, and which gives to the practice of homœopathy that tranquillizing certainty and trustworthiness in the treatment of diseases with highly dynamized attenuations of medicines in the smallest doses, whereby it vastly surpasses every other method of treatment,—our opponents, I say, on being informed of these extended experiments and observations of the author of this treatise, who has rendered such service to our art, can do nothing more than, as they have hitherto done, remain standing in amazement below the steps of the outer-court to the sanctuary of these health-bringing truths, and announce by a sceptical smile their inability to avail themselves of these beneficent revelations of the nature of things for the welfare of their patients. They wore the same sceptical smile when I some thirty and odd years ago pointed out the efficacy of the millionth part of a grain of belladonna in scarlet-fever; they can now also do nothing more when they read of the dematerialization of sulphur up to the thousandth potency, that it still displays a powerful medicinal action on the human body. Their Bœotian smiling however will not stay the eagle-flight of the new beneficent healing-art, and in the meantime they remain as they deserve to do, deprived of its blessings.[1]

However, it must be borne in mind, that the chief use of these experiments, was to demonstrate how high medicinal attenuations might be potentized without their action on man's state of health being reduced to nothing, and for this, these experiments are invaluable; but for the homœopathic treatment of patients it is advisable, in preparing all kinds of medicines, not to go higher than the decillionth attenuation and dynamization (X),

---

[1] One might apply to these gentlemen Goethe's words:

" Daran erkenn' ich die gelehrten Herrn!
Was ihr nicht tastet, steht euch Meilen fern;
Was ihr nicht fasst, das fehlt euch ganz und gar;
Was ihr nicht rechnet, glaubt ihr, sei nicht wahr;
Was ihr nicht wägt, hat für euch kein Gewicht;
Was ihr nicht münzt, das, meint ihr, gelte nicht."

(*Faust*, 2ter Theil.)

in order that homœopathic physicians may be able to assure themselves of uniform results in their practice.[1]

II. I can scarcely believe that the carefully discriminating Graf von Korsakoff can regard the subdivision and dynamization peculiar to homœopathy as complete at the millionth and billionth development [3d and 6th dilution], and incapable of any further disembodiment and spiritualization of their medicinal powers to an even greater degree by further trituration of the dry and further succussion of the fluid attenuations—the occurrence of which cannot be doubted—or that he actually looks upon them as weaker, as he seems to imply. Who can say that in the millionth or billionth development the small particles of the medicinal substances have arrived at the state of atoms not susceptible of further division, of whose nature we can form not the slightest conception? For if the living human organism shews an ever stronger reaction to the more highly dynamized attenuations when they are used medicinally (as experience teaches, and as the author himself admits), it follows that such higher medicinal preparations must be regarded as stronger, inasmuch as there can be no standard for measuring the degree of dynamic potency of a medicine, except the degree of the reaction of the vital force against it.

Thus much, however, is deducible from his experiments, that, since a single dry globule imbibed with a high medicinal dynamization, communicates to 13,500 unmedicated globules, with which it is shaken for five minutes, medicinal power fully equal to what it possesses itself, without suffering any diminution of power itself, it seems that this marvellous communication takes

---

[1] [In 1829 he wrote to Dr. Schreter thus (*Brit. Jour. of Hom.*, Vol. v, p. 398) : "I do not approve of your dynamizing the medicines higher (as for instance, up to XII and XX, (36th and 60th dilutions]). There must be some end to the thing, it cannot go on to infinity. By laying it down as a rule that all homœopathic remedies be attenuated and dynamized up to X [30th dil.], we have a uniform mode of procedure in treatment of all homœopathists, and when they describe a cure, we can repeat it, as they and we operate with the same tools. In one word, we would do well to go forward uninterruptedly in the beaten path. Then our enemies will not be able to reproach us with having nothing fixed—no normal standard." In 1833 he speaks more favourably of the higher attenuations, such as the 60th, 150th, and 300th dilutions (*Organon*, § CCLXXXVII, 2d note,) ascribing to them a more rapid and penetrating, but likewise a shorter action. Again in 1838 (*Chr. Kr.*, part v, preface), he speaks approvingly of the 50th dilution. As a rule, he seems to have used chiefly the 30th dilution, still we find from the cases sent to Dr. Bönninghausen, which I give farther on, that he occasionally gave other preparations, and in the letter of which a fac-simile is given in this work, he desires Dr. Lehmann to send him the 3d trituration of certain medicines, whether for therapeutic use or for further dilution it is impossible to say.]

place by means of proximity and contact, and is a sort of infection, bearing a strong resemblance to the infection of healthy persons by a contagion brought near or in contact with them— a perfectly novel, ingenious and probable idea, for which we are indebted to the Graf.

The communication or infection appears to take place by means of the power which is perpetually spreading around, like an exhalation or emanation from such bodies, even though they are dry, just like those globules the size of a mustard seed that had previously been moistened with a fluid medicine which we employ for the cure of patients by olfaction. A globule of this kind, e. g., of *staphisagria* X, which, in the course of twenty years, had been smelt several hundreds of times after opening the bottle in which it was, for a certain symptom that always recurred of the same character, possesses at this hour medicinal power of equal strength as at first, which could not be the case did it not continually exhale its medicinal power in an inexhaustible manner.

The supposition of our author that *dry* globules that have been impregnated with a certain degree of development of power can be further dynamized and their medicinal power increased in their bottles by shaking, or carrying about in the pocket, like medicinal fluids further shaken, is not borne out by any fact, and will appear to me incredible until it is supported by proper experimental proofs.

On the whole we owe many thanks to this ingenious and indefatigable investigator for his present valuable communication.

Cöthen, 30th May, 1832.

CASES ILLUSTRATIVE OF HOMŒOPATHIC PRACTICE.

Many persons of my acquaintance but half converted to homœopathy have begged of me from time to time to publish still more exact directions as to how this doctrine may be actually applied in practice, and how we are to proceed. I am astonished that after the very peculiar directions contained in the *Organon of medicine* more special instruction can be wished for.

I am also asked, "How are we to examine the disease in every

---

[1] From the *Reine Arzneimittellehre*, pt. ii, 3d. edit. 1833. [The cases here given originally appeared about 1817 in the first edition of the *R. A. M. L.*, but the notes and most of the preliminary matter are of the date we have given, and we may therefore consider the whole to represent Hahnemann's opinion and practice, with the exception of the dose in these two cases, of the latter period.]

particular case?" As if special enough directions were not to be found in the book just mentioned.

As in homœopathy the treatment is not directed towards any supposed or illusory internal causes of disease, nor yet towards any names of diseases invented by man which do not exist in nature, and as every case of non-miasmatic disease is a distinct individuality, independent, peculiar, differing in nature from all others, never compounded of a hypothetical arrangement of symptoms, so no particular directions can be laid down for them (no schema, no table), except that the physician, in order to effect a cure, must oppose to every aggregate of morbid symptoms in a case a group of similar medicinal symptoms as exact as it is to be met with in any single known medicine, for this doctrine cannot admit of more than a single medicinal substance (whose effects have been accurately tested) to be given at once (see *Organon of medicine,* § 271, 272).

Now we can neither enumerate all the possible aggregates of symptoms of all concrete cases of disease, nor indicate *a priori* the homœopathic medicines for these (*a priori* undefinable) possibilities. For every individual given case (and every case is an individuality, differing from all others) the homœopathic medical practitioner must himself find them, and for this end he must be acquainted with the medicines that have till now been investigated in respect of their positive action, or consult them for every case of disease; but besides this he must do his endeavour to prove on himself or on other healthy individuals medicines that have not yet been investigated as regards the morbid alterations they are capable of producing, in order thereby to increase our store of *known* remedial agents,[1] so that the choice of a remedy for every one of the infinite variety of cases of disease (for the combatting of which we can never possess enough of suitable tools and weapons) may become all the more easy and accurate.

That man is far from being animated with the true spirit of the homœopathic system, is no true disciple of this beneficent doctrine, who makes the slightest objections to institute *on himself* careful experiments for the investigation of the peculiar effects of the medicines which have remained unknown for 2500 years, without which investigation (and unless their pure patho-

---

[1] Before the discovery of Homœopathy, medicinal substances were known only in respect to their natural history, and besides their names nothing was known regarding them but their presumed qualities, which were either imaginary or altogether false.

genetic action on the healthy individual has previously been ascertained) all treatment of disease must continue to be not only a foolish, but even a criminal operation, a dangerous attack upon human life.

It is somewhat too much to expect us to work merely for the benefit of such self-interested individuals as will contribute nothing to the complete and indispensable building up of the indispensable edifice, who only seek to make money by what has been discovered and investigated by the labours of others, and to furnish themselves with the means of squandering the income derived from the capital of science, to the accumulation of which they do not evince the slightest inclination to contribute.

All who feel a true desire to assist in elucidating the peculiar effects of medicines—our sole instruments, the knowledge of which has for so many centuries remained uninvestigated, and which is yet so indispensable for enabling us to cure the sick, will find the directions how these pure experiments with medicines should be conducted in the *Organon of medicine*, § 118—142.

In addition to what has been there stated I shall only add, that as the experimenter cannot, any more than any other human being, be absolutely and perfectly healthy, he must, should slight ailments to which he was liable appear during these provings of the powers of medicines, place these between brackets, thereby indicating that they are not confirmed, or dubious. But this will not often happen, seeing that during the action upon a previously healthy person of a sufficiently strong dose of the medicine, he is under the influence of the medicine alone, and it is seldom that any other symptom can shew itself during the first days but what must be the effect of the medicine. Further, that in order to investigate the symptoms of medicines for chronic diseases, for example, in order to develop the cutaneous diseases, abnormal growths and so forth, to be expected from the medicine, we must not be contented with taking one or two doses of it only, but we must continue its use for several days, to the amount of two adequate doses daily, that is to say, of sufficient size to cause us to perceive its action, whilst at the same time we continue to observe the diet and regimen indicated in the work alluded to.

The mode of preparing the medicinal substances for use in homœopathic treatment will be found in the *Organon of medicine*, § 267—271, and also in the *Chronic diseases*. I would only observe here, that for the proving of medicines on healthy individuals, dilutions and dynamizations are to be employed as high as are used for the treatment of disease, namely, globules moistened with the decillionth development of power.

The request of some friends, halting half-way on the road to this method of treatment, to detail some examples of this treatment, is difficult to comply with, and no great advantage can attend a compliance with it. Every cured case of disease shews only how that case has been treated. The internal process of the treatment depends always on those principles which are already known, and they cannot be rendered concrete and definitely fixed for each individual case, nor can they become at all more distinct from the history of a single cure than they previously were when these principles were enunciated. Every case of non-miasmatic disease is peculiar and special, and it is the special in it that distinguishes it from every other case, that pertains to it alone, but that cannot serve as a guide to the treatment of other cases. Now if it is wished to describe a complicated case of disease consisting of many symptoms, in such a pragmatical manner that the reasons that influence us in the choice of the remedy shall be clearly revealed, this demands details laborious at once for the recorder and for the reader.

In order, however, to comply with the desires of my friends in this also, I may here detail two of the slightest cases of homœopathic treatment.

Sch—, a washerwoman, somewhat above 40 years old, had been more than three weeks unable to pursue her avocations, when she consulted me on the 1st September, 1815.

1. On any movement, especially at every step, and worst on making a false step, she has a shoot in the scrobiculus cordis, that comes, as she avers, every time from the left side.

2. When she lies she feels quite well, then she has no pain anywhere, neither in the side nor in the scrobiculus.

3. She cannot sleep after three o'clock in the morning.

4. She relishes her food, but when she has ate a little she feels sick.

5. Then the water collects in her mouth and runs out of it, like the water-brash.

6. She has frequently empty eructations after every meal.

7. Her temper is passionate, disposed to anger.—Whenever the pain is severe she is covered with perspiration.—The catamenia were quite regular a fortnight since.

In other respects her health is good.

Now, as regards Symptom 1, *belladonna*, *china*, and *rhus toxi-*

49

codendron cause shootings in the scrobiculus, but none of them *only on motion*, as is the case here. *Pulsatilla* (see Symp. 387) certainly causes shootings in the scrobiculus on making a false step, but only as a rare alternating action, and has neither the same digestive derangements as occur here at 4 compared with 5 and 6, nor the same state of the disposition.

Bryonia alone has among its chief alternating actions, as the whole list of its symptoms demonstrates, pains *from movement* and especially shooting pains, as also stitches beneath the sternum (in the scrobiculus) on raising the arm (448), and on making a false step it occasions shooting in other parts (520, 574).

The negative symptom 2 met with here answers especially to *bryonia* (558?); few medicines (with the exception, perhaps, of *nux vomica* and *rhus toxicodendron* in their alternating action—neither of which, however, are suitable for the other symptoms) shew a complete relief to pains during rest and when lying; *bryonia* does, however, in an especial manner (558, and many other bryonia-symptoms).

Symptom 3 is met with in several medicines, and also in *bryonia* (694).

Symptom 4 is certainly, as far as regards "sickness after eating," met with in several other medicines (*ignatia, nux vomica, mercurius, ferrum, belladonna, pulsatilla, cantharis*), but neither so constantly and usually, nor with relish for food, as in *bryonia* (279).

As regards Symptom 5 several medicines certainly cause a flow of saliva like water-brash, just as well as *bryonia* (282); the others, however, do not produce the remaining symptoms in a very similar manner. Hence bryonia is to be preferred to them in this point.

Empty eructation (of wind only) after eating (Symptom 6) is found in few medicines, and in none so constantly, so usually, and to such a great degree, as in *bryonia* (255, 239).

To 7.—One of the chief symptoms in diseases (see *Organon of Medicine*, § 213) is the "state of the disposition," and as *bryonia* (778) causes this symptom also in an exactly similar manner—*bryonia* is for all these reasons to be preferred in this case to all other medicines as the homœopathic remedy.

Now, as this woman was very robust, and the force of the disease must accordingly have been very considerable, to prevent her by its pain from doing any work, and as her vital forces, as has been observed, were not consensually affected, I gave her one of the strongest homœopathic doses, a full drop of the pure juice of bryonia root,[1] to be taken immediately, and bade her come to me again in 48 hours. I told my friend E., who was present, that within that time the woman would be quite cured, but he, being but half a convert to homœopathy, expressed his doubts about it. Two days afterwards he came again to ascertain the result, but the woman did not return then, and, in fact, never came back again. I could only allay the impatience of my friend by telling him her name and that of the village where she lived, about three miles off, and advising him to seek her out and ascertain for himself how she was. This he did, and her answer was: "What was the use of my going back? The very next day I was quite well, and could again commence my washing, and the day following I was as well as I am still. I am extremely obliged to the doctor, but the like of us have no time to leave off our work; and for three weeks previously my illness prevented me earning anything."

W—e, a weakly, pale man of 42 years, who was constantly kept by his business at his desk, came to me on the 27th December, 1815, having been already ill five days.

1. The first evening he became, without manifest cause, sick and giddy, with much eructation.

2. The following night (about 2 a. m.) sour vomiting.

3. The subsequent nights severe eructation.

4. To-day also sick eructation of fetid and sourish taste.

5. He felt as if the food lay crude and undigested in his stomach.

6. In his head he felt vacant, hollow and confused, and as if sensitive therein.

7. The least noise was painful to him.

8. He is of a mild, soft, patient disposition.

Here I may observe:—

To 1. That several medicines cause vertigo with nausea, as well as *pulsatilla* (3), which produces its vertigo in the *evening* also (7), a circumstance that has been observed from very few others.

To 2. *Stramonium* and *nux vomica* cause vomiting of sour and sour-smelling mucus, but, as far as is known, not at night. *Valerian* and *cocculus* cause vomiting at night, but not of sour stuff. *Iron* alone causes vomiting at night (61, 62), and can

---

[1] According to the most recent development of our new system the ingestion of a single, minutest globule, moistened with the decillionth ($\overline{x}$) potential development would have been quite adequate to effect an equally rapid and complete recovery; indeed, equally certain would have been the mere olfaction of a globule the size of a mustard seed moistened with the same dynamization, so that the drop of pure juice given by me in the above case to a robust person, should not be imitated.

also cause sour vomiting (66), but not the other symptoms observed here.

Pulsatilla, however, causes not only sour vomiting in the evening (349, 356) and nocturnal vomiting in general, but also the other symptoms of this case not found among those of *iron*.

To 3. Nocturnal eructations is peculiar to *pulsatilla* (296, 297).

To 4. Feted, putrid (249) and sour eructations (301, 302) are peculiar to *pulsatilla*.

To 5. The sensation of indigestion of the food in the stomach is produced by few medicines, and by none in such a perfect and striking manner as by *pulsatilla* (321, 322, 327).

To 6. With the exception of *ignatia* (2) which, however, cannot produce the other ailments, the same state is only produced by *pulsatilla* (39 compared with 40, 81).

To 7. *Pulsatilla* produces the same state (995), and it also causes over-sensitiveness of other organs of the senses, for example, of the sight (107). And although intolerance of noise is also met with in *nux vomica, ignatia,* and *aconite,* yet these medicines are not homœopathic to the other symptoms and still less do they possess symptom 8, the mild character of the disposition, which, as stated in the preface to *pulsatilla*, is particularly indicative of this plant.

This patient, therefore, could not be cured by anything in a more easy, certain and permanent manner than by *pulsatilla*, which was accordingly given to him immediately, but on account of his weakly and delicate state only in a very minute dose, *i. e.*, half-a-drop of the quadrillionth of a strong drop of pulsatilla. This was done in the evening.

The next day he was free from all ailments, his digestion was restored, and a week thereafter, as I was told by him, he remained free from complaint and quite well.

The investigation in such a slight case of disease, and the choice of the homœopathic remedy for it, is *very speedily* effected by the practitioner who has had only a little experience in it, and who either has the symptoms of the medicine in his memory, or who knows where to find them readily; but to give in writing all the reasons *pro* and *con* (which would be perceived by the mind in a few seconds) gives rise, as we see, to tedious prolixity.

For the convenience of treatment, we require merely to indi-

---

[1] According to our present knowledge and experience the same object would have been attained by taking one of the smallest globules of pulsatilla x (decillionth potency) and with equal certainty a single olfaction of a globule the size of a mustard seed of the same potency of pulsatilla.

cate for each symptom all the medicines which can produce the same symptoms by a few letters (*e. g.,* Ferr., Chin., Rheum, Puls.), and also to bear in mind the circumstances under which they occur, that have a determining influence on our choice and in the same way with all the other symptoms, by what medicine each is excited, and from the list so prepared we shall be able to perceive which of the medicines homœopathically covers the most of the symptoms present, especially the most peculiar and characteristic ones,—and this is the remedy sought for.

TWO CASES FROM HAHNEMANN'S NOTE BOOK.[1]

CASE I.

Julie M. a country girl; 14 years old; not yet menstruated. 12th September, 1842. A month previously she had slept in the sun. Four days after this sleeping in the sun, the frightful idea took possession of her that she saw a wolf, and six days thereafter she felt as if she had received a great blow on the head. She now spoke irrationally; became as if mad; wept much; had sometimes difficulty in breathing; spat white mucus; could not tell any of her sensations.

She got *Belladonna*,[2] weakened dynamization, in seven table-spoonfuls of water; of this, after it was shaken, a tablespoonful in a glass of water, and after stirring this, one teaspoonful to be taken in the morning.

16th.—Somewhat quieter; she can blow her nose, which she was unable to do during her madness; she still talks as much nonsense, but does not make so many grimaces while talking. She wept much last night. Good motion. Tolerable sleep. She is still very restless, but was more so before the Belladonna. The white of the eye full of red vessels. She seems to have a pain in the nape of the neck.

From the glass in which one tablespoonful was stirred, one teaspoonful is to be taken and stirred in a second glassful of water, and of this from two to four teaspoonfuls (increasing the dose daily by one teaspoonful) are to be taken in the morning.

20th.—Much better; speaks more rationally; works a little; recognises and names me; and wishes to kiss a lady present. She now begins to shew her amorous propensities; is easily put

---

[1] Communicated by letter, dated 24th April, 1843, to Dr. Von Bönninghausen, and published in the *Neues Archiv*, Vol. i. 1844.

[2] [Dr. B. tells us that whenever the dilution is not indicated, it is understood that the 60th dilution was administered.]

in a passion, and takes things in bad part; sleeps well; weeps very often; becomes angry about a trifle; eats more than usual; when she comes to her senses she likes to play, but only just as a little child would.

Belladonna, a globule of a higher potency: seven tablespoonfuls shaken in two glasses, 6 teaspoonfuls from the second glass early in the morning.[1]

28th.— On the 22d, 23d and 24, very much excited day and night; great lasciviousness in her actions and words; she pulls up her clothes and seeks to touch the genitals of others; she readily gets into a rage and beats every one.

Hyoscyamus X°, seven tablespoonfuls, &c., one tablespoonful in one tumblerful of water; in the morning a teaspoonful.

5th October. For five days she would eat nothing; complains of belly-ache; for the last few days less malicious and less lascivious; stools rather loose; itching all over the body, especially on her genitals; sleep, good.

Sacch. Lactis for seven days, in seven tablespoonfuls, &c.

10th.—On the 7th, fit of excessive anger; she sought to strike every one. The next day, the 8th, attack of fright and fear, almost like the commencement of her illness (fear of an imaginary wolf;) fear lest she should be burnt. Since then she has become quiet, and talks rationally and nothing indecent for the last two days.

Sacch. Lactis, &c.

14th.—Quite good and sensible.

18th.—The same, but severe headache; inclination to sleep by day; not so cheerful.

New *sulphur* (new dynamization of the smallest material portion) one globule in three tumblers; in the morning one teaspoonful.

22d.—Very well; very little headache.

Sulphur, the next dynamization in two tumblers.

She went on with the *sulphur* occasionally until November, at which time she was and still remains a healthy, rational, amiable girl.

CASE II.

O—t, an actor, 33 years old, married. 14th January, 1843. For several years he had been *frequently* subject to sore throat,

---

[1] [The meaning of these directions, which is not very obvious, seems to be that the globule shall be dissolved in seven tablespoonfuls of water, and of this a tablespoonful is to be stirred in a second tumbler of water, and from this second glass a teaspoonful is to be given for six successive mornings.]

as also now for a month past. The previous sore throat had lasted six weeks. On swallowing his saliva, a pricking sensation; feeling of contraction and excoriation.

When he has not the sore throat he suffers from a pressure in the anus, with violent excoriative pains; the anus is then inflamed, swollen and constricted; it is only with a great effort that he can then pass his fæces, when the swollen hæmorrhoidal vessels protude.

On the 15th January, he took, in the morning before breakfast a teaspoonful of a solution of one globule of *belladonna* X^0 then the lowest dynamization, dissolved in seven tablespoonfuls of water, of which a tablespoonful was well stirred up in a tumblerful of water.

15th.—In the evening aggravation of the sore throat.

16th.—Sore throat gone, but the affection of the anus returned as above described; an open fissure with excoriative pain, inflammation, swelling, throbbing pain and constriction;—also in the evening a painful motion.

He confessed having had a chancre eight years previously, which had been, as usual, destroyed by caustics, after which all the above affections had appeared.

18th.—*Merc. viv.* one globule of the lowest new dynamization I, (which contains a vastly smaller amount of matter than the usual kind), prepared in the same manner, and to be taken in the same way as the belladonna (the bottle being shaken each time), one spoonful in a tumberful of water well stirred.

20th.—Almost no sore throat. Anus better, but he still feels there excoriation pain after a motion; he has however no more throbbing, no more swelling of the anus, and no inflammation; anus less contracted.

One globule of *merc. viv.* ($^2|_0$) the second dynamization of the same kind; prepared in the same way, and taken in the morning.

25th.—Throat almost quite well; but in the anus, raw pain and *severe shootings;* great pain in the anus after a motion; still some contraction of it and heat.

30th.—In the afternoon, the last dose (one teaspoonful). On the 28th the anus was better; sore throat returned; pretty severe excoriation pain in the throat.

On globule in milk-sugar for seven days; prepared and taken in the same manner.

7th February.—Severe ulcerative pain in the threat. Belly-ache, but good stools; several in succession, with great thirst In the anus all is right.

Sulphur ²|₀ in seven tablespoonfuls, as above.

13th.—Had ulcerative pain in the throat, especially on swallowing his saliva, of which he has now a large quantity, especially copious on the 11th and 12th. Severe contraction of the anus, especially since yesterday.

He now smelt here *merc.*, and got to take as before *merc. v.* ²|₀, one globule in seven tablespoonfuls of water, and half a spoonful of brandy.

20th.—Throat better since the 18th; he has suffered much with the anus; the motion causes pain when it is passing; less thirst.

Milk-sugar in seven tablespoonfuls.

3d March.—No more sore throat. On going to stool a bloodless hæmorrhoidal knot comes down (formerly this was accompanied with burning and raw pain), now with merely itching on the spot.

To smell *acid. nitri.* and then to have milk-sugar in seve

Almost no more pain after a motion; yesterday some blood along with the motion (an old symptom). Throat well; only a little sensitive when drinking cold water.

Olfaction of *acid. nitri.* (olfaction is performed by opening small bottle containing an ounce of alcohol or brandy where one globule is dissolved, and smelt for an instant or two.

He remained permanently cured.[1]

---

[1] [The following account of an illness with which Hahnemann was attacked, which he gives in a letter to the same correspondent, dated 28th April, 1833, will be read with interest.

"Although I kept myself very calm, yet the annoyance I received from * * * * * may have contributed to bring upon me the suffocative catarrh, that for seven days before and 14 days after the 10th of April [Hahnemann's birthday], threatened to choke me, with instantaneous attacks of intolerable itching in the glottis, that would have caused spasmodic cough, had it not deprived me of breath altogether; irritation of the fauces with the finger, so as to cause sickness, was the only thing that restored the breathing, and that but slowly; there were besides other severe symptoms—very great shortness of breath (without constriction of the chest), total loss of appetite for food and drink, disgust at tobacco, bruised feeling and weariness of all the limbs, constant drowsiness, inability to do the least work, presentiment of death, &c.' The whole neighbourhood proved their great affection for me by sending so frequently to inquire how I was, that I felt quite ashamed. It is only within these four days that I have felt myself out of danger; I obtained relief by two olfactions, of *coff. cr.* X° first, and then of *calc.*; *ambra* too was of use. And so the Great Protector of all that is true and good will grant me as much more life upon this earth as seemeth good to his wisdom.']

GENERAL INDEX.